Handbook of
Experimental Pharmacology

Volume 174

Editor-in-Chief

K. Starke, Freiburg i. Br.

Stem Cells

Contributors

M.R. Alison, C. Badorff, N. Benvenisty, B. Berninger, N. Beyer
Nardi, A. Branzi, M. Brittan, P. Budde, G.A. Colvin, H. Darr,
C. Denning, S. Dimmeler, F. Dönmez, M.S. Dooner,
R. Enseñat-Waser, L.J. Field, M. Götz, G. Grenier, M. Hack,
R. Harris, J. Jones, T. León-Quinto, M. Lovell, C. Mummery,
R. Passier, G. Paul, P.J. Quesenberry, J.A. Reig, E. Roche,
S. Rose-John, M. Rubart, M.A. Rudnicki, H. Sauer, L. da Silva
Meirelles, B. Soria, N.D. Theise, C. Ventura, M. Wartenberg,
G. Weitzer, N.A. Wright

Editors

Anna M. Wobus and Kenneth R. Boheler

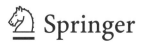 Springer

Professor
Anna M. Wobus, PhD
In Vitro Differentiation Group
Dept. of Cytogenetics
Leibnitz Institute of Plant Genetics
and Crop Plant Research (IPK)
Corrensstr. 3
D-06466 Gatersleben
Germany
wobusam@ipk-gatersleben.de

Kenneth R. Boheler, PhD
Investigator
Laboratory of Cardiovascular Science
Gerontology Research Program
National Institute on Aging, NIH
5600 Nathan Shock Drive
Baltimore, MD 21224
USA
bohelerk@grc.nia.nih.gov

With 53 Figures and 24 Tables

ISSN 0171-2004

ISBN-10 3-540-26133-8 Springer Berlin Heidelberg New York

ISBN-13 978-3-540-26133-9 Springer Berlin Heidelberg New York

Springer is a part of Springer Science + Business Media
springeronline.com

© Springer-Verlag Berlin Heidelberg 2006
Printed in Germany

The use of general descriptive names, registered names, trademarks, etc. in this publication does not imply, even in the absence of a specific statement, that such names are exempt from the relevant protective laws and regulations and therefore free for general use.

Product liability: The publishers cannot guarantee the accuracy of any information about dosage and application contained in this book. In every individual case the user must check such information by consulting the relevant literature.

Editor: S. Rallison
Editorial Assistant: S. Dathe
Cover design: design&production GmbH, Heidelberg, Germany
Typesetting and production: LE-TEX Jelonek, Schmidt & Vöckler GbR, Leipzig, Germany
Printed on acid-free paper   27/3151-YL - 5 4 3 2 1 0

Preface

Significant advances in stem cell research and their potentials for therapeutic applications have attracted the attention of the scientific community and captured the imagination of society as a whole. Not so long ago, the study of most stem cells, other than those that regenerated the haematopoietic system, was rather obscure and limited to a relatively small number of researchers and laboratories. The uproar over stem cells really began in 1998 with the successful derivation of pluripotent human embryonic stem (ES) cells by James Thomson and co-workers. This breakthrough and the subsequent generation of specialized human cells in vitro led to a paradigm shift within the scientific community, which transformed this specialized endeavour from a topic of scientific interest to a line of investigation with the potential to generate cells capable of treating serious ailments, including diabetes, cardiovascular diseases and neurodegenerative disorders. Thus the dawn of regenerative medicine has spawned from the somewhat esoteric study of stem cells.

Since 1998, extensive research endeavours have been devoted to the study of both embryonic and adult stem cells. Early reports suggested that adult stem cells had a higher plasticity than previously believed, perhaps even comparable with that demonstrated by embryonic stem cells, but several observations of the so-called transdifferentiation capacity and plasticity of adult stem cells have not been repeated. These reports, however, encouraged on-going debates about the capacity of adult versus embryonic stem cells and their potential use in regenerative medicine. Although at times controversial, these research efforts led to a better, although still limited, understanding of stem cells with respect to their identification, isolation, and developmental capacities.

Importantly, stem cells do not represent static entities that do not differ between embryos and adults. In fact, embryonic stem cells in early embryos represent basic units of life in higher organisms, while adult stem cells in somatic tissues represent cellular stores capable of regenerating tissue and maintaining organ functions. Regardless of these differences in potential, all stem cells derived from the embryo or adult are characterized by unique properties that permit accurate cell copying in vivo in a process termed self-renewal. Additionally, all stem cells retain the capacity to differentiate into more mature cell types. It is the degree of self-renewal and differentiation potential that differs among the various stem cell populations and cell lines.

These common traits have led to vigorous scientific and ethical debates, which are likely to persist for many years. Adding to the scientific and ethical dilemmas surrounding stem cells was the successful transfer of human somatic nuclei into fertilized human oocytes in a process known as nuclear transfer (nt), and the creation through a process known as therapeutic cloning of human ntES cell lines by South Korean scientists in 2004. This has recently (May 2005) been followed by the efficient generation of patient-derived ntES cell lines, which will likely influence the ethical debate and growth of stem cell research in the future. For the first time and as a consequence of these developments, stem cell research coupled with molecular biology and tissue engineering techniques constitute a potential basis for rational therapeutic strategies of regenerative medicine. Moreover, human ES-derived somatic cells may represent innovative pharmacological tools for drug screening, the identification of new drug targets and cell-based compound delivery systems. Finally, these cells may facilitate an unravelling of the hitherto inaccessible paradigms of human development.

In 2004, during one of the most contentious periods of debate with respect to the scientific, ethical and legal issues of stem cell research, the Board of Editors at the Handbook of Experimental Pharmacology approached us to edit a special volume devoted to stem cells. The idea was attractive because it would give us the chance to solicit and combine in one volume a body of work encompassing the rapidly advancing developments of stem cell research with a state-of-the-art view of stem cell biology. We invited leading experts in the fields of embryonic and adult stem cells to submit chapters for this volume, and although it proved impossible for everyone to submit a manuscript within the designated time frame, this volume is a compilation of their and our efforts to assemble an overview of the important aspects and issues surrounding stem cell research.

The first two chapters are dedicated to molecular mechanisms regulating self-renewal and differentiation of human (Darr and Benvenisty) and mouse (Weitzer) ES cells. In the latter, the author describes how ES cell research, through the in vitro use of the embryoid body model, reflects early developmental processes in vivo (Weitzer), and in the following contribution, Wartenberg et al. demonstrate how the in vitro model system can be employed for the study of angiogenesis and tumour-induced angiogenesis. The following chapters review the present state of knowledge with respect to mouse and human ES cell-derived cardiac (Rubart and Field; Passier et al.) and pancreatic (Roche et al.) cells and their potential application in tissue repair of heart diseases and diabetes, respectively. Ventura and Branzi describe autocrine and intracrine signalling pathways implicated in ES-derived cardiogenesis and how pharmacological approaches may facilitate this process.

The subsequent chapters deal mainly, but not exclusively, with adult stem cells, and the authors discuss mechanisms and potential applications of these cells in regenerative medicine. A unique concept of stem cell regulation based on haematopoietic stem cells (Quesenberry et al.) and a detailed overview that reflects the importance of markers in adult tissue-based stem cells (Alison et al.) are the perfect introduction to this set of chapters. Next, the chapters describe how haematopoietic stem/progenitor cells (Rose-John) or mesenchymal stem cells (Beyer Nardi and da Silva Meirelles) isolated from bone marrow may be isolated and manipulated by ex vivo expansion for tissue regeneration. Neovascularization and cardiac repair by bone marrow-derived stem cells (Badorff and Dimmeler) and the use of different stem/progenitor cells for myogenic tissue repair (Grenier and Rudnicki) are the topics of the following contributions. Neural stem cells, their properties and implications for the treatment of neurodegenerative diseases are extensively described and critically discussed by Berninger, Hack and Götz. The experimental studies described in the special issue are then complemented by a detailed description of the present state of a stem cell therapy with respect to patients with Parkinson's disease (Paul).

To end this special volume, we have selected a chapter dedicated to the future of stem cell research. Theise and Harris present a stimulating discussion on how unexpected and controversial findings of adult stem cell research may open up new perspectives to foster our understanding of cell biology.

We are deeply grateful to all the contributors for their active participation and significant contributions to this volume. We are aware that this volume could not and does not cover all topics and aspects of stem cell research. In fact, and during the past few years, stem cell research has metamorphosed into distinct and specialized avenues of research; however, we believe that this volume presents in a single book many novel aspects of stem cell biology with respect to scientific endeavours and future applications. Of particular note are the pharmacological issues that have been compiled, which have never been adequately addressed in the past.

We also would like to thank Mrs. Susanne Dathe, desk editor biomedicine at Springer, and Mrs. Kathrin Seiffert, IPK Gatersleben, for their support and expert editorial help.

In conclusion, we hope that this volume will be valued by researchers in the field, and by those who are engaged in the future developments of stem cell research and the applications of stem cells in regenerative medicine.

Gatersleben, Germany,   Anna M. Wobus
Baltimore, MD,   Kenneth R. Boheler
May 2005

List of Contents

List of Contributors

Addresses given at the beginning of respective chapters

Alison, M.R.   185

Badorff, C.   283
Benvenisty, N.   1
Berninger, B.   319
Beyer Nardi, N.   249
Branzi, A.   123
Brittan, M.   185
Budde, P.   53

Colvin, G.A.   169

Darr, H.   1
Denning, C.   101
Dimmeler, S.   283
Dönmez, F.   53
Dooner, M.S.   169

Enseñat-Waser, R.   147

Field, L.J.   73

Götz, M.   319
Grenier, G.   299

Hack, M.   319
Harris, R.   389

Jones, J.   147

León-Quinto, T.   147
Lovell, M.   185

Mummery, C.   101

Passier, R.   101
Paul, G.   361

Quesenberry, P.J.   169

Reig, J.A.   147
Roche, E.   147
Rose-John, S.   229
Rubart, M.   73
Rudnicki, M.A.   299

Sauer, H.   53
Silva Meirelles, L. da   249
Soria, B.   147

Theise, N.D.   389

Ventura, C.   123

Wartenberg, M.   53
Weitzer, G.   21
Wright, N.A.   185

HEP (2006) 174:1–19
© Springer-Verlag Berlin Heidelberg 2006

Factors Involved in Self-Renewal and Pluripotency of Embryonic Stem Cells

H. Darr · N. Benvenisty (✉)

Department of Genetics, The Life Sciences Institute, The Hebrew University,
91904 Jerusalem, Israel
nissimb@mail.ls.huji.ac.il

Abstract Embryonic stem (ES) cells are pluripotent cells derived from the inner cell mass of blastocyst stage embryos. These cells possess two unique characteristics: an indefinite self-renewal capacity and pluripotency, the ability to differentiate to cells from the three germ layers. Both human and mouse ES cells are currently at the center of intensive research. One of the burning issues in this research is the way in which these cells remain undifferentiated and maintain their pluripotency. In the past years, data has accumulated concerning the pathways responsible for the unique phenotype of these cells, in both human and mouse. This paper will review the main extrinsic factors and intrinsic transcriptional pathways currently implicated in the self-renewal and pluripotency of ES cells.

Keywords Embryonic stem (ES) cells · Self-renewal · Pluripotency

1
Introduction

Human embryonic stem (ES) cells are undifferentiated cells derived from the inner cell mass of blastocyst stage embryos (Thomson et al. 1998). They are unique in their capacity to self-renew indefinitely in culture, while maintaining a normal karyotype, and remaining pluripotent, namely, harboring the capacity to differentiate into multiple cell types of the three germ layers. Their differentiation potential has been demonstrated in vitro through the creation of embryonic bodies (EBs) (Itskovitz-Eldor et al. 2000; Schuldiner et al. 2000), which are cell aggregates comprised of multiple cell types. Alternatively, pluripotency was also demonstrated in vivo by injecting cells to immunodeficient mice, where they create teratomas, tumors composed of multiple cell types from the three germ layers (Thomson et al. 1998; Reubinoff et al. 2000). The definitive proof of the pluripotency of ES cells from mouse was obtained by injection of cells back into a blastocyst, which was followed by the formation of a chimera between the original embryo and the injected cells, including germ line transmission of the ES cell genetic content (Beddington and Robertson 1989).

Once ES cells had been derived from human (Thomson et al. 1998), they were proposed as a potential source for cell therapy, since they can differentiate into multiple cell types. It has been suggested that human ES cells could be used in future therapies of multiple diseases, including Parkinson's disease, heart diseases, diabetes mellitus, and more (Schuldiner and Benvenisty 2003). In addition, since these cells mimic to some extent the early stages of development, they can be used as a model for early human embryonic development after the implantation into the uterus (Dvash et al. 2004). This is extremely important since the early human embryo is inaccessible for research. It was also suggested that human ES cells may serve as a model for human diseases (Urbach et al. 2004). In mouse, the genetic manipulation of these cells has allowed an enormous advance in the study of gene function, since it enabled the creation of mutant mice for a large number of genes. In addition, ES cells have also been suggested as an in vitro model for the investigation of the mutagenicity, cytotoxicity, and embryotoxicity of substances on cells, either during their in-vitro differentiation or after the differentiation of the cells (Rohwedel et al. 2001).

So far three kinds of mammalian pluripotent stem cell types have been described: embryonic stem (ES) cells (Evans and Kaufman 1981; Martin 1981; Thomson et al. 1998), embryonic germ (EG) cells (Matsui et al. 1992; Resnick et al. 1992; Shamblott et al. 1998) derived from primordial germ cells, and embryonal carcinoma (EC) cells (Martin and Evans 1974; Andrews et al. 1984) derived from teratocarcinomas. These three cell types possess the two unique features of self-renewal and pluripotency. Each of these cell types has its own distinct properties, probably due to the difference in their origin. However, since they share these unique properties, they also share other common features. These include similar expression of specific marker genes, as well as some common pathways and factors which act to maintain the cells in the undifferentiated state. The elucidation of the molecules responsible for the cells' unique phenotype is now at the center of much research and interest. Understanding the mechanisms by which pluripotency and self-renewal are gained and maintained will highlight these fascinating phenomena and provide an understanding of the molecular pathways working in concert, to decide whether the cell will remain pluripotent or will differentiate. However, although the knowledge of the molecules governing this cell fate decision is beginning to unravel, there is more yet to be discovered. In addition, after the derivation of HESCs, it has become clear that not all the knowledge acquired from mouse ES cells is valid for human ES cells. This paper will review currently available knowledge regarding factors and mechanisms by which self-renewal and pluripotency are maintained in human and mouse ES cells. We will review both the extrinsic factors and the intrinsic transcriptional pathways governing the self-renewal of ES cells.

2
Extrinsic Factors Governing Maintenance of the Undifferentiated State of ES Cells

2.1
Leukemia Inhibitory Factor

When lines of mouse ES cells (MESCs) were first derived in the early 1980s, the cells were derived and propagated as co-culture with a layer of feeder cells (Evans and Kaufman 1981; Martin 1981). This methodology was adopted from the protocols established for embryonal carcinoma (EC) cells. It was found that the feeder cells support ES cells through the secretion of a signal that prevents differentiation, since the need for co-culture could be replaced by addition of media conditioned by feeder cells. Fractionation of conditioned media (CM) has allowed the identification of the active factor in it as leukemia inhibitory factor (LIF), and addition of LIF to the growth media could substitute the need for co-culture (see Table 1) (Smith et al. 1988; Williams et al. 1988).

LIF belongs to the family of interleukin 6 (IL-6)-type cytokines (Rose-John 2002). This family of cytokines stimulates cells through the gp130 receptor, which works as a heterodimer together with a ligand specific receptor (such as LIF-R). gp130 is expressed in all cells of the body, while the specific subunits are expressed in a cell-specific manner. Following the discovery of LIF as the active factor in the CM, it was shown that oncostatin M (OSM) (Rose et al. 1994) and ciliary neutrophic factor (CNF) (Conover et al. 1993), which also belong to the IL-6 cytokine family, can also substitute the need for CM. Their similar effect seems to be attributed to their shared downstream effectors.

Table 1 Cytokines required for ES self-renewal

Protein	Mutant mice	Role in MESCs	Role in HESC maintenance
LIF	Develop to term, fertile, essential for embryo implantation (Stewart et al. 1992)	Replaces the need for feeder cells. (Smith et al. 1998; Williams et al. 1998)	No apparent role in self-renewal (Daheron et al. 2004)
BMP4	Do not proceed beyond egg cylinder stage. Failure of gastrulation and mesoderm formation (Winnier et al. 1995)	Replaces the need for serum presence (Ying et al. 2003)	Drives HESCs to trophectoderm differentiation (Xu et al. 2004)
bFGF	Viable with defects in neural development and function (Dono et al. 1998)	Not required for their propagation	Required for propagation in serum replacement media (Amit et al. 2000)

Activation of gp130 leads to the activation of the Janus associated tyrosine kinase (JAK) and to activation of signal transducer and activator of transcription (STAT) proteins, their translocation to the nucleus, binding to DNA and subsequent activation of transcription. It has been shown that the ability of LIF to prevent differentiation of MESCs is dependent upon activation of STAT3. Concurrently, STAT3 activation even in the absence of LIF is sufficient to enable the propagation of the cells (Matsuda et al. 1999). In addition to the activation of STAT3, which is involved in the maintenance of the undifferentiated state, LIF also induces additional signals, among them the activation of ERKs (extracellular receptor kinases) (Burdon et al. 1999). The activation of ERKs promotes differentiation. Thus, the balance between the activation of STAT3 to the activation of ERK signals determines the fate of the dividing undifferentiated ES cell. Therefore, signals that control the activation of ERKs also have an important role in maintaining the undifferentiated state (see Fig. 1). Lately, it has been shown that inhibition of PI3K (phosphoinositide 3-kinase) leads to differentiation of MESCs (Paling et al. 2004). The PI3K signaling pathway is also induced by LIF, and the differentiation observed upon its inhibition is a result of augmented levels of activated ERKs. An additional report suggests another pathway that is activated by LIF in MESCs. This pathway involves the activation of the Src family of nonreceptor tyrosine kinases, and specifically its member cYes (Anneren et al. 2004). Inhibition of this family decreases the growth and expression of ES cell markers, both in MESCs and HESCs. The activity of cYes in MESCs is regulated both by LIF and by serum and it is down-regulated upon differentiation. However, it seems that cYes does not have a central function in vivo, since mice mutated in cYes are viable and fertile (Stein et al. 1994).

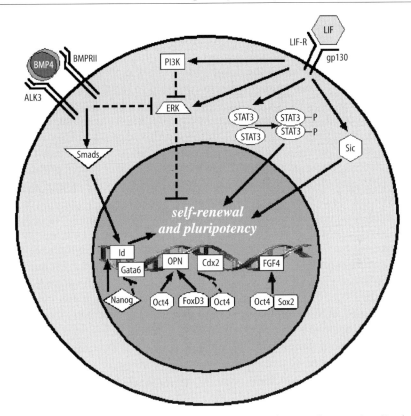

Fig. 1 Major pathways involved in mouse ES cell self-renewal. LIF and BMP4 signaling have been shown to be required for propagation of undifferentiated MESCs. Binding of BMP4 to its receptors activates two downstream pathways which prevent their differentiation: (a) activation of Smads, which leads to transcription of Id genes, which in turn mediate BMPs involvement in self-renewal; (b) inhibition of ERK, which drives the cells to differentiation. The binding of LIF to its receptors leads simultaneously to activation of differentiating and anti-differentiating signals. The differentiation signals include activation of ERK, while signals important for self-renewal include the activation of STAT3, activation of Src, and also the activation of PI3K (which inhibits ERK). The main transcription factors known so far as important for self-renewal in mouse are Oct4 and Nanog. Oct4 works in cooperation with several transcription factors to regulate transcription of its target genes. This cooperation is established through binding to different sites on enhancers of their target genes. Shown are examples of co-regulators and examples of putative target genes regulated by different combinations of regulators

In contrast to the vital role that LIF holds in vitro, knockout studies revealed that LIF signaling is dispensable during normal early embryonic development. Mice mutated in LIF develop to term and are fertile, although it is essential for embryo implantation (Stewart et al. 1992); mice mutated in LIF-R die within 24 h of birth (Li et al. 1995; Ware et al. 1995) and mice mutated in gp130 die progressively from day 12.5 dpc (Yoshida et al. 1996). Sequential studies suggested that although LIF is not required during normal early embryonal development, it is needed during a process called diapause (Nichols et al. 2001). This is the process in which the development of the embryo is arrested in late blastocyst stage before implantation in response to lactation. This arrest can take place for several weeks, during which the pluripotent compartment of the ICM has to be kept in an undifferentiated state. Embryos mutated in gp130 are unable to resume development following this arrest and they lose their pluripotent compartment. Therefore, it may be that the role LIF has taken in vitro reflects an aberrant condition, in which the normal transient proliferation of the ICM is artificially prolonged in culture, much like the extension of the proliferation state observed during diapause.

Human ES cells (HESCs) also require co-culture with feeders, but in human cells this requirement cannot be substituted by the addition of LIF (from human or mouse origin). Mouse LIF does not act on human cells (Layton et al. 1994) and therefore cannot be the protein secreted from the MEF cells that maintains HESCs pluripotency. In HESCs, just as in MESCs, the co-culture with feeders can be substituted by the addition of CM, and prolonged feeder-free culture can be maintained in the presence of certain extracellular matrixes (like matrigel or laminin) together with CM (Xu et al. 2001). When exploring the reason for the lack of responsiveness of HESCs to LIF, it was first hypothesized that this was a result of low or absent expression of LIF-R (Rose-John 2002). However, when this hypothesis was examined, it was observed that a variety of LIF-R expression levels can be found in different HESC lines (Ginis et al. 2004), ranging from low or absent to significant levels of expression. In addition, recent papers have shown that the reason for lack of LIF effect on HESCs is not the inability of the cells to respond to LIF signaling, but rather that activation of STAT3 in HESCs, which in MESCs is sufficient for self-renewal, does not prevent differentiation of HESCs (Daheron et al. 2004; Humphrey et al. 2004). Additionally, in the undifferentiated state of HESCs, the STAT3 pathway is not activated. While in undifferentiated MESCs a high level of phosphorylated STAT3 (which is the active form) can be found, this activated form is not seen in undifferentiated HESCs.

2.2
BMP4

BMP4, a member of the TGF-beta superfamily of polypeptide signaling mole-cules, was recently suggested to be involved in the prevention of MESC differ-entiation as well (Ying et al. 2003). Although LIF is sufficient to prevent MESC differentiation in the presence of serum, when serum is removed, even in the presence of LIF, neural differentiation occurs. Since serum contains many unknown factors, it seems that at least some of them prevent ES cell differenti-ation. Addition of BMP4 to the media enables serum-free culture (see Table 1).

This is possible only in the presence of LIF, since otherwise differentiation to non-neural lineages takes place. Withdrawal of both BMP4 and LIF results in neural differentiation. Therefore LIF is needed to maintain the undifferentiating capacity of BMP4, which in the absence of LIF actually drives the cells to differentiate. Thus, it seems that while BMP4 acts to prevent differentiation to neural lineages, LIF works to inhibit differentiation to non-neural lineages. Mouse embryos deficient in zygotic BMP4, BMPR-1a or Smad4 develop normally until early egg cylinder stages (Winnier et al. 1995; Mishina et al. 1995; Sirard et al. 1998), but later show reduced proliferation of the epiblast and failure of gastrulation. However, it may be that the reduced proliferation is the result of a defect in the differentiation of the visceral endoderm, and not intrinsic to the epiblast (Sirard et al. 1998).

BMP4 supports self-renewal of MESCs through the activation of Smad proteins. They in turn activate Id genes, which are negative bHLH factors. MESCs transfected with Ids can grow in a serum-free culture in the absence of BMP4. Serum was also shown to induce Id gene expression through multiple pathways, and MESCs grown in the presence of serum with no BMP4 addition show expression of Id genes (Ying et al. 2003). Another report showed that BMP4 also supports self-renewal by inhibition of ERK and p38 mitogen-activated protein kinase (MAPK) (Qi et al. 2004) (see Fig. 1). Furthermore, it was possible to show that by inhibiting the p38 pathway, Alk3 null embryos can be used for derivation of ES cells lines, which normally fail to expand in culture.

In HESCs, however, the addition of BMP4 to the media does not enhance self-renewal of the cells, as was observed for the MESCs. Actually BMP4 drives the cells to differentiate to trophoblast cells (Xu et al. 2002). This is in contrary to MESCs, which do not seem to have the capacity to differentiate to this cell type. This difference in the abilities to create trophoblast has raised the notion that HESCs and MESCs may be derived from different stages in development, and thus their self-renewal capacity may be affected by different factors.

2.3
bFGF

bFGF has been shown to be required for the routine culture of HESCs in the presence of serum replacement (see Table 1) (Amit et al. 2000). In serum-free media not substituted with bFGF, the cells differentiate, while its addition makes the cells' morphology more compact and enables prolonged undifferentiated culture under these conditions. In addition, bFGF enhances the cloning efficiency of the cells (Amit et al. 2000). While the addition of bFGF is not required for the propagation of MESCs, it was shown to be important for different pluripotent cells, embryonic germ (EG) cells, in both human and mouse. bFGF is needed to convert the transient proliferating population of primordial germ cells to an indefinitely proliferating population of EG cells (Matsui et al. 1992; Resnick et al. 1992). However, in the case of mouse EG cells, once the EG cell culture is established, bFGF is no longer needed for their routine culture (Matsui et al. 1992). Investigations that examined the expression of different elements of signaling pathways in HESCs have shown the presence of elements of FGF signaling, including all four FGF receptors and certain components of their downstream cascade, which are enriched in undifferentiated HESCs in comparison to their differentiated derivatives (Bhattacharya et al. 2004; Brandenberger et al. 2004; Dvash et al. 2004; Ginis et al. 2004; Rao and Stice 2004). bFGF is expressed by HESCs, but apparently its level is not enough to prevent differentiation.

2.4
Other Suggested Factors

Since neither LIF and BMP4 support self-renewal of HESCs, the search for other factors that can replace CM in HESCs continues. Even in MESCs there is evidence of self-renewal pathways that are independent of LIF or STAT3 activation (Berger and Sturm 1997; Dani et al. 1998). This coincides with the observation that LIF does not seem to be fundamental for the creation of pluripotency in vivo in mouse. For these reasons, it is plausible that another physiological pathway is fundamental for both human and mouse pluripotency. There have been several reports claiming the discovery of factors replacing the need for CM in HESCs. One report has implicated the Wnt pathway as able to maintain HESC self-renewal for a short period of time (Sato et al. 2004). Another report suggested that TGFβ1, in combination with fibronectin and LIF are sufficient for feeder and CM-free culture (Amit et al. 2004). However, neither of these protocols is used routinely to grow HESCs in feeder-independent cultures.

3
Intrinsic Factors Governing Maintenance of the Undifferentiated State of Embryonic Stem Cells

Several factors have been implicated in the maintenance of the pluripotent nature of ES cells, and much more research is being conducted to reveal additional factors.

3.1
Oct4

Oct4 is a transcription factor belonging to the POU transcription factor family that possesses an octamer recognition sequence, an 8-bp sequence found in the promoters and enhancers of many ubiquitously expressed and cell-specific genes. One of the unique features of Oct4 is its expression pattern, which seems to be restricted to pluripotent lineages (Palmieri et al. 1994; Yeom et al. 1996), although its reactivation in some cancers has been reported (Tai et al. 2004). It is expressed in the mouse embryo from the early stages of 4- to 8-cell stage embryos until the epiblast begins to differentiate, with expression persisting in germ cells. Mouse embryos with a mutated Oct4 die following implantation due to a lack of an ICM (Nichols et al. 1998), and these embryos are composed solely of trophoblast (see Table 2). MESCs in which Oct4 is down-regulated differentiate to trophoblast cells (a cell lineage that otherwise has not been shown to be produced by MESCs) (Niwa et al. 2000). In addition, increase of the expression level of Oct4 in MESCs by as little as twofold also caused the cells to differentiate, but in this case the cells adopted an extraembryonic endoderm and mesoderm fate. It is assumed that while Oct4 represses differentiation to trophoblast, it works in conjugation with other transcription factors or co-regulators, and the ratio between the concentrations of these factors determines the effect on cell fate. The role of Oct4 in maintaining HESC pluripotency is in concordance with its role in MESCs. As was shown in MESCs, down-regulation

Table 2 Major transcription factors involved in ES self-renewal

Gene	Mutant mice	Role in MESCs	Expression in HESCs and role in self-renewal
Oct4	Die following implantation due to lack of ICM	Required to prevent differentiation to trophoblast.	Expressed in multiple ES cell lines
		Overexpression leads to differentiation to extraembryonic endoderm and ectoderm	Role in self-renewal has been shown to be as in the MESCs
Nanog	Consisted only of disorganized extraembryonic tissues with no epiblast or extraembryonic ectoderm	Required to prevent differentiation to primitive endoderm. Overexpression enables LIF independent growth	Expressed in multiple ES cell lines
Sox2	Fail to survive shortly after implantation. Develop a normal ICM, but later lack egg cylinder structure and fail to maintain their epiblast	MESCs from null embryos cannot be established. Initially their outgrowths seem normal, but later produce only trophectoderm and parietal endoderm cells	Expressed in multiple ES cell lines
Foxd3	Die shortly after implantation. The size of their epiblast is reduced and the primitive streak is absent	MESCs from null embryos cannot be established, although initially their outgrowths seem normal. Have expansion of the extraembryonic ectoderm	Expressed only in some ES cell lines and therefore seems dispensable

of Oct4 in HESCs also leads to differentiation of the cells to trophoblast cells (Matin et al. 2004).

The target genes of Oct4 activity and the regulators it works with are not fully identified, but this information is beginning to unravel, especially in MESCs. Different target genes have been suggested based on different lines of evidence. The genes identified include Fgf4 (Ambrosetti et al. 1997), the transcriptional co-factor Utf-1 (Nishimoto et al. 1999), the zinc finger protein Rex-1 (Ben-Shushan et al. 1998), platelet-derived growth factor α receptor (Kraft et al. 1996), osteopontin (OPN) (Botquin et al. 1998), Fbx15 (Tokuzawa et al. 2003), and more. Oct4 has also been reported to repress several genes expressed in trophoblast, such as human chorionic gonadotropin α in human choriocarcinoma cells (Liu and Roberts 1996; Liu et al. 1997). The way in which the activation of Oct4 target genes establishes and maintains pluripotency is still unknown, partly because not all the targets are known or studied, and partly because the target genes that have been studied so far, did not prevent the establishment of the ICM when they were disrupted. An example of an Oct4 target gene is Fgf4. Although Fgf4 knockout embryos undergo implantation, their ICM fails to proliferate and they die shortly thereafter (Feldman et al. 1995).

By combining with different co-factors, Oct4 can act both as a transcriptional activator and as a transcriptional repressor (see Fig. 1). Oct4 has few known co-factors, including the adeno virus E1A (Scholer et al. 1991), the Sry-related factor Sox-2 (Yuan et al. 1995), Foxd3 (Guo et al. 2002), and HMG-1 (Butteroni et al. 2000). A squelching phenomenon was observed for the cooperation of Oct4 with some of its co-factors (Scholer et al. 1991). It was shown that the quantitative balance between Oct4 and its transactivators is of importance for the proper activation of their targets, at least in some of the targets, and a rise in the level of Oct4, or for example E1A, prevents the formation of an active transcriptional complex. Such a phenomenon can be seen in Rex1, which is repressed by high levels of Oct4 (Ben-Shushan et al. 1998). However, this is not the case for all of Oct4 targets, and this phenomenon is not observed for targets co-regulated by Sox-2, such as Fgf-4.

Oct4 co-factors are expressed at different expression patterns in pluripotent cells. For example, while Sox-2 is expressed both in the ICM and the primitive ectoderm (Collignon et al. 1996), ELA (E1A-like activity, which is present in undifferentiated ES cells) is expressed only in the ICM (Suemori et al. 1988). This may also be the reason for different expression patterns of Oct4 targets, since their transcription may rely on presence of different co-factors.

3.2
Sox2

Sox2 is a member of the Sox (SRY-related HMG box) gene family that encodes transcription factors with a single HMG DNA-binding domain. Like Oct-4, it is expressed in the pluripotent lineages of the early mouse embryo, the

ICM, epiblast, and germ cells. But unlike Oct4, it is also expressed in the multipotential cells of the extraembryonic ectoderm (Avilion et al. 2003) and has also been shown to mark neural progenitors of the central nervous system and be important for the maintenance of their identity (Graham et al. 2003). Its down-regulation is correlated with a commitment to differentiate. Sox2-null mouse embryos seem normal at the blastocyst stage, but fail to survive shortly after implantation (Avilion et al. 2003). These embryos lack egg cylinder structures and lack the epithelial cells typical of the epiblast. When cultured in vitro to produce ES cell lines, Sox2 null blastocysts progress normally in the first days, but later do not show the normal differentiation into the ICM, and the only cells observed are trophectoderm and parietal endoderm cells. Therefore, although in vivo the role of Sox2 manifests by knockout only after implantation, it does have a role in maintaining the pluripotent population of cells in the earlier embryonic stages from which ES cells are derived, namely the ICM and epiblast. Early embryos have substantial levels of maternal Sox2 protein, which unlike most of the maternal gene products persists until implantation. Even in Sox2-null embryos, maternal Sox2 protein persists until the blastocyst stage. Therefore, the reason that the mutated embryos survive until implantation may be the sufficient levels of maternal Sox2 protein until that stage. Hence, it may be that Sox2 does indeed have a role in maintaining or creating pluripotency in earlier stages, but this role cannot be detected in simple knockout experiments due to the presence of the maternal protein. In addition, Sox2 also has a role in the maintenance of trophoblast stem cells, and in the absence of Sox2 these cells cannot be generated.

3.3
Foxd3

Foxd3 (originally called genesis) belongs to the forkhead family genes. It is not expressed in unfertilized oocytes or one-cell stage fertilized embryos, but its transcripts are detected in blastocyst stage embryos (Hanna et al. 2002). Foxd3-null embryos die around the time of gastrulation with a loss of the epiblast and an expansion of extraembryonic ectoderm and endoderm (Hanna et al. 2002). However, in the blastocyst stage their ICM appears normal, with normal expression of ICM markers. When cultured in vitro, Foxd3-null blastocysts seem normal initially, but later their ICM fails to expand. Chimeric rescue experiments have shown that Foxd3-null cells are able to differentiate into many cell types. Thus, it seems that Foxd3 may be required for the regulation of either a secreted factor or a cell-surface signaling molecule.

The roles of Sox2 and Foxd3 have not been examined yet in HESCs (see Table 2). Sox2 is clearly expressed in undifferentiated HESCs. On the other hand, while in some human ES cell lines Foxd3 is expressed, in others it is not (Ginis et al. 2004). Thus, it seems dispensable for the self-renewal of human ES cells. However, since Foxd3-null embryos are defected in a stage after the creation of the pluripotent compartment of the ICM, it is unclear how much this difference in expression pattern can be attributed to differences in the maintenance of pluripotency between the two species.

3.4
Nanog

An additional gene recently described as involved in self-renewal of ES cells is Nanog (Chambers et al. 2003; Mitsui et al. 2003). Nanog is a homeobox transcription factor, which does not belong to any known group of home-obox genes. It is expressed in the mouse in the inner cells of the compacted morula and blastocyst, early germ cells, ES cells, embryonic germ cells (EGs), and embryonic carcinoma cells (ECs), and is absent from differentiated cells (Chambers et al. 2003; Mitsui et al. 2003). Nanog was named after the mytho-logical Celtic land of the ever young, Tir nan Og, since overexpression of Nanog in MESCs renders the cells independent of LIF supply. Although the cells self-renew and remain pluripotent in the absence of LIF, their self-renewal capacity is reduced. Therefore, Nanog overexpression does not completely relieve the cells from LIF dependence, but when these two factors are combined, they work together synergistically. The Nanog overexpression effect is not medi-ated through the activation of Stat3, and vice-versa (Chambers et al. 2003), and therefore Stat3 and Nanog pathways would seem to act independently of each other. Nanog overexpressing cells can also be propagated in serum-free media in the absence of BMP (Ying et al. 2003), and it appears that the overexpression of Nanog maintains a substantial constitutive level of Id expression. However, Nanog overexpression does not overcome the need for Oct4 activity (Cham-bers et al. 2003), and both Nanog and Oct4 are required for MESC self-renewal. Nanog disruption in MESCs results in differentiation to extraembryonic en-doderm lineages (Mitsui et al. 2003). Nanog knockout embryos develop to the blastocyst stage, but when cultured on gelatin their ICM differentiates completely to parietal endoderm-like cells (see Table 2). Therefore, Nanog is essential for the maintenance of pluripotency of the ICM at one stage later than the initial requirement for Oct4. Consequently, if Oct4 operates to inhibit the differentiation of ES cells to trophoblast, Nanog works to inhibit the transi-tion of the cells to primitive endoderm, which is the next cell fate decision in the embryo. Nevertheless, unlike Oct4 whose primary role is to prevent dif-ferentiation (to trophectoderm), Nanog not only prevents differentiation (to extraembryonic endoderm) but also actively works to maintain pluripotency.

The target genes that Nanog works to activate or repress are still unknown. Nonetheless, the DNA sequence that it binds has been identified using SELEX, and target genes have been suggested based on the presence of this sequence upstream to their transcription initiation site (Mitsui et al. 2003). One such gene is GATA6, and it seems that Nanog may repress its expression, since forced expression of GATA6 is sufficient for differentiation to extraembryonic endoderm (see Fig. 1) (Fujikura et al. 2002), the same phenotype observed in Nanog-null cells. However, Nanog also contains two domains capable of activating transcription (Pan and Pei 2004) and therefore might also positively regulate ES specific genes, on top of repressing extraembryonic endoderm genes.

Human Nanog is expressed in HESCs, EC and EG cells, germ cells, and in several tumors (Mitsui et al. 2003). When human Nanog was overexpressed in MESCs, partial release from LIF dependency was observed (Chambers et al. 2003). This may indicate that the Nanog pathway in human and mouse share functional homology, but this issue is yet to be examined.

3.5
miRNA

MicroRNAs (miRNAs) are additional regulators suggested to be involved in maintaining ES cell identity. These short RNA molecules are known to be involved in translational regulation, mostly by repressing translation and in some cases by directing mRNA to degradation (Elbashir et al. 2001). Recent studies have aimed at identifying such molecules, both in-silico and by examining miRNA libraries. One such study conducted in MESCs (Houbaviy et al. 2003) found novel miRNAs expressed specifically in undifferentiated ES cells, as well as several previously identified miRNAs, which are enriched in undifferentiated ES cells compared to their differentiated counterparts. Since one of the important functions of some miRNAs is the regulation of development, it has been suggested that these molecules might have a role in the maintenance of ES cell pluripotency. A similar study conducted in HESCs identified 17 novel miRNAs enriched in undifferentiated cells, 11 of which were homologous to those described in MESCs (Suh et al. 2004). Therefore, it may be that the role of these molecules will turn out to be conserved in mammalian embryonic development.

4
Summary

When examining self-renewal and pluripotency in ES cells, we have to bear in mind that this is a population that exists in vivo only transiently, and does not proceed for long in the embryo. This is also reflected in vitro, since usually an ES cell culture contains differentiated cells, in addition to the majority of cells, which are undifferentiated. Since ES cells differentiate very readily, it is not surprising that the pluripotent phenotype of the ES cells has to be actively maintained by exogenous signals from the environment. LIF is known in vivo to prolong the period the pluripotent lineage exists. LIF and BMP4 each prevent the differentiation of the cells to different cell fates. It may be that the fact that the cells remain undifferentiated is the result of the balance between different differentiation and anti-differentiation signals. The differentiation signals work on the pluripotency transcriptional pathways established already in the pluripotent cells and are required for them to maintain this feature. These pathways have been established earlier and include components that seem to be unique to pluripotent cells (like Oct4 and Nanog). It may also be that one of the roles of these transcriptional pathways is to enhance the maintenance of this pluripotent state. The fact that the level of the transcription factors involved in self-renewal is crucial to the determination of cell fate (as in the case of Oct4 and Nanog) also establishes that a very intricate interplay is involved in the cell fate decision in each cell division.

One of the important issues regarding self-renewal and pluripotency is the examination of the level of similarities by which these processes are governed in human vs mouse ES cells. While examining the response of the cells to exogenous factors, more discrepancies are uncovered than similarities. This observation is valid to the role of both LIF and BMP4. In contrast, when examining the role of the endogenous transcription factors that are unique to the pluripotent state, it seems that in this area the similarity is more pronounced. Although less research has been conducted so far on HESCs than on MESCs, the research published to date has not contradicted the MESCs results. The role of Oct4 is similar in both mouse and human, and the roles of Nanog and also Sox2, although not examined yet in human, may be similar, since in human as in mouse, these are genes with an expression pattern mostly restricted to pluripotent cells. Therefore, it may be that the pathways that establish the pluripotent state and are essential for its self-renewal will turn out to be common among these two species. On the other hand, the extrinsic signals and the pathways they activate, which are not exclusive to pluripotent cells, are different.

Acknowledgements   We thank Dr. Rachel Eiges and Yoav Mayshar for critical review of the manuscript. This research was partially supported by funds from Israel Science Foundation (grant no. 672/02–1) and by an NIH grant.

References

Ambrosetti DC, Basilico C, Dailey L (1997) Synergistic activation of the fibroblast growth factor 4 enhancer by Sox2 and Oct-3 depends on protein-protein interactions facilitated by a specific spatial arrangement of factor binding sites. Mol Cell Biol 17:6321–6329

Amit M, Carpenter MK, Inokuma MS, Chiu CP, Harris CP, Waknitz MA, Itskovitz-Eldor J, Thomson JA (2000) Clonally derived human embryonic stem cell lines maintain pluripotency and proliferative potential for prolonged periods of culture. Dev Biol 227:271–278

Amit M, Shariki C, Margulets V, Itskovitz-Eldor J (2004) Feeder layer- and serum-free culture of human embryonic stem cells. Biol Reprod 70:837–845

Andrews PW, Damjanov I, Simon D, Banting GS, Carlin C, Dracopoli NC, Fogh J (1984) Pluripotent embryonal carcinoma clones derived from the human teratocarcinoma cell line Tera-2. Differentiation in vivo and in vitro. Lab Invest 50:147–162

Anneren C, Cowan CA, Melton DA (2004) The Src family of tyrosine kinases is important for embryonic stem cell self-renewal. J Biol Chem 279:31590–31598

Avilion AA, Nicolis SK, Pevny LH, Perez L, Vivian N, Lovell-Badge R (2003) Multipotent cell lineages in early mouse development depend on SOX2 function. Genes Dev 17:126–140

Beddington RS, Robertson EJ (1989) An assessment of the developmental potential of embryonic stem cells in the midgestation mouse embryo. Development 105:733–737

Ben-Shushan E, Thompson JR, Gudas LJ, Bergman Y (1998) Rex-1, a gene encoding a transcription factor expressed in the early embryo, is regulated via Oct-3/4 and Oct-6 binding to an octamer site and a novel protein, Rox-1, binding to an adjacent site. Mol Cell Biol 18:1866–1878

Berger CN, Sturm KS (1997) Self renewal of embryonic stem cells in the absence of feeder cells and exogenous leukaemia inhibitory factor. Growth Factors 14:145–159

Bhattacharya B, Miura T, Brandenberger R, Mejido J, Luo Y, Yang AX, Joshi BH, Ginis I, Thies RS, Amit M, Lyons I, Condie BG, Itskovitz-Eldor J, Rao MS, Puri RK (2004) Gene expression in human embryonic stem cell lines: unique molecular signature. Blood 103:2956–2964

Botquin V, Hess H, Fuhrmann G, Anastassiadis C, Gross MK, Vriend G, Scholer HR (1998) New POU dimer configuration mediates antagonistic control of an osteopontin preimplantation enhancer by Oct-4 and Sox-2. Genes Dev 12:2073–2090

Brandenberger R, Wei H, Zhang S, Lei S, Murage J, Fisk GJ, Li Y, Xu C, Fang R, Guegler K, Rao MS, Mandalam R, Lebkowski J, Stanton LW (2004) Transcriptome characterization elucidates signaling networks that control human ES cell growth and differentiation. Nat Biotechnol 22:707–716

Burdon T, Stracey C, Chambers I, Nichols J, Smith A (1999) Suppression of SHP-2 and ERK signalling promotes self-renewal of mouse embryonic stem cells. Dev Biol 210:30–43

Butteroni C, De Felici M, Scholer HR, Pesce M (2000) Phage display screening reveals an association between germline-specific transcription factor Oct-4 and multiple cellular proteins. J Mol Biol 304:529–540

Chambers I, Colby D, Robertson M, Nichols J, Lee S, Tweedie S, Smith A (2003) Functional expression cloning of Nanog, a pluripotency sustaining factor in embryonic stem cells. Cell 113:643–655

Collignon J, Sockanathan S, Hacker A, Cohen-Tannoudji M, Norris D, Rastan S, Stevanovic M, Goodfellow PN, Lovell-Badge R (1996) A comparison of the properties of Sox-3 with Sry and two related genes, Sox-1 and Sox-2. Development 122:509–520

Conover JC, Ip NY, Poueymirou WT, Bates B, Goldfarb MP, DeChiara TM, Yancopoulos GD (1993) Ciliary neurotrophic factor maintains the pluripotentiality of embryonic stem cells. Development 119:559–565

Daheron L, Opitz SL, Zaehres H, Lensch WM, Andrews PW, Itskovitz-Eldor J, Daley GQ (2004) LIF/STAT3 signaling fails to maintain self-renewal of human embryonic stem cells. Stem Cells 22:770–778

Dani C, Chambers I, Johnstone S, Robertson M, Ebrahimi B, Saito M, Taga T, Li M, Burdon T, Nichols J, Smith A (1998) Paracrine induction of stem cell renewal by LIF-deficient cells: a new ES cell regulatory pathway. Dev Biol 203:149–162

Dvash T, Mayshar Y, Darr H, McElhaney M, Barker D, Yanuka O, Kotkow KJ, Rubin LL, Benvenisty N, Eiges R (2004) Temporal gene expression during differentiation of human embryonic stem cells and embryoid bodies. Hum Reprod 19:2875–2883

Elbashir SM, Harborth J, Lendeckel W, Yalcin A, Weber K, Tuschl T (2001) Duplexes of 21-nucleotide RNAs mediate RNA interference in cultured mammalian cells. Nature 411:494–498

Evans MJ, Kaufman MH (1981) Establishment in culture of pluripotential cells from mouse embryos. Nature 292:154–156

Feldman B, Poueymirou W, Papaioannou VE, DeChiara TM, Goldfarb M (1995) Requirement of FGF-4 for postimplantation mouse development. Science 267:246–249

Fujikura J, Yamato E, Yonemura S, Hosoda K, Masui S, Nakao K, Miyazaki Ji J, Niwa H (2002) Differentiation of embryonic stem cells is induced by GATA factors. Genes Dev 16:784–789

Ginis I, Luo Y, Miura T, Thies S, Brandenberger R, Gerecht-Nir S, Amit M, Hoke A, Carpenter MK, Itskovitz-Eldor J, Rao MS (2004) Differences between human and mouse embryonic stem cells. Dev Biol 269:360–380

Graham V, Khudyakov J, Ellis P, Pevny L (2003) SOX2 functions to maintain neural progenitor identity. Neuron 39:749–765

Guo Y, Costa R, Ramsey H, Starnes T, Vance G, Robertson K, Kelley M, Reinbold R, Scholer H, Hromas R (2002) The embryonic stem cell transcription factors Oct-4 and FoxD3 interact to regulate endodermal-specific promoter expression. Proc Natl Acad Sci U S A 99:3663–7

Hanna LA, Foreman RK, Tarasenko IA, Kessler DS, Labosky PA (2002) Requirement for Foxd3 in maintaining pluripotent cells of the early mouse embryo. Genes Dev 16:2650–2661

Houbaviy HB, Murray MF, Sharp PA (2003) Embryonic stem cell-specific microRNAs. Dev Cell 5:351–358

Humphrey RK, Beattie GM, Lopez AD, Bucay N, King CC, Firpo MT, Rose-John S, Hayek A (2004) Maintenance of pluripotency in human embryonic stem cells is STAT3 independent. Stem Cells 22:522–530

Itskovitz-Eldor J, Schuldiner M, Karsenti D, Eden A, Yanuka O, Amit M, Soreq H, Benvenisty N (2000) Differentiation of human embryonic stem cells into embryoid bodies comprising the three embryonic germ layers [In Process Citation]. Mol Med 6:88–95

Kraft HJ, Mosselman S, Smits HA, Hohenstein P, Piek E, Chen Q, Artzt K, van Zoelen EJ (1996) Oct-4 regulates alternative platelet-derived growth factor alpha receptor gene promoter in human embryonal carcinoma cells. J Biol Chem 271:12873–12878

Layton MJ, Owczarek CM, Metcalf D, Clark RL, Smith DK, Treutlein HR, Nicola NA (1994) Conversion of the biological specificity of murine to human leukemia inhibitory factor by replacing 6 amino acid residues. J Biol Chem 269:29891–29896

Li M, Sendtner M, Smith A (1995) Essential function of LIF receptor in motor neurons. Nature 378:724–727

Liu L, Roberts RM (1996) Silencing of the gene for the beta subunit of human chorionic gonadotropin by the embryonic transcription factor Oct-3/4. J Biol Chem 271:16683–16689

Liu L, Leaman D, Villalta M, Roberts RM (1997) Silencing of the gene for the alpha-subunit of human chorionic gonadotropin by the embryonic transcription factor Oct-3/4. Mol Endocrinol 11:1651–1658

Martin GR (1981) Isolation of a pluripotent cell line from early mouse embryos cultured in medium conditioned by teratocarcinoma stem cells. Proc Natl Acad Sci U S A 78:7634–7638

Martin GR, Evans MJ (1974) The morphology and growth of a pluripotent teratocarcinoma cell line and its derivatives in tissue culture. Cell 2:163–172

Matin MM, Walsh JR, Gokhale PJ, Draper JS, Bahrami AR, Morton I, Moore HD, Andrews PW (2004) Specific knockdown of Oct4 and beta2-microglobulin expression by RNA interference in human embryonic stem cells and embryonic carcinoma cells. Stem Cells 22:659–668

Matsuda T, Nakamura T, Nakao K, Arai T, Katsuki M, Heike T, Yokota T (1999) STAT3 activation is sufficient to maintain an undifferentiated state of mouse embryonic stem cells. EMBO J 18:4261–4269

Matsui Y, Zsebo K, Hogan BL (1992) Derivation of pluripotential embryonic stem cells from murine primordial germ cells in culture. Cell 70:841–847

Mishina Y, Suzuki A, Ueno N, Behringer RR (1995) Bmpr encodes a type I bone morphogenetic protein receptor that is essential for gastrulation during mouse embryogenesis. Genes Dev 9:3027–3037

Mitsui K, Tokuzawa Y, Itoh H, Segawa K, Murakami M, Takahashi K, Maruyama M, Maeda M, Yamanaka S (2003) The homeoprotein Nanog is required for maintenance of pluripotency in mouse epiblast and ES cells. Cell 113:631–642

Nichols J, Zevnik B, Anastassiadis K, Niwa H, Klewe-Nebenius D, Chambers I, Scholer H, Smith A (1998) Formation of pluripotent stem cells in the mammalian embryo depends on the POU transcription factor Oct4. Cell 95:379–391

Nichols J, Chambers I, Taga T, Smith A (2001) Physiological rationale for responsiveness of mouse embryonic stem cells to gp130 cytokines. Development 128:2333–2339

Nishimoto M, Fukushima A, Okuda A, Muramatsu M (1999) The gene for the embryonic stem cell coactivator UTF1 carries a regulatory element which selectively interacts with a complex composed of Oct-3/4 and Sox-2. Mol Cell Biol 19:5453–5465

Niwa H, Miyazaki J, Smith AG (2000) Quantitative expression of Oct-3/4 defines differentiation, dedifferentiation or self-renewal of ES cells. Nat Genet 24:372–376

Paling NR, Wheadon H, Bone HK, Welham MJ (2004) Regulation of embryonic stem cell self-renewal by phosphoinositide 3-kinase-dependent signaling. J Biol Chem 279:48063–48070

Palmieri SL, Peter W, Hess H, Scholer HR (1994) Oct-4 transcription factor is differentially expressed in the mouse embryo during establishment of the first two extraembryonic cell lineages involved in implantation. Dev Biol 166:259–267

Pan G, Pei D (2004) The stem cell pluripotency factor Nanog activates transcription with two unusually potent subdomains at its C-terminus. J Biol Chem 280:1401–1407

Qi X, Li TG, Hao J, Hu J, Wang J, Simmons H, Miura S, Mishina Y, Zhao GQ (2004) BMP4 supports self-renewal of embryonic stem cells by inhibiting mitogen-activated protein kinase pathways. Proc Natl Acad Sci U S A 101:6027–6032

Rao RR, Stice SL (2004) Gene expression profiling of embryonic stem cells leads to greater understanding of pluripotency and early developmental events. Biol Reprod 71:1772–1778

Resnick JL, Bixler LS, Cheng L, Donovan PJ (1992) Long-term proliferation of mouse primordial germ cells in culture. Nature 359:550–551

Reubinoff BE, Pera MF, Fong CY, Trounson A, Bongso A (2000) Embryonic stem cell lines from human blastocysts: somatic differentiation in vitro. Nat Biotechnol 18:399–404

Rohwedel J, Guan K, Hegert C, Wobus AM (2001) Embryonic stem cells as an in vitro model for mutagenicity, cytotoxicity and embryotoxicity studies: present state and future prospects. Toxicol In Vitro 15:741–753

Rose TM, Weiford DM, Gunderson NL, Bruce AG (1994) Oncostatin M (OSM) inhibits the differentiation of pluripotent embryonic stem cells in vitro. Cytokine 6:48–54

Rose-John S (2002) GP130 stimulation and the maintenance of stem cells. Trends Biotechnol 20:417–419

Sato N, Meijer L, Skaltsounis L, Greengard P, Brivanlou AH (2004) Maintenance of pluripo-
    tency in human and mouse embryonic stem cells through activation of Wnt signaling
    by a pharmacological GSK-3-specific inhibitor. Nat Med 10:55–63
Scholer HR, Ciesiolka T, Gruss P (1991) A nexus between Oct-4 and E1A: implications for
    gene regulation in embryonic stem cells. Cell 66:291–304
Schuldiner M, Benvenisty N (2003) Factors controlling human embryonic stem cell differ-
    entiation. Methods Enzymol 365:446–461
Schuldiner M, Yanuka O, Itskovitz-Eldor J, Melton DA, Benvenisty N (2000) Effects of eight
    growth factors on the differentiation of cells derived from human embryonic stem cells.
    Proc Natl Acad Sci U S A 97:11307–11312
Shamblott MJ, Axelman J, Wang S, Bugg EM, Littlefield JW, Donovan PJ, Blumenthal PD,
    Huggins GR, Gearhart JD (1998) Derivation of pluripotent stem cells from cultured
    human primordial germ cells. Proc Natl Acad Sci U S A 95:13726–13731
Sirard C, de la Pompa JL, Elia A, Itie A, Mirtsos C, Cheung A, Hahn S, Wakeham A, Schwartz L,
    Kern SE, Rossant J, Mak TW (1998) The tumor suppressor gene Smad4/Dpc4 is required
    for gastrulation and later for anterior development of the mouse embryo. Genes Dev
    12:107–119
Smith AG, Heath JK, Donaldson DD, Wong GG, Moreau J, Stahl M, Rogers D (1988) Inhibition
    of pluripotential embryonic stem cell differentiation by purified polypeptides. Nature
    336:688–690
Stein PL, Vogel H, Soriano P (1994) Combined deficiencies of Src, Fyn, and Yes tyrosine
    kinases in mutant mice. Genes Dev 8:1999–2007
Stewart CL, Kaspar P, Brunet LJ, Bhatt H, Gadi I, Kontgen F, Abbondanzo SJ (1992) Blastocyst
    implantation depends on maternal expression of leukaemia inhibitory factor. Nature
    359:76–79
Suemori H, Hashimoto S, Nakatsuji N (1988) Presence of the adenovirus E1A-like activity
    in preimplantation stage mouse embryos. Mol Cell Biol 8:3553–3555
Suh MR, Lee Y, Kim JY, Kim SK, Moon SH, Lee JY, Cha KY, Chung HM, Yoon HS, Moon SY,
    Kim VN, Kim KS (2004) Human embryonic stem cells express a unique set of microRNAs.
    Dev Biol 270:488–498
Tai MH, Chang CC, Olson LK, Trosko JE (2005) Oct4 expression in adult human stem cells:
    evidence in support of the stem cell theory of carcinogenesis. Carcinogenesis 26:495–502
Thomson JA, Itskovitz-Eldor J, Shapiro SS, Waknitz MA, Swiergiel JJ, Marshall VS, Jones JM
    (1998) Embryonic stem cell lines derived from human blastocysts. Science 282:1145–1147
Tokuzawa Y, Kaiho E, Maruyama M, Takahashi K, Mitsui K, Maeda M, Niwa H, Yamanaka S
    (2003) Fbx15 is a novel target of Oct3/4 but is dispensable for embryonic stem cell
    self-renewal and mouse development. Mol Cell Biol 23:2699–2708
Urbach A, Schuldiner M, Benvenisty N (2004) Modeling for Lesch-Nyhan disease by gene
    targeting in human embryonic stem cells. Stem Cells 22:635–641
Ware CB, Horowitz MC, Renshaw BR, Hunt JS, Liggitt D, Koblar SA, Gliniak BC, McKenna HJ,
    Papayannopoulou T, Thoma B et al. (1995) Targeted disruption of the low-affinity
    leukemia inhibitory factor receptor gene causes placental, skeletal, neural and metabolic
    defects and results in perinatal death. Development 121:1283–1299
Williams RL, Hilton DJ, Pease S, Willson TA, Stewart CL, Gearing DP, Wagner EF, Met-
    calf D, Nicola NA, Gough NM (1988) Myeloid leukaemia inhibitory factor maintains the
    developmental potential of embryonic stem cells. Nature 336:684–687
Winnier G, Blessing M, Labosky PA, Hogan BL (1995) Bone morphogenetic protein-4 is
    required for mesoderm formation and patterning in the mouse. Genes Dev 9:2105–116
Xu C, Inokuma MS, Denham J, Golds K, Kundu P, Gold JD, Carpenter MK (2001) Feeder-free
    growth of undifferentiated human embryonic stem cells. Nat Biotechnol 19:971–974

Xu RH, Chen X, Li DS, Li R, Addicks GC, Glennon C, Zwaka TP, Thomson JA (2002) BMP4 initiates human embryonic stem cell differentiation to trophoblast. Nat Biotechnol 20:1261–1264

Yeom YI, Fuhrmann G, Ovitt CE, Brehm A, Ohbo K, Gross M, Hubner K, Scholer HR (1996) Germline regulatory element of Oct-4 specific for the totipotent cycle of embryonal cells. Development 122:881–894

Ying QL, Nichols J, Chambers I, Smith A (2003) BMP induction of Id proteins suppresses differentiation and sustains embryonic stem cell self-renewal in collaboration with STAT3. Cell 115:281–292

Yoshida K, Taga T, Saito M, Suematsu S, Kumanogoh A, Tanaka T, Fujiwara H, Hirata M, Yamagami T, Nakahata T, Hirabayashi T, Yoneda Y, Tanaka K, Wang WZ, Mori C, Shiota K, Yoshida N, Kishimoto T (1996) Targeted disruption of gp130, a common signal transducer for the interleukin 6 family of cytokines, leads to myocardial and hematological disorders. Proc Natl Acad Sci U S A 93:407–411

Yuan H, Corbi N, Basilico C, Dailey L (1995) Developmental-specific activity of the FGF-4 enhancer requires the synergistic action of Sox2 and Oct-3. Genes Dev 9:2635–2645

HEP (2006) 174:21–51
© Springer-Verlag Berlin Heidelberg 2006

Embryonic Stem Cell-Derived Embryoid Bodies: An In Vitro Model of Eutherian Pregastrulation Development and Early Gastrulation

G. Weitzer

Max F. Perutz Laboratories, Department of Medical Biochemistry, Division of Molecular Cell Biology, University Institutes at the Vienna Biocenter, Medical University of Vienna, Dr. Bohrgasse 9, 1030 Vienna, Austria
georg.weitzer@univie.ac.at

Abstract In this review, I describe the dawn of embryoid body research and the influence of stem cell properties on embryoid body development. I will focus on the in vitro differentiation of embryonic stem cells in embryoid bodies. I summarize and combine published data for embryo-like development of embryoid bodies, and based on these findings, I will discuss open questions, concerns, and possible future directions of this still emerging field of research. I hope to provide new perspectives and experimental approaches that go beyond the current state of the art to foster an understanding of eutherian embryogenesis and provide clues for the efficient production of somatic cells for cell therapy.

Keywords Embryoid body · Gastrulation · Morphogenesis · Embryogenesis

1
Introduction

Embryoid bodies represent a unique tool to investigate developmental processes. They seem to mimic the development of eutherian embryos during stages of pregastrulation development and early gastrulation, and serve as surrogates of eutherian embryos, which are generally inaccessible following implantation of late blastocysts into the uterine wall of the mother. Embryoid body research should therefore facilitate an understanding of embryonic development at the molecular and cellular level, and based on this the comparative phylogeny of species. Establishment of a reliable model of in vitro embryogenesis may also contribute to a reduction in the number of animal experiments required for tests in the medical and pharmacological field. This research may significantly contribute to the direct differentiation of embryonic and somatic stem cells towards a specific cell type useful for therapeutic applications and for unravelling the cascade of molecular events that lead to the development of a certain somatic cell type, and inversely, how to exclude the development of other cell lineages. Last but most importantly, these studies will provide means to extinguish residual uncommitted cells, which are the source of tumours that would arise during tissue regeneration after injection of embryonic stem cell-derived somatic cells (Czyz et al. 2003). In this review, I focus on the developmental processes initiated in embryoid bodies upon aggregation of embryonic stem cells, and I will ask whether this in vitro model indeed represents a faithful recapitulation of early eutherian embryogenesis. Based on these data, I shall discuss future developments, limits, and consequences of this still evolving field of research.

2
The Genesis of the Embryoid Body

Embryoid bodies are aggregates of stem cells, the development of which is reminiscent of early eutherian embryogenesis. Embryoid bodies were first observed and described in the second half of the nineteenth century by the German anatomist Heinrich Wilhelm Gottfried von Waldeyer-Hartz and by the German gynaecologist Hans Herrmann Johannes Pfannenstiel (Young 2004) as an in vivo phenomenon in ovarian tumours. The name "embryoid body" was likely given by the French scientist Albert Peyron who described them in testicular tumours (Masson 1970; Peyron 1939). Much later, embryoid bodies were reported to arise in experimentally induced teratomas and teratocarcinomas in mice (Pierce et al. 1960; Stevens 1958, 1959, 1960), and with the exception of one manuscript demonstrating the developmental potential of clonal embryonic carcinoma cells in 1964 (Kleinsmith and Pierce 1964), another 15 years passed before embryoid bodies became the subject of in vitro studies. Arnold Levine generated embryoid bodies from teratoma cells in 1974 (Levine et al. 1974), immediately followed by Gail Martin and J.F. Nicolas in 1975, who generated embryoid bodies from teratocarcinoma cells (Evans 1981; Martin and Evans 1975; Martin et al. 1977; Nicolas et al. 1975). In 1980, embryoid bodies were generated from a human ovarian teratocarcinoma-derived cell line (Zeuthen et al. 1980), and finally from embryonic stem cells, isolated from the inner cell mass of murine blastocysts (Evans and Kaufman 1981; Martin 1981). These were the first cells shown to contribute to chimeric mice and finally to the germ line of an animal (Bradley et al. 1984, 1998). Two years later, embryonic stem cells were successfully used for the first time as vectors to introduce a transgene into the germ line of mice (Robertson et al. 1986). In the meantime, Thomas Doetschman and Rolf Kemler reported that embryonic stem cells spontaneously differentiate into derivatives of all three germ lines in vitro (Doetschman et al. 1985), and since then, innumerable data have been obtained providing evidence that embryoid body-derived somatic cells may be used as the point of origin for cell therapy, and that embryoid bodies may represent a useful in vitro model for early eutherian embryonic development. In 1992, primordial germ cells were also isolated and shown to form embryoid bodies (Resnick et al. 1992). It also became evident that embryoid bodies represented a good tool to study homozygous null alleles (Robertson et al. 1992) with subtle phenotypes that were either hidden in vivo (Bagutti et al. 1996; Fässler et al. 1996; Milner et al. 1996; Weitzer et al. 1995) or caused early embryonic lethality (Di Cristofano et al. 1998; Fässler et al. 1995; Rohwedel et al. 1998).

The development of embryoid bodies was dependent on the type and potential of stem cells, and the species from which these cells were derived. Early embryoid body research, employing different teratocarcinoma cell lines such as the F9, P19, PC13, C145A12, OC15S1, P10, etc. (Dyban 1984; Martin 1980; McBurney and Strutt 1980), gave useful information on developmental processes that somehow recapitulated certain aspects of early embryogenesis (Martin 1980). Due to the different origin of these cell lines and their divergent developmental potential, a common theme could not be established that provided a uniform picture of in vitro embryonic development. Publication of articles in French, Russian and German contributed to this mainly cell line-based Babylonian confusion of tongues. The main prerequisite for the establishment of an in vitro model of early eutherian embryogenesis was, and still is, the isolation and in vitro maintenance of embryonic stem cells. These issues proved to be the rate limiting steps to scientific progress in this field of research. After four decades of research, embryonic stem cells could only be isolated from a dozen or so species, and all but the murine embryonic stem cells failed to contribute to the germ line in chimeric animals (Table 1).

Probably due to the continued failure to isolate and adequately maintain embryonic stem cells in culture, progress in embryonic stem cell research, and correspondingly in embryoid body research, was very sluggish until 1990 (Fig. 1). This research area developed more quickly between 1990 and 1997, a period accompanied by the description of embryonic stem cells and primordial germ cell-like cells. Nonetheless, at the end of 1997, only a total of 260 papers were published in English that mentioned embryoid bodies in their abstracts. This was a frustratingly small number of publications, when compared

Table 1 Establishment of pluripotent stem cell lines from vertebrate species

Cell type	Year	Species	Reference[a]
Teratocarcinoma cell lines			
	1972	Mouse (*Mus musculum*)	Evans 1972
	1980	Human (*Homo sapiens*)	Zeuthen et al. 1980
Primordial germ cells			
	1992	Mouse (*Mus musculum*)	Matsui et al. 1992; Resnick et al. 1992
	1997	Rabbit (*Oryctolagus cuniculus*)	Moens et al. 1997
	1997	Chicken (*Gallus domesticus*)	Chang et al. 1997
	1997	Pig, Hampshire x Yorkshire (*Sus scrofa*)	Piedrahita et al. 1998; Shim et al. 1997
	1998	Human (*Homo sapiens*)	Shamblott et al. 1998
Embryonic stem cells			
	1981	Mouse (*Mus musculum*)	Evans and Kaufman 1981; Martin 1981
	1983	Mouse, from haploid blastocyst	Kaufman et al. 1983
	1983	Mouse, from parthenogenetic blastocyst	Allen et al. 1994; Robertson et al. 1983
	1988	Golden hamster (*Mesocricetus auratus*)	Doetschman et al. 1988
	1990	Mouse, from androgenetic blastocyst	Mann et al. 1990
	1991	Sheep (*Ovis dalli*)	Notarianni et al. 1991; Wells et al. 1997
	1992	American mink (*Mustela vison*)	Sukoyan et al. 1992; Sukoyan et al. 1993
	1993	Rabbit (*Oryctolagus cuniculus*)	Graves et al. 1993; Schoonjans et al. 1996
	1994	Rat (*Rattus norvegicus*)[b]	Iannaccone et al. 1994
	1994	Pig (*Sus scrofa*)	Li et al. 2003; Wheeler 1994
	1995	Rhesus monkey (*Macaca mulatta*)	Pau and Wolf 2004; Thomson et al. 1995
	1996	Cattle (*Bos taurus*)	Mitalipova et al. 2001; Stice et al. 1996
	1996	Common marmoset (*Callithrix jacchus*)	Thomson et al. 1996, 1998
	1996	Chicken (*Gallus domesticus*)	Pain et al. 1996; Petitte et al. 2004
	1998	Medaka (*Oryzias latipes*)	Hong et al. 1998a, 1998b
	1998	Human (*Homo sapiens*)	Thomson et al. 1998
	2002	Horse (*Equus* sp., Hokkaido native pony)	Saito et al. 2002

Table 1 (continued)

Cell type	Year	Species	Reference[a]
	2002	Cynomolgus monkey (*M. afascicularis*)	Nakatsuji et al. 2002; Suemori et al. 2003
	2004	Mouse (*Mus spretus x Mus musculum*)	Hochepied et al. 2004
	2004	Dog (*Canis familiaris*)	http://swri.ca/scientists/G-L/hough
	2004	Human, from cloned blastocyst	Hwang et al. 2004
	2004	Human, from parthenogenetic blastocyst	Chen and Li 2004

[a] Selected references indicate only the first reported isolation of stem cells for each species
[b] Isolation of embryonic stem cells from rat could not be repeated

to other fields of research such as on the role of tubulin, which produced 8,474 papers in the same period of time. Embryoid body research obtained a boost, and perhaps a logarithmic increase in research interest, after the isolation of human embryonic stem cells (Thomson et al. 1998), which, similar to mouse cells, could contribute to all three germ layers in teratomas induced in mice. In parallel, pluripotent stem cells were derived from cultured human primordial germ cells (Park et al. 2004; Shamblott et al. 1998). Shortly thereafter, human embryonic stem cell-derived embryoid bodies were shown to have a potential comparable to that of murine embryoid bodies (Itskovitz Eldor et al. 2000; Schuldiner et al. 2000). Finally, in 2004 a Korean group succeeded in generating

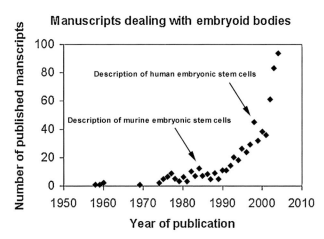

Fig. 1 Historical development of the field of embryoid body research. Data were obtained from PUBMED, http://www.ncbi.nlm.nih.gov/entrez/query.fcgi covering the time period of 1.1.1900 to 26.11.2004

embryonic stem cells from cloned human blastocysts (Hwang et al. 2004). For ethical and practical reasons (or at least experiments were not published), it is unclear whether any of these human embryonic stem and embryonic germ cells would contribute to the germ line in chimeric animals (Prelle et al. 2002); however, these cells were most certainly pluripotent.

The generation of human embryonic stem cells was a step in the development of a basic science field, which originated from the observation of naturally occurring teratomas. The generation of human embryonic stem cell lines ushered embryonic stem cell and embryoid body research to the medical field, and put it squarely in the centre of public awareness. Research on human embryonic stem cells has led to the expectations of possible therapies (Wobus and Boheler 2005), but it has also raised the specter of serious ethical issues pertaining to the status and role of these cells in human ontogeny and, for religious people, in creation. Hypothetically, humans could for the first time view themselves as a group of cells influenced by an unforeseeable number of factors and stochastic events. Research on eutherian and, in particular on human embryos, embryonic stem cells and embryoid bodies may lead to new therapeutic strategies that will revolutionize medicine, but the inevitable price for these advances will involve philosophical and ethical questions pertaining to human self-perception (Nusslein-Volhard 2004).

3
The Influence of Embryonic Stem Cell Lines on Embryoid Body Development

To date, embryonic stem cells have only been isolated from the inner cell mass of blastocysts from a few eutherian species (Table 1), and it is probable that many unpublished attempts to generate embryonic stem cell lines from other species have only met with failure. From our own attempts to isolate new cell lines from different strains of mice, we learned that embryonic stem cell lines could be readily obtained from 38% of the explanted blastocysts from 129Sv x C57BL/6J and C3H mouse strains, but only 1% of C57BL/6J inner cell masses gave rise to an embryonic stem cell line. It has proved impossible so far to isolate a single embryonic stem cell line from FVB blastocysts. These highly variable rates of success, with respect to the generation of embryonic stem cell lines from different mouse strains performed under identical conditions, suggest that the genetic background and perhaps even minor epigenetic differences between strains and perhaps profound differences among species might predetermine whether the inner cell masses can survive on feeder cells in the presence of leukaemia inhibitory factor or not. These strain- and species-dependent characteristics became even more pronounced when the cultivation of human embryonic stem cells lines were found to be independent of leukaemia inhibitory factor (Humphrey et al. 2004).

Many researchers who have acquired embryonic stem cell lines from other labs have unfortunately discovered that these cells do not always behave as their own cell lines, and even worse, some of these lines give rise to unexpected phenotypes in embryoid bodies. Self-renewal capacity, plasticity and differentiation control, often comprehended as potency, is therefore highly variable among even isogenic embryonic stem cell lines generated in different laboratories. Embryoid body development is not only influenced by the genetic background of embryonic stem cells, but also by the complex conditions under which these embryonic stem cell lines have been generated.

Additional parameters that influence embryonic stem cell potential and embryoid body differentiation include the developmental stage of the embryo at the time of embryonic stem cell generation, the time required to reach confluency of embryonic stem cells in vitro, the type of feeder cells, the source and batch of foetal calf serum, and last but not least, the handling of the cells by the investigator. The influence of serum components such as growth factors and cytokines, in particular, of leukaemia inhibitory factor on pluripotency and differentiation has been the subject of intense investigation (Burdon et al. 2002; Schuldiner et al. 2000). Furthermore, self-renewal capacity (Chambers and Smith 2004) strongly influences embryoid body development. The initial proliferation of embryonic stem cells, for example, determines the number of embryonic stem cells which aggregate to form embryoid bodies, and the final number of cells in the compact embryoid body strongly influences cardiomyogenesis and haematopoietic cell development (Bader et al. 2001; Dang et al. 2002, 2004). Thus embryonic stem cell proliferation and maintenance of pluripotency significantly contribute to their differentiation potential in embryoid bodies later on.

Gene microarray analysis of various embryonic stem cell clones also support the notion that established embryonic stem cell lines have a highly divergent plasticity and differentiation potential. Fortunel et al. (Fortunel et al. 2003) demonstrated that apart from a very small core of common stemness genes, such as Oct-3/4, Tdgf1 (cripto) and Nanog, expression of other genes is extremely heterogeneous. Currently these findings are insufficient to predict genes that are necessary or sufficient to maintain pluripotency and self-renewal capacity of embryonic stem cells by gene array analysis (Bhattacharya et al. 2004; Carpenter et al. 2003, 2004; Ginis et al. 2004; Ivanova et al. 2002; Ramalho Santos et al. 2002; Sato et al. 2003; Zeng et al. 2004).

So far, too little data have been published with respect to how predifferentiation parameters, other than the genetic background and cell cycle control, influence differentiation potential and elicit certain phenotypes in embryoid bodies. Among many explanations for the differential survival of embryonic stem cells in vitro is the suggestion that rapid loss of the POU domain transcription factor Oct-3/4 in explanted inner cell masses is responsible for the failure to generate stable embryonic stem cell lines (Buehr et al. 2003). In addition, premature or delayed downregulation of Oct-3/4 differentially influences embryoid body development, in particular, that of extra-embryonic lineages (Niwa et al. 2000). Alternatively, the time when zygotic transcription starts will surely determine the availability of receptors for developmentally important growth factors, and thus may either foster or hamper the isolation and maintenance of embryonic stem cells.

Contradictory results and a lack of understanding of the molecular mechanism that influence embryonic stem cell behaviour abet the notion that generation and/or maintenance of embryonic stem cells somehow cause an unforeseeable variability in plasticity and differentiation control. Embryonic stem cell isolation per se might be prone to uncontrollable epigenetic events or other stochastic processes that predispose the differentiation potential of embryonic stem cell lines. For sure, the first contact of an inner cell mass cell with a feeder layer, trophectodermal cells or primitive endodermal cells, which are located at the upper surface of the inner cell mass, facing the blastocoel and later on the culture medium, will predetermine the differentiation potential of these cells. Developmental stage-dependent differences in isogenic embryonic stem cell lines and clonal embryonic stem cell lines, derived from single inner cell masses, respectively, are also responsible for the different developmental potentials of embryoid bodies and the commitment of their primitive ectodermal cells to certain somatic lineages (Lauss et al. 2005) Even uniform expression of "stemness" genes (Ramalho Santos et al. 2002) does not guarantee a foreseeable differentiation potential of newly derived embryonic stem cell lines and inversely, lack of expression of those genes does not exclude the differentiation of cells to certain cell lines.

Differential differentiation potentials of isogenic embryonic stem cell lines has led to the notion, previously discussed (Lake et al. 2000; Stern and Canning 1990), that the inner cell mass is a heterogeneous population of cells. Considering that cells of the inner cell mass are surrounded by an inhomogeneous environment composed of trophectoderm and blastocoel, respectively, and feeder cells and medium later on, it is probable that embryonic stem cells are generated stochastically from one or a few of these cells during a narrow time frame; consequently, these cells will have a defined, but unpredictable differentiation potential. Since the genetic background does not significantly contribute to variations in the differentiation potential (i.e. the differentiation potential varies more between isogenic twins of embryonic stem cell lines than between different genotypes; Lauss et al. 2005), we need to consider developmental differences of the inner cell mass at the blastocyst stage. In other words, when all parameters of embryonic stem cell isolation are effectively identical and the differentiation potential and differentiation control in isogenic embryonic stem cells differ, we must conclude that inner cell mass cells must correspond to a heterogeneous population with different potentials. Embryonic stem cells, which stochastically are generated from one or a few of these cells, therefore must have a defined but unpredictable differentiation potential.

The inherent epigenetic instability of embryonic stem cells (Humpherys et al. 2001) may also influence embryonic stem cell differentiation potential. It is generally accepted that embryonic stem cells are reprogrammed to delete all epigenetic modifications (Dean et al. 2003; Reik et al. 2001); however, examples of epigenetic inheritance exist, which may additionally contribute to the divergence of the differentiation potential observed in embryoid body development (Chong and Whitelaw 2004). Austin Smith places the lack of a physiological rationale for epiblast cells to have a potential for sustained self-renewal on their transient role and existence in vivo (Smith 2001a, 2001b), and furthermore suggests that embryonic stem cell generation may be an "accidental" feature (Buehr and Smith 2003) that occurs only when a certain balance is attained between genetic factors and the facility for epigenetic reprogramming.

Parallel studies with a large set of different human and murine embryonic stem cell lines, e.g. by tagging candidate developmental genes in a stage-specific manner during the development of embryoid bodies (Xiong et al. 1998), will certainly help define a common theme underlying their in vitro development and will provide means to correlate divergent differentiation potentials with the expression of certain sets of genes. Nevertheless questions remain, concerning variability of the differentiation potential, that may be further clarified by cloning several embryonic stem cell lines from individual inner cell mass cells of a single embryo and then determining their differentiation potential. The origin, generation and properties of embryonic stem cells have been most recently and extensively reviewed in an 800-page book edited by Robert Lanza (Lanza 2004a); however, this review does not touch upon phenomena such as divergent developmental potentials of isogenic embryonic stem cell clones or transcriptional noise in embryonic stem cells upon the onset of differentiation.

4
Pregastrulation-Like Development of Embryoid Bodies

Eutherian development requires the implantation of the blastocyst into the maternal uterus. Compaction of the eight-cell morula and three to four further rounds of cell division generate the first cell lineage, the trophectoderm, which contributes to the placenta (Tanaka et al. 1998). The inner cell mass, covered by the trophectoderm, then gives rise to the second differentiating lineage, the primitive endoderm or hypoblast (Watson and Barcroft 2001). The remaining pluripotent primitive ectoderm constitutes the epiblast. During implantation, primitive endoderm differentiates into two extra-embryonic lineages, the visceral endoderm and the parietal endoderm, both of which form the yolk sac (Gardner 1985). Specific cell fates depend on whether primitive endoderm remains on top of the epiblast or migrates along the Reichert's membrane formed by trophectoderm and lining the blastocoele surface (Murray and Edgar 2001b). While visceral endoderm forms a closely associated polarized epithelium, parietal endoderm migrates along the inner side of the trophectodermal bubble and undergoes the first epithelial-mesenchymal transition in embryonic development (Veltmaat et al. 2000; Verheijen and Defize 1999) (see also Fig. 4). These three extra-embryonic endodermal cell layers provide the first contact between the conceptus and the uterus, nurture the remaining central primitive ectoderm, and deliver signals preparing the epiblast for gastrulation (Coucouvanis and Martin 1999; Mummery et al. 1991).

Cell adhesion and cell recognition seem to stand at the dawn of embryogenesis, and indeed differentiation of embryonic stem cells can be induced by culturing cells on bacterial grade Petri dishes, tissue culture dishes, in methylcellulose gels, in liquid suspension cultures, or within gel droplets (Dang et al. 2004; Dang and Zandstra 2004; Gerecht-Nir et al. 2004) at high density in the absence of feeder cells and recombinant leukaemia inhibitory factor. Culturing embryonic stem cells in monolayers on Petri dishes, in the absence of additional influences, such as expression of a committing or selecting transgene, leads primarily to endoderm formation (Thompson and Gudas 2002; Verheijen and Defize 1999), and a much lower and seemingly irreproducible development of other lineages, such as neurons (Li et al. 1998) or cardiomyocytes (Weitzer, unpublished results). Experimental approaches using suspension cultures of embryoid bodies in combination with cell-specific selection procedures may well give rise to pure cell lines suitable for cell therapy; however, this will not allow one to study developmental processes that mimic embryogenesis because of the lack of a reproducible and uniform spatiotemporal organization of these cell aggregates, which requires, firstly, a uniform size of embryoid bodies, and secondly, an implantation-simulating attachment of embryoid bodies to a surface (Bader et al. 2001).

Reproducible aggregation of embryonic stem cells may be achieved in hanging drop cultures, which is much more laborious than suspension cultures; however, these cultures guarantee the generation of embryoid bodies with a uniform size and an equal number of embryonic stem cells. A sufficiently large number of aggregating embryonic stem cells are necessary to give rise to a critical mass of cells within embryoid bodies. Once formed, the cell mass fundamentally influences further development of embryoid bodies (Bader et al. 2001; Miki 1999; Nicolas et al. 1975); therefore, size uniformity of embryoid bodies is an inevitable prerequisite for studying embryogenesis-like developmental processes. It is of utmost importance to establish the correct microenvironment within an embryoid body to maintain or mimic intrinsic cell properties that are critical to the precise regulation of a developmental schedule. This is currently best achieved by a rigorous control of the size of embryoid bodies. Differentiation protocols that use varying numbers of embryonic stem cells, varying percentages of residual leukaemia inhibitory factor-producing feeder cells, or variations in the time that embryonic stem cells are allowed to aggregate, resulted in significant differences in cell lineage commitment. The successful development of rhythmically beating cardiomyocytes, for example, diverges greatly depending on the experimental conditions (Dang et al. 2002; Kuo et al. 2003; Maltsev et al. 1993; Sachinidis et al. 2003; Weitzer et al. 1995).

Mouse embryogenesis is recapitulated best in embryoid bodies when a culture regime is employed that temporally resembles zygote development in the fluid-like environment of the oviduct to the compacted 64 cell containing morula and early 128 cell blastocyst, followed by the implantation of the 128–256 cell blastocysts or early egg cylinder stage embryo into the uterine wall at day 4.5 postcoitum. In hanging drop cultures, embryonic stem cells aggregate within 24 h and form an early morula-like structure. The initial number of embryonic stem cells, however, must be significantly higher than the 16–64 cells of a morula to guarantee development of cells within an embryoid body into derivatives of all three germ layers (remove later on) (Bader et al. 2001; Dang et al. 2004); however, it is still questionable whether embryonic stem cell aggregation is a process that is truly comparable to morula aggregation and compaction, particularly since normally trophectoderm development does not follow compaction of embryoid bodies.

In many laboratories, the initial embryonic stem cell number required for appropriate aggregation and embryoid body formation ranges from 300 to 700 cells. Most likely many of these aggregating cells cannot attach to each other and die, due to damage suffered during trypsination, suspension of embryonic stem cells, or removal of feeder cells. Aggregation and further development is also influenced by the percentage of residual leukaemia inhibitory factor-secreting feeder cells (Bader et al. 2000). Feeder cells interfere with the formation of a morula-like aggregate of embryonic stem cells, because, firstly, they compete for cell–cell interactions with embryonic stem cells; secondly, they insulate communication between embryonic stem cells; and thirdly, they secrete leukaemia inhibitory factor, which negatively affects differentiation to both primitive endoderm and primitive ectoderm by sustaining Oct-3/4 expression in embryonic stem cells (Niwa et al. 2000; Pesce and Schöler 2001).

Once embryonic stem cells successfully aggregate to form small spheres roughly 50–100 µm in diameter, the irregular surface smoothens during the 2nd day of in vitro development to morphologically resemble the process of morula compaction (Fig. 2a). After 3 days, embryoid bodies have a diameter of 100–200 µm and the first primitive endoderm cells appear as refractive bubbles on the surface of the embryoid body (Adamson et al. 1985; Grover et al. 1983). Aggregation of stem cells per se induces primitive endoderm differentiation by downregulation of the stemness factor Nanog (Hamazaki et al. 2004), which is mediated by Ras and MAPK (Smith et al. 2004; Yoshida-Koide et al. 2004). At this time, the outermost cells of the embryoid bodies start to express alpha-fetoprotein (Miki 1999) and N-acetyl-galactosamine epitopes (Bader et al. 2001), and continue to emerge from the embryonic stem cell aggregate until the entire surface of the sphere is covered by primitive endoderm by day 4–5 (Li et al. 2003b; Smyth et al. 1999) (Fig. 2b, 2e).

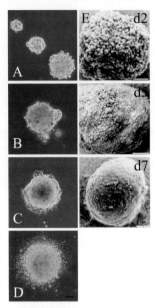

Fig. 2a–e The early development of embryoid bodies. Aggregation of embryonic stem cells and development to embryoid bodies consisting of a central epiblast-like primitive ectoderm and an enclosing hypoblast-like primitive endoderm. **a** The irregularly shaped embryonic stem cell aggregate that forms after 1 day (*upper left*) develops into a spherical embryoid body by day 2 (*middle*) that increases in size through the formation of an outer layer of primitive endoderm cells (bubble-like cells, *lower right*) and epithelialization of the primitive ectoderm (not visible). **b** A cystic embryoid body on day 4.5 with an early visceral endoderm bubble right before attachment to a collagen-coated culture dish. **c** An attached embryoid body on day 5 with migrating primitive endoderm cells that differentiate to parietal endoderm cells. **d** An embryoid body on day 6 with a uniform central mass of cells presumptively composed of primitive ectoderm and early mesoderm surrounded by parietal endoderm. Phase contrast images, bar 70 µm. **e** Scanning microscopy images of embryoid bodies in suspension culture at days 2, 5 and 7 after aggregation demonstrates increasing epithelialization of the extra-embryonic endoderm engulfing the embryoid bodies. Note that these embryoid bodies are composed of a larger initial number of embryonic stem cells, and that the size of embryoid bodies does not increase in suspension as much as when attached to a surface. Images were kindly provided by Dr. Anna Wobus (Wobus et al. 1997). Bars, 50 µm

Concomitantly, these cells start to secrete components of the extracellular matrix to form a basement membrane (Aumailley et al. 2000; Gao et al. 2004; Li et al. 2001, 2004; Murray and Edgar 2001b; Smyth et al. 1999), which effectively isolates the remaining embryonic stem cells from at least some environmental influences and consequently generates a new microenvironment for the emerging primitive ectoderm. The pattern of endodermal gene expression in embryoid bodies reflects the order found during murine embryogenesis in vivo (Abe et al. 1996; Leahy et al. 1999). At the inner side of the primitive endoderm, embryonic stem cells develop into primitive ectoderm that reorganizes into a columnar epithelium (Ikeda et al. 1999; Smyth et al. 1999) surrounding a central cavity. Expansion of the cysts proceeds either by apoptosis or by reorganization of the growing embryoid body (Miki 1999). This results in a functional analogue to the amniotic cavity of the peri-implantation embryo.

When embryoid bodies are removed from hanging drop cultures and placed on a collagen-coated surface at day 4.5, a time when murine blastocysts lose their zona pellucida and start to implant into the uterine wall, primitive endoderm attaches to the artificial extracellular matrix and starts to migrate (Fig. 2c). The collagen matrix, which substitutes for Reichert's membrane at the inner side of the trophectoderm of an embryo, facilitates attachment of primitive endoderm cells (Fig. 2d) and promotes the differentiation to parietal endoderm (Adamson et al. 1985; Casanova and Grabel 1988; Grabel and Casanova 1986; Grabel and Watts 1987; Grover et al. 1983) in a GATA-6-dependent manner (Fujikura et al. 2002; Li et al. 2004). Parietal endoderm migration is regulated by integrins (Jiang and Grabel 1995), and subsequently parietal endoderm undergoes an epithelial to mesenchymal transition at the distal part of the attached embryoid bodies (Cheng and Grabel 1997; Jiang et al. 1995; Murray and Edgar 2001b). Visceral endoderm develops as epithelial bubbles on top of the central cell mass (Bader et al. 2001; Conley et al. 2004a; Murray and Edgar 2001a). Indian hedgehog promotes development of visceral endoderm in F9 embryonic carcinoma cell-derived embryoid bodies (Becker et al. 1997; Coucouvanis and Martin 1999), whereas the transcription factor MyoR functions as a transcriptional repressor of endoderm development (Yu et al. 2004). Targeted disruption of either GATA-4 (Soudais et al. 1995) or fibroblast growth factor receptor 1 (Esner et al. 2002) blocks the development and maturation of visceral endoderm. Finally, bone morphogenetic protein signalling is required for the differentiation of visceral endoderm and the cavitation of embryoid bodies (Coucouvanis and Martin 1999). Cavitation defines the volume of liquid in the pro-amniotic cavity below the epithelium of primitive ectoderm in embryoid bodies. In F9-derived embryoid bodies, the volume of liquid functions as a signal for visceral endoderm differentiation, thus influencing the later fate of embryoid bodies (Miki 1999). Notably, until the stage of differentiation that resembles the implanted pre-egg cylinder state of a murine embryo, embryoid bodies maintain a three-dimensional point symmetry. Symmetry is disturbed when embryoid bodies are attached, in particular when cultured at a distance from their neighbours of less than 600 µm.

Removal of the primitive endoderm, at the time when embryoid bodies have formed a continuous layer at the outer side of the sphere, results in a significantly delayed attachment of embryoid bodies, and delays gastrulation-like development and mesoderm formation (Bader et al. 2001; Li et al. 2002); however, it did not irreversibly abolish any developmental process leading to cardiomyocytes. Because removal of primitive endoderm does not inhibit and only delays cardiomyogenesis, it may be reasoned that residual embryonic stem cells, or primitive ectoderm, still have the potential to form primitive endoderm, and that primitive endoderm secretes factors necessary for proper mesoderm development and cardiomyogenesis.

Formation of epithelial primitive endoderm is also necessary for the generation of the basement membrane on which primitive ectoderm undergoes epithelialization (Li et al. 2003b). The loss of the basement membrane in integrin-$\beta1^{-/-}$ (Aumailley et al. 2000; Li et al. 2002), laminin-$\gamma1^{-/-}$ (Aumailley et al. 2000; Li et al. 2002), and dominant negative fibroblast growth factor receptor expressing embryoid bodies (Chen et al. 2000) results in a total failure of epithelialization of the primitive ectoderm and cavitation of embryoid bodies (Li et al. 2003b). Thus primitive endoderm seems to be an indispensable requisite for proper development of primitive ectoderm and uninterrupted gastrulation-like processes. Epithelialization of primitive ectoderm in embryoid bodies depends also on the function of afadin, a key player in epithelial cell–cell interactions (Ikeda et al. 1999). It is essential for further embryo-like development of embryoid bodies, because apoptosis of primitive ectoderm but not of primitive endoderm was increased in afadin-null embryoid bodies before gastrulation.

Basement membrane proteins are necessary but not sufficient for the expression of ectoderm-specific genes in the epithelial primitive ectoderm. The role of extracellular factors evidently plays the major role in commitment of embryonic stem cells to certain lineages in embryoid bodies (Czyz and Wobus 2001). Thus both extracellular matrix components and soluble growth factors produced by the primitive endoderm cells and their derivatives, visceral endoderm and parietal endoderm, seem to be obligatory for full ectodermal development and further gastrulation-like processes in embryoid bodies (Bader et al. 2001; Murray and Edgar 2001a, 2001b; Schuldiner et al. 2000; Veltmaat et al. 2000; Verheijen and Defize 1999). Thus, while endodermal cells are necessary for the formation of basement membrane, on which epithelialization of the primitive ectoderm commences, other factors, partly produced by extra-embryonic and later by definitive endoderm, such as the transforming growth factor-β/bone morphogenetic protein, wnt, notch, fibroblast growth factor, and hedgehog family members and their respective receptors, are all necessary for gastrulation and formation of mesoderm (Brand 2003; Harland and Gerhart 1997; Pandur et al. 2002; Schultheiss et al. 1997; Wang et al. 2004). Epithelialization, as probably the first process of cell organization in the epiblast and hypoblast, both in vivo and in vitro, is immediately followed by an epithelial to mesenchymal transition of hypoblast-derived parietal endoderm, which further contributes to embryoid body development by the upregulation of growth factor expression in mesenchymal parietal endoderm (Stary et al., personal communication). In summary, embryoid body development perfectly recapitulates hypoblast development by producing primitive endoderm that gives rise to visceral endoderm and parietal endoderm; the latter undergoes an epithelial to mesenchymal transition to mature mesenchymal parietal endoderm and through these developmental processes provides the foundation for consecutive gastrulation-like development in embryoid bodies.

Most importantly, these processes lead to a highly ordered structure within embryoid bodies (Ikeda et al. 1999; Li et al. 2002, 2003b, 2004; Vallier et al. 2004), which can be seen in immunostained cross-sections of embryoid bodies. Patricia Murray and David Edgar were the first to point out a topographical regulation of the pregastrulation-like development of embryoid bodies (Murray and Edgar 2004), and they demonstrated that cellular asymmetry and polarity arises from the interaction of embryonic stem cells in an aggregate both by direct cell–cell interaction and via the extracellular matrix. Based on the simple point-symmetrical topography of the early cystic embryoid body, composed of primitive ectoderm and primitive endoderm, topographically predestined interactions built up structures that allow subsequent developmental processes such as gastrulation.

5
Gastrulation-Like Development in Embryoid Bodies

By day 4 to 5 post aggregation, the embryoid body resembles a point-symmetrical shell composed of an inner epiblast and an outer endoblast. The surrounding culture medium may function as a substitute for the blastocoel, and similarly the inner cavity of the embryoid body may serve as a surrogate for the pro-amniotic cavity. Once an embryoid body has attached via its primitive endoderm layer, and visceral endoderm and parietal endoderm have formed, the central mass composed of primitive ectoderm starts to proliferate and mesodermal cells expressing brachyury or haemoglobin appear within 2 days (Bader et al. 2001; Doetschman et al. 1985; Leahy et al. 1999). So far, a gastrulation-like process is only apparent from the expression of markers for mesoderm (Keller et al. 1993), definitive endoderm (Kubo et al. 2004), and definitive ectoderm (Lake et al. 2000; Lang et al. 2004; Pelton et al. 1998; Rathjen and Rathjen 2003). Despite the development of a variety of somatic cells of all three germ lineages in embryoid bodies, as extensively reviewed by Anna Wobus and Richard Mollard (Conley et al. 2004b; Czyz et al. 2003) and in other chapters of this book, there is no doubt that gastrulation-like processes take place in embryoid bodies, but thus far morphological cell movements resembling gastrulation (Keller et al. 2003) have not been described, and as such, embryoid body development is generally considered to be chaotic.

We have previously described a ring-like arrangement of brachyury-positive mesoderm, erythrocytes and cardiomyocytes situated around the centre of embryoid bodies (Bader et al. 2001). If embryoid bodies are handled carefully and individually placed on gelatin-coated culture dishes, a rudimentary morphogenetic development can be observed in a small percentage of embryoid bodies between days 6.5 and 9 (Fig. 3). From days 6 to 7, the two-dimensional point-symmetrical arrangement of the central portion of an embryoid body is disturbed by the formation of a wedge-like epithelial sheet of cells positioned on one side of the embryoid body. These cells are located between the inner cells, which are mainly composed of presumptive primitive ectoderm, and the outer flatted area, which is composed of parietal endoderm cells (Fig. 3a). At day 7, this cellular sheet increases in size; however, it always remains on one side of the embryoid body to establish a twofold axis (Fig. 3b). Axis formation becomes more evident between days 8 and 9 when a horseshoe-shaped, thick area of cells separates from the centre of the embryoid body and migrates or is pushed distally (Fig. 3c, d). This horseshoe-shaped area is lined at its distal side by visceral and parietal endoderm (Fig. 3e), and it contains somatic cells of mesodermal origin such as erythrocytes and fat cells (Fig. 3f, g). The devel-

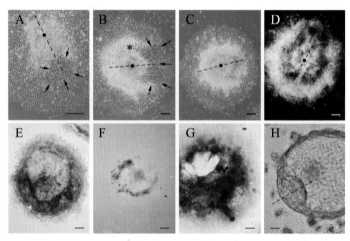

Fig. 3a–h Axis formation in attached embryoid bodies. **a** Formation of a flat epithelial cell sheet on one side of the embryoid body at day 6.5. **b** Increase in the size of the epithelial cell sheet at day 7 and beginning of the asymmetric separation of putative mesodermal cells from the centre of embryoid bodies. **c** Day-8 embryoid body with a clear horseshoe-shaped area of mesoderm containing cell layers. **d** Dark-field image of a day-9 embryoid body highlighting the elevated horseshoe shaped area. **e** visceral endoderm (*dark purple area*) located on top of the horseshoe-shaped area surrounded by epithelial parietal endoderm (*purple cells*) and more distally by mesenchymal parietal endoderm (*light purple cells*) in a day-9 embryoid body. Toluidine blue O-stained embryoid body. **f** Horseshoe-shaped location of erythropoietic cells in a day-8 embryoid body (*dark bluish areas*), Benzidine-stained embryoid body. **g** Day-9 embryoid body with the asymmetric position of the bright epithelial cell sheet negative for adipocytes that contain fat droplets. Sudan Red III-stained embryoid body. **h** First-axis formation in an E4.5 blastocyst by the differentiation of the inner cell mass into primitive ectoderm (*bright cells of the inner cell mass*), and primitive endoderm (*light brown cells of the inner cell mass*), the latter building the border towards the blastocoel. Phase contrast images (**a–c, h**); dark field image (**d**); bright field images (**e–g**). *Black dots*, centre of embryoid bodies; *dashed line*, putative axis; *arrows*, demarcation of the borders of the asymmetric epithelial cell area. Bars in **a–g**, 100 μm; in **h** 25 μm

opment of mesodermal cells in a restricted area of embryoid bodies suggests a gastrulation-like development and axis formation might be similar to the rostrocaudal axis superimposed on the primitive streak of the early mouse gastrula (Rossant and Tam 2002).

Symmetry and the axis are lost when embryoid bodies are cultured at high densities. Usually, embryoid bodies, placed at a distance closer than one to two diameters, develop in a stochastic manner. These chaotic events may be induced by the uncontrolled diffusion of secreted growth factors from one embryoid body to the next and are particularly pronounced when neighbouring embryoid bodies are at distinct developmental stages and thus secrete different growth factors, or when plates are moved and medium is changed, which effectively destroys established gradients of secreted growth factors.

Embryoid bodies, in all probability, express most if not all of the growth factors, cytokines, signal mediators and transcription factors necessary for the induction and regulation of embryogenesis in vivo (Czyz and Wobus 2001; Mummery et al. 1990; O'Shea 2004). The development of ordered structures in certain areas of the embryoid bodies may be the key event associated with reproducible cell–cell contacts and morphogen gradient formation, which are necessary to direct the spatiotemporal regulation of growth factors on developmental processes. Additionally, the formation of reproducible asymmetric structures in embryoid bodies provides clues with respect to how spatiotemporal development may occur. Thus the interaction of cells, the regulation of cell adhesion, the commitment to certain cell fates and the observation of rudimentary morphogenesis suggest that an intricate network of inductive interactions, which patterns and shapes the embryo in vivo, also commence in vitro, in embryoid bodies. Comparison of the morphology of a late egg cylinder-stage and early gastrula-stage embryo with the morphology of an attached embryoid body on day 7 indeed suggests that embryoid bodies may mimic early embryonic development (Fig. 4).

By analogy, the surface of the culture dish fulfils the role of Reichert's membrane on which the parietal endoderm migrates and differentiates, and the culture medium steps in for the liquid filled blastocoel (Watson and Barcroft 2001). Between these two environmental barriers, the hypoblast develops into visceral endoderm, which forms large yolk sac-like bubbles (Abe et al. 1996; Conley et al. 2004a) on top of the central mass of cells resembling the epiblast. In this region, the primitive ectoderm gives rise to embryonic endoderm, definitive ectoderm and mesoderm, the latter of which has been studied extensively because it seems to be a default pathway that generates rhythmically beating cardiomyocytes that appear between days 7 and 8 of in vitro differentiation (Doetschman et al. 1985). Ever since these initial findings, cardiomyogenesis in embryoid bodies has been studied in great detail by many research groups, including ours, and the results of these studies have led directly to the field of cell therapy of cardiac diseases, which are reviewed and discussed from different points of view by several authors in this book.

Egg cyliner stage embryo

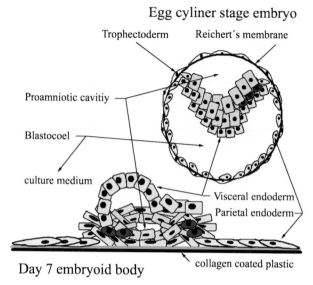

Fig. 4 Schematic comparison of cells and structures between an embryoid body on day 7 and an early egg cylinder stage mouse embryo. The embryoid body is attached to a collagen matrix (*green line*) that substitutes for Reichert's membrane (*black line*) via primitive endoderm (*green rectangular cells underneath the centre of the embryoid body*) and later on via parietal endoderm (*yellow cells*). The visceral endoderm (*green cells*), lining the primitive ectoderm (*purple cells*) in the embryo, forms epithelial cysts on top of the central cell mass of embryoid bodies, which is composed of primitive ectoderm (*purple cells*), mesodermal cells (*red elliptic cells*) and embryonic endoderm (*green cells*). The culture medium substitutes for the blastocoel, and central cyst in the embryoid body is analogous to the pro-amniotic cavity in the embryo

Other than the generation of somatic cells for cell therapy, which is beyond the scope of this review, the most stunning findings that have resulted from embryonic stem cell-derived embryoid body research have been the in vitro generation of germ cells. Embryoid body-derived oocytes can give rise to parthenogenetic blastocysts (Hubner et al. 2003), and embryoid body-derived male gametes have been successfully used to fertilize oocytes to produce diploid blastocysts (Geijsen et al. 2004; Lacham-Kaplan 2004). These results demonstrate that structural self-organization of cells indeed takes place in embryoid bodies, thus raising the possibility that viable and perhaps implantable blastocysts, which have no parents except the foster mother, can be generated from male embryonic stem cell-derived gametes and female embryonic stem cell-derived oocytes in vitro. This raises the possibility that embryos can be generated in vitro for the purpose of establishing new embryonic stem cell lines, which should be ethically less controversial and suitable for the study of germ cell development and fertilization in vitro. The "horror scenario", which alludes to the homunculus theme, has luckily not yet reached public awareness.

6
Developmental Noise or Chaos in Embryoid Bodies

The phenotype of any organism results from a combination of factors, including genotype, epigenetic parameters, and the environment (Rakyan et al. 2001), and it includes a poorly understood component termed "developmental noise". Developmental noise, also known as "intangible variation", is rarely discussed, even though it appears to contribute significantly to the variance of quantitative traits within a species. The molecular basis of developmental noise remains unknown, but it appears to be established in embryonic development and to be retained for the life of the organism. It has been proposed that the molecular basis of developmental noise is, at least in some instances, the epigenetic state of the genome (Blewitt et al. 2004). The stochastic nature for the establishment of an epigenetic state, combined with its heritability during mitosis, seems to provide all of the essential components for developmental noise during embryogenesis.

Stochastic patterning and developmental noise most-likely take place in embryoid bodies and may well be caused, firstly, by stochastic gene expression during differentiation processes that lead to intangible variations in the phenotype, secondly, to so called variegation, the mosaic expression of a gene within a given embryoid body, and thirdly, to random monoallelic expression, independent of parental origin. The possibility that epigenetic modifications are not fully or differentially reset in embryonic stem cell clones further increases the spectrum of phenotypes and fosters the somehow perfunctory notion that embryoid body development is mainly stochastic. These parameters, with currently unpredictable consequences, are interpreted as being chaotic. This somewhat pessimistic view, however, should not affect our continuous endeavour to understand the molecular mechanisms causing variation of phenotypes. Research on embryoid body development might significantly contribute to the discovery of mechanisms that act on top of the genetic program to finally determine the phenotype of each individual organism.

The distinct topographical regulation of very early embryoid body development (Murray and Edgar 2004) and the observation that a given embryonic stem cell line contributes equally well to the development of a certain somatic cell type over time stand in opposition to the notion that embryoid body development is completely chaotic. As an example of the latter, we have employed AB2.2 cells (Soriano et al. 1991) to generate cardiomyocytes from embryoid bodies for 12 years. On average, 86% of all the embryoid bodies produced during this period have yielded equal amounts of beating cardiomyocytes (Lauss et al. 2005), strongly suggesting that these events cannot be wholly chaotic. Transformation of a uniform spherical shell-like shaped embryoid body into a flattened disc with, at least initially, a twofold axis furthermore suggests the existence of intrinsic information for patterning in the cell aggregate. In summary, I have tried to put together the first "pieces of a puzzle" that may eventually clarify in vitro morphogenesis and in vitro embryogenesis-like development.

7
Perspectives

We are only now beginning to understand the morphological processes that occur during in vitro differentiation of embryoid bodies; consequently, many more issues remain to be solved than answers currently can be provided. I will conclude by focusing on three pending questions related to embryogenesis-like development of embryoid bodies.

First, why do embryonic stem cell aggregates fail to develop into blastocysts? The preceding description and discussion of pregastrulation development of the hypoblast-like domain in embryoid bodies clearly points out that primitive endoderm and not trophectoderm form on the surface of embryonic stem cell aggregates. Nonetheless, murine embryonic stem cells can differentiate to trophectoderm in an Oct-3/4-dependent manner (Rossant 2001), and human embryonic stem cells require Bmp-4 to generate trophoblasts (Xu et al. 2002). Lack of trophectoderm formation on the outer surface of embryonic stem cell aggregates may be due to the absence of the zona pellucida, which might contribute some important signals for trophectoderm development. Alternatively, loss of competence of embryonic stem cells to develop into trophectoderm might be a consequence of the morula to blastula transition and consecutive embryonic stem cell generation procedures. Isolation of embryonic stem cells from compacted morula, however, does not solve this problem because these cells differentiate to an inner cell mass indistinguishable from those derived from embryonic stem cell lines (Weitzer, unpublished results). Most-likely, morula-derived cells must first develop to inner cell mass cells in vitro before embryonic stem cells can be derived. This would also explain the extremely low frequency of successful derivation of embryonic stem cell lines from morula-stage embryos. Finally, primitive endoderm, which develops by default from even nonaggregated embryonic stem cells, may secrete factors that are nonpermissive for trophectoderm development, particularly since temporally trophectoderm development in vivo begins prior to primitive endoderm development.

Second, does the timing of in vitro embryogenesis in embryoid bodies mimic embryogenesis? It may well be that embryonic-like development in embryoid bodies is shifted or spread over time and space. In other words, do remnant self-renewing embryonic stem cells continuously "top up" the pool of some somatic lineages? This appears to be the case, because we have succeeded in isolating embryonic stem cell clones from 19-day-old embryoid bodies that have an in vitro differentiation potential indistinguishable from their ancestor embryonic stem cell line for at least 15 passages (Weitzer, unpublished results). Thus embryonic stem cells when encapsulated in perhaps cystic areas of embryoid bodies, where they are shielded against influences that induce their differentiation, can be maintained pluripotent and remain undifferentiated even under conditions that promote differentiation. Consequently, the timing of in vitro embryogenesis is disturbed by the continuous development of new cells. The development and longevity of a certain cell type in embryoid bodies thus may be protracted by continual commitment of embryonic stem cells to primitive ectoderm and subsequent development of somatic cells. This constitutes a major problem, because residual stem cells present in embryonic stem cell-derived somatic cells can give rise to tumours. Getting rid of these undifferentiated cells therefore remains a major obstacle in stem cell research that must be surmounted before stem cell-based therapies can be effectively realized.

Third, what are the mechanisms by which a morphogen gradient (Smith and Gurdon 2004) can be established and maintained in embryoid bodies, and is it possible to obtain morphogenetic development in three dimensions in vitro? Ways to increase the similarities between early embryos in vivo and embryonic-like development in embryoid bodies in vitro might include, firstly, the identification of a suitable substitute for the missing zona pellucida. Secondly, it may be necessary to provide a uterus-like substrate for embryoid bodies for pseudo-implantation. This would perhaps improve in vitro gastrulation by providing additional growth factors secreted from extra-embryonic or maternal compartments. And thirdly, it will be necessary to reduce or avoid serum supplementation, because in vivo, blastocysts do not come directly into contact with the maternal serum. Serum can also be cytotoxic, and it can inhibit developmental processes.

Finally, it will be interesting to determine whether somatic, so-called adult stem cells, have the potential to form embryoid bodies and give rise to all those somatic cell lines that can be generated from embryonic stem cell-derived embryoid bodies. This would provide further evidence that morphogenetic development is not a unique feature of the eutherian zygote.

8
Conclusions

In this review, I have focused on a single aspect of stem cell research and tried to demonstrate that the analysis of embryoid bodies may be useful, at the molecular and cellular level, to further our understanding of events that occur at the very beginning of eutherian embryogenesis. This review stands on the shoulders of several excellent reviews describing embryoid body development from different points of view. The most recent ones (Boheler et al. 2002; Conley et al. 2004b; Czyz et al. 2003; Daley 2003; Desbaillets et al. 2000; Edwards 2004; Hescheler et al. 1997; Lavon and Benvenisty 2003; Murray and Edgar 2004; Nakatsuji and Suemori 2002; O'Shea 2004; Prelle et al. 2002) culminated in a two-volume monograph that encompasses most aspects of stem cell biology (Lanza 2004a, 2004b) and range from the origin of stem cells to the therapeutic application of their somatic derivatives, and conclude with ethical considerations.

The field of stem cell research and with it embryoid body-related research is divided into two camps. The intentions of each camp in embryoid body studies, however, seem to compete for acceptance and are apparently contradictory. One camp focuses on ways to make embryonic stem cells differentiate into one cell type only and meet the demands of cell therapy. On that subject, a plethora of papers sufficient to fill another chapter of this book have been published since human embryonic stem cells were first described in 1998. This type of research has gained tremendous public awareness because of the hope and hype for novel approaches to treat many currently incurable diseases. The second much smaller camp has focused on the developmental biology of stem cells and has attempted to understand the orderly development of all cell types and tissues in vitro. This sounds like pure basic science, but in the long run these approaches will contribute to cell therapy – the first and generally more desirable aim with a clear societal and medical impact. Investigation of in vitro pregastrulation and gastrulation-like development in embryoid bodies will likely provide answers to how lineage commitment and propagation takes place in the eutherian embryo, and consequently, these basic science studies will satisfy not only the curiosity of scientists, but will contribute to a reduction in the number of otherwise necessary animal experiments, and more importantly, will provide hints on how differentiation of many types of stem cells can be deliberately directed to obtain pure somatic cells for future cell-based therapies.

Acknowledgements Special thanks are extended to Dr. Boheler for the significant improvement of the readability of this review and to Dr. Wobus for providing Fig. 2e.
The author's research is supported by grants from the Austrian Fonds zur Förderung der wissenschaftlichen Forschung, grant P15303, the Jubiläumsfonds der Österreichischen Nationalbank, grant 8437, the Hochschuljubiläumsstiftung der Stadt Wien, grant H-933/2003 and the Austrian Ministry of Science, bm:bwk.

References

Abe K, Niwa H, Iwase K, Takiguchi M, Mori M, Abe SI, Yamamura KI (1996) Endoderm-specific gene expression in embryonic stem cells differentiated to embryoid bodies. Exp Cell Res 229:27–34

Adamson ED, Strickland S, Tu M, Kahan B (1985) A teratocarcinoma-derived endoderm stem cell line (1H5) that can differentiate into extra-embryonic endoderm cell types. Differentiation 29:68–76

Allen ND, Barton SC, Hilton K, Norris ML, Surani MA (1994) A functional analysis of imprinting in parthenogenetic embryonic stem cells. Development 120:1473–1482

Aumailley M, Pesch M, Tunggal L, Gaill F, Fässler R (2000) Altered synthesis of laminin 1 and absence of basement membrane component deposition in (beta)1 integrin-deficient embryoid bodies. J Cell Sci 113:259–268

Bader A, Al-Dubai H, Weitzer G (2000) Leukemia inhibitory factor modulates cardiogenesis in embryoid bodies in opposite fashions. Circ Res 86:787–794

Bader A, Gruss A, Höllrigl A, Al Dubai H, Capetanaki Y, Weitzer G (2001) Paracrine promotion of cardiomyogenesis in embryoid bodies by LIF modulated endoderm. Differentiation 68:31–43

Bagutti C, Wobus AM, Fässler R, Watt FM (1996) Differentiation of embryonal stem cells into keratinocytes: comparison of wild-type and beta 1 integrin-deficient cells. Dev Biol 179:184–196

Becker S, Wang ZJ, Massey H, Arauz A, Labosky P, Hammerschmidt M, St-Jacques B, Bumcrot D, McMahon A, Grabel L (1997) A role for Indian hedgehog in extraembryonic endoderm differentiation in F9 cells and the early mouse embryo. Dev Biol 187:298–310

Bhattacharya B, Miura T, Brandenberger R, Mejido J, Luo Y, Yang AX, Joshi BH, Ginis I, Thies RS, Amit M, Lyons I, Condie BG, Itskovitz-Eldor J, Rao MS, Puri RK (2004) Gene expression in human embryonic stem cell lines: unique molecular signature. Blood 103:2956–2964

Blewitt ME, Chong S, Whitelaw E (2004) How the mouse got its spots. Trends Genet 20:550–554

Boheler KR, Czyz J, Tweedie D, Yang HT, Anisimov SV, Wobus AM (2002) Differentiation of pluripotent embryonic stem cells into cardiomyocytes. Circ Res 91:189–201

Bradley A, Evans M, Kaufman MH, Robertson E (1984) Formation of germ-line chimaeras from embryo-derived teratocarcinoma cell lines. Nature 309:255–256

Bradley A, Zheng B, Liu P (1998) Thirteen years of manipulating the mouse genome: a personal history. Int J Dev Biol 42:943–950

Brand T (2003) Heart development: molecular insights into cardiac specification and early morphogenesis. Dev Biol 258:1–19

Buehr M, Smith A (2003) Genesis of embryonic stem cells. Philos Trans R Soc Lond B Biol Sci 358:1397–1402

Buehr M, Nichols J, Stenhouse F, Mountford P, Greenhalgh CJ, Kantachuvesiri S, Brooker G, Mullins J, Smith AG (2003) Rapid loss of Oct-4 and pluripotency in cultured rodent blastocysts and derivative cell lines. Biol Reprod 68:222–229

Burdon T, Smith A, Savatier P (2002) Signalling, cell cycle and pluripotency in embryonic stem cells. Trends Cell Biol 12:432–438

Carpenter MK, Rosler E, Rao MS (2003) Characterization and differentiation of human embryonic stem cells. Cloning Stem Cells 5:79–88

Carpenter MK, Rosler ES, Fisk GJ, Brandenberger R, Ares X, Miura T, Lucero M, Rao MS (2004) Properties of four human embryonic stem cell lines maintained in a feeder-free culture system. Dev Dyn 229:243–258

Casanova JE, Grabel LB (1988) The role of cell interactions in the differentiation of teratocarcinoma-derived parietal and visceral endoderm. Dev Biol 129:124–139

Chambers I, Smith A (2004) Self-renewal of teratocarcinoma and embryonic stem cells. Oncogene 23:7150–7160

Chang IK, Jeong DK, Hong YH, Park TS, Moon YK, Ohno T, Han JY (1997) Production of germline chimeric chickens by transfer of cultured primordial germ cells. Cell Biol Int 21:495–499

Chen L, Li H (2004) [Progress in the studies of parthenogenetic embryonic stem cells]. Zhonghua Nan Ke Xue 10:55–58

Chen Y, Li X, Eswarakumar VP, Seger R, Lonai P (2000) Fibroblast growth factor (FGF) signaling through PI 3-kinase and Akt/PKB is required for embryoid body differentiation. Oncogene 19:3750–3756

Cheng L, Grabel LB (1997) The involvement of tissue-type plasminogen activator in parietal endoderm outgrowth. Exp Cell Res 230:187–196

Chong S, Whitelaw E (2004) Epigenetic germline inheritance. Curr Opin Genet Dev 14:692–696

Conley BJ, Trounson AO, Mollard R (2004a) Human embryonic stem cells form embryoid bodies containing visceral endoderm-like derivatives. Fetal Diagn Ther 19:218–223

Conley BJ, Young JC, Trounson AO, Mollard R (2004b) Derivation, propagation and differentiation of human embryonic stem cells. Int J Biochem Cell Biol 36:555–567

Coucouvanis E, Martin GR (1999) BMP signaling plays a role in visceral endoderm differentiation and cavitation in the early mouse embryo. Development 126:535–546

Czyz J, Wobus A (2001) Embryonic stem cell differentiation: the role of extracellular factors. Differentiation 68:167–174

Czyz J, Wiese C, Rolletschek A, Blyszczuk P, Cross M, Wobus AM (2003) Potential of embryonic and adult stem cells in vitro. Biol Chem 384:1391–1409

Daley GQ (2003) From embryos to embryoid bodies: generating blood from embryonic stem cells. Ann N Y Acad Sci 996:122–131

Dang SM, Zandstra PW (2004) Scalable production of embryonic stem cell-derived cells. Methods Mol Biol 290:353–364

Dang SM, Kyba M, Perlingeiro R, Daley GQ, Zandstra PW (2002) Efficiency of embryoid body formation and hematopoietic development from embryonic stem cells in different culture systems. Biotechnol Bioeng 78:442–453

Dang SM, Gerecht-Nir S, Chen J, Itskovitz-Eldor J, Zandstra PW (2004) Controlled, scalable embryonic stem cell differentiation culture. Stem Cells 22:275–282

Dean W, Santos F, Reik W (2003) Epigenetic reprogramming in early mammalian development and following somatic nuclear transfer. Semin Cell Dev Biol 14:93–100

Desbaillets I, Ziegler U, Groscurth P, Gassmann M (2000) Embryoid bodies: an in vitro model of mouse embryogenesis. Exp Physiol 85:645–651

Di Cristofano A, Pesce B, Cordon-Cardo C, Pandolfi PP (1998) Pten is essential for embryonic development and tumour suppression. Nat Genet 19:348–355

Doetschman TC, Eistetter H, Katz M, Schmidt W, Kemler R (1985) The in vitro development of blastocyst-derived embryonic stem cell lines: formation of visceral yolk sac, blood islands and myocardium. J Embryol Exp Morphol 87:27–45

Doetschman T, Williams P, Maeda N (1988) Establishment of hamster blastocyst-derived embryonic stem (ES) cells. Dev Biol 127:224–227

Dyban PA (1984) [Characteristics of the growth and differentiation of teratocarcinoma OC15S1 in syngeneic and allogeneic mice]. Biull Eksp Biol Med 97:71–72

Edwards RG (2004) Stem cells today: A. Origin and potential of embryo stem cells. Reprod Biomed Online 8:275–306

Esner M, Pachernik J, Hampl A, Dvorak P (2002) Targeted disruption of fibroblast growth factor receptor-1 blocks maturation of visceral endoderm and cavitation in mouse embryoid bodies. Int J Dev Biol 46:817–825

Evans MJ (1972) The isolation and properties of a clonal tissue culture strain of pluripotent mouse teratoma cells. J Embryol Exp Morphol 28:163–176

Evans M (1981) Origin of mouse embryonal carcinoma cells and the possibility of their direct isolation into tissue culture. J Reprod Fertil 62:625–631

Evans MJ, Kaufman MH (1981) Establishment in culture of pluripotential cells from mouse embryos. Nature 292:154–156

Fässler R, Pfaff M, Murphy J, Noegel AA, Johansson S, Timpl R, Albrecht R (1995) Lack of beta 1 integrin gene in embryonic stem cells affects morphology, adhesion, and migration but not integration into the inner cell mass of blastocysts. J Cell Biol 128:979–988

Fässler R, Rohwedel J, Maltsev V, Bloch W, Lentini S, Guan K, Gullberg D, Hescheler J, Addicks K, Wobus AM (1996) Differentiation and integrity of cardiac muscle cells are impaired in the absence of beta 1 integrin. J Cell Sci 109:2989–2999

Fortunel NO, Otu HH, Ng HH, Chen J, Mu X, Chevassut T, Li X, Joseph M, Bailey C, Hatzfeld JA, Hatzfeld A, Usta F, Vega VB, Long PM, Libermann TA, Lim B (2003) Comment on " 'Stemness': transcriptional profiling of embryonic and adult stem cells" and "a stem cell molecular signature". Science 302:393b

Fujikura J, Yamato E, Yonemura S, Hosoda K, Masui S, Nakao K, Miyazaki Ji J, Niwa H (2002) Differentiation of embryonic stem cells is induced by GATA factors. Genes Dev 16:784–789

Gao F, Shi HY, Daughty C, Cella N, Zhang M (2004) Maspin plays an essential role in early embryonic development. Development 131:1479–1489

Gardner RL (1985) Regeneration of endoderm from primitive ectoderm in the mouse embryo: fact or artifact? J Embryol Exp Morphol 88:303–326

Geijsen N, Horoschak M, Kim K, Gribnau J, Eggan K, Daley GQ (2004) Derivation of embryonic germ cells and male gametes from embryonic stem cells. Nature 427:148–154

Gerecht-Nir S, Cohen S, Itskovitz-Eldor J (2004) Bioreactor cultivation enhances the efficiency of human embryoid body (hEB) formation and differentiation. Biotechnol Bioeng 86:493–502

Ginis I, Luo Y, Miura T, Thies S, Brandenberger R, Gerecht-Nir S, Amit M, Hoke A, Carpenter MK, Itskovitz-Eldor J, Rao MS (2004) Differences between human and mouse embryonic stem cells. Dev Biol 269:360–380

Grabel LB, Casanova JE (1986) The outgrowth of parietal endoderm from mouse teratocarcinoma stem-cell embryoid bodies. Differentiation 32:67–73

Grabel LB, Watts TD (1987) The role of extracellular matrix in the migration and differentiation of parietal endoderm from teratocarcinoma embryoid bodies. J Cell Biol 105:441–448

Graves KH, Moreadith RW (1993) Derivation and characterization of putative pluripotential embryonic stem cells from preimplantation rabbit embryos. Mol Reprod Dev 36:424–433

Grover A, Oshima RG, Adamson ED (1983) Epithelial layer formation in differentiating aggregates of F9 embryonal carcinoma cells. J Cell Biol 96:1690–1696

Hamazaki T, Oka M, Yamanaka S, Terada N (2004) Aggregation of embryonic stem cells induces Nanog repression and primitive endoderm differentiation. J Cell Sci 117:5681–5686

Harland R, Gerhart J (1997) Formation and function of Spemann's organizer. Annu Rev Cell Dev Biol 13:611–667

Hescheler J, Fleischmann BK, Lentini S, Maltsev VA, Rohwedel J, Wobus AM, Addicks K (1997) Embryonic stem cells: a model to study structural and functional properties in cardiomyogenesis. Cardiovasc Res 36:149–162

Hochepied T, Schoonjans L, Staelens J, Kreemers V, Danloy S, Puimege L, Collen D, Van Roy F, Libert C (2004) Breaking the species barrier: derivation of germline-competent embryonic stem cells from Mus spretus x C57BL/6 hybrids. Stem Cells 22:441–447

Hong Y, Winkler C, Schartl M (1998a) Efficiency of cell culture derivation from blastula embryos and of chimera formation in the medaka (Oryzias latipes) depends on donor genotype and passage number. Dev Genes Evol 208:595–602

Hong Y, Winkler C, Schartl M (1998b) Production of medakafish chimeras from a stable embryonic stem cell line. Proc Natl Acad Sci U S A 95:3679–3684

Hubner K, Fuhrmann G, Christenson LK, Kehler J, Reinbold R, De La Fuente R, Wood J, Strauss JF 3rd, Boiani M, Scholer HR (2003) Derivation of oocytes from mouse embryonic stem cells. Science 300:1251–1256

Humphrey RK, Beattie GM, Lopez AD, Bucay N, King CC, Firpo MT, Rose-John S, Hayek A (2004) Maintenance of pluripotency in human embryonic stem cells is STAT3 independent. Stem Cells 22:522–530

Humpherys D, Eggan K, Akutsu H, Hochedlinger K, Rideout WM 3rd, Biniszkiewicz D, Yanagimachi R, Jaenisch R (2001) Epigenetic instability in ES cells and cloned mice. Science 293:95–97

Hwang WS, Ryu YJ, Park JH, Park ES, Lee EG, Koo JM, Jeon HY, Lee BC, Kang SK, Kim SJ, Ahn C, Hwang JH, Park KY, Cibelli JB, Moon SY (2004) Evidence of a pluripotent human embryonic stem cell line derived from a cloned blastocyst. Science 303:1669–1674

Iannaccone PM, Taborn GU, Garton RL, Caplice MD, Brenin DR (1994) Pluripotent embryonic stem cells from the rat are capable of producing chimeras. Dev Biol 163:288–292

Ikeda W, Nakanishi H, Miyoshi J, Mandai K, Ishizaki H, Tanaka M, Togawa A, Takahashi K, Nishioka H, Yoshida H, Mizoguchi A, Nishikawa S, Takai Y (1999) Afadin: a key molecule essential for structural organization of cell–cell junctions of polarized epithelia during embryogenesis. J Cell Biol 146:1117–1131

Itskovitz Eldor J, Schuldiner M, Karsenti D, Eden A, Yanuka O, Amit M, Soreq H, Benvenisty N (2000) Differentiation of human embryonic stem cells into embryoid bodies comprising the three embryonic germ layers. Mol Med 6:88–95

Ivanova NB, Dimos JT, Schaniel C, Hackney JA, Moore KA, Lemischka IR (2002) A stem cell molecular signature. Science 298:601–604

Jiang R, Grabel LB (1995) Function and differential regulation of the alpha 6 integrin isoforms during parietal endoderm differentiation. Exp Cell Res 217:195–204

Jiang R, Kato M, Bernfield M, Grabel LB (1995) Expression of syndecan-1 changes during the differentiation of visceral and parietal endoderm from murine F9 teratocarcinoma cells. Differentiation 59:225–233

Kaufman MH, Robertson EJ, Handyside AH, Evans MJ (1983) Establishment of pluripotential cell lines from haploid mouse embryos. J Embryol Exp Morphol 73:249–261

Keller G, Kennedy M, Papayannopoulou T, Wiles MV (1993) Hematopoietic commitment during embryonic stem cell differentiation in culture. Mol Cell Biol 13:473–486

Keller R, Davidson LA, Shook DR (2003) How we are shaped: the biomechanics of gastrulation. Differentiation 71:171–205

Kleinsmith LJ, Pierce GB Jr (1964) Multipotentiality of single embryonal carcinoma cells. Cancer Res 24:1544–1551

Kubo A, Shinozaki K, Shannon JM, Kouskoff V, Kennedy M, Woo S, Fehling HJ, Keller G (2004) Development of definitive endoderm from embryonic stem cells in culture. Development 131:1651–1662

Kuo HC, Pau KY, Yeoman RR, Mitalipov SM, Okano H, Wolf DP (2003) Differentiation of monkey embryonic stem cells into neural lineages. Biol Reprod 68:1727–1735

Lacham-Kaplan O (2004) In vivo and in vitro differentiation of male germ cells in the mouse. Reproduction 128:147–152

Lake J, Rathjen J, Remiszewski J, Rathjen PD (2000) Reversible programming of pluripotent cell differentiation. J Cell Sci 113:555–566

Lang KJ, Rathjen J, Vassilieva S, Rathjen PD (2004) Differentiation of embryonic stem cells to a neural fate: a route to re-building the nervous system? J Neurosci Res 76:184–192

Lanza R (2004a) Handbook of stem cells. Elsevier, Academic Press, Amsterdam

Lanza R (2004b) Handbook of stem cells. Elsevier, Academic Press, Amsterdam

Lauss M, Stary M, Tischler J, Egger G, Puz S, Bader-Allmer A, Seiser C, Weitzer G (2005) Single inner cell masses yield embryonic stem cell lines differing in life expression and their developmental potential. Biochem Biophys Res Commun 331:1577–1586

Lavon N, Benvenisty N (2003) Differentiation and genetic manipulation of human embryonic stem cells and the analysis of the cardiovascular system. Trends Cardiovasc Med 13:47–52

Leahy A, Xiong JW, Kuhnert F, Stuhlmann H (1999) Use of developmental marker genes to define temporal and spatial patterns of differentiation during embryoid body formation. J Exp Zool 284:67–81

Levine AJ, Torosian M, Sarokhan AJ, Teresky AK (1974) Biochemical criteria for the in vitro differentiation of embryoid bodies produced by a transplantable teratoma of mice. The production of acetylcholine esterase and creatine phosphokinase by teratoma cells. J Cell Physiol 84:311–317

Li L, Arman E, Ekblom P, Edgar D, Murray P, Lonai P (2004) Distinct GATA6- and laminin-dependent mechanisms regulate endodermal and ectodermal embryonic stem cell fates. Development 131:5277–5286

Li M, Pevny L, Lovell Badge R, Smith A (1998) Generation of purified neural precursors from embryonic stem cells by lineage selection. Curr Biol 8:971–974

Li S, Harrison D, Carbonetto S, Fassler R, Smyth N, Edgar D, Yurchenco PD (2002) Matrix assembly, regulation, and survival functions of laminin and its receptors in embryonic stem cell differentiation. J Cell Biol 157:1279–1290

Li M, Zhang D, Hou Y, Jiao L, Zheng X, Wang WH (2003a) Isolation and culture of embryonic stem cells from porcine blastocysts. Mol Reprod Dev 65:429–434

Li S, Edgar D, Fassler R, Wadsworth W, Yurchenco PD (2003b) The role of laminin in embryonic cell polarization and tissue organization. Dev Cell 4:613–624

Li X, Chen Y, Scheele S, Arman E, Haffner Krausz R, Ekblom P, Lonai P (2001) Fibroblast growth factor signaling and basement membrane assembly are connected during epithelial morphogenesis of the embryoid body. J Cell Biol 153:811–822

Maltsev VA, Rohwedel J, Hescheler J, Wobus AM (1993) Embryonic stem cells differentiate in vitro into cardiomyocytes representing sinusnodal, atrial and ventricular cell types. Mech Dev 44:41–50

Mann JR, Gadi I, Harbison ML, Abbondanzo SJ, Stewart CL (1990) Androgenetic mouse embryonic stem cells are pluripotent and cause skeletal defects in chimeras: implications for genetic imprinting. Cell 62:251–260

Martin GR (1980) Teratocarcinomas and mammalian embryogenesis. Science 209:768–776

Martin GR (1981) Isolation of a pluripotent cell line from early mouse embryos cultured in medium conditioned by teratocarcinoma stem cells. Proc Natl Acad Sci U S A 78:7634–7638

Martin GR, Evans MJ (1975) Differentiation of clonal lines of teratocarcinoma cells: formation of embryoid bodies in vitro. Proc Natl Acad Sci U S A 72:1441–1445

Martin GR, Wiley LM, Damjanov I (1977) The development of cystic embryoid bodies in vitro from clonal teratocarcinoma stem cells. Dev Biol 61:230–244

Masson P (1970) Human tumors, histology, diagnosis and technique, http://www.navi.net/~rsc/cancer/masson01.txt edn. Wayne State University Press

Matsui Y, Zsebo K, Hogan BL (1992) Derivation of pluripotential embryonic stem cells from murine primordial germ cells in culture. Cell 70:841–847

McBurney MW, Strutt BJ (1980) Genetic activity of X chromosomes in pluripotent female teratocarcinoma cells and their differentiated progeny. Cell 21:357–364

Miki K (1999) Volume of liquid below the epithelium of an F9 cell as a signal for differentiation into visceral endoderm. J Cell Sci 112:3071–3080

Milner DJ, Weitzer G, Tran D, Bradley A, Capetanaki Y (1996) Disruption of muscle architecture and myocardial degeneration in mice lacking desmin. J Cell Biol 134:1255–1270

Mitalipova M, Beyhan Z, First NL (2001) Pluripotency of bovine embryonic cell line derived from precompacting embryos. Cloning 3:59–67

Moens A, Flechon B, Degrouard J, Vignon X, Ding J, Flechon JE, Betteridge KJ, Renard JP (1997) Ultrastructural and immunocytochemical analysis of diploid germ cells isolated from fetal rabbit gonads. Zygote 5:47–60

Mummery CL, van den Eijnden-van Raaij AJ, Feijen A, Freund E, Hulskotte E, Schoorlemmer J, Kruijer W (1990) Expression of growth factors during the differentiation of embryonic stem cells in monolayer. Dev Biol 142:406–413

Mummery CL, van Achterberg TA, van den Eijnden-van Raaij AJ, van Haaster L, Willemse A, de Laat SW, Piersma AH (1991) Visceral-endoderm-like cell lines induce differentiation of murine P19 embryonal carcinoma cells. Differentiation 46:51–60

Murray P, Edgar D (2001a) The regulation of embryonic stem cell differentiation by leukaemia inhibitory factor (LIF). Differentiation 68:227–234

Murray P, Edgar D (2001b) Regulation of the differentiation and behaviour of extra-embryonic endodermal cells by basement membranes. J Cell Sci 114:931–939

Murray P, Edgar D (2004) The topographical regulation of embryonic stem cell differentiation. Philos Trans R Soc Lond B Biol Sci 359:1009–1020

Nakatsuji N, Suemori H (2002) Embryonic stem cell lines of nonhuman primates. Sci World J 2:1762–1773

Nicolas JF, Dubois P, Jakob H, Gaillard J, Jacob F (1975) [Mouse teratocarcinoma: differentiation in cultures of a multipotential primitive cell line (author's transl)]. Ann Microbiol (Paris) 126:3–22

Niwa H, Miyazaki J, Smith AG (2000) Quantitative expression of Oct-3/4 defines differentiation, dedifferentiation or self-renewal of ES cells. Nat Genet 24:372–376

Notarianni E, Galli C, Laurie S, Moor RM, Evans MJ (1991) Derivation of pluripotent, embryonic cell lines from the pig and sheep. J Reprod Fertil Suppl 43:255–260

Nusslein-Volhard CN (2004) Von Genen und Embryonen. Reclam Verlag, Leipzig

O'Shea KS (2004) Self-renewal vs. differentiation of mouse embryonic stem cells. Biol Reprod 71:1755–1765

Pain B, Clark ME, Shen M, Nakazawa H, Sakurai M, Samarut J, Etches RJ (1996) Long-term in vitro culture and characterisation of avian embryonic stem cells with multiple morphogenetic potentialities. Development 122:2339–2348

Pandur P, Lasche M, Eisenberg LM, Kuhl M (2002) Wnt-11 activation of a non-canonical Wnt signalling pathway is required for cardiogenesis. Nature 418:636–641

Park JH, Kim SJ, Lee JB, Song JM, Kim CG, Roh S 2nd, Yoon HS (2004) Establishment of a human embryonic germ cell line and comparison with mouse and human embryonic stem cells. Mol Cells 17:309–315

Pau KY, Wolf DP (2004) Derivation and characterization of monkey embryonic stem cells. Reprod Biol Endocrinol 2:41

Pelton TA, Bettess MD, Lake J, Rathjen J, Rathjen PD (1998) Developmental complexity of early mammalian pluripotent cell populations in vivo and in vitro. Reprod Fertil Dev 10:535–549

Pesce M, Scholer HR (2001) Oct-4: gatekeeper in the beginnings of mammalian development. Stem Cells 19:271–278

Petitte JN, Liu G, Yang Z (2004) Avian pluripotent stem cells. Mech Dev 121:1159–1168
Peyron A (1939) Faits nouveaux relatifs à l'origine et à l'histogénèse des embryomes. Bull Assoc Franc étude cancer 28:658–681
Piedrahita JA, Moore K, Oetama B, Lee CK, Scales N, Ramsoondar J, Bazer FW, Ott T (1998) Generation of transgenic porcine chimeras using primordial germ cell-derived colonies. Biol Reprod 58:1321–1329
Pierce GB Jr, Dixon FJ Jr, Verney EL (1960) Teratocarcinogenic and tissue-forming potentials of the cell types comprising neoplastic embryoid bodies. Lab Invest 9:583–602
Prelle K, Zink N, Wolf E (2002) Pluripotent stem cells—model of embryonic development, tool for gene targeting, and basis of cell therapy. Anat Histol Embryol 31:169–186
Rakyan VK, Preis J, Morgan HD, Whitelaw E (2001) The marks, mechanisms and memory of epigenetic states in mammals. Biochem J 356:1–10
Ramalho Santos M, Yoon S, Matsuzaki Y, Mulligan RC, Melton DA (2002) "Stemness": transcriptional profiling of embryonic and adult stem cells. Science 298:597–600
Rathjen J, Rathjen PD (2003) Lineage specific differentiation of mouse ES cells: formation and differentiation of early primitive ectoderm-like (EPL) cells. Methods Enzymol 365:3–25
Reik W, Dean W, Walter J (2001) Epigenetic reprogramming in mammalian development. Science 293:1089–1093
Resnick JL, Bixler LS, Cheng L, Donovan PJ (1992) Long-term proliferation of mouse primordial germ cells in culture. Nature 359:550–551
Robertson EJ, Evans MJ, Kaufman MH (1983) X-chromosome instability in pluripotential stem cell lines derived from parthenogenetic embryos. J Embryol Exp Morphol 74:297–309
Robertson E, Bradley A, Kuehn M, Evans M (1986) Germ-line transmission of genes introduced into cultured pluripotential cells by retroviral vector. Nature 323:445–448
Robertson EJ, Conlon FL, Barth KS, Costantini F, Lee JJ (1992) Use of embryonic stem cells to study mutations affecting postimplantation development in the mouse. Ciba Found Symp 165:237–250; discussion 250–255
Rohwedel J, Guan K, Zuschratter W, Jin S, Ahnert-Hilger G, Furst D, Fassler R, Wobus AM (1998) Loss of beta1 integrin function results in a retardation of myogenic, but an acceleration of neuronal, differentiation of embryonic stem cells in vitro. Dev Biol 201:167–184
Rossant J (2001) Stem cells from the mammalian blastocyst. Stem Cells 19:477–482
Rossant J, Tam PPL (2002) Mouse development. Academic Press, London
Sachinidis A, Fleischmann BK, Kolossov E, Wartenberg M, Sauer H, Hescheler J (2003) Cardiac specific differentiation of mouse embryonic stem cells. Cardiovasc Res 58:278–291
Saito S, Ugai H, Sawai K, Yamamoto Y, Minamihashi A, Kurosaka K, Kobayashi Y, Murata T, Obata Y, Yokoyama K (2002) Isolation of embryonic stem-like cells from equine blastocysts and their differentiation in vitro. FEBS Lett 531:389–396
Sato N, Sanjuan IM, Heke M, Uchida M, Naef F, Brivanlou AH (2003) Molecular signature of human embryonic stem cells and its comparison with the mouse. Dev Biol 260:404–413
Schoonjans L, Albright GM, Li JL, Collen D, Moreadith RW (1996) Pluripotential rabbit embryonic stem (ES) cells are capable of forming overt coat color chimeras following injection into blastocysts. Mol Reprod Dev 45:439–443
Schuldiner M, Yanuka O, Itskovitz-Eldor J, Melton DA, Benvenisty N (2000) Effects of eight growth factors on the differentiation of cells derived from human embryonic stem cells. Proc Natl Acad Sci U S A 97:11307–11312
Schultheiss TM, Burch JB, Lassar AB (1997) A role for bone morphogenetic proteins in the induction of cardiac myogenesis. Genes Dev 11:451–462

Shamblott MJ, Axelman J, Wang S, Bugg EM, Littlefield JW, Donovan PJ, Blumenthal PD, Huggins GR, Gearhart JD (1998) Derivation of pluripotent stem cells from cultured human primordial germ cells. Proc Natl Acad Sci U S A 95:13726–13731

Shim H, Gutierrez-Adan A, Chen LR, BonDurant RH, Behboodi E, Anderson GB (1997) Isolation of pluripotent stem cells from cultured porcine primordial germ cells. Biol Reprod 57:1089–1095

Smith A (2001a) Embryonic stem cells. Cold Spring Harbor Laboratory Press, New York

Smith AG (2001b) Embryo-derived stem cells: of mice and men. Annu Rev Cell Dev Biol 17:435–462

Smith ER, Smedberg JL, Rula ME, Xu XX (2004) Regulation of Ras-MAPK pathway mitogenic activity by restricting nuclear entry of activated MAPK in endoderm differentiation of embryonic carcinoma and stem cells. J Cell Biol 164:689–699

Smith JC, Gurdon JB (2004) Many ways to make a gradient. Bioessays 26:705–706

Smyth N, Vatansever HS, Murray P, Meyer M, Frie C, Paulsson M, Edgar D (1999) Absence of basement membranes after targeting the LAMC1 gene results in embryonic lethality due to failure of endoderm differentiation. J Cell Biol 144:151–160

Soriano P, Montgomery C, Geske R, Bradley A (1991) Targeted disruption of the c-src proto-oncogene leads to osteopetrosis in mice. Cell 64:693–702

Soudais C, Bielinska M, Heikinheimo M, MacArthur CA, Narita N, Saffitz JE, Simon MC, Leiden JM, Wilson DB (1995) Targeted mutagenesis of the transcription factor GATA-4 gene in mouse embryonic stem cells disrupts visceral endoderm differentiation in vitro. Development 121:3877–3888

Stern CD, Canning DR (1990) Origin of cells giving rise to mesoderm and endoderm in chick embryo. Nature 343:273–275

Stevens LC (1958) Studies on transplantable testicular teratomas of strain 129 mice. J Natl Cancer Inst 20:1257–1275

Stevens LC (1959) Embryology of testicular teratomas in strain 129 mice. J Natl Cancer Inst 23:1249–1295

Stevens LC (1960) Embryonic potency of embryoid bodies derived from a transplantable testicular teratoma of the mouse. Dev Biol 2:285–297

Stice SL, Strelchenko NS, Keefer CL, Matthews L (1996) Pluripotent bovine embryonic cell lines direct embryonic development following nuclear transfer. Biol Reprod 54:100–110

Suemori H, Nakatsuji N (2003) Growth and differentiation of cynomolgus monkey ES cells. Methods Enzymol 365:419–429

Sukoyan MA, Golubitsa AN, Zhelezova AI, Shilov AG, Vatolin SY, Maximovsky LP, Andreeva LE, McWhir J, Pack SD, Bayborodin SI (1992) Isolation and cultivation of blastocyst-derived stem cell lines from American mink (Mustela vison). Mol Reprod Dev 33:418–431

Sukoyan MA, Vatolin SY, Golubitsa AN, Zhelezova AI, Semenova LA, Serov OL (1993) Embryonic stem cells derived from morulae, inner cell mass, and blastocysts of mink: comparisons of their pluripotencies. Mol Reprod Dev 36:148–158

Tanaka S, Kunath T, Hadjantonakis AK, Nagy A, Rossant J (1998) Promotion of trophoblast stem cell proliferation by FGF4. Science 282:2072–2075

Thomson JA, Marshall VS (1998) Primate embryonic stem cells. Curr Top Dev Biol 38:133–165

Thompson JR, Gudas LJ (2002) Retinoic acid induces parietal endoderm but not primitive endoderm and visceral endoderm differentiation in F9 teratocarcinoma stem cells with a targeted deletion of the Rex-1 (Zfp-42) gene. Mol Cell Endocrinol 195:119–133

Thomson JA, Kalishman J, Golos TG, Durning M, Harris CP, Becker RA, Hearn JP (1995) Isolation of a primate embryonic stem cell line. Proc Natl Acad Sci U S A 92:7844–7848

Thomson JA, Kalishman J, Golos TG, Durning M, Harris CP, Hearn JP (1996) Pluripotent cell lines derived from common marmoset (Callithrix jacchus) blastocysts. Biol Reprod 55:254–259

Thomson JA, Itskovitz Eldor J, Shapiro SS, Waknitz MA, Swiergiel JJ, Marshall VS, Jones JM (1998) Embryonic stem cell lines derived from human blastocysts. Science 282:1145–1147

Vallier L, Reynolds D, Pedersen RA (2004) Nodal inhibits differentiation of human embryonic stem cells along the neuroectodermal default pathway. Dev Biol 275:403–421

Veltmaat JM, Orelio CC, Ward Van Oostwaard D, Van Rooijen MA, Mummery CL, Defize LH (2000) Snail is an immediate early target gene of parathyroid hormone related peptide signaling in parietal endoderm formation. Int J Dev Biol 44:297–307

Verheijen MH, Defize LH (1999) Signals governing extraembryonic endoderm formation in the mouse: involvement of the type 1 parathyroid hormone-related peptide (PTHrP) receptor, p21Ras and cell adhesion molecules. Int J Dev Biol 43:711–721

Wang QT, Piotrowska K, Ciemerych MA, Milenkovic L, Scott MP, Davis RW, Zernicka-Goetz M (2004) A genome-wide study of gene activity reveals developmental signaling pathways in the preimplantation mouse embryo. Dev Cell 6:133–144

Watson AJ, Barcroft LC (2001) Regulation of blastocyst formation. Front Biosci 6: D708–D730

Weitzer G, Milner DJ, Kim JU, Bradley A, Capetanaki Y (1995) Cytoskeletal control of myogenesis: a desmin null mutation blocks the myogenic pathway during embryonic stem cell differentiation. Dev Biol 172:422–439

Wells DN, Misica PM, Day TA, Tervit HR (1997) Production of cloned lambs from an established embryonic cell line: a comparison between in vivo- and in vitro-matured cytoplasts. Biol Reprod 57:385–393

Wheeler MB (1994) Development and validation of swine embryonic stem cells: a review. Reprod Fertil Dev 6:563–568

Wobus AM, Boheler KR (2005) Embryonic stem cells: prospects for developmental biology and cell therapy. Physiol Rev 85:635–678

Wobus AM, Rohwedel J, Strübing C, Jin S, Adler K, Maltsev V, Hescheler J (1997) In vitro differentiation of embryonic stem cells. Blackwell, Berlin, pp 1–17

Xiong JW, Battaglino R, Leahy A, Stuhlmann H (1998) Large-scale screening for developmental genes in embryonic stem cells and embryoid bodies using retroviral entrapment vectors. Dev Dyn 212:181–197

Xu RH, Chen X, Li DS, Li R, Addicks GC, Glennon C, Zwaka TP, Thomson JA (2002) BMP4 initiates human embryonic stem cell differentiation to trophoblast. Nat Biotechnol 20:1261–1264

Yoshida-Koide U, Matsuda T, Saikawa K, Nakanuma Y, Yokota T, Asashima M, Koide H (2004) Involvement of Ras in extraembryonic endoderm differentiation of embryonic stem cells. Biochem Biophys Res Commun 313:475–481

Young RH (2004) A brief history of the pathology of the gonads. Mod Pathol doi:10.1038/modpathol.3800305:1–15

Yu L, Sangster N, Perez A, McCormick PJ (2004) The bHLH protein MyoR inhibits the differentiation of early embryonic endoderm. Differentiation 72:341–347

Zeng X, Miura T, Luo Y, Bhattacharya B, Condie B, Chen J, Ginis I, Lyons I, Mejido J, Puri RK, Rao MS, Freed WJ (2004) Properties of pluripotent human embryonic stem cells BG01 and BG02. Stem Cells 22:292–312

Zeuthen J, Norgaard JO, Avner P, Fellous M, Wartiovaara J, Vaheri A, Rosen A, Giovanella BC (1980) Characterization of a human ovarian teratocarcinoma-derived cell line. Int J Cancer 25:19–32

HEP (2006) 174:53–71
© Springer-Verlag Berlin Heidelberg 2006

Embryonic Stem Cells: A Novel Tool for the Study of Antiangiogenesis and Tumor-Induced Angiogenesis

M. Wartenberg[1] · F. Dönmez[2] · P. Budde[2] · H. Sauer[3] (✉)

[1]Department of Cell Biology, GKSS Research Center Teltow, Teltow, Germany

[2]Center of Physiology and Pathophysiology, University of Cologne, Cologne, Germany

[3]Department of Physiology, Justus Liebig University Giessen, Aulweg 129, 35392 Giessen, Germany
heinrich.sauer@physiologie.med.uni-giessen.de

Abstract Major research initiatives in antiangiogenesis research have been undertaken to control angiogenic diseases such as polyarthritis, psoriasis, endometriosis, and diabetic retinopathy, and inhibition of tumor-induced angiogenesis has emerged as one of the most promising anti-cancer therapies currently available. Although several quantitative in vivo (i.e., animal models) as well as in vitro (i.e., pure endothelial cell cultures) angiogenesis assays have been described, the development of novel angiogenesis assays with organotypic culture systems that take into account oxygen and nutrient gradients, depth-dependent changes in intracellular pH and a redox state similar to that found in a natural tissue microenvironment are necessary to investigate blood vessel growth. Embryonic stem cells of mouse and human origin have the capacity to develop into three-dimensional tissues with functional capillaries, and this model system represents an excellent in vitro model for antiangiogenesis research. Upon confrontation of stem cells by co-culture with multicellular tumor spheroids, tumor-induced angiogenesis, i.e., the invasion of endothelial host-derived cells into a tumor tissue, can also be monitored. The current review provides an overview of embryonic stem cells as novel tools for antiangiogenesis research and outlines the use of confrontation cultures for the study of tumor-induced angiogenesis.

Keywords Embryonic stem cell · Embryoid body · Angiogenesis · Vasculogenesis · Tumor-induced angiogenesis

1
Introduction

Increasing numbers of angiogenesis assays have been developed in recent years to investigate the molecular events of angiogenesis, and it has become evident that combinations of assays are necessary to investigate the complex cellular and molecular events associated with in vivo angiogenesis (Jain et al. 1997; Auerbach et al. 2003; Staton et al. 2004). The ideal assay would be reliable, technically straightforward, easily quantifiable, and physiologically relevant (Staton et al. 2004), but most of the currently available assays meet only one of these criteria, principally because of the complexity of blood vessel formation in embryos and adult organisms. In vivo, the adult vasculature system is formed from a network of blood vessels that develops during embryogenesis in a process called vasculogenesis. By definition, vasculogenesis means de novo blood vessel formation from endothelial cell precursors. These endothelial cell precursors, i.e., the angioblasts, proliferate and coalesce into a primitive network of blood vessels, thereby forming the primary capillary plexus. From this endothelial cell lattice, angiogenesis (i.e., the sprouting and anastomosis of blood vessels from preexisting ones) subsequently occurs (Papetti et al. 2002; Jain 2003). Thus, the endothelial cell is central to the angiogenic process, but it is not the only cell type involved. In vivo angiogenesis is regulated by several supporting cells, e.g., pericytes, smooth muscle cells, and fibroblast. Furthermore, circulating blood with its cellular and humoral components and the mechanical force that it exerts onto the vascular wall are critical to the process of angiogenesis. This is especially true for arteriogenesis, which refers to the growth of preexisting collateral arterioles and the formation of large conductance arteries that are able to compensate for the loss of function of occluded arteries. The process of arteriogenesis is initiated when shear stresses increase in preexisting collateral pathways upon narrowing of a main artery. The increased shear stress leads to an upregulation of cell adhesion molecules for circulating monocytes, which accumulate subsequently around the proliferating arteries to provide essential cytokines and growth factors (van Royen et al. 2001). An absence of all these adjuvant factors essential to endothelial cell growth and lumen formation limits the reliability of many in vitro angiogenesis assays, which are routinely based on pure endothelial cell cultures grown in either two- or three-dimensions.

In vivo angiogenesis requires that mural cells, i.e., pericytes, be released from the sprouting blood vessel before branching can proceed. Subsequently, basement membrane and extracellular matrix are degraded by matrix-metalloproteinases (MMPs), and stromal cells synthesize new matrix to promote migration and proliferation of endothelial cells (Nguyen et al. 2001). This process is supported by several soluble growth factors, which either positively or negatively guide the complex phenomenon of blood vessel growth. Since endothelial cells in most in vitro assays are removed from their natural tissue microenvironment, no in vitro assay is currently available that fully simulates the fine-tuned set of events that occur during in vivo angiogenesis.

This gap in angiogenesis research can be bridged through the use of embryonic stem (ES) cells grown as multicellular embryoid bodies. Embryoid bodies are cultivated either in hanging drops (Robertson 1987; Wobus et al. 2002), in semisolid (methylcellulose-containing) media (Wiles et al. 1991), or in spinner flasks (Wartenberg et al. 1998b), where they attain sizes of 1–2 mm. Since ES cells spontaneously differentiate into cell types of all three germ layers, all progenic and angiogenic factors normally present in vivo should be available and accessible for scientific investigation in this system. Hence, the embryoid body model provides high reliability, technical novelty, easy handling, and quantification as well as physiological relevance, all of which are prerequisites for an ideal angiogenesis assay that is useful for routine and rapid throughput screening of pro- and antiangiogenic agents in pharmaceutical research.

2
Current Methods for Assaying Angiogenesis In Vitro

Several in vitro models of angiogenesis applicable to the study of endothelial cell proliferation and migration have been developed over the years (Auerbach et al. 2003; Jain et al. 1997; Staton et al. 2004). The most frequently employed test is the Boyden chamber assay in which endothelial cells are placed on the upper layer of a cell-permeable filter and permitted to migrate in response to pro- as well as antiangiogenic factors dissolved in the medium below the filter (Glaser et al. 1980). The formation of three-dimensional structures (i.e., tube formation) is generally studied on supports of extracellular matrix components established in culture dishes coated with collagen and/or fibrin. When endothelial cells are seeded on matrigel, which is a matrix-enriched substance prepared from Engelbreth–Holm–Swarm (EHS) tumor cells that predominantly contains laminin (Madri et al. 1988), tube formation occurs within 24 h. Through the use of the matrigel assay, many fundamental molecular events of tube formation and sprouting have been unraveled; however, angiogenesis assays based on pure endothelial cell lines suffer from two major disadvantages: (a) antiangiogenic effects of compounds cannot be discriminated from nonspecific toxic effects, and (b) dose–response relationships may differ from in vivo angiogenesis. Furthermore, angiogenesis in vivo involves more than one cell type, which renders in vitro experiments largely incommensurate to the in vivo situation.

To achieve experimental conditions more indicative of in vivo angiogenesis, in vitro assays based on organ culture have been developed. The most widely used organ culture model is the rat aortic ring assay(Nicosia et al. 1990). This assay employs cut segments of rat aorta placed in an extracellular matrix containing culture medium to investigate whether pro/antiangiogenic agents affect the outgrowth of endothelial cells from the explant. Quantification of endothelial cell outgrowth and vessel abundance is performed by computer-assisted image analysis of transmission images or after fluorescence staining of cells with endothelial cell-specific markers. Recently, the aortic ring assay was refined in co-cultures with rat inferior vena cava embedded in collagen gel to study arteriovenous anastomosis formation (Nicosia et al. 2005). In another modification, the chick aortic arch assay was developed, which investigated the outgrowth of endothelial cells from aortic arches of 12- to 14-day-old chick embryos. Although of nonmammalian origin, this system may be of benefit under circumstances when antiangiogenic agents, e.g., thalidomide, that have been shown to be ineffective in mammalian systems are studied (Auerbach et al. 2003).

Although many fundamental investigations on the complex set of events that occur during angiogenesis have been performed through the use of in vitro angiogenesis assays, some caveats and cautions need to be considered. These include:

1. The absence of a variety of known (and unknown) factors that regulate angiogenesis in vivo;

2. The inability of cells to differentiate into specific endothelial cell types (e.g., tumor-specific vasculature; microvascular cells);

3. The absence of hematopoietic cells in sprouting capillaries;

4. The lack of heterospecific interactions of endothelial cells with other neighboring cells;

5. The inability to study the role of endothelial precursor cells in angiogenesis.

All of these limitations can be overcome through the use of embryonic stem cells in angiogenesis research. This in vitro model system has the ability to form different proangiogenic cell types and release cytokines and growth factors required for angiogenesis in vitro as well as form blood vessel in vivo.

3
Angiogenesis in Embryonic Stem Cell-Derived Embryoid Bodies

In 1985, Doetschman and colleagues first reported the differentiation of hematopoietic precursor cells surrounded by endothelial cells from mouse ES cells (Doetschman et al. 1985). In a subsequent study, the development of blood vessels from in situ differentiating endothelial cells of blood islands was induced by injecting ES cells into the peritoneal cavity of syngeneic mice (Risau et al. 1988). Endothelial cells, which developed in ES cell-derived embryoid bodies, formed vascular channels containing hematopoietic cells. These findings led to the conclusion that not only primary differentiation of endothelial cells but also some aspects of vascular maturation are intrinsic to this cell culture system (Wang et al. 1992). The ES cell model was subsequently used by Vittet et al. to unravel several successive maturation stages during differentiation into the endothelial cell lineage (Vittet et al. 1996). ES cell-derived endothelial cells express a variety of endothelial cell-specific markers, including Flk-1, PECAM-1, and VE-cadherin. Kabrun et al. demonstrated that Flk-1 is expressed on an early population of hematopoietic precursors coincident with the onset of embryonic hematopoiesis (Kabrun et al. 1997). The three-dimensional structure of an embryoid body does not seem, however, to be absolutely necessary for vascular differentiation, because it was recently demonstrated that Flk1$^+$ cells derived from ES cells in two-dimensional cell cultures differentiate into both endothelial and mural cells, which effectively reproduced the vascular organization process. VEGF promoted endothelial cell differentiation, whereas mural cells were induced by platelet-derived growth factor-BB (PDGF-BB). Furthermore, vascular cells derived from Flk1$^+$ cells could organize into vessel-like structures consisting of endothelial tubes supported by mural cells in three-dimensional culture (Yamashita et al. 2000). In vivo, interactions between endothelial cells and mural cells (pericytes and vascular smooth muscle) are essential for vascular development and maintenance. During embryogenesis, endothelial cells arise from Flk1-expressing (Flk1$^+$) mesoderm cells, whereas mural cells are believed to be derived from mesoderm, neural crest, or epicardial cells and migrate to form the vessel wall. In the ES cell model, the developmental differentiation of endothelial precursors as well as mural cells requires Pim-1 activity, which may act as a downstream Flk-1 effector in vasculogenesis (Zippo et al. 2004). Pim-1 is a serine/threonine kinase that is able to phosphorylate and regulate the activity of transcription factors (Leverson et al. 1998; Winn et al. 2003). Recently, time-lapse imaging of green fluorescent protein (GFP)-expressing vessels derived from stem cells was used to analyze dynamic aspects of vascular sprout formation and to determine how the VEGF receptor flt-1 affects sprouting. Interestingly, loss of flt-1 led to decreased sprout formation and migration, which resulted in reduced vascular branching (Kearney et al. 2004). Furthermore, VEGF-mediated vascular morphogenesis has been studied in mouse ES cells through the use of wild type and *VEGF*-null cell lines. *VEGF*-null ES cells contained PECAM-1-positive endothelial cells, which, however, did not participate in vascular morphogenesis. Using gene expression microarray analysis, genes downstream of VEGF function that may be involved in VEGF-mediated vascular morphogenesis have also been analyzed (Ng et al. 2004).

The availability of human ES cells has raised interest in the use of this system for blood vessel tissue engineering and therapeutic angiogenesis. The potential applicability of this system has already been demonstrated with mouse ES cells, which can be used to tissue engineer blood vessels on biodegradable scaffolds (Shen et al. 2003). Several publications have recently reported that human ES cells, similar to mouse ES cells, can form blood vessels upon differentiation induction. Isolated embryonic PECAM-1-positive cells, grown in culture, displayed characteristics consistent with vessel endothelium. The cells expressed endothelial cell markers in a pattern similar to human umbilical vein endothelial cells, the cell junctions were correctly organized, and the cells had high rates of metabolism for acetylated low-density lipoprotein. In addition, the human cells were able to differentiate and form tube-like structures when cultured on matrigel. When transplanted into SCID mice, the cells appeared to form microvessels containing mouse blood cells (Levenberg et al. 2002), and using a bioengineering approach, the same group demonstrated that biodegradable polymer scaffolds promoted human ES cell growth and differentiation, and formation of 3D structures. Complex structures with features of various committed embryonic tissues were generated, in vitro, through the use of early differentiating human ES cells that were further differentiated in a supportive 3D environment containing poly(lactic-co-glycolic acid)/poly(L-lactic acid) polymer scaffolds. Human ES cell differentiation and organization could be influenced by the scaffold and directed by growth factors such as retinoic acid, transforming growth factor beta, activin-A, or insulin-like growth factor (Levenberg et al. 2003).

In a recent study, gene expression patterns of vascular cells were investigated. Changes in gene expression concomitant with the development of human embryoid bodies for 4 weeks were studied by large-scale gene screening. Two main clusters of genes were identified—one with reduced expression (POU5, NANOG, TDGF1/Cripto [TDGF, teratocarcinoma-derived growth factor-1], LIN28, CD24, TERF1 [telomeric repeat binding factor-1], LEFTB [left-right determination, factor B]), and a second with enhanced expression (TWIST, WNT5A, WT1, AFP, ALB, NCAM1). Genes known to be involved in vasculogenesis and angiogenesis were explored further, and the authors described a set of up-regulated genes that included vasculogenic growth factors such as VEGFA, VEGFC, FIGF (VEGFD), ANG1, ANG2, TGFβ3, and PDGFB, as well as the related receptors Flt1, Flt4, PDGFRB, TGFβR2, and TGFβR3, other markers such as CD34, VCAM1, PECAM-1, VE-CAD, and transcription factors TAL1, GATA2, and GATA3 (Gerecht-Nir et al. 2005). Altogether, these analyses indicate that human ES cells differentiating in vitro produce many, if not all, of the factors necessary for vasculogenesis and angiogenesis.

4
Embryonic Stem Cell-Derived Embryoid Bodies as a Tool for Antiangiogenesis Research

Since ES cells differentiate into cells of all three germ layers, they potentially possess the capacity to mimic the complex events of blood vessel formation that occur in vivo. In mouse ES cells, capillary structures differentiated in embryoid bodies are functional and improve the diffusion properties of the vascularized tissue (Wartenberg et al. 1998b). When ES cells aggregate to form multicellular embryoid bodies, they are avascular for the first 4 days of culture. This results in a gradient of oxygen and presumably a deficit of nutrients toward the center of the spheroidal multicellular tissue. Central embryoid body hypoxia induces upregulation of hypoxia-inducible factor-1α (HIF-1α), and since VEGF expression is under the control of HIF-1α, a concomitant upregulation of VEGF and initiation of vasculogenesis can be observed after day 5 of cell culture. With the onset of vasculogenesis in embryoid bodies, oxygen gradients are dissipated, and both HIF-1α and VEGF expression are downregulated. This results in cessation of angiogenesis after approximately 8 days of mouse embryoid body culture (Wartenberg et al. 2001a) (see Fig. 1). Endothelial cell lineage differentiation of vascular smooth muscle cells also occurs in embryoid bodies after treatment with retinoic acid and db-cAMP (Drab et al. 1997), which indicates that ES cells may form not only capillaries but also precapillary arterioles and postcapillary venules. In vivo, a mutual interaction occurs among

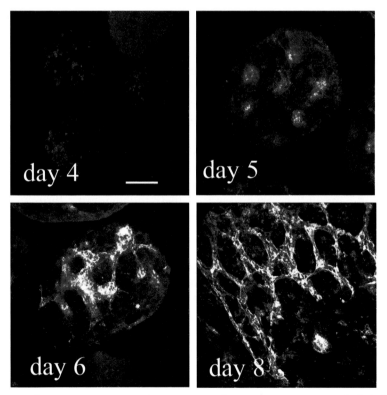

Fig. 1 Vasculogenesis/angiogenesis in mouse ES cells. PECAM-1-positive endothelial cells were visualized by confocal laser scanning microscopy in 4-, 5-, 6-, and 8-day-old embryoid bodies. Angioblast-like structures were obvious on day 5. During subsequent days, capillary sprouting occurred, which resulted in a vascular plexus on day 8 of differentiation. Bar, 150 μm

blood vessel growth, hematopoiesis, and blood circulation, and comparable mechanisms may prevail in ES cells, since blood vessels differentiated from ES cells contain red blood cells (Wang et al. 1992). Furthermore, it has been demonstrated that hematopoiesis and differentiation to various hematopoietic cell types occur in ES cells. Embryoid bodies cultivated in semisolid methylcellulose medium contain visible erythropoietic cells (i.e., red with hemoglobin), and upon addition of cytokines, e.g., IL-3 alone or in combination with IL-1 and M-CSF or GM-CSF, ES cells differentiate to form macrophages, mast cells, and in some instances neutrophils, in addition to cells of the erythroid cell lineage (Wiles et al. 1991; Keller et al. 1993). Because vasculogenesis based on the differentiation of angioblasts as defined in the embryonic stages is not applicable in the adult, the differentiation of white blood cells may be critical to adult neovascularization in vivo. It has therefore been suggested that monocytes/macrophages produce tunnels within the tissue as a consequence of their protease-dependent migration into the extracellular matrices, which are then colonized by precursor endothelial cells (Moldovan 2003).

Given the capacity of ES cells to differentiate into all cell types required for angiogenesis and to synthesize proangiogenic factors, the ES cell-derived embryoid body model has proved superior to all other in vitro models of antiangiogenesis research currently employed. Specifically, sprouting angiogenesis from mouse ES cells can be observed when growing embryoid bodies are plated into type I collagen matrix. Sprouting and tube formation also can be promoted by the addition of exogenous VEGF and inhibited by known angiostatic agents (Feraud et al. 2001). ES cells grown in spinner flasks spontaneously form thousands of embryoid bodies that can be used for routine screening of antiangiogenic agents. Several known antiangiogenic agents, i.e., Suramin, tamoxifen, tetrahydrocortisol, and a combination of tetrahydrocortisol and heparin have been tested for their antiangiogenic capacity in the embryoid body system, and these compounds efficiently inhibit endothelial differentiation in vitro (Wartenberg et al. 1998b). Inhibition of capillary formation significantly reduced the diffusion of the anti-cancer agent doxorubicin as well as a fluorescence-labeled dextran into the tissue, which indicated that the embryoid body model may also be suitable for drug penetration studies designed to examine avascular and vascularized tissue (Wartenberg et al. 1998b) (see Fig. 2). Inhibition of angiogenesis in embryoid bodies resulted in central necrosis, a typical feature of avascular micrometastases and avascular regions of solid tumors in vivo (Brown 2002). In solid tumors, central necrosis occurs due to gradients in oxygen, which consequently results in upregulation of HIF-1α and VEGF and induction of a proangiogenic phenotype.

The use of embryoid bodies as a tool to study antiangiogenic agents facilitates the analysis of changes in protein expression as well as physiologic parameters, e.g., the pericellular oxygen tension, intracellular pH, calcium, and reactive oxygen species (ROS) generation that may occur following treatment with antiangiogenic agents. The antiangiogenic activity of the teratogenic

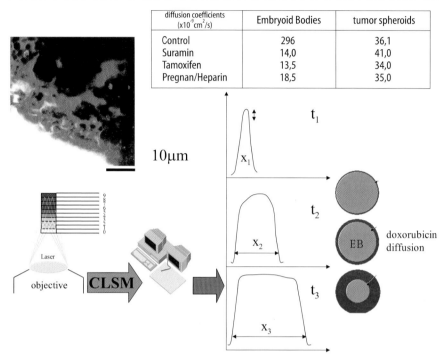

diffusion coefficients $(\times 10^{-9} cm^2/s)$	Embryoid Bodies	tumor spheroids
Control	296	36,1
Suramin	14,0	41,0
Tamoxifen	13,5	34,0
Pregnan/Heparin	18,5	35,0

Fig. 2 Diffusion studies in vascularized embryoid bodies and embryoid bodies treated with antiangiogenic agents as performed by confocal laser scanning microscopy-based optical probe technique. Embryoid bodies are immersed in a fluorescent solution (*upper left*, fluorescence-labeled dextran solution), which diffuses into the tissue through vascular channels. Subsequently, optical sections at different depths of the tissue are performed by confocal laser scanning microscopy (*lower left*). From the fluorescence information obtained at different depths over time, dye diffusion curves can be monitored (*lower right*) and diffusion coefficients calculated (*upper right*). Note that treatment of vascularized embryoid bodies with antiangiogenic agents resulted in a significant loss of diffusion of the tracer substance, doxorubicin, which proved similar in magnitude to those findings observed in avascular multicellular tumor spheroids. Bar, 10 μm

agent thalidomide is due to the generation of highly reactive hydroxyl radicals, since the antiangiogenic effect could be reversed by specific hydroxyl radical scavengers (Sauer et al. 2000). A similar mechanism of action was shown for the antiangiogenic activity of the anti-malaria agent artemisinin, which comparably to thalidomide raised intracellular levels of ROS in embryoid bodies. Artemisinin treatment impaired organization of the extracellular matrix component laminin and altered expression patterns of MMPs 1, 2, and 9 during the time course of embryoid body differentiation. Consequently, accelerated penetration kinetics of the fluorescent anthracycline doxorubicin occurred within the tissue, indicating increased tissue permeability. Furthermore, artemisinin downregulated HIF-1α and VEGF expression, which together control endothelial cell growth (Wartenberg et al. 2003c). Recently, the embryoid body model was used to clarify whether endothelial progenitor cell differentiation is involved in the mechanism of antiangiogenic effect of vitamin B(6), and it was found that vitamin B(6) compounds significantly inhibited vasculogenesis (Matsubara et al. 2004).

5
Embryonic Stem Cell-Derived Embryoid Bodies to Study Tumor-Induced Angiogenesis

From the pioneering studies of Folkman and colleagues, it became clear that the growth of avascular tumors cannot proceed beyond a mass of approximately 1–3 mm^3 without access to host vasculature (Gimbrone et al. 1972; Holleb et al. 1972; Folkman 1972). Up to this size, cells are supplied by oxygen and nutrients through simple diffusion. With ongoing growth, central hypoxia occurs in the center of the tumor, and cells in the depth of the tissue exit the cell cycle and become multidrug-resistant. A number of cellular stress factors such as hypoxia, nutrient deprivation, or inducers of ROS are important stimuli of angiogenic signaling. These factors mediate upregulation of proangiogenic factors in the hypoxic tumor tissue as a stress response. This notion is underscored by observations reporting an association of HIF-1α with angiogenesis, and expression of bFGF, PDGF-BB, and EGFR in invasive breast cancer (Bos et al. 2005). Furthermore, the expression of the proangiogenic factors VEGF and interleukin-8/CXCL8 by human breast carcinomas has been shown to be responsive to nutrient deprivation and endoplasmic reticulum stress (Abcouwer et al. 2002; Marjon et al. 2004). VEGF expression is well known to be regulated by HIF-1α (Forsythe et al. 1996), which is upregulated both in avascular hypoxic micrometastases (Fang et al. 2001) and in avascular regions of large solid tumors (Kimura et al. 2004; Buchler et al. 2003). The upregulation of angiogenic factors is not sufficient for a tumor to enter the proangiogenic state. To initiate the angiogenic switch, which results in attraction of host-derived blood vessels toward the tumor tissue, distinct angiostatic factors that inhibit vascular growth have to be downregulated. If a preponderance of angiogenic factors in the local milieu of the tumor tissue prevails, the neovasculature may form capillaries and/or arterioles and venules. However, in the presence of a surplus of angiostatic factors the neovessels within the tumor can regress (Gupta et al. 2003). Besides eliciting the invasion of endothelial cells from preexisting capillaries, tumor cells can grow around an existing vessel and, at least initially, do not need adequate vascularization for proper supply with oxygen and nutrients (Holash et al. 1999). In addition to the sprouting and co-option of neighboring preexisting vessels, tumor angiogenesis is supported by the mobilization and functional incorporation of endothelial progenitor cells that are mobilized from bone marrow (Ribatti 2004). The recruitment of endothelial progenitor cells to tumor angiogenesis represents a multistep process, including (Ribatti 2004):

1. Active arrest and homing of the circulating cells within the angiogenic microvasculature

2. Transendothelial extravasation into the interstitial space

3. Extravascular formation of cellular clusters

4. Creation of vascular sprouts and cellular networks

5. Incorporation into a functional microvasculature

The involvement of endothelial progenitor cells in tumor-induced angiogenesis was demonstrated through the use of a class of embryonic cells (Tie-2$^+$, c-Kit$^+$, Sca-1$^+$, and Flk-1-/low), which were isolated at E7.5 of mouse development at the onset of vasculogenesis and which retained the ability to contribute to tumor angiogenesis in the adult. Using intravital fluorescence videomicroscopy, it was observed that circulating endothelial progenitor cells were specifically arrested in "hot spots" within the tumor microvasculature, extravasated into the interstitium, formed multicellular clusters, and incorporated into functional vascular networks. Expression analysis and in vivo blocking experiments provided evidence that the initial cell arrest of endothelial progenitor cell homing is mediated by E- and P-selectin and P-selectin glycoprotein ligand 1 (Vajkoczy et al. 2003). In endothelial progenitor cells, the protease cathepsin L (CathL) is highly expressed as opposed to endothelial cells, and it is essential for matrix degradation and invasion by endothelial progenitor cells in vitro. CathL-deficient mice displayed impaired functional recovery following hind limb ischemia, supporting the concept of a crucial role for CathL in postnatal neovascularization. Infused CathL-deficient progenitor cells neither homed to sites of ischemia nor augmented neovascularization. Forced expression of CathL in mature endothelial cells considerably enhanced their invasive activity and sufficed to confer their capacity for neovascularization in vivo (Urbich et al. 2005). However, the percentage of endothelial cells incorporation is generally low and depends on the nature of the tumor, supporting the concept that most tumor neovascularization occurs via tumor-induced angiogenesis (Ribatti 2004).

The study of tumor-induced angiogenesis has mainly involved in vivo models. In the corneal assay, neoangiogenesis is monitored by implantation of multicellular tumor spheroids or tumor-fragment spheroids onto the avascular cornea of either the rabbit or mouse eye. To test inhibitors of angiogenesis, their effect on the locally (i.e., by the tumor) induced angiogenic reaction can be monitored by direct observation through a slit lamp (for rabbits) or a stereomicroscope (for mice). The test inhibitors can be administered locally or systemically, the latter either by bolus injection, or through use of a sustained release method such as implantation of osmotic pumps loaded with the test inhibitor (Auerbach et al. 2003). Other animal models to study tumor-induced angiogenesis include chronic transparent chambers (e.g., rabbit ear chamber; dorsal skinfold chamber in mice, rats, hamsters, and rabbits; cranial windows in mice and rats), exterior tissue preparations (e.g., hamster cheek pouch; mouse, rat, or rabbit mesentery), and subcutaneous or peritoneal implantation of tumor spheroids or tumor fragment spheroids (Jain et al. 1997). However, all in vivo animal models suffer from inflammation and graft-versus-host rejection of implanted tumor tissues as well as from insufficiently defined pharmacokinetics of the applied agents. Furthermore, microphysiological analysis, e.g., imaging of signal transduction molecules and investigation of gene expression is not possible in animal experiments.

For many years, no suitable in vitro models were available to study tumor-induced angiogenesis in vitro. Recently, hanging drop multicellular spheroids that were co-cultivated with human umbilical vein endothelial cells were introduced as a model of tumour angiogenesis, and it may be of some interest in antiangiogenesis research (Timmins et al. 2004). Multicellular tumor spheroids represent a widely accepted in vitro model of avascular micrometastases and avascular regions of vascularized solid tumors. These spheroids, which consist of peripheral proliferating cells, intermediate layers of quiescent cells, and a central necrotic core (Sutherland et al. 1971), have been extensively used for studies on P-glycoprotein-mediated multidrug resistance (Wartenberg et al. 1998a, 2001b, 2003b, 2005), nutrient (Walenta et al. 2000), lactate, oxygen (Sutherland et al. 1986a, 1986b), and pH (Gorlach et al. 1994) gradients as well as cancer drug response (Nicholson et al. 1997; Kerr et al. 1988). Multicellular tumor spheroids express VEGF in central regions, similar to the in vivo situation where solid tumors attract blood vessels from the host by secreting proangiogenic growth factors (Waleh et al. 1995; Shweiki et al. 1995). In a more straightforward approach, confrontation cultures were tested with multicellular tumor spheroids and mouse ES cell-derived embryoid bodies (Wartenberg et al. 2001a). To achieve close tissue contact, multicellular tumor spheroids and embryoid bodies were allowed to coalesce in hanging drops for 48 h. Early in this process, endothelial cells, which were positive for the endothelial-specific cell marker PECAM-1, appeared in the contact region between the tumor spheroid and the embryoid bodies. In the contact region, increased expression of VEGF was observed, which may attract endothelial cells toward the tumor tissue. During the following days, sprouting of capillary-like structures occurred from the contact region toward more central parts of the embryoid body and the tumor spheroid. Within 5 days of confrontation culture, extended areas of capillary networks were observed in the embryoid bodies and the tumor spheroids (see Figs. 3, 4). Treatment of the confrontation object with the antiangiogenic agent SU5614, a VEGF receptor antagonist, resulted in significant inhibition of angiogenesis in the embryoid body. Tumor-induced angiogenesis in the tumor spheroid was completely absent under these experimental condi-

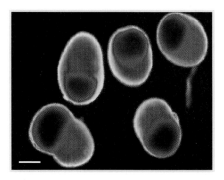 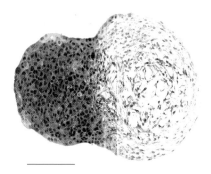

Fig. 3 Confrontation cultures of embryoid bodies and multicellular tumor spheroids. *Left*, transmission image of confrontation cultures (bar, 500 μm). The embryoid body appears dark due to a higher optical density of the tissue. *Right*, paraffin section of a representative confrontation culture after hematoxylin/eosin staining (bar, 500 μm). The tumor tissue appears dark relative to the embryoid body

tions. Interestingly, confrontation culture resulted in an increased steepness of the oxygen gradients in the vascularized tumor tissue. This may be due to the proliferation stimulus usually seen following tumor vascularization. Re-entry of quiescent cells in the depth of the tumor tissue into the cell cycle results in increased oxygen consumption of the proliferating cancer cells with ongoing central hypoxia, VEGF expression and maintenance of the proangiogenic phenotype. Indeed, confrontation culture resulted in an increased growth of the tumor tissue and disappearance of central necrosis, which is characteristic for solid avascular tumors.

Reactive oxygen species are known to regulate various growth factor and cytokine-mediated signaling cascades (Sauer et al. 2001), and ROS is increased in confrontation cultures (Wartenberg et al. 2003a). Recently it was demonstrated that VEGF stimulates a Rac1-dependent NAD(P)H oxidase to produce ROS that are involved in VEGF-R2 autophosphorylation and angiogenic-related responses in endothelial cells (Ikeda et al. 2005; Ushio-Fukai et al. 2002). Furthermore, the expression of MMPs has been shown to be activated by either exogenous ROS or cytokines and growth factors that involve ROS within their signal transduction cascade (Siwik et al. 2001; Yoon et al. 2002; Zhang et al. 2002). In confrontation cultures, upregulation of MMP-1, MMP-2, and MMP-9 expression, which is generally associated with the process of tumor vascularization, has been observed. The first MMP to be upregulated after confrontation culture was MMP-9, followed by MMP-1 and MMP-2. MMP-1 and MMP-2 expression as well as tumor-induced angiogenesis in confrontation cultures was inhibited by acteoside, baicalein, berberine, and epicatechin, which exert antioxidative capacity and are ingredients of Chinese herbal medicine.

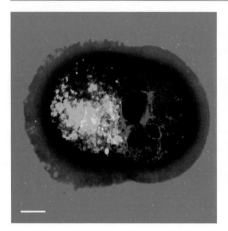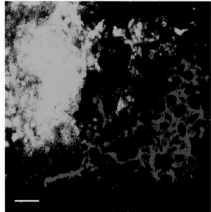

Fig. 4 Tumor-induced angiogenesis in confrontation cultures. The tumor tissue was labeled with the long-term cell tracker dye CMFDA. After 5 days of confrontation culture, the tissue was fixed and immunolabeled using an antibody directed against endothelial cell-specific PECAM-1. The *left image* shows an overlay between a transmission image (*blue*), CMFDA fluorescence of tumor tissue (*green*), and PECAM-1 fluorescence of capillary-like structures (*red*). Note that endothelial cells have entered the tumor tissue in the process of tumor-induced angiogenesis. Bar, 100 μm. The *right image* shows the region of interaction of tumor tissue (*green*) with capillary-like structures from the embryoid body tissue (*red*). Bar, 50 μm

6
Conclusions and Outlook

In general, stem cell-derived vasculogenesis and angiogenesis is discussed most often with respect to tissue repair and tissue engineering (Zwaginga et al. 2003). Besides the potential use of ES cells for patient treatment, this model system has also proven useful for numerous in vitro assays, including toxicological drug testing (Rolletschek et al. 2004; Rohwedel et al. 2001) using cardiotoxic (Na et al. 2003), neurotoxic (Rolletschek et al. 2001), pancreotoxic (Blyszczuk et al. 2003), and antiangiogenic (Wartenberg et al. 1998b) agents, and an embryotoxicity test (EST) (Scholz et al. 1999; Seiler et al. 2002), which may be extended to human ES cells in the future. With the finding that endothelial precursor cells contribute to tumor-induced angiogenesis, there is renewed interest in the ES cells as an in vitro model system for the study of tumor vascularization. In contrast to all currently applied in vitro angiogenesis assays, this model facilitates the study of blood vessel growth and maturation within a multicellular tissue context that closely resembles the tissue microarchitecture, oxygen and nutrient gradients, as well as cytokine and growth factor expression found in vivo. Furthermore, the ES cell model allows detailed analysis of changes in gene and protein expression as well as changes in diffusion properties that occur during the vascularization of a growing embryonic tissue and the invasion process of capillary-like cells into tumor tissue. In conclusion, the mouse ES cell system has proven its utility for routine testing of antiangiogenic agents known to inhibit angiogenesis in humans, and the availability of human ES cells will lead to refinements in the mouse system that should significantly reduce the risk of inadequate transferability of in vitro data to the human patient.

References

Abcouwer SF, Marjon PL, Loper RK, Vander Jagt DL (2002) Response of VEGF expression to amino acid deprivation and inducers of endoplasmic reticulum stress. Invest Ophthalmol Vis Sci 43:2791–2798

Auerbach R, Lewis R, Shinners B, Kubai L, Akhtar N (2003) Angiogenesis assays: a critical overview. Clin Chem 49:32–40

Blyszczuk P, Czyz J, Kania G, Wagner M, Roll U, St Onge L, Wobus AM (2003) Expression of Pax4 in embryonic stem cells promotes differentiation of nestin-positive progenitor and insulin-producing cells. Proc Natl Acad Sci U S A 100:998–1003

Bos R, van Diest PJ, de Jong JS, van der Groep P, van der Valk P, van der Wall E (2005) Hypoxia-inducible factor-1alpha is associated with angiogenesis, and expression of bFGF, PDGF-BB, and EGFR in invasive breast cancer. Histopathology 46:31–36

Brown JM (2002) Tumor microenvironment and the response to anticancer therapy. Cancer Biol Ther 1:453–458

Buchler P, Reber HA, Buchler M, Shrinkante S, Buchler MW, Friess H, Semenza GL, Hines OJ (2003) Hypoxia-inducible factor 1 regulates vascular endothelial growth factor expression in human pancreatic cancer. Pancreas 26:56–64

Doetschman TC, Eistetter H, Katz M, Schmidt W, Kemler R (1985) The in vitro development of blastocyst-derived embryonic stem cell lines: formation of visceral yolk sac, blood islands and myocardium. J Embryol Exp Morphol 87:27–45

Drab M, Haller H, Bychkov R, Erdmann B, Lindschau C, Haase H, Morano I, Luft FC, Wobus AM (1997) From totipotent embryonic stem cells to spontaneously contracting smooth muscle cells: a retinoic acid and db-cAMP in vitro differentiation model. FASEB J 11:905–915

Fang J, Yan L, Shing Y, Moses MA (2001) HIF-1alpha-mediated up-regulation of vascular endothelial growth factor, independent of basic fibroblast growth factor, is important in the switch to the angiogenic phenotype during early tumorigenesis. Cancer Res 61:5731–5735

Feraud O, Cao Y, Vittet D (2001) Embryonic stem cell-derived embryoid bodies development in collagen gels recapitulates sprouting angiogenesis. Lab Invest 81:1669–1681

Folkman J (1972) Anti-angiogenesis: new concept for therapy of solid tumors. Ann Surg 175:409–416

Forsythe JA, Jiang BH, Iyer NV, Agani F, Leung SW, Koos RD, Semenza GL (1996) Activation of vascular endothelial growth factor gene transcription by hypoxia-inducible factor 1. Mol Cell Biol 16:4604–4613

Gerecht-Nir S, Dazard JE, Golan-Mashiach M, Osenberg S, Botvinnik A, Amariglio N, Domany E, Rechavi G, Givol D, Itskovitz-Eldor J (2005) Vascular gene expression and phenotypic correlation during differentiation of human embryonic stem cells. Dev Dyn 232:487–497

Gimbrone MA Jr, Leapman SB, Cotran RS, Folkman J (1972) Tumor dormancy in vivo by prevention of neovascularization. J Exp Med 136:261–276

Glaser BM, D'Amore PA, Seppa H, Seppa S, Schiffmann E (1980) Adult tissues contain chemoattractants for vascular endothelial cells. Nature 288:483–484

Gorlach A, Acker H (1994) pO2- and pH-gradients in multicellular spheroids and their relationship to cellular metabolism and radiation sensitivity of malignant human tumor cells. Biochim Biophys Acta 1227:105–112

Gupta MK, Qin RY (2003) Mechanism and its regulation of tumor-induced angiogenesis. World J Gastroenterol 9:1144–1155

Holash J, Maisonpierre PC, Compton D, Boland P, Alexander CR, Zagzag D, Yancopoulos GD, Wiegand SJ (1999) Vessel cooption, regression, and growth in tumors mediated by angiopoietins and VEGF. Science 284:1994–1998

Holleb AI, Folkman J (1972) Tumor angiogenesis. CA Cancer J Clin 22:226–229

Ikeda S, Ushio-Fukai M, Zuo L, Tojo T, Dikalov S, Patrushev NA, Alexander RW (2005) Novel role of ARF6 in vascular endothelial growth factor-induced signaling and angiogenesis. Circ Res 96:467–475

Jain RK (2003) Molecular regulation of vessel maturation. Nat Med 9:685–693

Jain RK, Schlenger K, Hockel M, Yuan F (1997) Quantitative angiogenesis assays: progress and problems. Nat Med 3:1203–1208

Kabrun N, Buhring HJ, Choi K, Ullrich A, Risau W, Keller G (1997) Flk-1 expression defines a population of early embryonic hematopoietic precursors. Development 124:2039–2048

Kearney JB, Kappas NC, Ellerstrom C, DiPaola FW, Bautch VL (2004) The VEGF receptor flt-1 (VEGFR-1) is a positive modulator of vascular sprout formation and branching morphogenesis. Blood 103:4527–4535

Keller G, Kennedy M, Papayannopoulou T, Wiles MV (1993) Hematopoietic commitment during embryonic stem cell differentiation in culture. Mol Cell Biol 13:473–486

Kerr DJ, Wheldon TE, Hydns S, Kaye SB (1988) Cytotoxic drug penetration studies in multicellular tumour spheroids. Xenobiotica 18:641–648

Kimura S, Kitadai Y, Tanaka S, Kuwai T, Hihara J, Yoshida K, Toge T, Chayama K (2004) Expression of hypoxia-inducible factor (HIF)-1alpha is associated with vascular endothelial growth factor expression and tumour angiogenesis in human oesophageal squamous cell carcinoma. Eur J Cancer 40:1904–1912

Levenberg S, Golub JS, Amit M, Itskovitz-Eldor J, Langer R (2002) Endothelial cells derived from human embryonic stem cells. Proc Natl Acad Sci U S A 99:4391–4396

Levenberg S, Huang NF, Lavik E, Rogers AB, Itskovitz-Eldor J, Langer R (2003) Differentiation of human embryonic stem cells on three-dimensional polymer scaffolds. Proc Natl Acad Sci U S A 100:12741–12746

Leverson JD, Koskinen PJ, Orrico FC, Rainio EM, Jalkanen KJ, Dash AB, Eisenman RN, Ness SA (1998) Pim-1 kinase and p100 cooperate to enhance c-Myb activity. Mol Cell 2:417–425

Madri JA, Pratt BM, Tucker AM (1988) Phenotypic modulation of endothelial cells by transforming growth factor-beta depends upon the composition and organization of the extracellular matrix. J Cell Biol 106:1375–1384

Marjon PL, Bobrovnikova-Marjon EV, Abcouwer SF (2004) Expression of the pro-angiogenic factors vascular endothelial growth factor and interleukin-8/CXCL8 by human breast carcinomas is responsive to nutrient deprivation and endoplasmic reticulum stress. Mol Cancer 3:4

Matsubara K, Mori M, Akagi R, Kato N (2004) Anti-angiogenic effect of pyridoxal 5'-phosphate, pyridoxal and pyridoxamine on embryoid bodies derived from mouse embryonic stem cells. Int J Mol Med 14:819–823

Moldovan NI (2003) Tissular insemination of progenitor endothelial cells: the problem, and a suggested solution. Adv Exp Med Biol 522:99–113

Na L, Wartenberg M, Nau H, Hescheler J, Sauer H (2003) Anticonvulsant valproic acid inhibits cardiomyocyte differentiation of embryonic stem cells by increasing intracellular levels of reactive oxygen species. Birth Defects Res A Clin Mol Teratol 67:174–180

Ng YS, Ramsauer M, Loureiro RM, D'Amore PA (2004) Identification of genes involved in VEGF-mediated vascular morphogenesis using embryonic stem cell-derived cystic embryoid bodies. Lab Invest 84:1209–1218

Nguyen M, Arkell J, Jackson CJ (2001) Human endothelial gelatinases and angiogenesis. Int J Biochem Cell Biol 33:960–970

Nicholson KM, Bibby MC, Phillips RM (1997) Influence of drug exposure parameters on the activity of paclitaxel in multicellular spheroids. Eur J Cancer 33:1291–1298

Nicosia RF, Ottinetti A (1990) Growth of microvessels in serum-free matrix culture of rat aorta. A quantitative assay of angiogenesis in vitro. Lab Invest 63:115–122

Nicosia RF, Zhu WH, Fogel E, Howson KM, Aplin AC (2005) A new ex vivo model to study venous angiogenesis and arterio-venous anastomosis formation. J Vasc Res 42:111–119

Papetti M, Herman IM (2002) Mechanisms of normal and tumor-derived angiogenesis. Am J Physiol Cell Physiol 282:C947–C970

Ribatti D (2004) The involvement of endothelial progenitor cells in tumor angiogenesis. J Cell Mol Med 8:294–300

Risau W, Sariola H, Zerwes HG, Sasse J, Ekblom P, Kemler R, Doetschman T (1988) Vasculogenesis and angiogenesis in embryonic-stem-cell-derived embryoid bodies. Development 102:471–478

Robertson EJ (1987) Embryo-derived stem cell lines. Teratocarcinoma and embryonic stem cells—a practical approach. Oxford: IRL Press. pp 71–112

Rohwedel J, Guan K, Hegert C, Wobus AM (2001) Embryonic stem cells as an in vitro model for mutagenicity, cytotoxicity and embryotoxicity studies: present state and future prospects. Toxicol In Vitro 15:741–753

Rolletschek A, Chang H, Guan K, Czyz J, Meyer M, Wobus AM (2001) Differentiation of embryonic stem cell-derived dopaminergic neurons is enhanced by survival-promoting factors. Mech Dev 105:93–104

Rolletschek A, Blyszczuk P, Wobus AM (2004) Embryonic stem cell-derived cardiac, neuronal and pancreatic cells as model systems to study toxicological effects. Toxicol Lett 149:361–369

Sauer H, Gunther J, Hescheler J, Wartenberg M (2000) Thalidomide inhibits angiogenesis in embryoid bodies by the generation of hydroxyl radicals. Am J Pathol 156:151–158

Sauer H, Wartenberg M, Hescheler J (2001) Reactive oxygen species as intracellular messengers during cell growth and differentiation. Cell Physiol Biochem 11:173–186

Scholz G, Pohl I, Genschow E, Klemm M, Spielmann H (1999) Embryotoxicity screening using embryonic stem cells in vitro: correlation to in vivo teratogenicity. Cells Tissues Organs 165:203–211

Seiler A, Visan A, Pohl I, Genschow E, Buesen R, Spielmann H (2002) [Improving the embryonic stem cell test (EST) by establishing molecular endpoints of tissue specific development using murine embryonic stem cells (D3 cells)]. ALTEX 19 Suppl 1:55–63

Shen G, Tsung HC, Wu CF, Liu XY, Wang XY, Liu W, Cui L, Cao YL (2003) Tissue engineering of blood vessels with endothelial cells differentiated from mouse embryonic stem cells. Cell Res 13:335–341

Shweiki D, Neeman M, Itin A, Keshet E (1995) Induction of vascular endothelial growth factor expression by hypoxia and by glucose deficiency in multicell spheroids: implications for tumor angiogenesis. Proc Natl Acad Sci U S A 92:768–772

Siwik DA, Pagano PJ, Colucci WS (2001) Oxidative stress regulates collagen synthesis and matrix metalloproteinase activity in cardiac fibroblasts. Am J Physiol Cell Physiol 280:C53–C60

Staton CA, Stribbling SM, Tazzyman S, Hughes R, Brown NJ, Lewis CE (2004) Current methods for assaying angiogenesis in vitro and in vivo. Int J Exp Pathol 85:233–248

Sutherland RM, McCredie JA, Inch WR (1971) Growth of multicell spheroids in tissue culture as a model of nodular carcinomas. J Natl Cancer Inst 46:113–120

Sutherland R, Freyer J, Mueller-Klieser W, Wilson R, Heacock C, Sciandra J, Sordat B (1986a) Cellular growth and metabolic adaptations to nutrient stress environments in tumor microregion. Int J Radiat Oncol Biol Phys 12:611–615

Sutherland RM, Sordat B, Bamat J, Gabbert H, Bourrat B, Mueller-Klieser W (1986b) Oxygenation and differentiation in multicellular spheroids of human colon carcinoma. Cancer Res 46:5320–5329

Timmins NE, Dietmair S, Nielsen LK (2004) Hanging-drop multicellular spheroids as a model of tumour angiogenesis. Angiogenesis 7:97–103

Urbich C, Heeschen C, Aicher A, Sasaki KI, Bruhl T, Farhadi MR, Vajkoczy P, Hofmann WK, Peters C, Pennacchio LA, Abolmaali ND, Chavakis E, Reinheckel T, Zeiher AM, Dimmeler S (2005) Cathepsin L is required for endothelial progenitor cell-induced neovascularization. Nat Med 11:206–213

Ushio-Fukai M, Tang Y, Fukai T, Dikalov SI, Ma Y, Fujimoto M, Quinn MT, Pagano PJ, Johnson C, Alexander RW (2002) Novel role of gp91(phox)-containing NAD(P)H oxidase in vascular endothelial growth factor-induced signaling and angiogenesis. Circ Res 91:1160–1167

Vajkoczy P, Blum S, Lamparter M, Mailhammer R, Erber R, Engelhardt B, Vestweber D, Hatzopoulos AK (2003) Multistep nature of microvascular recruitment of ex vivo-expanded embryonic endothelial progenitor cells during tumor angiogenesis. J Exp Med 197:1755–1765

Van Royen N, Piek JJ, Buschmann I, Hoefer I, Voskuil M, Schaper W (2001) Stimulation of arteriogenesis; a new concept for the treatment of arterial occlusive disease. Cardiovasc Res 49:543–553

Vittet D, Prandini MH, Berthier R, Schweitzer A, Martin-Sisteron H, Uzan G, Dejana E (1996) Embryonic stem cells differentiate in vitro to endothelial cells through successive maturation steps. Blood 88:3424–3431

Waleh NS, Brody MD, Knapp MA, Mendonca HL, Lord EM, Koch CJ, Laderoute KR, Sutherland RM (1995) Mapping of the vascular endothelial growth factor-producing hypoxic cells in multicellular tumor spheroids using a hypoxia-specific marker. Cancer Res 55:6222–6226

Walenta S, Doetsch J, Mueller-Klieser W, Kunz-Schughart LA (2000) Metabolic imaging in multicellular spheroids of oncogene-transfected fibroblasts. J Histochem Cytochem 48:509–522

Wang R, Clark R, Bautch VL (1992) Embryonic stem cell-derived cystic embryoid bodies form vascular channels: an in vitro model of blood vessel development. Development 114:303–316

Wartenberg M, Frey C, Diedershagen H, Ritgen J, Hescheler J, Sauer H (1998a) Development of an intrinsic P-glycoprotein-mediated doxorubicin resistance in quiescent cell layers of large, multicellular prostate tumor spheroids. Int J Cancer 75:855–863

Wartenberg M, Gunther J, Hescheler J, Sauer H (1998b) The embryoid body as a novel in vitro assay system for antiangiogenic agents. Lab Invest 78:1301–1314

Wartenberg M, Donmez F, Ling FC, Acker H, Hescheler J, Sauer H (2001a) Tumor-induced angiogenesis studied in confrontation cultures of multicellular tumor spheroids and embryoid bodies grown from pluripotent embryonic stem cells. FASEB J 15:995–1005

Wartenberg M, Ling FC, Schallenberg M, Baumer AT, Petrat K, Hescheler J, Sauer H (2001b) Down-regulation of intrinsic P-glycoprotein expression in multicellular prostate tumor spheroids by reactive oxygen species. J Biol Chem 276:17420–17428

Wartenberg M, Budde P, De Marees M, Grunheck F, Tsang SY, Huang Y, Chen ZY, Hescheler J, Sauer H (2003a) Inhibition of tumor-induced angiogenesis and matrix-metalloprotein-ase expression in confrontation cultures of embryoid bodies and tumor spheroids by plant ingredients used in traditional Chinese medicine. Lab Invest 83:87–98

Wartenberg M, Ling FC, Muschen M, Klein F, Acker H, Gassmann M, Petrat K, Putz V, Hescheler J, Sauer H (2003b) Regulation of the multidrug resistance transporter P-glycoprotein in multicellular tumor spheroids by hypoxia-inducible factor (HIF-1) and reactive oxygen species. FASEB J 17:503–505

Wartenberg M, Wolf S, Budde P, Grunheck F, Acker H, Hescheler J, Wartenberg G, Sauer H (2003c) The antimalaria agent artemisinin exerts antiangiogenic effects in mouse em-bryonic stem cell-derived embryoid bodies. Lab Invest 83:1647–1655

Wartenberg M, Gronczynska S, Bekhite MM, Saric T, Niedermeier W, Hescheler J, Sauer H (2005) Regulation of the multidrug resistance transporter P-glycoprotein in multicellular prostate tumor spheroids by hyperthermia and reactive oxygen species. Int J Cancer 113:229–240

Wiles MV, Keller G (1991) Multiple hematopoietic lineages develop from embryonic stem (ES) cells in culture. Development 111:259–267

Winn LM, Lei W, Ness SA (2003) Pim-1 phosphorylates the DNA binding domain of c-Myb. Cell Cycle 2:258–262

Wobus AM, Guan K, Yang HT, Boheler KR (2002) Embryonic stem cells as a model to study cardiac, skeletal muscle, and vascular smooth muscle cell differentiation. Methods Mol Biol 185:127–156

Yamashita J, Itoh H, Hirashima M, Ogawa M, Nishikawa S, Yurugi T, Naito M, Nakao K, Nishikawa S (2000) Flk1-positive cells derived from embryonic stem cells serve as vas-cular progenitors. Nature 408:92–96

Yoon SO, Park SJ, Yoon SY, Yun CH, Chung AS (2002) Sustained production of H_2O_2 activates pro-matrix metalloproteinase-2 through receptor tyrosine kinases/phosphat-idylinositol 3-kinase/NF-kappa B pathway. J Biol Chem 277:30271–30282

Zhang HJ, Zhao W, Venkataraman S, Robbins ME, Buettner GR, Kregel KC, Oberley LW (2002) Activation of matrix metalloproteinase-2 by overexpression of manganese super-oxide dismutase in human breast cancer MCF-7 cells involves reactive oxygen species. J Biol Chem 277:20919–20926

Zippo A, De Robertis A, Bardelli M, Galvagni F, Oliviero S (2004) Identification of Flk-1 target genes in vasculogenesis: Pim-1 is required for endothelial and mural cell differentiation in vitro. Blood 103:4536–4544

Zwaginga JJ, Doevendans P (2003) Stem cell-derived angiogenic/vasculogenic cells: possible therapies for tissue repair and tissue engineering. Clin Exp Pharmacol Physiol 30:900–908

HEP (2006) 174:73–100
© Springer-Verlag Berlin Heidelberg 2006

Cardiac Repair by Embryonic Stem-Derived Cells

M. Rubart · L. J. Field (✉)

Wells Center for Pediatric Research and Krannert Institute of Cardiology, Indiana University School of Medicine, 1044 West Walnut Street, Indianapolis IN, 46202–5225, USA
ljfield@iupui.edu

Abstract Cell transplantation approaches offer the potential to promote regenerative growth of diseased hearts. It is well established that donor cardiomyocytes stably engraft into recipient hearts when injected directly into the myocardial wall. Moreover, the transplanted donor cardiomyocytes participate in a functional syncytium with the host myocardium. Thus, transplantation of donor cardiomyocytes resulted in at least partial restoration of lost muscle mass. It is also well established that embryonic stem (ES) cells differentiate into cells of ecto-, endo-, and mesodermal lineages when cultured under appropriate conditions in vitro. Robust cardiomyogenic differentiation was frequently observed in spontaneously differentiating ES cultures. Cellular, molecular and physiologic analyses indicated that ES-derived cells were bona fide cardiomyocytes, with in vitro characteristics typical for cells obtained from early stages of cardiac development. Thus, ES-derived cardiomyocytes constitute a viable source of donor cells for cell transplantation therapies.

Keywords Cell transplantation · Cardiac regeneration · Heart disease · Embryonic stem cell · Cardiomyocytes

1
Introduction

Many forms of cardiovascular disease result in cardiomyocyte death due to necrosis, oncosis, and/or apoptosis. Although there is an intrinsic capacity for adult cardiomyocytes to re-enter the cell cycle (Rumiantsev 1991; Anversa and Kajstura 1998; Soonpaa and Field 1998), this process is insufficient to reverse pathology in severely injured hearts. Thus a number of strategies have emerged to facilitate replacement of lost cardiac mass. These include efforts to reactivate cell cycle activity in surviving cardiomyocytes (Pasumarthi and Field 2002; Dowell et al. 2003a), mobilization of myogenic stem cells (Anversa and Nadal-Ginard 2002), and direct transplantation of cardiomyocytes or myogenic cells (Reinlib and Field 2000; Dowell et al. 2003b). Of these, cell transplantation approaches are currently the most advanced, with skeletal myoblast and bone marrow-derived cell transplantation already in early clinical trials.

This review will examine the use of cell transplantation for heart repair. The use of fetal cardiomyocytes, skeletal myoblasts, or adult-derived stem cells as donors is discussed. This is followed by a discussion of the characteristics of ES-derived cardiomyocytes, as well as potential strategies to enhance cardiomyogenic differentiation and yield in ES cultures. Finally, experiences to date wherein ES-derived cardiomyocytes have been transplanted into normal or diseased hearts are discussed. It is hoped that this review will provide the reader with a suitable introduction into the field of cardiac cell transplantation, as well as spur the reader's interest in the potential utility of ES-derived cells for therapeutic applications in cardiovascular disease.

2
Cell Transplantation for Cardiac Repair

2.1
Cardiomyocytes

The notion of employing cell transplantation as a means to replace lost myocardial mass can be traced back to experiments performed in the early 1990s. A priori, it was thought that cardiomyocytes likely constituted the ideal donor cell for intracardiac transplantation therapies since they express all of the requisite ion channels, junctional complex proteins, and myofiber components required for functional integration with the host myocardium. The initial proof of concept study utilized AT-1 cardiomyocytes, an immortalized tumor cell line derived from the left atrium of transgenic mice expressing the SV40 Large T Antigen oncoprotein under the regulation of the atrial natriuretic factor promoter (Steinhelper et al. 1990). When injected directly into the left ventricle of anesthetized, intubated syngeneic animals, AT-1 cells formed a stable graft comprised of differentiated, proliferating cardiomyocytes (Koh et al. 1993b).

The initial positive result prompted a second series of experiments to determine if fetal cardiomyocytes also formed stable intracardiac grafts. To monitor donor cell fate, transgenic mice expressing a cardiomyocyte-restricted, nuclear localized beta-galactosidase reporter construct were produced. Fetal cardiomyocytes prepared from the transgenic mice were transplanted into the

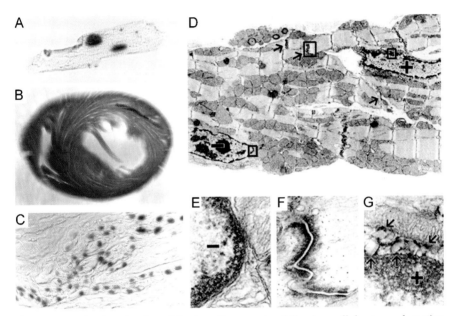

Fig. 1a–g Monitoring the fate of fetal cardiomyocytes following cellular transplantation into adult hearts. **a** Single, bi-nucleated cardiomyocyte isolated from an adult transgenic mouse (designated MHC-n LAC) expressing the enzyme beta-galactosidase exclusively in cardiomyocyte nuclei. Section was stained with X-GAL, a chromogenic dye that produces blue staining in the presence of beta-galactosidase activity. This assay demonstrates the specificity of the reporter transgene. **b** Survey photomicrograph of a coronal section of a heart following transplantation of fetal cardiomyocytes isolated from an MHC-n LAC embryo; section was stained with X-GAL. Reporter transgene activity readily identifies the transplanted donor cardiomyocytes. **c** Thin section of a heart following transplantation of fetal cardiomyocytes isolated from an MHC-n LAC embryo; section was stained with X-GAL. **d–g**) Transmission electron microscopy analysis of fetal cardiomyocyte grafts reveals the presence of intercalated discs between donor and host cells. **d** Transmission electron microscopy of a host cardiomyocyte juxtaposed to an engrafted fetal cardiomyocyte; − indicates the nucleus of the host cardiomyocyte and + indicates the nucleus of the donor MHC-nLAC cardiomyocyte. *Arrows* indicate an intercalated disk that connects the two cells. **e** High-power view of the host cardiomyocyte nucleus shown in **d**; note the complete absence of crystalloid X-gal reaction product in the perinuclear region. **f** High-power view of a region of the intercalated disk (boxed in **d**) that connects the host and fetal cardiomyocytes. **g** High-power view of the MHC-nLAC fetal cardiomyocyte nucleus shown in **d**; note the presence of crystalloid X-gal reaction product (*arrows*) in the perinuclear region. (Modified after Soonpaa et al. 1994)

hearts of nontransgenic recipients, and their fate was monitored by staining with a chromogenic beta-galactosidase substrate (X-GAL; see Fig. 1). Light and ultrastructural analyses revealed that the transplanted fetal cardiomyocytes underwent terminal differentiation and were stably integrated with the host myocardium (Soonpaa et al. 1994). Donor cells were well aligned with host cardiomyocytes. Moreover, intercalated discs with desmosomes, fascia adherens, and gap junctions were observed to connect donor and host cardiomyocytes (Koh et al. 1995), suggesting that these cells were functionally coupled. Numerous subsequent studies demonstrated that fetal and neonatal cardiomyocytes could successfully be transplanted into normal and damaged myocardium (Dowell et al. 2003b).

Although improvement in left ventricular function was observed in several studies where fetal cardiomyocytes were transplanted into injured hearts, the mechanism underlying the improvement was not obvious (Muller-Ehmsen et al. 2002; Roell et al. 2002). This was particularly true in instances where donor cell density was low, suggesting that the donor cells might have exerted a beneficial effect on the myocardium independent of participation in a functional syncytium. Direct proof of functional coupling between donor and host cardiomyocytes required the development of an imaging system capable of monitoring function in individual cells within intact hearts. The system employed two photon molecular excitation laser scanning microscopes to monitor intracellular calcium transients in intact hearts (Rubart et al. 2003b). This assay system was used to monitor calcium transients in transplanted, green fluorescent protein (EGFP)-expressing fetal donor cardiomyocytes and the adjacent host cardiomyocytes (Rubart et al. 2003a). The calcium transients were observed to occur simultaneously in donor and host cardiomyocytes, indicating that the donor cells formed a functional syncytium with the host myocardium (see Fig. 2). Collectively these studies indicated that donor cardiomyocytes survived following transplantation into normal or injured hearts, that they were able to functionally couple with host cardiomyocytes, and that they might also have a beneficial impact on host heart function independent of their contractile activity.

2.2
Skeletal Myoblasts

Skeletal myoblasts (SMBs) constituted an alternative source of myogenic donor cells for cardiac transplantation. When grown in serum-rich media, SMBs isolated from adult animals were readily amplified in an undifferentiated state. When cultured in serum-poor media, SMB exited the cell cycle and fused, resulting in the formation of differentiated, albeit electrically isolated, multinucleated myotubes. The initial study demonstrating that skeletal myoblasts survived and differentiated following transplantation into the heart utilized the C2C12 SMB cell line (Koh et al. 1993a). Once again, light microscopic anal-

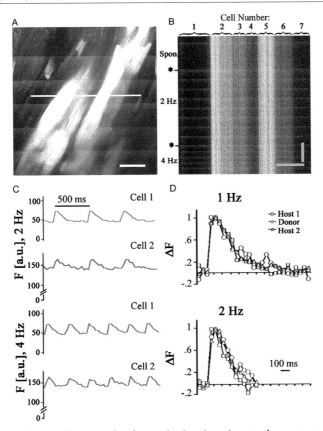

Fig. 2a–d Use of two photon molecular excitation imaging to demonstrate functional coupling between donor and host cardiomyocytes. **a** Enhanced green fluorescent protein (EGFP)-expressing fetal cardiomyocytes were transplanted into a nontransgenic adult heart. The image shown was acquired in full-frame mode 37 days after cellular transplantation; the heart was loaded with the calcium-sensitive fluorophore rhod-2 and continuously paced at 2 Hz. Action potential-evoked increases in rhod-2 fluorescence impose as ripple-like wave fronts and are visible in both engrafted cardiomyocytes (*bright cells*) and host (*dark calls*) cardiomyocytes. The *white bar* indicates the position of line-scan mode data acquisition. **b** Line-scan mode image of the region in panel **a** indicated by the *white line*. The image shows vertically stacked line scans that traverse 7 cardiomyocytes. Cells 1, 4, and 7 are host cardiomyocytes and cells 2, 3, 5, and 6 are EGFP-expressing donor cardiomyocytes. The preparation was paced via point stimulation at a remote site at the rates indicated. *Spon.* indicates spontaneous intracellular calcium ($[Ca^{2+}]_i$) transients. Scale bars, 20 μm horizontally, 1,000 ms vertically. **c** Spatially integrated traces of the changes in rhod-2 fluorescence for cardiomyocyte no. 1 (host) and cardiomyocyte no. 2 (donor). The signal across the entire cell was averaged. The traces were recorded during pacing at 2 and 4 Hz as indicated. **d** Superimposed tracings of electrically evoked changes in rhod-2 fluorescence as a function of time from host (*squares* and *triangles*) and donor (*circles*) cardiomyocytes. For each cell, the relative changes in fluorescence were normalized such that 0 represents the prestimulus fluorescence intensity and 1 represents the peak fluorescence intensity. Traces were recorded with pacing at a rate of 1 and 2 Hz as indicated. (Modified after Rubart et al. 2003a)

yses revealed that the donor-derived myocytes were well aligned with host cardiomyocytes (see Fig. 3). Ultrastructural analyses revealed marked undulations in the cell membrane of transplanted myotubes; the appearance of the donor cells was reminiscent of myocytes in "contracture," and suggested that the donor skeletal myotubes were not coupled with host cardiomyocytes. Similar results were obtained with primary skeletal myoblasts.

Numerous studies subsequently demonstrated that SMBs formed large, stable grafts following transplantation into normal or injured hearts (Dowell et al. 2003b). In some cases, SMB transplantation had a positive impact on cardiac function in injured hearts (Taylor et al. 1998). It appeared that functional improvement resulted largely from decreased postinjury ventricular remodeling. Indeed, in vitro contractility (Murry et al. 1996), dye transfer (Leobon et al. 2003), intracellular calcium imaging studies (Rubart et al. 2004) with hearts harboring SMB grafts strongly suggested that the donor-derived skeletal myotubes were not functionally coupled with the host myocardium. The observed positive impact on cardiac function in animal models (despite the absence of overt cardiomyogenic differentiation) promoted clinical trials with SMBs for the treatment of heart failure. Preliminary results have indicated that autologous SMBs survived and differentiated following transplantation in humans

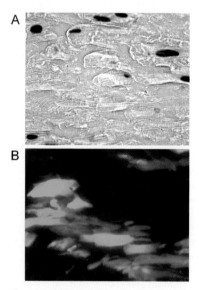

Fig. 3a, b Skeletal myoblasts form grafts comprising predominately nascent skeletal myotubes following cellular transplantation. EGFP-expressing C2C12 skeletal myoblasts were transplanted into an MHC-nLAC heart. **a** Brightfield micrograph of a thin section prepared from a heart following cellular transplantation; section was stained with X-GAL and host cardiomyocytes can readily be identified by virtue of their nuclear localized beta-galactosidase activity (*black nuclei*). **b** Epifluorescence micrograph of the same section depicted in a; EGFP-positive myotubes (*white cytoplasm*) are readily seen

(Hagege et al. 2003; Herreros et al. 2003; Menasche et al. 2003; Pagani et al. 2003; Smits et al. 2003).

Although the protocol appeared to be safe, episodic ventricular tachyarrhythmias were observed in some patients (Menasche et al. 2003; Smits et al. 2003). Interestingly, SMBs were observed to form heterokaryons with host cardiomyocytes at a very low frequency following transplantation into mouse hearts (Reinecke et al. 2004; Rubart et al. 2004; Fig. 4). Moreover, SMB/cardiomyocyte heterokaryon formation was accompanied with abnormal intracellular calcium transients (Rubart et al. 2004, Fig. 5); such a mechanism might underlie the arrhythmias seen in some patients receiving this treatment. Collectively, these data indicated that skeletal myoblasts form stable grafts comprised of differentiated, electrically isolated myotubes following transplantation into normal or injured hearts. Although the engrafted cells did not participate in a functional syncytium with the myocardium, transplantation nonetheless had

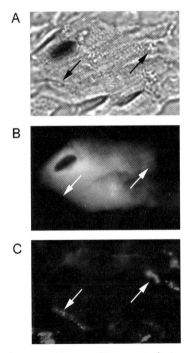

Fig. 4a–c Myocytes arising from myoblast-cardiomyocyte fusion events form gap junctions with neighboring host cardiomyocytes. Sections prepared from MHC-nLAC hearts transplanted with EGFP-expressing skeletal myoblasts were stained with X-Gal and reacted with an anti-connexin43 antibody, followed by a fluorophore-conjugated secondary antibody. Cells arising from myocyte–cardiomyocyte fusion events are identified by the presence of nuclear beta galactosidase staining (**a**) and cytoplasmic EGFP fluorescence (**b**). *Arrows* mark punctuate connexin43 signal (**c**), indicating the presence of gap junctions between the fusion-derived heterokaryon and a host cardiomyocyte. (From Rubart et al. 2004)

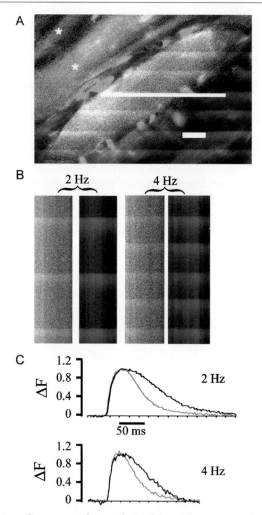

Fig. 5a–c Myoblast-cardiomyocyte fusion-derived heterokaryons are functionally coupled to the host myocardium and exhibit abnormal $[Ca^{2+}]_i$ transients. **a** Full-frame mode image of a rhod-2 loaded heart 28 days following transplantation of EGFP-expressing skeletal myoblasts. Only the EGFP-expressing myocyte (*white cytoplasm*) that is immediately juxtaposed to host cardiomyocytes (*black cytoplasm*) exhibits action potential-evoked $[Ca^{2+}]_i$ transients in synchrony with the host cardiomyocytes, whereas other donor-derived myocytes (*asterisks*) do not. The heart was point stimulated at a rate of 4 Hz. *White bar* indicates the position of the line-scan mode data acquisition. **b** Stacked line-scan image depicting $[Ca^{2+}]_i$ transients during pacing at 2 and 4 Hz in the indicated regions in **a**. **c** Superimposed tracings of changes in rhod-2 fluorescence as a function of time from the donor-derived EGFP-positive myocyte and resident host EGFP-negative cardiomyocytes in **b**. For each cell, spatially averaged changes in rhod-2 fluorescence were obtained and normalized such that 0 represents the fluorescence intensity before the $[Ca^{2+}]_i$ transient and 1 represents the peak fluorescence intensity. The heterokaryon $[Ca^{2+}]_i$ transient duration is prolonged as compared to that in the neighboring host cardiomyocyte

a positive impact on heart function (presumably through indirect effects, as for example enhanced angiogenesis or altered postinjury remodeling).

2.3
Adult-Derived Stem Cells

Recent studies have suggested that adult stem cells harbored a greater capacity to "trans-differentiate" into other cell lineages than was previous anticipated. Several bone marrow transplantation studies suggested that hematopoietic progenitor cells were recruited to the myocardium following injury and underwent cardiomyogenic differentiation (Bittner et al. 1999; Jackson et al. 2001). Subsequent studies revealed that fusion events between marrow-derived cells and cardiomyocytes was the likely source of these trans-differentiation events (Alvarez-Dolado et al. 2003). Other studies have suggested that hematopoietic stem cells were cardiomyogenic following direct transplantation (Orlic et al. 2001a) or cytokine-mediated mobilization (Orlic et al. 2001b) into the infarcted myocardium, although these experiments have not readily been replicated by other groups (Agbulut et al. 2003; Balsam et al. 2004; Murry et al. 2004; Nygren et al. 2004). The basis for these differential results was not clear, but likely reflected differences in the approaches used to isolate the stem cell population and/or differences in the experimental read-out used to document cardiomyogenic differentiation. Nonetheless, the early successes with marrow-derived cell transplantation in small animals prompted several clinical trials, some of which suggested a benefit resulting from the treatment (Assmus et al. 2002; Perin et al. 2003; Messina et al. 2004; Wollert et al. 2004). Finally, several laboratories have identified cardiomyogenic cells within the adult heart (Hierlihy et al. 2002; Beltrami et al. 2003; Oh et al. 2003; Martin et al. 2004). Collectively, the cardiomyogenic adult stem cell literature to date has been extremely interesting; however, the results were somewhat confusing, as in most cases mutually exclusive criteria were used to isolate the stem cell population. If circulating or cardiac-resident adult stem cells were capable of bona fide cardiomyogenic differentiation, and if they were able to be amplified (either in vitro or in vivo with cytokine treatment), they would constitute ideal cells for transplantation-based therapies.

3
Cardiomyogenic Differentiation in Embryonic Stem Cells

3.1
Spontaneous Cardiomyogenic Differentiation

Doetschman and colleagues (Doetschman et al. 1985) made the initial observation that when grown in suspension culture and under conditions favorable for differentiation, mouse ES cells aggregated to form spherical structures called embryoid bodies (EBs). Stochastic differentiation within EBs resulted in the juxtaposition of different developmental fields, thereby mimicking induction cues that occurred during normal embryogenesis. As a consequence, cell lineages of endo-, ecto-, and mesodermal origin were observed to appear in differentiating EBs. Prominent cardiomyogenesis occurred during EB differentiation, as evidenced by the presence of well-formed myofibers (Fig. 6) as well as spontaneous contractile activity. Thus differentiating ES cells might provide a surrogate source of donor cardiomyocytes for therapeutic cell transplantation.

Cardiomyocytes derived from EBs have been studied in great detail (Boheler et al. 2002; Caspi and Gepstein 2004). Studies with mouse ES-derived cardiomyocytes revealed that cardiomyogenic differentiation in EBs closely paralleled that observed for early stages of heart development in vitro (Doevendans et al. 2000), and that cardiomyocytes with characteristics typical of the primitive heart tube and early chamber myocardium could be readily identified (Fijnvandraat et al. 2003b, 2003c). The temporal and phenotypic

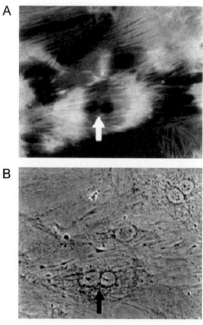

Fig. 6a,b ES-derived cardiomyocytes are highly differentiated. **a** Immune cytologic localization of sarcomeric myosin in ES-derived cardiomyocytes. Myosin was detected by MF-20 immune cytology; the signal was developed with a fluorophore-conjugated secondary antibody and visualized under epifluorescence illumination. Multiple myocytes with well-developed myofibers are seen. **b** Image of the same microscopic field viewed under phase contrast. *Arrows* in **a** and **b** denote a bi-nucleated cardiomyocyte. (From Klug et al. 1995)

changes in myofiber structure in ES-derived cardiomyocytes closely paralleled that seen for cardiomyocytes in vivo (Guan et al. 1999). Similarly, ES-derived cardiomyocytes exhibited a temporal pattern of cell cycle withdraw and multi-nucleation similar to that seen in vivo (Klug et al. 1995). Treatment of cultures with cytokines and growth factors that induce sarcomeric organization in fetal cardiomyocytes had a similar effect on ES-derived cardiomyocytes (Guan et al. 1999). Electrophysiological studies revealed that cells with characteristics of atrial, ventricular, and sinus-nodal cardiomyocytes were present following terminal differentiation of ES-derived cells (Maltsev et al. 1993), a result that was confirmed via molecular analyses (Miller-Hance et al. 1993). The developmental changes in the electrophysiological properties of ES-derived cardiomyocytes from initial cardiomyoblast commitment (Kolossov et al. 1998) through formation of three-dimensional, spontaneously contracting structures (Maltsev et al. 1993; Banach et al. 2003) have been well characterized.

The isolation of human ES cells by Thompson and colleagues (Thomson et al. 1998) permitted analyses of in vitro generated human cardiomyocytes. When cultured in suspension, human ES cells also formed EBs, which underwent differentiation and exhibited spontaneous contractile activity (Kehat et al. 2001; Odorico et al. 2001; Xu et al. 2002). Molecular, immune cytologic, and electrophysiologic studies indicated that human ES cells differentiated into bona fide cardiomyocytes (Kehat et al. 2001). Human ES-derived cardiomyocytes underwent terminal differentiation as evidenced by cell cycle withdrawal and myofiber maturation (Snir et al. 2003), albeit over a longer time frame as compared to that observed for mouse-derived cells (Klug et al. 1995). As was observed in the mouse studies cited above, electrophysiological analyses revealed that cardiomyocytes of atrial, ventricular, and nodal lineages were present in cultures of in vitro differentiated human ES cells (He et al. 2003). Characterization of the ion currents and action potential profiles in dissociated cell preparations revealed that the Nav1.5 Na^+ channel was important for initiating spontaneous excitability in human ES-derived cardiomyocytes (Satin et al. 2004). Collectively these data indicated that bona fide cardiomyocytes can be obtained from spontaneously differentiating mouse and human ES cultures.

3.2
Identification of Factors That Enhance Cardiomyogenic Differentiation

The reproducible differentiation observed in cultured EBs has been exploited to identify factors capable of enhancing cardiomyogenic induction. For example, a number of studies have implicated signaling of BMP and Wnt family members in cardiomyogenic differentiation of ES cells (Winnier et al. 1995; Czyz and Wobus 2001; Behfar et al. 2002; Kawai et al. 2004; Terami et al. 2004). In addition, signaling through the FGF (Dell'Era et al. 2003; Kawai et al. 2004), IGF-II (Morali et al. 2000), Crypto (Parisi et al. 2003), PDGF-BB (Sachinidis et al. 2003), CT-1 (Sauer et al. 2004), TGF-beta (Behfar et al. 2002), and dynorphin B (Ventura et al. 2003) pathways enhanced cardiomyogenesis during EB differentiation. Perhaps not unexpectedly, cytokine/growth factor treatments were occasionally observed to promote cardiomyogenic differentiation via rather indirect mechanisms. For example, LIF (leukemia inhibitory factor) regulated cardiomyogenesis in ES cultures indirectly via its effect on parietal endoderm differentiation (Bader et al. 2000; Bader et al. 2001). Thus, altering the relative content of other cell lineages that subsequently provided cardiomyogenic-inducing factors enhanced the yield of cardiomyocytes.

In some cases, treatment with cytokines appeared to have contrasting effects on cardiomyogenic differentiation, depending on the culture conditions. For example, retinoic acid (Wobus et al. 1997) has been shown to accelerate differentiation, although it was not clear if there was an overall enhancement of total cardiomyocyte yield. Interestingly, treatment with retinoic acid resulted in an increase in cardiomyoblast differentiation toward the ventricular lineage in EBs cultured under high serum conditions (Wobus et al. 1997; Hidaka et al. 2003), with a concomitant reduction in differentiation toward the atrial lineage. Paradoxically, depletion of retinoic acid in low serum cultures enhanced cardiomyogenic differentiation (Gajovic et al. 1997), presumably due to effects on other cell lineages.

In addition to these defined factors, co-culture experiments revealed that precardiac endoderm contained factors capable of enhancing ES cell cardiomyogenic differentiation (Rudy-Reil and Lough 2004). Similarly, Mummery and colleagues have shown that a factor secreted by mouse endoderm cells enhanced cardiomyogenic differentiation of human ES cells (Mummery et al. 2002, 2003). Inorganic compounds such as nitric oxide (Kanno et al. 2004), lithium (Schmidt et al. 2001), reactive oxygen species (Sauer et al. 2000), and a novel butyric and retinoic acid linked ester of hyaluronan (Ventura et al. 2004) also increased cardiomyocyte content in cultured EBs. Finally, a number of compounds were identified that promoted cardiomyogenic differentiation in embryonic carcinoma cell lines. These include Wnt-11 (Pandur et al. 2002), dimethysulfoxide (Rudnicki et al. 1990), and oxytocin (Paquin et al. 2002). There is a high probability that these factors would have similar effects on ES cell differentiation.

Gene transfer experiments identified additional pathways that enhanced cardiomyogenic differentiation in ES cells. For example, overexpression of GATA-4 (Arceci et al. 1993; Grepin et al. 1997) or alpha-1,3-Fucosyltransferase (Sudou et al. 1997) resulted in increased yields of cardiomyocytes in differentiating EB cultures. Similarly, overexpression of TBX5 (Fijnvandraat et al. 2003a) and opioid peptide (Ventura and Maioli 2000) enhanced cardiomyogenic differentiation in embryonic carcinoma cells. Conversely, loss of beta-1 integrin (Fassler et al. 1996) or alternatively overexpression of Rac-1 (Puceat et al. 2003) decreased the levels of cardiomyogenesis in differentiating ES cells. Thus a large number of cytokines, inorganic molecules, and genes have been identified that influenced the ability of ES cells to generate cardiomyocytes.

The above-mentioned studies were largely candidate experiments designed to assess the effects of a specific factor or gene on cardiomyogenic differentiation. In contrast, there have been several studies wherein systematic screens were performed to identify compounds that were able to promote cardiomyocyte differentiation. For example, Takahashi and colleagues screened a chemical library for compounds that were able to directly promote cardiomyogenesis in cultured ES cells (Takahashi et al. 2003). The screen utilized ES cells that carried a cardiac-restricted reporter transgene that encoded EGFP. Of the 880 compounds screened, one (ascorbic acid) was observed to enhance EGFP expression in the ES cells. In other studies, Wu and colleagues screened a library of heterocyclic compounds designed around kinase-directed molecular scaffolds in an effort to identify compounds that induced cardiomyogenesis in P19 embryonic carcinoma cells. The cells contained a reporter transgene comprised of a cardiac-restricted reporter transgene that targeted expression of luciferase (Wu et al. 2004). Subsequent studies showed that a compound identified in the screen, which was designated cardiogenol A-D, promoted high levels of cardiomyogenic differentiation in ES cells.

Collectively, the studies described above identified a host of molecules that increased cardiomyocyte content in differentiating ES cultures. In some instances, the signaling cascades were revealed through analysis of cardiac differentiation in genetically modified ES cells. Information obtained from such studies can in turn be exploited to enhance the production of ES-derived cardiomyocytes for clinical applications.

4
Experiences with Embryonic Stem-Derived Cardiomyocyte Transplantation

The observation that fetal cardiomyocytes formed stable grafts and participated in a functional syncytium with the host myocardium following transplantation into adult hearts, and that differentiating ES cells gave rise to bona fide cardiomyocytes, prompted additional studies wherein ES-derived cardiomyocytes were used for cardiac cell transplantation. The initial study employed a relatively simple genetic selection approach to generate pure cultures of cardiomyocytes for transplantation (Klug et al. 1996). A fusion gene comprised of a cardiac-restricted promoter and sequences encoding aminoglycoside phosphotransferase was stably transfected into mouse ES cells. The resulting cells were differentiated in vitro and then were treated with G418, an analog to the antibiotic neomycin. Cardiomyocytes derived from the ES cells expressed the aminoglycoside phosphotransferase transgene (due to the use of a cardiomyocyte-restricted promoter) and thus survived treatment with G418. In contrast, noncardiomyocytes derived from the ES cells did not express the aminoglycoside phosphotransferase transgene and were killed by G418 treatment (see Fig. 7).

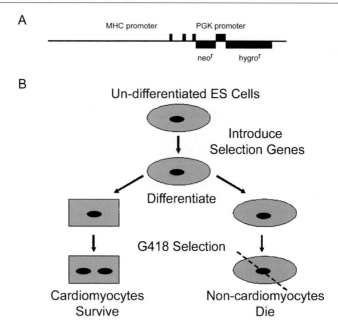

Fig. 7a,b Strategy for the generation of pure ES-derived cardiomyocyte cultures. **a** Structure of the MHC-neo^r/PGK-hygro^r transgene. **b** Scheme for in vitro selection of ES-derived cardiomyocytes. ES cells are transfected with the MHC-neo^r/PGK-hygro^r transgene, and allowed to differentiate. For cardiomyocyte selection, the differentiated cultures are grown in the presence of G418

Cultures generated in this way were comprised of highly differentiated cardiomyocytes (>99% pure). The purified ES-derived cardiomyocytes were transplanted into the hearts of adult mdx recipients. These mice, a genetic model for Duchenne's muscular dystrophy, harbored a mutation in the dystrophin gene and failed to express the dystrophin protein. In contrast, the donor ES-derived cardiomyocytes were not mutant and expressed normal levels of dystrophin. The fate of the engrafted cells was thus monitored by anti-dystrophin immune reactivity. Donor ES-derived cardiomyocytes formed stable grafts and were observed to be well aligned with host cardiomyocytes (see Fig. 8). Although this study demonstrated ES-derived cardiomyocytes survived intracardiac transplantation and were structurally well integrated with the host myocardium, the potential impact on cardiac function was not assessed.

ES-derived cardiomyocytes have also been transplanted into hearts with myocardial infarction. For example, Yang and colleagues micro-dissected beating regions of cultured EBs and transplanted the cells (which were enriched for cardiomyocyte content) into infarcts 15 min after permanent coronary artery occlusion. Cardiac function was observed to be improved at 6 weeks following transplantation in hearts treated with cells as compared to hearts with me-

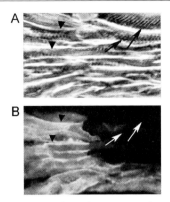

Fig. 8a,b Genetically-selected ES-derived cardiomyocytes form stable grafts following cellular transplantation. Phase-contrast image (**a**) and anti-dystrophin immune fluorescence (**b**), respectively, of a dystrophin-deficient heart engrafted with G418-selected ES-derived cardiomyocytes. The same field is depicted in both panels, and dystrophin immune reactivity appears as white signal in **b**. *Arrows* indicate myofiber-containing host cells (dystrophin negative), while *arrowheads* indicate myofiber-containing donor cells (dystrophin positive). (From Klug et al. 1996)

dia injection alone (Yang et al. 2002). Cardiac function was further enhanced when the donor cells were genetically engineered to express vascular endothelial growth factor, and a concomitant increase in vessel density was observed. Although the donor cells expressed an EGFP reporter gene under the regulation of a ubiquitously active promoter, identification of stem-cell derived cardiomyocyte content in hearts with cell transplants was hampered due to the reliance of fluorescent-based assays. Given this, and the lack of a systematic measurement of donor cell content within the infarcted tissue, it was difficult to ascertain if improved cardiac function resulted from direct contractile activity of the donor cells or from indirect effects (i.e., enhanced vessel formation).

In other studies, Behfar and colleagues injected undifferentiated ES cells expressing enhanced cyan fluorescent protein (ECFP) under the regulation of a muscle specific promoter. The cells were delivered along the infarct border in mice immediately following permanent coronary artery ligation. Cardiomyogenic differentiation was observed, as evidenced by the induction of ECFP expression. In addition, ECFP expression was observed to co-localize with anti-myosin light chain 2V immune reactivity (Behfar et al. 2002). Echocardiographic analyses revealed greater left ventricular ejection fraction in the mice receiving cell transplants as compared to those receiving media. Once again, no systematic assessment of stem cell-derived cardiomyocyte content was performed; thus it was difficult to determine the mechanistic basis for the observed physiologic effects. It was nonetheless interesting that a propensity for cardiomyogenic differentiation was observed in this study, despite the fact that undifferentiated ES cells were transplanted. Unfortunately, the percentage of ES-derived cells that exhibited a cardiomyogenic phenotype was not quantitated, so it was impossible to determine if enhanced cardiomyogenic differentiation occurred.

Mouse ES-derived cardiomyocytes have also been transplanted into rats with experimental myocardial infarction. For example, Min and colleagues isolated enriched cultures of ES-derived cardiomyocytes via micro-dissection, and transplanted the cells at the infarct border zone in rats 30 min following coronary artery ligation. Analysis of pressure volume loops obtained using an intraventricular catheter, as well as echocardiographic analyses, revealed enhanced cardiac function at 6 weeks after infarction in rats that received cell transplants (Min et al. 2002). The cells were labeled with reporter transgene expressing green fluorescent protein (GFP) under the regulation of a ubiquitous promoter, and GFP-expressing cardiomyocytes were observed at 6 weeks after transplantation. The authors indicated that more than 7% of the cells isolated from the injected hearts were GFP-expressing cardiomyocytes; however, the cardiomyocyte content (as opposed to nonmyocytes) was difficult to ascertain in the histologic sections shown. This study was nonetheless interesting in that mouse ES-derived cardiomyocytes appeared to survive in infarcted rat hearts in the absence of immune suppression.

Several other groups have performed xenogenic transplantation with mouse ES-derived cardiomyocytes. For example, Hodgson and colleagues differenti-ated ES cells carrying an actin-promoter ECFP reporter transgene in vitro, and the resulting ES-derived cardiomyocytes were enriched from nonmyocytes via Percoll density gradient centrifugation (Hodgson et al. 2004). The ES-derived cardiomyocytes were transplanted into infarcted rat hearts 8 weeks following permanent coronary artery occlusion. A marked and sustained improvement in cardiac function was observed from 3–12 weeks following cell transplanta-tion, as evidenced by echocardiographic analyses. ES-derived cardiomyocytes were detected, as well as a remarkable reduction in infarct size. However, this latter observation must be viewed with caution, as the number of animal an-alyzed was quite small in this study. No evidence for donor cell rejection was noted. Absence of immune rejection was also observed following transplanta-tion of mouse ES-derived cardiomyocytes into Wistar rats with concomitant cyclosporin administration (Naito et al. 2004).

Xenogenic cell transplants have recently been performed using cardiomy-ocytes isolated from differentiating human ES cells. Kehat and colleagues (Kehat et al. 2004) injected micro-dissected regions of adherent EBs exhibiting spontaneous contractile activity and transplanted these cells into pigs with complete heart block (surgically induced via his bundle ablation). Pacing ac-tivity originating from the site of cell delivery was observed at 1–3 weeks after transplantation, as evidenced by both surface electrocardiograms and EP mapping techniques. This observation suggested that the ES-derived car-diomyocytes were functionally coupled and able to drive electrical activity in the heart. The animals received cyclosporin and prednisolone over the course of the experiment, and no rejection was evident. The observation that only a relatively small number of donor-derived myocytes were present at the graft site raised interesting questions regarding the mass of cells needed to drive ventricular depolarization.

A similar result was reported by Xue and colleagues (Xue et al. 2005), wherein beating EBs were transplanted into the left ventricle of guinea pig hearts. The hearts were harvested 72 h later, and subjected to cryoablation of the atrioventricular node so as to eliminate all intrinsic pacing activity. The hearts were then placed into a perfused imaging chamber, and epicardial optical mapping revealed propagating action potential waves that originated from the site of cell engraftment. No histologic evaluation of the engraftment site was presented in this latter study, despite the use of EGFP-labeled cells.

Several other reports with ES-derived cells should be mentioned. For example, Wang and colleagues injected undifferentiated ES cells and encephalomyocarditis virus into the tail vein of mice. The presence of ES cells enhanced the survival rate and lessened the incidence of inflammatory cell infiltration and myocardial lesions (Wang et al. 2002). ES-derived cardiomyocytes were also detectable in the heart. Although interesting, the mechanism for the observed phenotypes was unclear in this study. ES cells have also been used to impregnate biomaterials. Kofidis and colleagues seeded matrigel with undifferentiated ES cells carrying a reporter transgene that expressed EGFP under a ubiquitous promoter. The mixture was delivered into the ischemic region of a heterotrophic heart transplant. Two weeks later, ES-derived cells were observed in the transplant region, although the cardiomyocyte content was not quantitated. The presence of the ES-derived cells nonetheless had a positive impact on wall motion in the engrafted, heterotrophic heart transplants. Given these results, it would be of considerable interest to determine the suitability of ES-derived cardiomyocytes for other biomaterials-based cell delivery systems. The collagen cast system developed by Zimmermann and colleagues might be particularly suitable for such applications (Zimmermann et al. 2002). Finally, ES-derived stem cells have been transplanted at ectopic sites in vivo. The transplanted cells exhibited spontaneous contractile activity for 30 days after delivery, and acquired many structural traits typical of myocardial tissue (Johkura et al. 2003). Transplantation at ectopic sites might permit more rapid assessment of the effects of factors and/or genes on the behavior of ES-derived cardiomyocytes in vivo.

Collectively these data supported the notion that ES-derived cardiomyocytes were able to form stable grafts following transplantation into normal or injured hearts. In many cases, the donor cardiomyocytes were observed to be well aligned with the host myocardium, and indirect evidence suggested that the cells were functionally coupled and under certain conditions able to pace the host myocardium. Improvement in left ventricular function was observed in several studies wherein cells were delivered into injured hearts; however, the mechanism underlying functional improvement remained unclear.

5
Large-Scale Generation of Embryonic Stem-Derived Cardiomyocytes

The data reviewed above suggests that cell transplantation could have a beneficial effect in injured hearts, and furthermore that ES-derived cardiomyocytes might constitute ideal donor cells. These studies relied on laboratory-scale production of donor cells, and typically no more than 10^6 cells were used (and in many cases, significantly fewer cells were used). In contrast, the human left ventricle has been estimated to contain 5.8×10^9 cardiomyocytes (Kajstura et al. 1998). Given the low seeding rate and relatively limited proliferation observed for transplanted cells, therapeutic application of ES-derived cardiomyocytes for treating severely injured hearts would require the production of a large number of donor cells. Several groups have developed systems that permitted the generation of large-scale cultures of ES-derived cells.

As indicated above, differentiation of ES cells is typically initiated by growing the cells in suspension, which promoted the formation of EBs. Ideal differentiation was observed if EBs initially comprised aggregates of approximately 200 cells. If cultured at too high of a cell concentration, large aggregates formed, which subsequently failed to differentiate. Maltsev and colleagues developed the hanging drop technique, which permitted reproducible generation of uniformly sized EBs (Maltsev et al. 1993). Dang and colleagues subsequently showed that cell–cell interactions in EBs was largely mediated by E-cadherin, and furthermore that E-cadherin expression decreased as EBs began to differentiate (Dang et al. 2002, 2004). Zandstra and colleagues took advantage of these observations: EBs generated with the hanging drop technique and subsequently transferred into stirred suspension cultures yielded high-density cultures comprised of well-differentiated cells (Zandstra et al. 2003). These authors performed similar studies with ES cells that expressed the cardiomyocyte restricted G418-resistance transgenes described above (Klug et al. 1996); treatment of the high-density suspension cultures with G418 resulted in the formation of spherical structure (termed cardiac bodies, or CBs), which were comprised of cardiomyocytes (the G418 having effectively killed essentially all of the noncardiomyocytes in the culture; see Fig. 9). Yields of 8×10^4 cardiomyocytes per milliliter (2×10^7 total cardiomyocytes per 250 ml of culture) were obtained (Zandstra et al. 2003). In subsequent studies, these authors allowed ES cells to aggregate in suspension culture for 24 h, and then microencapsulated the cells within agarose hydrogel capsules. The encapsulated ES cells were then seeded into stirred suspension cultures, where they differentiated in the absence of aggregation (Dang et al. 2004). Cardiomyocyte differentiation was not quantitated in this latter experiment.

The studies described above permitted the generation of intermediate-size cultures of ES-derived cells, but required at least two cell culture steps to avoid EB aggregation. Zweigerdt and colleagues adopted a somewhat different approach to develop a single-step culture for generation of ES-derived cells. Initial

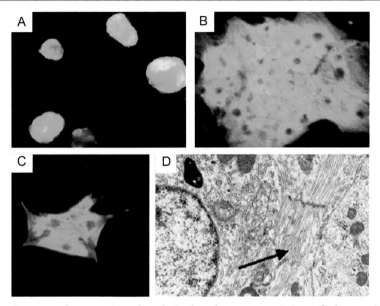

Fig. 9a–d Large-scale generation of ES-derived cardiomyocytes. Spinner flasks were inoculated with EBs and after 9 days of culture G418 was added to kill noncardiomyocytes. **a, b** Epifluorescent images of G418-selected cardiac bodies generated in spinner flasks; the parental ES cells expressed an EGFP reporter transgene. Panel **a** shows a gross cardiac body image, while **b** shows a section through a cardiac body. **c** Antisarcomeric myosin (MF-20) immune fluorescent staining of dissociated cardiomyocytes generated in spinner flasks; the parental ES cells did not express a reporter transgene. **d** Transmission electron micrographic image of a cardiac body; mature sarcomeric organization and Z-banding (*arrow*) are readily seen

studies revealed that rotating suspension culture could be used to generate large numbers of individual EBs within standard-sized culture dishes. This procedure obviated the need to use hanging drop cultures (Zweigerdt et al. 2003a). Once again, ES cells carrying a cardiomyocyte restricted G418-resistance transgene were employed. Addition of G418 resulted in CB formation, with a yield of approximately 2×10^5 cardiomyocytes per milliliter after 10 days of selection. These observations suggested that fluid dynamics could be exploited to block EB aggregation, thereby permitting the isolation of ES-derived cells in a single-step culture system. Accordingly, a single cell suspension of ES cells carrying a cardiomyocyte restricted G418-resistance transgene were inoculated directly into a fully controlled, stirred 2-l bioreactor. The bioreactor employed a pitched-blade-turbine, which permitted optimal cell expansion, EB formation, and efficient ES cell differentiation (Schroeder et al., in press; Zweigerdt et al. 2003b). After 9 days of differentiation, G418 was added to the EBs, which were then cultured for an additional 9 days. The protocol resulted in the generation of essentially pure cardiomyocyte cultures, with a yield of 6.4×10^5 cardiomyocytes per milliliter. In terms of total yield, 1.28×10^9 cardiomyocytes were obtained from a single 2-l bioreactor run initially seeded with 2×10^8 undifferentiated ES cells (Schroeder et al., in press; Zweigerdt et al. 2003b). Collectively these data indicated that relatively large-scale production of ES-derived cardiomyocytes was possible, and that use of the G418 selection technique resulted in essentially pure cultures.

6
Conclusions

Cell transplantation approaches have emerged as potential therapies for heart disease, with several clinical trials already initiated. These procedures hold the potential for a curative treatment of heart diseases that are character-ized by progressive cardiomyocyte loss, provided that the underlying cause of cell loss is also addressed. At present, a variety of donor cells have been tested, with varied and sometimes conflicting results obtained for the level of cardiomyogenic differentiation and functional integration, particularly in the case of adult-derived stem cell transplantation. However, it is clear from the studies reviewed here that cardiomyocytes, and in particular ES-derived cardiomyocytes, formed stable grafts following transplantation into either nor-mal or injured hearts. The transplanted cells exhibited highly differentiated phenotypes and frequently appeared structurally integrated with the host my-ocardium, and attributes required for functional integration (i.e., intercalated discs) were readily detected. Both direct and indirect evidence for functional coupling between donor and host cardiomyocytes have been reported.

Additional studies are needed to ascertain the potential value of cell trans-plantation as a treatment for heart disease. In the case of cardiomyocyte trans-plantation, preclinical studies using dispersed cell preparations from fetal hearts indicated that the number of total cells which successfully seeded the heart following transplantation was quite low, and the number of seeded car-diomyocytes was undoubtedly markedly lower (Yao et al. 2003). Additional development of biomaterials approaches might enhance the seeding capacity of donor cells (Zimmermann et al. 2002; Kofidis et al. 2004). Other studies indicated that donor cell death was prevalent during the period immediately following transplantation (Zhang et al. 2001). Treatment with cell-survival fac-tors might greatly enhance donor cell viability after transplantation (Mangi et al. 2003; Bock-Marquette et al. 2004). Tritiated thymidine incorporation stud-ies revealed relatively rapid cell cycle withdrawal following transplantation of fetal cardiomyocytes (Soonpaa and Field 1994) and during ES cardiomyogenic differentiation in vitro (Klug et al. 1995). Interventions aimed at enhancing donor cardiomyocyte cell cycle activity might circumvent this issue, and result in the formation of larger grafts (Nakajima et al. 2004; Pasumarthi et al. 2005).

It is also imperative to determine if the functional improvement observed in some studies resulted from donor cell participation in a functional syncytium with the host myocardium, or alternatively from secondary effects of the donor cells (as for example secretion of angiogenic and/or survival factors). This concern was heightened by the observation that cells that a priori would not differentiate into cardiomyocytes and/or would not functionally couple with the host myocardium nonetheless appeared to enhance cardiac function following transplantation into injured hearts (Dowell et al. 2003b; Hassink et al. 2003). In the case of ES-derived cardiomyocyte, while the presence of pacemaker activity originating from sites of ES-derived cardiomyocyte transplantation suggested that those cells were functionally coupled to the host myocardium, other explanations for the activity could be envisioned. Definitive proof of functional coupling between ES-derived cardiomyocytes and the host myocardium requires analyses performed at the single cell level in intact hearts (Rubart et al. 2003a, 2003b).

Despite the requirements for additional experimentation and optimization, there are many reasons to be optimistic for the therapeutic potential of cell transplantation. In the event that ES-derived cardiomyocytes prove to be the ideal donor for cell transplantation therapies, the studies described here will have direct relevance to their use. Conversely, if an adult stem cell-derived cardiomyocyte becomes the ideal donor cell, many of the technologies developed for the isolation, in vitro amplification, in vivo delivery, and analysis of ES-derived cardiomyocytes will likely be applicable to those cells as well. The evolution of this field over the next 5 years should be both interesting and informative.

Acknowledgements We thank the National Institutes of Health for support.

References

Agbulut O, Menot ML, Li Z, Marotte F, Paulin D, Hagege AA, Chomienne C, Samuel JL, Menasche P (2003) Temporal patterns of bone marrow cell differentiation following transplantation in doxorubicin-induced cardiomyopathy. Cardiovasc Res 58:451–459

Alvarez-Dolado M, Pardal R, Garcia-Verdugo JM, Fike JR, Lee HO, Pfeffer K, Lois C, Morrison SJ, Alvarez-Buylla A (2003) Fusion of bone-marrow-derived cells with Purkinje neurons, cardiomyocytes and hepatocytes. Nature 425:968–973

Anversa P, Kajstura J (1998) Ventricular myocytes are not terminally differentiated in the adult mammalian heart. Circ Res 83:1–14

Anversa P, Nadal-Ginard B (2002) Myocyte renewal and ventricular remodelling. Nature 415:240–243

Arceci RJ, King AA, Simon MC, Orkin SH, Wilson DB (1993) Mouse GATA-4: a retinoic acid-inducible GATA-binding transcription factor expressed in endodermally derived tissues and heart. Mol Cell Biol 13:2235–2246

Assmus B, Schachinger V, Teupe C, Britten M, Lehmann R, Dobert N, Grunwald F, Aicher A, Urbich C, Martin H, Hoelzer D, Dimmeler S, Zeiher AM (2002) Transplantation of progenitor cells and regeneration enhancement in acute myocardial infarction (TOPCARE-AMI). Circulation 106:3009–3017

Bader A, Al-Dubai H, Weitzer G (2000) Leukemia inhibitory factor modulates cardiogenesis in embryoid bodies in opposite fashions. Circ Res 86:787–794

Bader A, Gruss A, Hollrigl A, Al-Dubai H, Capetanaki Y, Weitzer G (2001) Paracrine promotion of cardiomyogenesis in embryoid bodies by LIF modulated endoderm. Differentiation 68:31–43

Balsam LB, Wagers AJ, Christensen JL, Kofidis T, Weissman IL, Robbins RC (2004) Haematopoietic stem cells adopt mature haematopoietic fates in ischaemic myocardium. Nature 428:668–673

Banach K, Halbach MD, Hu P, Hescheler J, Egert U (2003) Development of electrical activity in cardiac myocyte aggregates derived from mouse embryonic stem cells. Am J Physiol Heart Circ Physiol 284:H2114–H2123

Behfar A, Zingman LV, Hodgson DM, Rauzier JM, Kane GC, Terzic A, Puceat M (2002) Stem cell differentiation requires a paracrine pathway in the heart. FASEB J 16:1558–1566

Beltrami AP, Barlucchi L, Torella D, Baker M, Limana F, Chimenti S, Kasahara H, Rota M, Musso E, Urbanek K, Leri A, Kajstura J, Nadal-Ginard B, Anversa P (2003) Adult cardiac stem cells are multipotent and support myocardial regeneration. Cell 114:763–776

Bittner RE, Schofer C, Weipoltshammer K, Ivanova S, Streubel B, Hauser E, Freilinger M, Hoger H, Elbe-Burger A, Wachtler F (1999) Recruitment of bone-marrow-derived cells by skeletal and cardiac muscle in adult dystrophic mdx mice. Anat Embryol (Berl) 199:391–396

Bock-Marquette I, Saxena A, White MD, Dimaio JM, Srivastava D (2004) Thymosin beta4 activates integrin-linked kinase and promotes cardiac cell migration, survival and cardiac repair. Nature 432:466–472

Boheler KR, Czyz J, Tweedie D, Yang HT, Anisimov SV, Wobus AM (2002) Differentiation of pluripotent embryonic stem cells into cardiomyocytes. Circ Res 91:189–201

Caspi O, Gepstein L (2004) Potential applications of human embryonic stem cell-derived cardiomyocytes. Ann N Y Acad Sci 1015:285–298

Czyz J, Wobus A (2001) Embryonic stem cell differentiation: the role of extracellular factors. Differentiation 68:167–174

Dang SM, Kyba M, Perlingeiro R, Daley GQ, Zandstra PW (2002) Efficiency of embryoid body formation and hematopoietic development from embryonic stem cells in different culture systems. Biotechnol Bioeng 78:442–453

Dang SM, Gerecht-Nir S, Chen J, Itskovitz-Eldor J, Zandstra PW (2004) Controlled, scalable embryonic stem cell differentiation culture. Stem Cells 22:275–282

Dell'Era P, Ronca R, Coco L, Nicoli S, Metra M, Presta M (2003) Fibroblast growth factor receptor-1 is essential for in vitro cardiomyocyte development. Circ Res 93:414–420

Doetschman TC, Eistetter H, Katz M, Schmidt W, Kemler R (1985) The in vitro development of blastocyst-derived embryonic stem cell lines: formation of visceral yolk sac, blood islands and myocardium. J Embryol Exp Morphol 87:27–45

Doevendans PA, Kubalak SW, An RH, Becker DK, Chien KR, Kass RS (2000) Differentiation of cardiomyocytes in floating embryoid bodies is comparable to fetal cardiomyocytes. J Mol Cell Cardiol 32:839–851

Dowell JD, Field LJ, Pasumarthi KB (2003a) Cell cycle regulation to repair the infarcted myocardium. Heart Fail Rev 8:293–303

Dowell JD, Rubart M, Pasumarthi KB, Soonpaa MH, Field LJ (2003b) Myocyte and myogenic stem cell transplantation in the heart. Cardiovasc Res 58:336–350

Fassler R, Rohwedel J, Maltsev V, Bloch W, Lentini S, Guan K, Gullberg D, Hescheler J, Addicks K, Wobus AM (1996) Differentiation and integrity of cardiac muscle cells are impaired in the absence of beta 1 integrin. J Cell Sci 109:2989–2999

Fijnvandraat AC, Lekanne Deprez RH, Christoffels VM, Ruijter JM, Moorman AF (2003a) TBX5 overexpression stimulates differentiation of chamber myocardium in P19C16 embryonic carcinoma cells. J Muscle Res Cell Motil 24:211–218

Fijnvandraat AC, van Ginneken AC, de Boer PA, Ruijter JM, Christoffels VM, Moorman AF, Lekanne Deprez RH (2003b) Cardiomyocytes derived from embryonic stem cells resemble cardiomyocytes of the embryonic heart tube. Cardiovasc Res 58:399–409

Fijnvandraat AC, van Ginneken AC, Schumacher CA, Boheler KR, Lekanne Deprez RH, Christoffels VM, Moorman AF (2003c) Cardiomyocytes purified from differentiated embryonic stem cells exhibit characteristics of early chamber myocardium. J Mol Cell Cardiol 35:1461–1472

Gajovic S, St-Onge L, Yokota Y, Gruss P (1997) Retinoic acid mediates Pax6 expression during in vitro differentiation of embryonic stem cells. Differentiation 62:187–192

Grepin C, Nemer G, Nemer M (1997) Enhanced cardiogenesis in embryonic stem cells overexpressing the GATA-4 transcription factor. Development 124:2387–2395

Guan K, Furst DO, Wobus AM (1999) Modulation of sarcomere organization during embryonic stem cell-derived cardiomyocyte differentiation. Eur J Cell Biol 78:813–823

Hagege AA, Carrion C, Menasche P, Vilquin JT, Duboc D, Marolleau JP, Desnos M, Bruneval P (2003) Viability and differentiation of autologous skeletal myoblast grafts in ischaemic cardiomyopathy. Lancet 361:491–492

Hassink RJ, Dowell JD, Brutel de la Riviere A, Doevendans PA, Field LJ (2003) Stem cell therapy for ischemic heart disease. Trends Mol Med 9:436–441

He JQ, Ma Y, Lee Y, Thomson JA, Kamp TJ (2003) Human embryonic stem cells develop into multiple types of cardiac myocytes: action potential characterization. Circ Res 93:32–39

Herreros J, Prosper F, Perez A, Gavira JJ, Garcia-Velloso MJ, Barba J, Sanchez PL, Canizo C, Rabago G, Marti-Climent JM, Hernandez M, Lopez-Holgado N, Gonzalez-Santos JM, Martin-Luengo C, Alegria E (2003) Autologous intramyocardial injection of cultured skeletal muscle-derived stem cells in patients with non-acute myocardial infarction. Eur Heart J 24:2012–2020

Hidaka K, Lee JK, Kim HS, Ihm CH, Iio A, Ogawa M, Nishikawa S, Kodama I, Morisaki T (2003) Chamber-specific differentiation of Nkx2.5-positive cardiac precursor cells from murine embryonic stem cells. FASEB J 17:740–742

Hierlihy AM, Seale P, Lobe CG, Rudnicki MA, Megeney LA (2002) The post-natal heart contains a myocardial stem cell population. FEBS Lett 530:239–243

Hodgson DM, Behfar A, Zingman LV, Kane GC, Perez-Terzic C, Alekseev AE, Puceat M, Terzic A (2004) Stable benefit of embryonic stem cell therapy in myocardial infarction. Am J Physiol Heart Circ Physiol 287:H471–H479

Jackson KA, Majka SM, Wang H, Pocius J, Hartley CJ, Majesky MW, Entman ML, Michael LH, Hirschi KK, Goodell MA (2001) Regeneration of ischemic cardiac muscle and vascular endothelium by adult stem cells. J Clin Invest 107:1395–1402

Johkura K, Cui L, Suzuki A, Teng R, Kamiyoshi A, Okamura S, Kubota S, Zhao X, Asanuma K, Okouchi Y, Ogiwara N, Tagawa Y, Sasaki K (2003) Survival and function of mouse embryonic stem cell-derived cardiomyocytes in ectopic transplants. Cardiovasc Res 58:435–443

Kajstura J, Leri A, Finato N, Di Loreto C, Beltrami CA, Anversa P (1998) Myocyte proliferation in end-stage cardiac failure in humans. Proc Natl Acad Sci U S A 95:8801–8805

Kanno S, Kim PK, Sallam K, Lei J, Billiar TR, Shears LL, 2nd (2004) Nitric oxide facilitates cardiomyogenesis in mouse embryonic stem cells. Proc Natl Acad Sci U S A 101:12277–12281

Kawai T, Takahashi T, Esaki M, Ushikoshi H, Nagano S, Fujiwara H, Kosai K (2004) Efficient cardiomyogenic differentiation of embryonic stem cell by fibroblast growth factor 2 and bone morphogenetic protein 2. Circ J 68:691–702

Kehat I, Kenyagin-Karsenti D, Snir M, Segev H, Amit M, Gepstein A, Livne E, Binah O, Itskovitz-Eldor J, Gepstein L (2001) Human embryonic stem cells can differentiate into myocytes with structural and functional properties of cardiomyocytes. J Clin Invest 108:407–414

Kehat I, Khimovich L, Caspi O, Gepstein A, Shofti R, Arbel G, Huber I, Satin J, Itskovitz-Eldor J, Gepstein L (2004) Electromechanical integration of cardiomyocytes derived from human embryonic stem cells. Nat Biotechnol 22:1282–1289

Klug MG, Soonpaa MH, Field LJ (1995) DNA synthesis and multinucleation in embryonic stem cell-derived cardiomyocytes. Am J Physiol 269:H1913–H1921

Klug MG, Soonpaa MH, Koh GY, Field LJ (1996) Genetically selected cardiomyocytes from differentiating embryonic stem cells form stable intracardiac grafts. J Clin Invest 98:216–224

Kofidis T, de Bruin JL, Hoyt G, Lebl DR, Tanaka M, Yamane T, Chang CP, Robbins RC (2004) Injectable bioartificial myocardial tissue for large-scale intramural cell transfer and functional recovery of injured heart muscle. J Thorac Cardiovasc Surg 128:571–578

Koh GY, Klug MG, Soonpaa MH, Field LJ (1993a) Differentiation and long-term survival of C2C12 myoblast grafts in heart. J Clin Invest 92:1548–1554

Koh GY, Soonpaa MH, Klug MG, Field LJ (1993b) Long-term survival of AT-1 cardiomyocyte grafts in syngeneic myocardium. Am J Physiol 264:H1727–H1733

Koh GY, Soonpaa MH, Klug MG, Pride HP, Cooper BJ, Zipes DP, Field LJ (1995) Stable fetal cardiomyocyte grafts in the hearts of dystrophic mice and dogs. J Clin Invest 96:2034–2042

Kolossov E, Fleischmann BK, Liu Q, Bloch W, Viatchenko-Karpinski S, Manzke O, Ji GJ, Bohlen H, Addicks K, Hescheler J (1998) Functional characteristics of ES cell-derived cardiac precursor cells identified by tissue-specific expression of the green fluorescent protein. J Cell Biol 143:2045–2056

Leobon B, Garcin I, Menasche P, Vilquin JT, Audinat E, Charpak S (2003) Myoblasts transplanted into rat infarcted myocardium are functionally isolated from their host. Proc Natl Acad Sci U S A 100:7808–7811

Maltsev VA, Rohwedel J, Hescheler J, Wobus AM (1993) Embryonic stem cells differentiate in vitro into cardiomyocytes representing sinusnodal, atrial and ventricular cell types. Mech Dev 44:41–50

Mangi AA, Noiseux N, Kong D, He H, Rezvani M, Ingwall JS, Dzau VJ (2003) Mesenchymal stem cells modified with Akt prevent remodeling and restore performance of infarcted hearts. Nat Med 9:1195–1201

Martin CM, Meeson AP, Robertson SM, Hawke TJ, Richardson JA, Bates S, Goetsch SC, Gallardo TD, Garry DJ (2004) Persistent expression of the ATP-binding cassette transporter, Abcg2, identifies cardiac SP cells in the developing and adult heart. Dev Biol 265:262–275

Menasche P, Hagege AA, Vilquin JT, Desnos M, Abergel E, Pouzet B, Bel A, Sarateanu S, Scorsin M, Schwartz K, Bruneval P, Benbunan M, Marolleau JP, Duboc D (2003) Autologous skeletal myoblast transplantation for severe postinfarction left ventricular dysfunction. J Am Coll Cardiol 41:1078–1083

Messina E, De Angelis L, Frati G, Morrone S, Chimenti S, Fiordaliso F, Salio M, Battaglia M, Latronico MV, Coletta M, Vivarelli E, Frati L, Cossu G, Giacomello A (2004) Isolation and expansion of adult cardiac stem cells from human and murine heart. Circ Res 95:911–921

Miller-Hance WC, LaCorbiere M, Fuller SJ, Evans SM, Lyons G, Schmidt C, Robbins J, Chien KR (1993) In vitro chamber specification during embryonic stem cell cardiogenesis. Expression of the ventricular myosin light chain-2 gene is independent of heart tube formation. J Biol Chem 268:25244–25252

Min JY, Yang Y, Converso KL, Liu L, Huang Q, Morgan JP, Xiao YF (2002) Transplantation of embryonic stem cells improves cardiac function in postinfarcted rats. J Appl Physiol 92:288–296

Morali OG, Jouneau A, McLaughlin KJ, Thiery JP, Larue L (2000) IGF-II promotes mesoderm formation. Dev Biol 227:133–145

Muller-Ehmsen J, Peterson KL, Kedes L, Whittaker P, Dow JS, Long TI, Laird PW, Kloner RA (2002) Rebuilding a damaged heart: long-term survival of transplanted neonatal rat cardiomyocytes after myocardial infarction and effect on cardiac function. Circulation 105:1720–1726

Mummery C, Ward D, van den Brink CE, Bird SD, Doevendans PA, Opthof T, Brutel de la Riviere A, Tertoolen L, van der Heyden M, Pera M (2002) Cardiomyocyte differentiation of mouse and human embryonic stem cells. J Anat 200:233–242

Mummery C, Ward-van Oostwaard D, Doevendans P, Spijker R, van den Brink S, Hassink R, van der Heyden M, Opthof T, Pera M, de la Riviere AB, Passier R, Tertoolen L (2003) Differentiation of human embryonic stem cells to cardiomyocytes: role of coculture with visceral endoderm-like cells. Circulation 107:2733–2740

Murry CE, Wiseman RW, Schwartz SM, Hauschka SD (1996) Skeletal myoblast transplantation for repair of myocardial necrosis. J Clin Invest 98:2512–2523

Murry CE, Soonpaa MH, Reinecke H, Nakajima H, Nakajima HO, Rubart M, Pasumarthi KB, Virag JI, Bartelmez SH, Poppa V, Bradford G, Dowell JD, Williams DA, Field LJ (2004) Haematopoietic stem cells do not transdifferentiate into cardiac myocytes in myocardial infarcts. Nature 428:664–668

Naito H, Nishizaki K, Yoshikawa M, Yamada T, Satoh H, Nagasaka S, Kiji T, Taniguchi S (2004) Xenogeneic embryonic stem cell-derived cardiomyocyte transplantation. Transplant Proc 36:2507–2508

Nakajima H, Nakajima HO, Tsai SC, Field LJ (2004) Expression of mutant p193 and p53 permits cardiomyocyte cell cycle reentry after myocardial infarction in transgenic mice. Circ Res 94:1606–1614

Nygren JM, Jovinge S, Breitbach M, Sawen P, Roll W, Hescheler J, Taneera J, Fleischmann BK, Jacobsen SE (2004) Bone marrow-derived hematopoietic cells generate cardiomyocytes at a low frequency through cell fusion, but not transdifferentiation. Nat Med 10:494–501

Odorico JS, Kaufman DS, Thomson JA (2001) Multilineage differentiation from human embryonic stem cell lines. Stem Cells 19:193–204

Oh H, Bradfute SB, Gallardo TD, Nakamura T, Gaussin V, Mishina Y, Pocius J, Michael LH, Behringer RR, Garry DJ, Entman ML, Schneider MD (2003) Cardiac progenitor cells from adult myocardium: homing, differentiation, and fusion after infarction. Proc Natl Acad Sci U S A 100:12313–12318

Orlic D, Kajstura J, Chimenti S, Bodine DM, Leri A, Anversa P (2001a) Transplanted adult bone marrow cells repair myocardial infarcts in mice. Ann N Y Acad Sci 938:221–229; discussion 229–230

Orlic D, Kajstura J, Chimenti S, Limana F, Jakoniuk I, Quaini F, Nadal-Ginard B, Bodine DM, Leri A, Anversa P (2001b) Mobilized bone marrow cells repair the infarcted heart, improving function and survival. Proc Natl Acad Sci U S A 98:10344–10349

Pagani FD, DerSimonian H, Zawadzka A, Wetzel K, Edge AS, Jacoby DB, Dinsmore JH, Wright S, Aretz TH, Eisen HJ, Aaronson KD (2003) Autologous skeletal myoblasts transplanted to ischemia-damaged myocardium in humans. Histological analysis of cell survival and differentiation. J Am Coll Cardiol 41:879–888

Pandur P, Lasche M, Eisenberg LM, Kuhl M (2002) Wnt-11 activation of a non-canonical Wnt signalling pathway is required for cardiogenesis. Nature 418:636–641

Paquin J, Danalache BA, Jankowski M, McCann SM, Gutkowska J (2002) Oxytocin induces differentiation of P19 embryonic stem cells to cardiomyocytes. Proc Natl Acad Sci U S A 99:9550–9555

Parisi S, D'Andrea D, Lago CT, Adamson ED, Persico MG, Minchiotti G (2003) Nodal-dependent Cripto signaling promotes cardiomyogenesis and redirects the neural fate of embryonic stem cells. J Cell Biol 163:303–314

Pasumarthi KB, Field LJ (2002) Cardiomyocyte cell cycle regulation. Circ Res 90:1044–1054

Pasumarthi KB, Nakajima H, Nakajima HO, Soonpaa MH, Field LJ (2005) Targeted expression of cyclin D2 results in cardiomyocyte DNA synthesis and infarct regression in transgenic mice. Circ Res 96:110–118

Perin EC, Dohmann HF, Borojevic R, Silva SA, Sousa AL, Mesquita CT, Rossi MI, Carvalho AC, Dutra HS, Dohmann HJ, Silva GV, Belem L, Vivacqua R, Rangel FO, Esporcatte R, Geng YJ, Vaughn WK, Assad JA, Mesquita ET, Willerson JT (2003) Transendocardial, autologous bone marrow cell transplantation for severe, chronic ischemic heart failure. Circulation 107:2294–2302

Puceat M, Travo P, Quinn MT, Fort P (2003) A dual role of the GTPase Rac in cardiac differentiation of stem cells. Mol Biol Cell 14:2781–2792

Reinecke H, Minami E, Poppa V, Murry CE (2004) Evidence for fusion between cardiac and skeletal muscle cells. Circ Res 94:e56–e60

Reinlib L, Field L (2000) Cell transplantation as future therapy for cardiovascular disease?: A workshop of the National Heart, Lung, and Blood Institute. Circulation 101:E182–E187

Roell W, Lu ZJ, Bloch W, Siedner S, Tiemann K, Xia Y, Stoecker E, Fleischmann M, Bohlen H, Stehle R, Kolossov E, Brem G, Addicks K, Pfitzer G, Welz A, Hescheler J, Fleischmann BK (2002) Cellular cardiomyoplasty improves survival after myocardial injury. Circulation 105:2435–2441

Rubart M, Pasumarthi KB, Nakajima H, Soonpaa MH, Nakajima HO, Field LJ (2003a) Physiological coupling of donor and host cardiomyocytes after cellular transplantation. Circ Res 92:1217–1224

Rubart M, Wang E, Dunn KW, Field LJ (2003b) Two-photon molecular excitation imaging of Ca^{2+} transients in Langendorff-perfused mouse hearts. Am J Physiol Cell Physiol 284:C1654–C1668

Rubart M, Soonpaa MH, Nakajima H, Field LJ (2004) Spontaneous and evoked intracellular calcium transients in donor-derived myocytes following intracardiac myoblast transplantation. J Clin Invest 114:775–783

Rudnicki MA, Jackowski G, Saggin L, McBurney MW (1990) Actin and myosin expression during development of cardiac muscle from cultured embryonal carcinoma cells. Dev Biol 138:348–358

Rudy-Reil D, Lough J (2004) Avian precardiac endoderm/mesoderm induces cardiac myocyte differentiation in murine embryonic stem cells. Circ Res 94:e107–e116

Rumiantsev PP (1991) Growth and hyperplasia of cardiac muscle cells. Harwood Academic, London

Sachinidis A, Gissel C, Nierhoff D, Hippler-Altenburg R, Sauer H, Wartenberg M, Hescheler J (2003) Identification of plateled-derived growth factor-BB as cardiogenesis-inducing factor in mouse embryonic stem cells under serum-free conditions. Cell Physiol Biochem 13:423–429

Satin J, Kehat I, Caspi O, Huber I, Arbel G, Itzhaki I, Magyar J, Schroder EA, Perlman I, Gepstein L (2004) Mechanism of spontaneous excitability in human embryonic stem cell derived cardiomyocytes. J Physiol 559:479–496

Sauer H, Rahimi G, Hescheler J, Wartenberg M (2000) Role of reactive oxygen species and phosphatidylinositol 3-kinase in cardiomyocyte differentiation of embryonic stem cells. FEBS Lett 476:218–223

Sauer H, Neukirchen W, Rahimi G, Grunheck F, Hescheler J, Wartenberg M (2004) Involvement of reactive oxygen species in cardiotrophin-1-induced proliferation of cardiomyocytes differentiated from murine embryonic stem cells. Exp Cell Res 294:313–324

Schmidt MM, Guan K, Wobus AM (2001) Lithium influences differentiation and tissue-specific gene expression of mouse embryonic stem (ES) cells in vitro. Int J Dev Biol 45:421–429

Schroeder M, Niebruegge S, Werner A, Willbold E, Burg M, Ruediger M, Field LJ, Lehmann J, Zweigerdt R, Embryonic Stem Cell Differentiation and Lineage Selection in a Stirred Bench Scale Bioreactor with Automated Process Control. Biotechnol and Bioengin, in press

Smits PC, van Geuns RJ, Poldermans D, Bountioukos M, Onderwater EE, Lee CH, Maat AP, Serruys PW (2003) Catheter-based intramyocardial injection of autologous skeletal myoblasts as a primary treatment of ischemic heart failure: clinical experience with six-month follow-up. J Am Coll Cardiol 42:2063–2069

Snir M, Kehat I, Gepstein A, Coleman R, Itskovitz-Eldor J, Livne E, Gepstein L (2003) Assessment of the ultrastructural and proliferative properties of human embryonic stem cell-derived cardiomyocytes. Am J Physiol Heart Circ Physiol 285:H2355–H2363

Soonpaa MH, Field LJ (1994) Assessment of cardiomyocyte DNA synthesis during hypertrophy in adult mice. Am J Physiol 266:H1439–H1445

Soonpaa MH, Field LJ (1998) Survey of studies examining mammalian cardiomyocyte DNA synthesis. Circ Res 83:15–26

Soonpaa MH, Koh GY, Klug MG, Field LJ (1994) Formation of nascent intercalated disks between grafted fetal cardiomyocytes and host myocardium. Science 264:98–101

Steinhelper ME, Lanson NA Jr, Dresdner KP, Delcarpio JB, Wit AL, Claycomb WC, Field LJ (1990) Proliferation in vivo and in culture of differentiated adult atrial cardiomyocytes from transgenic mice. Am J Physiol 259:H1826–H1834

Sudou A, Muramatsu H, Kaname T, Kadomatsu K, Muramatsu T (1997) Le(X) structure enhances myocardial differentiation from embryonic stem cells. Cell Struct Funct 22:247–251

Takahashi T, Lord B, Schulze PC, Fryer RM, Sarang SS, Gullans SR, Lee RT (2003) Ascorbic acid enhances differentiation of embryonic stem cells into cardiac myocytes. Circulation 107:1912–1916

Taylor DA, Atkins BZ, Hungspreugs P, Jones TR, Reedy MC, Hutcheson KA, Glower DD, Kraus WE (1998) Regenerating functional myocardium: improved performance after skeletal myoblast transplantation. Nat Med 4:929–933

Terami H, Hidaka K, Katsumata T, Iio A, Morisaki T (2004) Wnt11 facilitates embryonic stem cell differentiation to Nkx2.5-positive cardiomyocytes. Biochem Biophys Res Commun 325:968–975

Thomson JA, Itskovitz-Eldor J, Shapiro SS, Waknitz MA, Swiergiel JJ, Marshall VS, Jones JM (1998) Embryonic stem cell lines derived from human blastocysts. Science 282:1145–1147

Ventura C, Maioli M (2000) Opioid peptide gene expression primes cardiogenesis in embryonal pluripotent stem cells. Circ Res 87:189–194

Ventura C, Zinellu E, Maninchedda E, Fadda M, Maioli M (2003) Protein kinase C signaling transduces endorphin-primed cardiogenesis in GTR1 embryonic stem cells. Circ Res 92:617–622

Ventura C, Maioli M, Asara Y, Santoni D, Scarlata I, Cantoni S, Perbellini A (2004) Butyric and retinoic mixed ester of hyaluronan. A novel differentiating glycoconjugate affording a high throughput of cardiogenesis in embryonic stem cells. J Biol Chem 279:23574–23579

Wang JF, Yang Y, Wang G, Min J, Sullivan MF, Ping P, Xiao YF, Morgan JP (2002) Embryonic stem cells attenuate viral myocarditis in murine model. Cell Transplant 11:753–758

Winnier G, Blessing M, Labosky PA, Hogan BL (1995) Bone morphogenetic protein-4 is required for mesoderm formation and patterning in the mouse. Genes Dev 9:2105–2116

Wobus AM, Kaomei G, Shan J, Wellner MC, Rohwedel J, Ji G, Fleischmann B, Katus HA, Hescheler J, Franz WM (1997) Retinoic acid accelerates embryonic stem cell-derived cardiac differentiation and enhances development of ventricular cardiomyocytes. J Mol Cell Cardiol 29:1525–1539

Wollert KC, Meyer GP, Lotz J, Ringes-Lichtenberg S, Lippolt P, Breidenbach C, Fichtner S, Korte T, Hornig B, Messinger D, Arseniev L, Hertenstein B, Ganser A, Drexler H (2004) Intracoronary autologous bone-marrow cell transfer after myocardial infarction: the BOOST randomised controlled clinical trial. Lancet 364:141–148

Wu X, Ding S, Ding Q, Gray NS, Schultz PG (2004) Small molecules that induce cardiomyogenesis in embryonic stem cells. J Am Chem Soc 126:1590–1591

Xu C, Police S, Rao N, Carpenter MK (2002) Characterization and enrichment of cardiomyocytes derived from human embryonic stem cells. Circ Res 91:501–508

Xue T, Cho HC, Akar FG, Tsang SY, Jones SP, Marban E, Tomaselli GF, Li RA (2005) Functional integration of electrically active cardiac derivatives from genetically engineered human embryonic stem cells with quiescent recipient ventricular cardiomyocytes: insights into the development of cell-based pacemakers. Circulation 111:11–20

Yang Y, Min JY, Rana JS, Ke Q, Cai J, Chen Y, Morgan JP, Xiao YF (2002) VEGF enhances functional improvement of postinfarcted hearts by transplantation of ESC-differentiated cells. J Appl Physiol 93:1140–1151

Yao M, Dieterle T, Hale SL, Dow JS, Kedes LH, Peterson KL, Kloner RA (2003) Long-term outcome of fetal cell transplantation on postinfarction ventricular remodeling and function. J Mol Cell Cardiol 35:661–670

Zandstra PW, Bauwens C, Yin T, Liu Q, Schiller H, Zweigerdt R, Pasumarthi KB, Field LJ (2003) Scalable production of embryonic stem cell-derived cardiomyocytes. Tissue Eng 9:767–778

Zhang M, Methot D, Poppa V, Fujio Y, Walsh K, Murry CE (2001) Cardiomyocyte grafting for cardiac repair: graft cell death and anti-death strategies. J Mol Cell Cardiol 33:907–921

Zimmermann WH, Schneiderbanger K, Schubert P, Didie M, Munzel F, Heubach JF, Kostin S, Neuhuber WL, Eschenhagen T (2002) Tissue engineering of a differentiated cardiac muscle construct. Circ Res 90:223–230

Zweigerdt R, Burg M, Willbold E, Abts H, Ruediger M (2003a) Generation of confluent cardiomyocyte monolayers derived from embryonic stem cells in suspension: a cell source for new therapies and screening strategies. Cytotherapy 5:399–413

Zweigerdt R, Schroeder M, Werner A, Lehmann J, Zandstra PW, Field LJ, Abts H, Ruediger M, Burg M (2003b) Clinical scale generation of enriched embryonic stem cell derived cardiomyocytes (abstract 3083). In: Keystone Symposia: From Stem Cells to Therapy, Steamboat Springs, CO, pp 136

HEP (2006) 174:101–122

Cardiomyocytes from Human Embryonic Stem Cells

R. Passier[1] · C. Denning[2] · C. Mummery[1] (✉)

[1]Hubrecht Laboratory and Interuniversity Cardiology Institute of the Netherlands,
Uppsalalaan 8, 3584 CT Utrecht, The Netherlands
christin@niob.knaw.nl

[2]Institute of Genetics, University of Nottingham, Queens Medical Centre, Nottingham UK

Abstract Terminal heart failure is characterized by a significant loss of cardiac myocytes. Stem cells represent a possibility for replacing these lost myocytes but the question of which stem cells are most ideally suited for cell transplantation therapies is still being addressed. Here, we consider human embryonic stem cells (HESC), derived from human embryos in this context. We review the methods used to induce their differentiation to cardiomyocytes in culture, their properties in relation to primary human cardiomyocytes and their ability to integrate into host myocardium. In addition, issues regarding their safety that need addressing before use in cell transplantation therapies, both generally and specifically in relation to the heart, are considered.

Keywords Embryonic stem cells · Cardiomyocyte · Human · Mouse · Differentiation · Human embryonic stem cells · Heart development · Cell therapy

1
Introduction

Human embryonic stem cells (HESCs) are diploid-cultured cell lines derived from the inner cell mass of blastocyst-stage embryos surplus to requirements for assisted reproduction. They can be grown indefinitely in an undifferentiated state yet are also capable of differentiating to all somatic cell types of the adult body as well as extraembryonic tissue. Among the specialist cell types that can form in culture, cardiomyocytes are particularly striking, forming rhythmically contracting structures containing cells highly reminiscent of normal human heart cells (reviewed by Passier and Mummery 2003). Progressive heart failure that is secondary to ventricular remodeling after myocardial infarction is a major medical problem worldwide (Caplice and Gersh 2003). Since there is a shortage of donor hearts for transplantation, it is becoming a matter of urgency to consider alternative therapies such as cardiac cell replacement. This would involve transplantation of appropriate heart cells to the infarcted area of the myocardium, which would augment contractile function by replacing those cardiomyocytes lost as a result of injury. HESC-derived cardiomyocytes are candidates for application in cardiac cell therapy as they represent a renewable source of multiple heart cell types that could in principle be produced in large numbers as required. However, aside from ethical issues associated with their origin in human embryos, there are a number of scientific issues that will need to be addressed before they would be suitable even for clinical trials. These include evidence of their ability to improve long-term cardiac function in animals that have undergone cardiac injury, semi-industrial upscale to cell numbers that would be sufficient for treating a human heart, and issues of safety, both in terms of the potential of transplanted cells to cause arrhythmias in the host heart and for any residual stem cells to give rise to tumours. Solutions to some of these problems might be found in a deeper understanding of the molecular control of cardiomyocyte differentiation as it takes place in the developing embryo. In this review we first consider aspects of early embryonic development relevant to heart cell formation by stem cells and then review the present state of knowledge on HESC-derived cardiomyocytes. Finally, we consider how current obstacles to clinical application might be addressed.

2
Development of the Mammalian Heart

2.1
Differentiation and Early Morphogenesis

Heart formation is initiated in vertebrate embryos soon after gastrulation when the three embryonic germ layers, ectoderm, endoderm and mesoderm, are established in the primitive streak. The heart is derived from the mesoderm and is the first definitive organ to form in development. Its morphogenesis, growth and integrated function are essential for survival of the embryo even by mid-gestation. Cardiac progenitor cells are for the most part localized in the anterior primitive streak. Different populations of precursor cells are distributed within the streak (in relation to the organizing center, or node) in the same anterior–posterior order that they are later found in the tubular heart (Garcia-Martinez and Schoenwolf 1993). As a result, cells furthest from the node end up in the atrium; those nearer the node end up in the ventricle, whilst those nearest the node later form the outflow tract. In addition to precursors in the primitive streak, there are also precursors bilaterally distributed in the epiblast directly adjacent to the streak. As development proceeds, the precursor population of precardiac mesoderm emigrates from the streak in an anterolateral direction, giving rise to the heart-forming fields on either side of the streak. These heart fields then harbour not only progenitors of the atrial, ventricular and outflow tract lineages, but also endocardial progenitor cells. The axial distribution is maintained as the fields migrate to fuse and form the cardiac crescent. Cells of the cardiac crescent then adopt a definitive cardiac fate in response to cues from adjacent anterior endoderm (Olson and Schneider 2003). Anterior endoderm in particular appears to have an instructive function in cardiogenesis in various species (reviewed in Brand 2003). Ablation of anterior endoderm in amphibians results in loss of myocardial specification (Nascone and Mercola 1995), whilst explants of posterior, blood-forming mesoderm in chick are reprogrammed to express cardiac instead of blood-restricted marker genes if combined with anterior endoderm (Schultheiss et al. 1995). After cardiac mesoderm has been specified, it is then directed towards the midline where the heart fields fuse and form a single heart tube. In mutant mouse and zebrafish in which this fails to take place, two tube-like structures form (cardiac bifida), which both acquire contractile activity (Molkentin et al. 1997; Roebroek et al. 1998; Saga et al. 1999; Reiter et al. 1999). These mutants include several that lack endodermal tissue. Thus, the endoderm is not only important for differentiation of cardiac precursors but is also essential for cardiac mesoderm migration, although it is clear that tube formation also involves a cell autonomous function of cardiac mesoderm itself.

Once this process of primary cardiac induction is complete, cells are then recruited from lateral plate mesoderm, medial to the primary heart field, to give rise to the secondary, anterior heart field (AHF). The cells recruited contribute to the primitive right ventricle and the outflow tract (Kelly and Buckingham 2002). Whilst the heart tube is initially almost straight, the ventricular segment at this stage starts to bulge ventrally, flips to the right and begins to form a C-shaped heart. Left–right asymmetry thus becomes evident and cardiac looping morphogenesis has commenced. Through a series of "ballooning" steps and morphogenetic movements, the four-chambered heart eventually forms (Christoffels et al. 2000).

Understanding the molecular control of heart development in vertebrates can provide essential clues on which signal transduction pathways might direct differentiation of HESCs towards specific cardiac lineages. The sequential activation of the transcription factors that results in the formation of nascent then precardiac mesoderm, and eventually determines cardiac cell fate, is likely to be controlled in HESCs as in embryos in vivo. The signals may be known or novel, in either case emanating from the endoderm, node or acting cell autonomously in mesoderm. In the following section, some of the most relevant aspects of this molecular control are considered.

2.2
Molecular Control of Cardiac Development

Three families of peptide growth factors have been studied most intensely for their positive and negative effects on cardiogenesis. These are the bone morphogenetic proteins (BMPs), members of the transforming growth factor β superfamily, the wnts and the fibroblast growth factors (FGFs). Members of all of these families or their inhibitors are expressed in endoderm. Disrupted expression of these ligands, receptors or their downstream target genes has dramatic and distinct effects on cardiac development that are highly conserved between species (reviewed by Olson and Schneider 2003). In general, BMP signaling promotes cardiogenesis in vertebrates (Zaffran and Frasch 2002; Schneider et al. 2003; Schultheiss et al. 1997; Shi et al. 2000; Krishnan et al. 2001; Gaussin et al. 2002) and is also required to generate mesoderm/cardiac muscle cells from mouse teratocarcinoma stem cells and ES cells in culture (Gaussin et al. 2002; Johansson and Wiles 1995).

Wingless in *Drosophila* and related wnt proteins in vertebrates are involved in cardiac specification although their function is complex. Wnts were initially considered suppressive of heart formation, but both induction and inhibition have since been reported (Olson and Schneider 2003). Results have not yet been reconciled but may relate to distinct effects of the canonical (acting via β-catenin/GSK3 to repress cardiogenesis) vs noncanonical (acting via PKC/JNK to promote cardiogenesis) signalling pathways, and/or indirect effects in certain model systems (for example, induction, expansion or augmentation of BMP-producing endoderm-like cells). Finally, limited studies in chick and zebrafish have implicated a cardioinductive role for FGFs (Lough et al. 1996; Barron et al. 2000; Alsan and Schultheiss 2002), although in *Drosophila*, FGFs appear to provide positional cues to cells for specification. It is of interest that BMP2 is able to upregulate FGF8 ectopically and that BMP2 and FGF8 probably synergize to drive mesodermal cells into myocardial differentiation. These three signaling pathways are essential not only for primary cardiogenesis but are also involved in secondary (AHF) cardiogenesis (Brand 2003).

Once anterior mesoderm cells have received appropriate signals, such as those described above, they switch on a set of cardiac-restricted transcription factors that interact in combination to control downstream genes in the cardiac pathway. The homeodomain transcription factor Nkx2.5 (Lints et al. 1993) and the T-box protein Tbx5 (Bruneau et al. 1999; Horb and Thomsen 1999) are among the earliest markers of the cardiac lineage and are activated shortly after cells have formed the heart fields. Nkx2.5 is thought to be required in mice specifically for left ventricular chamber development (Yamagishi et al. 2001), whilst loss of Tbx5 results in severe hypoplasia of both the atrial and left ventricular compartments (Bruneau et al. 2001) and may thus be important for the formation of both. Nkx2.5 and Tbx 5 associate with members of the GATA family of zinc finger transcription factors and with serum response factor (SRF) to activate cardiac structural genes, such as actin, myosin light chain (MLC), myosin heavy chain (MHC), troponins and desmin. Tbx5 can also cooperate with Nkx2.5 to activate expression of ANF and the junctional protein connexin 40 (Bruneau et al. 2001; Habets et al. 2002). Members of the myocyte enhancer factor 2 (MEF2) family of transcription factors also play key roles in cardiomyocyte differentiation by switching on cardiac muscle structural genes. In addition, association of SRF with a nuclear protein myocardin, activates cardiac-specific promoters (Wang et al. 2001). HOP, a cardiac homeodomain protein, which affects cardiomyocyte proliferation and differentiation (Shin et al. 2002), also associates with SRF and inhibits myocardin transcriptional activity (Wang et al. 2002). Thus multiple complex interactions take place between various transcription factors to control initial differentiation and maturation of cardiomyocytes. Apart from their functional role, many of these factors serve as excellent markers of cardiomyocytes in differentiating cultures of HESC and mES (see Table 1) and can be useful in identifying the degree of maturity of specific cardiac cells and the kinetics with which differentiation is taking place because their normal expression is under tight temporal control. A recent addition to this list is Isl1, a LIM homeodomain transcription factor, which identifies a cardiac progenitor population that proliferates prior to differentiation and contributes the majority of cells to the heart (Cai et al. 2003). Unlike skeletal muscle cells, where differentiation and proliferation are mutually exclusive, embryonic cardiac myocytes differentiate and assemble sarcomeres even while they proliferate, although organization is much greater postnatally. The prospect of using Isl1 as a marker for the undifferentiated cardiac progenitor state is exciting and cell sorting of differentiating HESCs on the basis of Isl1 expression could allow further characterization and expansion in culture. This could provide a very useful contribution to upscaling cardiomyocyte production for transplantation.

Table 1 Markers for hES-CM characterization

Marker	HESC line(s)	Method(s) of detection	Expression in HESC-CM	References
Transcription factors				
NK2 transcription factor-related locus 5 (Nkx2.5)	H1, H7, H9, H9.1, H9.2	RT-PCR	+	Kehat et al. 2001; Xu et al. 2002
GATA4	H1, H7, H9, H9.1, H9.2	RT-PCR, IF, W	+	Kehat et al. 2001; Xu et al. 2002
Myocyte enhancer factor 2 (Mef-2)	H1, H7, H9, H9.1, H9.2	IF	+	Xu et al. 2002
Structural elements				
Cardiac troponin I (cTnI)	H1, H7, H9, H14, H9.1, H9.2	IF, W, RT-PCR	+	Xu et al. 2002; Snir et al. 2003; He et al. 2003; Kehat et al. 2001
Cardiac troponin T (cTnT)	H1, H7, H9, H9.1, H9.2	RT-PCR, IF	+	Kehat et al. 2001; Xu et al. 2002
α-myosin heavy chain (α-MHC)	H1, H7, H9, H9.1, H9.2	RT-PCR, IF	+	Kehat et al. 2001; Xu et al. 2002
β-myosin heavy chain (β-MHC)	H1, H7, H9, H9.1, H9.2	IF	+	Xu et al. 2002
Sarcomeric myosin heavy chain (sMHC)	H1, H7, H9, H9.1, H9.2, H14	IF	+	He et al. 2003; Xu et al. 2002
Myosin light chain 2a (MLC-2a)	H9.2, HES-2	RT-PCR, IF	+	Kehat et al. 2001; Mummery et al. 2003
Myosin light chain 2v (MLC-2v)	H9.2, HES-2	RT-PCR, IF	+	Kehat et al. 2001; Mummery et al. 2003
α-actinin	H1, H7, H9, H9.1, H9.2H14, HES-2	RT-PCR, IF	+	He et al. 2003; Mummery et al. 2003; Kehat et al. 2001; Xu et al. 2002
Tropomyosin	H1, H7, H9, H9.1, H9.2, HES-2	IF	+	Mummery et al. 2003; Xu et al. 2002

Table 1 (continued)

Marker	HESC line(s)	Method(s) of detection	Expression in HESC-CM	References
Desmin	H1, H7, H9, H9.1, H9.2	IF	+	Kehat et al. 2001; Xu et al. 2002
Smooth muscle actin (SMA)	H1, H7, H9, H9.1, H9.2	IF	+	Xu et al. 2002
Receptors & regulatory elements				
Atrial natriuretic factor (ANF)	H1, H7, H9, H9.1, H9.2, HES-2	RT-PCR, IF	+	Kehat et al. 2001; Mummery et al. 2003; Xu et al. 2002
Phospholamban (PLN)	HES-2	RT-PCR	+	Mummery et al. 2003
Ryanodine receptor (RyR)	HES-2	IF	+	Mummery et al. 2003
Creatine kinase-MB (CK-MB)	H1, H7, H9, H9.1, H9.2	IF	+	Xu et al. 2002
Myoglobin	H1, H7, H9, H9.1, H9.2	IF	+	Xu et al. 2002
α1-Adrenoceptors	H1, H7, H9, H9.1, H9.2, HES-2	IF, phenylephrine (ph.)	+	Xu et al. 2002; Mummery et al. 2003; Kehat et al. 2001; He et al. 2003
β1-Adrenoceptors	H1, H7, H9, H9.1, H9.2, HES-2	IF, isoprenaline (ph.)	+	Xu et al. 2002; Mummery et al. 2003; Kehat et al. 2001
β2-Adrenoceptors	H1, H7, H9, H9.1, H9.2	IF, clenbuterol (ph.)	+	Xu et al. 2002
Muscarinic receptors	HES-2	Carbachol (ph.)	+	Mummery et al. 2003
Phosphodiesterase	H1, H7, H9, H9.1, H9.2	IBMX (ph.)	+	Xu et al. 2002; Kehat et al. 2001
Adenylate cyclase	H9.2	Forskolin (ph.)	+	Kehat et al. 2001
Ki67 (cell division)	H1, H7, H9, H9.1, H9.2	IF	+	Xu et al. 2002; Snir et al. 2003

Table 1 (continued)

Marker	HESC line(s)	Method(s) of detection	Expression in HESC-CM	References
Gap junction and adhesion proteins				
Connexin 43	H9.2, HES-2	IF	+	Kehat et al. 2002; Mummery et al. 2003
Connexin 45	H9.2	IF	+	Kehat et al. 2002
Connexin 40	H9.2	IF	+	Kehat et al. 2002
N-cadherin	H1, H7, H9, H9.1, H9.2	IF	+	Xu et al. 2002
Ion channels				
L-type Ca^{2+} channel; I_{Ca-L} ($\alpha 1c$)	H1, H7, H9, H9.1, H9.2, HES-2	RT-PCR, IF, diltiazem (ph.)	+	Mummery et al. 2003; Xu et al. 2002
Transient outward K^+ channel I_{TO} (*Kv4.3*)	HES-2	RT-PCR	+	Mummery et al. 2003
Slow delayed rectifier K^+ channel I_{Ks} (*KvLQT1*)	HES-2	RT-PCR	+	Mummery et al. 2003
Slow delayed rectifier K^+ channel I_{Kr} (*HERG*)	H9, H14	E4031 (ph.)	+	He et al. 2003
Noncardiac proteins				
Myogenin (skeletal muscle)	H1, H7, H9, H9.1, H9.	IF	–	Xu et al. 2002
Nebulin (skeletal)	H9.2	IF	–	Kehat et al. 2001
α-Fetal protein (AFP; endodermal)	H1, H7, H9, H9.1, H9.2	IF	–	Xu et al. 2002
β-Tubulin III (neuronal)	H1, H7, H9, H9.1, H9.2	IF	–	Xu et al. 2002

Methods of detection are RT-PCR, reverse transcriptase-polymerase chain reaction; IF, immunofluorescence; W, Western blot analysis; pharmacological agents are given as agent name (ph.)

3
Cardiomyocytes from Embryonic Stem Cells

3.1
In Vitro Differentiation of Mouse Embryonic Stem Cells to Cardiomyocytes

Pluripotent mouse embryonal carcinoma (EC) stem cells derived from tera-tocarcinomas and mouse embryonic stem (mES) cells derived from mouse blastocysts (Martin 1981; Evans and Kaufman 1981) retain the capacity to form derivatives of the three germ layers in culture. In vitro differentiation usually requires an initial aggregation to form structures termed embryoid bodies (EBs). After a few days of culture under appropriate conditions of cell density, culture medium and serum supplement, cardiomyocytes form between an outer epithelial layer of the EB with characteristics of visceral endoderm and basal mesenchymal cells become readily identifiable by spontaneous contraction (review by Boheler et al. 2002; for a general review of lineage determination in mES, see Loebel et al. 2003). Differentiation may be enhanced by culture supplements such as DMSO or retinoic acid or co-culture with endoderm-like cells (Mummery et al. 2002; Rathjen et al. 1999; Rathjen and Rathjen 2001). Wnt11, which activates the noncanonical wnt pathway, induced GATA4 and Nkx2.5 expression in P19 EC cells (Pandur et al. 2002) and repressed the canonical pathway although wnt-3a, acting through the canonical pathway, promoted cardiomyogenesis in a P19 subclone (Nakamura et al. 2003). The effects of wnt signalling on cardiomyogenesis of mES have not been described. Cardiomyocyte differentiation in mEBs recapitulates the programmed expression of cardiac genes observed in the mouse embryo in vivo both in the kinetics and the sequence in which genes are upregulated. GATA-4 and Nkx2.5 transcripts appear before mRNAs encoding ANF, MLC-2v, α-MHC and β-MHC. Sarcomeric proteins are also established in a manner similar to that seen in normal myocardial development. The electrical properties and phenotype of cardiomyocytes derived from mouse EB cultures have been examined in some detail (reviewed by Boheler et al. 2002). The rate of contraction decreases with differentiation and maturation in culture, as in normal mouse development, and their differentiation as such can be divided into three developmental stages: early (pacemaker-like or primary myocardial-like cells) intermediate, and terminal (atrial-, ventricular-, nodal-, His-, and Purkinje-like cells) (Hescheler et al. 1997). In early stages, the nascent myofibrils are sparse and irregular but myofibrillar and sarcomeric organization increases with maturation. Functional gap junctions develop between cells and eventually their phenotype resembles that of neonatal rat myocytes. Likewise, the electrophysiological properties of mES cardiomyocytes (mES-CMs) develop, with differentiation in a manner reminiscent of their development in the mouse embryo (Boheler et al. 2002). Fully differentiated mES-CMs are responsive to β-adrenergic stimulation, whilst early mES-CMs are not (Maltsev et al. 1999).

They also exhibit many features of excitation–contraction coupling found in isolated fetal or neonatal cardiomyocytes.

Several of the features described above in combination with the amenability of mES to genetic manipulation have made it possible to develop strategies for genetic selection of cardiomyocytes from mixed populations of differentiating cells. In the absence of cell-surface antibodies recognizing cardiomyocytes or their precursors, this has been important for initiating studies to transplant pure cell populations of specific cardiac lineages to the adult mouse heart. The first study of this type was carried out using mES expressing a fusion gene composed of the α-MHC promoter and a neo^R cassette (Klug et al. 1996). After selection in G418, the percentage of cardiomyocytes increased from 3%–5% to almost 100%. Similar studies have been carried out using the MLC-2v or α-cardiac alpha-actin promoter coupled with either neo^R or GFP for selection (Meyer et al. 2000; Muller et al. 2000; Kolossov et al. 1998). Unfortunately in the adult heart after transplantation, survival of mES-CM is poor ($\sim$5% survival) and many undergo apoptosis (Klug et al. 1996), a potential problem to be addressed before cell transplantation therapy is likely to be effective. In addition, an estimated 10^8–10^9 cells lost during myocardial infarction would be required per patient for effective therapy. A useful step towards upscaling was recently made when 10^9 mES-CM were produced by genetic selection in combination with a cardiac-specific promoter on EBs grown in a bioreactor (Zandstra et al. 2003).

3.2
In Vitro Differentiation of Human Embryonic Stem Cells to Cardiomyocytes

Several groups have shown the differentiation from HESCs to cardiomyocytes (Table 1). The first report of cardiomyocytes from HESCs (Kehat et al. 2001) appeared almost 3 years after HESCs were first derived (Thomson et al. 1998). To induce cardiomyocyte differentiation, HESCs (cell line H9.2) were dispersed using collagenase IV into small clumps (3–20 cells) and grown for 7–10 days in suspension to form EB-like structures like mES but without the distinct outer layer of endoderm cells. After plating these EBs onto gelatin-coated culture dishes, beating areas were first observed in the outgrowths 4 days after plating (i.e. 11–14 days after the start of the differentiation protocol). A maximum in the number of beating areas was observed 20 days after plating (27–30 days of differentiation), with 8.1% of 1884 EBs scored beating. This spontaneous differentiation to cardiomyocytes in aggregates was also observed by others using different cell lines e.g. H1, H7, H9, H9.1 and H9.2 (Xu et al. 2002). However, in this case approximately 70% of the embryoid bodies displayed beating areas after 20 days of differentiation. On day 8 of their differentiation protocol (growth in suspension followed by plating in culture dishes), 25% of the EBs were beating. A third group also demonstrated spontaneous derivation of cardiomyocytes from HESC lines H1, H7, H9 and H14 but in this case 10%–

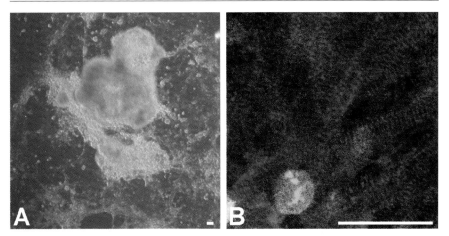

Fig. 1a HESC differentiating towards cardiomyocytes, co-cultured on END-2 cells (phase-contrast microscopy, ×5 magnification). **b** Dissociated beating areas of HESC-END-2 co-cultures stained for the cardiac-specific α-actinin (*red*) and a marker for proliferation Ki67 (*green*) (fluorescent microscopy, magnification ×63). Bar, 100 μm

25% of the embryoid bodies were beating after 30 days of differentiation (He et al. 2003). The reasons for these apparent differences in efficiency are not clear. In addition, counting beating EBs may not accurately reflect the conversion of HESCs to cardiomyocytes, since EBs may contain significantly different numbers of cardiac cells. Recently, the differentiation of two independent HESC lines BG01 and BG02 has been described (Zeng et al. 2004). Following dissociation of HESCs by collagenase IV into small clumps, cells were grown for 7 days as EBs and cultured on adherent plates for another 7 days. In this case, immunoreactivity was demonstrated for the cardiac marker cardiac troponin I (cTnI).

An alternative method for the derivation of cardiomyocytes from HESCs was described by Mummery et al. (2002, 2003). Beating areas were observed following co-culture of HESCs with a mouse visceral endoderm-like cell-line (END-2) (Fig. 1). As described above, endoderm plays an important role in the differentiation of cardiogenic precursor cells in the adjacent mesoderm in vivo. Earlier co-culture of END-2 cells with mouse P19 embryonal carcinoma (EC), a mouse embryonal carcinoma cell line with pluripotent differentiation properties, and ES cells already showed that beating areas appeared in aggregated cells (van den Eijnden-van Raaij et al. 1991). For the derivation of cardiomyocytes from HESCs, mitotically inactivated END-2 cells were seeded on a 12-well plate and co-cultured with the HESC line HES-2. This resulted in beating areas in approximately 35% of the wells after 12 days in co-culture (Mummery et al. 2003).

Whilst these methods appear to be effective, all produce cardiomyocytes at low efficiency and in insufficient numbers to treat adult human patients. In addition, it will be important to reduce the risk of teratoma formation from residual undifferentiated HESCs by developing sensitive assays for their detection prior to transplantation. Significant upscale will be required before HESC cardiomyocytes have any clinical applications. This could involve increasing the efficiency of cardiomyocyte differentiation, promoting proliferation of the emerging cardiomyocytes or developing methods of purificaton of the required cardiac cell type. Following manual dissection and dissociation of beating areas from HESCs, between 2% and 70% of the cells are positively stained for cardiac markers (He et al. 2003; Mummery et al. 2003). The only enrichment method described to date for HESC cardiomyocytes used discontinuous Percoll gradient purification (40.5% over 58.5%) (Xu et al. 2002). This resulted in approximately fourfold enrichment (70% positively stained for cardiac markers) in a particular cell fraction compared with the initial differentiated cell suspension. FACS analysis and sorting would be a useful approach to quantification and selection and a significant improvement on counting beating EBs or physical selection methods. The fact that it has not been widely used reflects the lack of specific cell-surface markers for cardiomyocytes. Genetically marked cardiac derivatives of HESCs that have been described in mice (Klug et al. 1996; Meyer et al. 2000; Muller et al. 2000) have not yet been described.

3.3
Improving Cardiomyocyte Differentiation from Human Embryonic Stem Cells

Although there are differences in the morphology, growth characteristics and molecular signalling pathways between mES and HESCs, studies on cardiomyocyte differentiation from mouse ES cells (reviewed in Boheler et al. 2002; Sachinidis et al. 2003a) may nevertheless help identify conserved properties including methods promoting the conversion of the stem cells to cardiomyocytes. In addition, P19 EC cells have also been useful in understanding cardiomyocyte differentiation (van der Heyden and Defize 2003). Using these cells and embryo explants in culture, it has been shown that a variety of well described proteins control cardiogenesis, just as described above in studies of mutant embryos. For example, both BMP-2 and BMP-4 can induce cardiac differentiation in chick explant studies from a tissue that normally does not give rise to cardiac tissue (Schultheiss et al. 1997). The importance of BMP-2 for cardiac differentiation has also been shown in mES (Behfar et al. 2002). Retinoic acid and DMSO are well known factors which are able to enhance or promote cardiac differentiation in mES or P19 EC cells (Wobus et al. 1997; McBurney et al. 1982; Ventura and Maioli 2000). Oxytocin, a nonapeptide originally recognized as a female reproductive hormone, has been recently found to increase cardiomyocyte differentiation in P19 EC cells (Paquin et al. 2002). Other factors that have been shown to play an important role in cardiac differentiation are members of TGFβ, FGF and Wnt families (reviewed in Boheler et al. 2002; Sachinidis et al. 2003a).

Several of these potential cardiogenic factors have been tested in HESCs. No significant improvement in cardiomyocyte differentiation has been achieved by adding DMSO and retinoic acid (Kehat et al. 2001; Xu et al. 2002) or BMP-2 (Mummery et al. 2003). It is not clear whether these factors do not play a role in cardiac differentiation of HESCs, or whether differentiation protocols were not optimal. Variations in concentration, timing and combinatorial effects of potential cardiogenic factors in HESC differentiation methods may have a crucial effect on the outcome of cardiomyocyte differentiation. The only factor at present that shows enhanced cardiomyocyte differentiation of HESCs is 5-aza-2'deoxycytidine, a demethylating agent, which has been shown to stimulate cardiomyocyte differentiation in human mesenchymal stem cells (Makino et al. 1999). Treatment of HESCs with 5-aza-2'deoxycytidine showed a time- and concentration-dependent effect on cardiomyocyte differentiation. Upregulation of the expression of cardiac α myosin heavy chain, as determined by real-time RT-PCR, was up to twofold higher (Xu et al. 2002).

The presence of fetal calf serum during differentiation may also have effects on differentiation efficiency. In all reports to date, serum has been present in the culture medium, whilst there is evidence that serum contains stimulatory as well as inhibitory factors for cardiomyocyte differentiation. For example, Sachinidis et al. (2003b) observed a 4.5-fold upregulation in the percentage of beating mEBs after changing to a serum-free differentiation medium. In addition, a 24-fold increase in the number of beating areas was observed when HESCs co-cultured with END-2 cells were differentiated in the absence of serum instead of 20% fetal calf serum (Passier et al. 2005).

In addition to improving differentiation efficiency, it is also important to identify factors that control maturation, proliferation and electrophysiology. These aspects will be discussed below.

4
Characteristics of Human Embryonic Stem Cell-Derived Cardiomyocytes

The previous sections have described the current methods to promote spontaneous and induced differentiation of HESCs towards the cardiac lineage. Although functional cardiomyocytes can easily be identified in vitro by their beating phenotype, only more detailed interrogation can establish the specific cardiac cell types generated, the degree of maturation they achieve compared to in vivo cardiac development and whether they possess fully functional excitation–contraction coupling machinery that responds appropriately to pharmacological agents. To realize the scientific and therapeutic potential of HESC-derived cardiomyocytes (HESC-CM), comprehensive characterization is therefore required.

4.1
Transcriptional Profile of Human Embryonic Stem Cell-Derived Cardiomyocytes

Differentiation of HESC to the cardiac lineage creates a gene expression profile (Table 1) reminiscent of both mouse ES cell differentiation and the early stages of normal mouse heart development (Fijnvandraat et al. 2003). Analysis of HESC-CM RNA and proteins has demonstrated the presence of cardiac transcription factors including GATA-4, myocyte enhancer factor (MEF-2) and Nkx2 transcription factor related locus 5 (Nkx2.5) (Kehat et al. 2001; Xu et al. 2002). Correspondingly, structural components of the myofibres are appropriately expressed. These include α-, β- and sarcomeric-myosin heavy chain (MHC), atrial and ventricular forms of myosin light chain (MLC-2a and −2v), tropomyosin, α-actinin and desmin. Furthermore, HESC-CMs fail to react with antibodies from noncardiac lineages (Table 1).

Antibody reactivity to two members of the troponin complex, cardiac troponin T (cTnT), which binds to tropomyosin, and cardiac troponin I (cTnI), which provides a calcium-sensitive molecular switch for the regulation of striated muscle contraction, has been demonstrated. cTnI appears to be truly cardiac-specific as antibodies to this protein only react with cells arising from beating and not nonbeating regions. In addition, upregulation of atrial natriuretic factor (ANF), a hormone that is actively expressed in both atrial and ventricular cardiomyocytes in the developing heart, has also been observed during cardiac differentiation of HESCs. Moreover, these cells express creatine kinase-MB (CK-MB) and myoglobin (Xu et al. 2002). CK-MB is found to be involved in high-energy phosphate transfer and facilitates diffusion of high-energy phosphate from the mitochondria to myofibril in myocytes. Myoglobin is a cytosolic oxygen binding protein responsible for the storage and diffusion of oxygen in myocytes. Thus many of the transcription factors, structural proteins and metabolic regulators of cardiac development are found within HESC-CM.

These cardiomyocytes do, however, react with antibodies to smooth muscle actin, a protein found in embryonic and fetal, but not adult cardiomyocytes, suggesting a limited degree of maturation (Xu et al. 2002). Adding weight to this notion, single HESC cardiomyocytes, rather than showing the more defined rod shape of mature cells, display numerous different morphologies, including spindle, round, tri- or multi-angular shapes. Sarcomeric immunostaining reveals sarcomeric striations organized in separated bundles, which parallels the pattern seen in human fetal cardiomyocytes and not the highly organized parallel bundles seen in human adult cardiomyocytes (Mummery et al. 2003).

Ultramicroscopical analysis does, however, demonstrate HESC-CM maturation during extended culture. While during the early stages of differentiation ($\sim$10–20 days) cardiomyocytes have a large nucleus to cytoplasm ratio with disoriented myofibrils lacking sarcoplasmic pattern distributed throughout the cytoplasm in a random fashion, both numbers and organization of myofibrils increased at later times ($\sim$20–50 days) (Snir et al. 2003). During this time, cells elongated and Z-line assembly from periodically aligned Z-bodies was observed. At late stages ($>$50 days) a high degree of sarcomeric organization was observed and discrete A (dark) and I (light) bands could be seen in some sarcomeres. Furthermore, HESC-CMs progressively withdraw from the cell cycle during culture. However, although this developmental pattern is reminiscent of mES cell differentiation to cardiomyocytes, maturation of HESC cardiomyocytes proceeds more slowly, is more heterogeneous, and does not reach the level of maturity, typical of adult cardiomyocytes. This was manifested, for example, by the lack of a developed T tubule system (Snir et al. 2003). Thus, it has been suggested that maturation may be aided by the addition of prohypertrophic factors such as cardiotrophin. Alternatively, subjecting the HESC cardiomyocytes to oscillating mechanical load (Mummery et al. 2003; Capsi and Gepstein 2004) or culturing them in three-dimensional matrices may stimulate maturation. Considering that cardiomyocytes in the infarcted heart regress to an embryonic phenotype, it will be interesting to see whether HESC-CMs with an embryonic or adult phenotype are more suited to functional and electrical integration following transplantation.

4.2
A Functional Conduction System: Excitation–Contraction Coupling Machinery

Cardiomyocytes from HESCs have a beat rate of $\sim$30–130 bpm and respond appropriately to pharmacological agents. Ligand binding to the adrenoceptors (ARs) generates a signaling cascade that results in elevated cAMP levels. This activates cAMP-dependent protein kinase (PKA), which then phosphorylates and alters the function of a few cardiac proteins that have key effects on the overall cardiac function. The presence of α1- and β1-ARs in HESC-CMs has been demonstrated by immunocytochemical analysis. Pharmacological induction with phenylephrine (α1-AR agonist) resulted in a dose-dependent increase in contraction rate in both human fetal and HESC-CMs. Increases in beat rate and amplitude were observed after isoprenaline (β1-AR agonist) treatment (Xu et al. 2002; Mummery et al. 2003; Kehat et al. 2001; He et al. 2003). However, β2-AR agonists such as clenbuterol only elicited a response during late stages of in vitro differentiation (day 61–72) and not early stages (day 22 and 39) (He et al. 2003), consistent with the observation cardiac contractility to β-adrenergic stimulation changes during development (Wobus et al. 1991). Negative chronotropic responses to muscarinic agonists, such as carbachol, have also been observed, again consistent with data from mouse fetal and mES-CMs (Wobus et al. 1991; An et al. 1996). Alternatively, perturbation of pathways downstream of receptors can also modulate cardiac output. Inhibition of phosphodiesterase (which converts cAMP into 5$'$AMP) by isobutyl methylxanthine (IBMX) and activation of adenylate cyclase by forskolin, results in increased or decreased beat rate, respectively (Kehat et al. 2001).

Other known and unknown factors influence beat rate. HESC-CMs are exquisitely sensitive to temperature; reduced temperature correlates with decreased beat rate. In EBs, continuous and episodic beat patterns have been observed, with the latter being speculatively attributed to conduction block related to tissue geometry, impaired cell-to-cell coupling, reduced cellular excitability or an immature Ca^{2+} regulatory system. HESC-CMs do express adhesion molecules (N-cadherin), and the gap junction proteins connexins 43 and 45, but Cx45 usually only in early stages of in vivo development (Mummery et al. 2003; Kehat et al. 2002). They are also well coupled by functional gap junctions, as evidenced by visualizing Lucifer Yellow dye spread or Ca^{2+} movement between connected cells. However, visualization of Ca^{2+} ion transients via fura-2 fluorescence revealed the rate to peak concentration in each beat was significantly longer in the HESC-CMs (Kehat et al. 2002).

In heart muscle, the main currents involved in the action potential are influx of Ca^{2+} and Na^+ during depolarization (phase 0) and efflux or maintenance of K^+ during repolarization and resting potential (phases 1–4). Sodium channels are the major current of depolarization in atrial and ventricular cells but in pacemaker cells it is Ca^{2+} via L-type calcium channels (I_{Ca-L}). Molecularly, I_{Ca-L} channels are expressed in HESC-CMs (Mummery et al. 2003) and functionally they are inhibited, and hence also beat rate, in a dose-dependent manner by blockers such as diltiazem (Xu et al. 2002). Verapamil also inhibited action potential in human fetal and HESC-CMs. By contrast, mES-CMs at early stages of differentiation are nonresponsive despite the presence of I_{Ca-L} channels. Thus, while there are many similarities between human fetal or HESC-CMs and mES-CMs, their Ca^{2+} channel modulation resembles that of the adult mouse (Mummery et al. 2003).

The sarcoplasmic reticulum is also a major source of Ca^{2+} release in myocytes. Expression of ryanodine receptors (RyR; Ca^{2+} activated Ca^{2+} release) and phospholamban (PLN; regulation of SERCA2a-mediated Ca^{2+} uptake) has been demonstrated in HESC-CMs.

Repolarization is initiated by numerous K^+ channels. Among these are transient outward current (I_{TO1}; encoded by the genes *Kv4.2* and *Kv4.3*), which causes the early rapid repolarization seen in phase 1 of the action potential; slow activating current (I_{Ks}; encoded by *KvLQT1* with the *mink* subunit), which causes repolarization associated with phase 3 of the action potential. Mutations in *KvLQT1* are the cause of long QT syndrome in humans; the rapid component of delayed rectification (I_{Kr}; encoded by human *eag*-related gene [HERG]), which is involved in all phases of repolarization, but is most active during phase 3. Mutations in *HERG* have been linked to a congenital form of long QT syndrome. Furthermore, these channels are the target of anti-arrhythmic agents such as E4031.

RNA for *Kv4.3* and *KvLQT1* has been detected by RT-PCR in HESC-CMs (Mummery et al. 2003). However, while *Kv4.3* could be detected in differentiating cells several days before the onset of beating, *KvLQT1* was expressed in undifferentiated HESC but transcripts disappeared during early differentiation and reappeared later. Functionally, application of E-4031 lead to increased duration of phase 3 (terminal repolarization) and triggered early after depolarization (EAD)-based arrhythmias, providing pharmacological evidence that I_{Kr} contributes to repolarization in HESC-CM (He et al. 2003). Delayed after depolarizations (DADs) typically occur during Ca^{2+} overload such as that produced by injury or digitonin toxicity and were observed to occur spontaneously, possibly a result of microelectrode impalement or spontaneous Ca^{2+} release.

Interestingly, forced electrical stimulation at increasing frequencies resulted in action potential shortening adaptation in ventricular-like cardiomyocytes. This physiological response leads to systolic shortening at high heart rates, thereby maintaining diastolic time for ventricular filling, as shown in the ventricular myocardium of human embryos (He et al. 2003).

Based on electrophysiological characteristics of the action potential, such as resting potential, upstroke, amplitude and duration, it is possible to assign cell type (pacemaker, atrial, ventricular, nodal) to HESC-CMs in culture. Upstroke velocities, a measure of the rate of depolarization, were particularly low in the ventricular-like cells (average 8 V/s, (Mummery et al. 2003); 5–30 V/s, (He et al. 2003), which is comparable to cultured fetal ventricular cardiomyocytes but very different from the rapid upstroke of adult ventricular cells (~150–350 V/s; He et al. 2003). Similarly, the relatively positive resting potential of atrial- and ventricular-like HESC-CMs (approximately –40 to −50 mV) is comparable to early stages of fetal development. While some studies describe up to 85% of HESC-CMs being ventricular-like (Mummery et al. 2003), others report a lesser predominance of this cell type (He et al. 2003; Kehat et al. 2002). This may relate to the time of analysis since the cardiomyocyte composition of mES-derived embryoid bodies changes during culture duration (Hescheler et al. 1997). It may also reflect differences in the HESC cell lines or methods of differentiation used, or that the analysis by Mummery et al. (2003) used dissociated HESC-CMs rather than EBs.

5
Applications and Conclusions

It is clear that HESCs can be differentiated towards cardiomyocytes that appropriately respond to different stimuli, and this infers functional expression of many of the components required for excitation-coupling. However, while maturation of HESC-CMs does occur during prolonged culture, currently these cells fail to attain the characteristic of adult cardiomyocytes. It will be important to assess novel methods to stimulate maturation so in vitro produced cardiomyocytes with embryonic or adult characteristics are at the disposal of the scientific and clinical community. This would be potentially useful in drug discovery and testing. In addition, it might be possible to use HESCs to develop in vitro models for studying specific genetic cardiac diseases, such as channelopathies where specific ion channel mutations may cause fatal arrhythmias in asymptotic carriers. It is also important to be aware that while introduction of ectopic cardiac cells in mice might not cause arrhythmias because of the high heart rate and adaptive capacity of the mouse heart, this may not be the case in humans. Transplantation of skeletal myoblasts in patients has already caused serious clinical complications (reviewed in Menasche 2004) because of inadequate incorporation into the host myocardium. More recently, the first transplantation of HESC-derived cardiomyocytes into the hearts of pigs was described (Kehat et al. 2004). Since pig heart physiology is more reminiscent of human heart than rodents, the observation of ectopic pacemaker-like activity from the transplanted cells cautions against premature clinical application. On the other hand, there are few proven alternative sources of transplantable cardiomyocytes to replace those lost after infarct, although recent descriptions of cardiac progenitor cells are of major interest, particularly following reports that bone marrow-derived stem cells do not transdifferentiate to cardiomyocytes in the heart following transplantation, as originally thought (Murry et al. 2004; Balsam et al. 2004). Further research will be required before cardiac cell therapy becomes routine clinical practice.

References

Alsan BH, Schultheiss TM (2002) Regulation of avian cardiogenesis by Fgf8 signaling. Development 129:1935–1943

An RH, Davies MP, Doevendans PA, Kubalak SW, Bangalore R, Chien KR, Kass RS (1996) Developmental changes in beta-adrenergic modulation of L-type Ca^{2+} channels in embryonic mouse heart. Circ Res 78:371–378

Balsam LB, Wagers AJ, Christensen JL, Kofidis T, Weissman IL, Robbins RC (2004) Haematopoietic stem cells adopt mature haematopoietic fates in ischaemic myocardium. Nature 428:668–673

Barron M, Gao M, Lough J (2000) Requirement for BMP and FGF signaling during cardiogenic induction in non-precardiac mesoderm is specific, transient, and cooperative. Dev Dyn 218:383–393

Behfar A, Zingman LV, Hodgson DM, Rauzier JM, Kane GC, Terzic A, Puceat M (2002) Stem cell differentiation requires a paracrine pathway in the heart. FASEB J 16:1558–1566

Boheler KR, Czyz J, Tweedie D, Yang HT, Anisimov SV, Wobus AM (2002) Differentiation of pluripotent embryonic stem cells into cardiomyocytes. Circ Res 91:189–201

Brand T (2003) Heart development: molecular insights into cardiac specification and early morphogenesis. Dev Biol 258:1–19

Bruneau BG, Logan M, Davis N, Levi T, Tabin CJ, Seidman JG, Seidman CE (1999) Chamber-specific cardiac expression of Tbx5 and heart defects in Holt-Oram syndrome. Dev Biol 211:100–108

Bruneau BG, Nemer G, Schmitt JP, Charron F, Robitaille L, Caron S, Conner DA, Gessler M, Nemer M, Seidman CE, Seidman JG (2001) A murine model of Holt-Oram syndrome defines roles of the T-box transcription factor Tbx5 in cardiogenesis and disease. Cell 106:709–721

Cai CL, Liang X, Shi Y, Chu PH, Pfaff SL, Chen J, Evans S (2003) Isl1 identifies a cardiac progenitor population that proliferates prior to differentiation and contributes a majority of cells to the heart. Dev Cell 5:877–889

Caplice NM, Gersh BJ (2003) Stem cells to repair the heart: a clinical perspective. Circ Res 92:6–8

Christoffels VM, Habets PE, Franco D, Campione M, de Jong F, Lamers WH, Bao ZZ, Palmer S, Biben C, Harvey RP, Moorman AF (2000) Chamber formation and morphogenesis in the developing mammalian heart. Dev Biol 223:266–278

Evans MJ, Kaufman MH (1981) Establishment in culture of pluripotential cells from mouse embryos. Nature 292:154–156

Fijnvandraat AC, van Ginneken AC, Schumacher CA, Boheler KR, Lekanne Deprez RH, Christoffels VM, Moorman AF (2003) Cardiomyocytes purified from differentiated embryonic stem cells exhibit characteristics of early chamber myocardium. J Mol Cell Cardiol 35:1461–1472

Garcia-Martinez V, Schoenwolf GC (1993) Primitive-streak origin of the cardiovascular system in avian embryos. Dev Biol 159:706–719

Gaussin V, Van de Putte T, Mishina Y, Hanks MC, Zwijsen A, Huylebroeck D, Behringer RR, Schneider MD (2002) Endocardial cushion and myocardial defects after cardiac myocyte-specific conditional deletion of the bone morphogenetic protein receptor ALK3. Proc Natl Acad Sci U S A 99:2878–2883

Habets PE, Moorman AF, Clout DE, van Roon MA, Lingbeek M, van Lohuizen M, Campione M, Christoffels VM (2002) Cooperative action of Tbx2 and Nkx2.5 inhibits ANF expression in the atrioventricular canal: implications for cardiac chamber formation. Genes Dev 16:1234–1246

He JQ, Ma Y, Lee Y, Thomson JA, Kamp TJ (2003) Human embryonic stem cells develop into multiple types of cardiac myocytes: action potential characterization. Circ Res 93:32–39

Hescheler J, Fleischmann BK, Lentini S, Maltsev VA, Rohwedel J, Wobus AM, Addicks K (1997) Embryonic stem cells: a model to study structural and functional properties in cardiomyogenesis. Cardiovasc Res 36:149–162

Horb ME, Thomsen GH (1999) Tbx5 is essential for heart development. Development 126:1739–1751

Johansson BM, Wiles MV (1995) Evidence for involvement of activin A and bone morphogenetic protein 4 in mammalian mesoderm and hematopoietic development. Mol Cell Biol 15:141–151

Kehat I, Kenyagin-Karsenti D, Snir M, Segev H, Amit M, Gepstein A, Livne E, Binah O, Itskovitz-Eldor J, Gepstein L (2001) Human embryonic stem cells can differentiate into myocytes with structural and functional properties of cardiomyocytes. J Clin Invest 108:407–414

Kehat I, Gepstein A, Spira A, Itskovitz-Eldor J, Gepstein L (2002) High-resolution electrophysiological assessment of human embryonic stem cell-derived cardiomyocytes: a novel in vitro model for the study of conduction. Circ Res 91:659–661

Kehat I, Khimovich L, Caspi O, Gepstein A, Shofti R, Arbel G, Huber I, Satin J, Itskovitz-Eldor J, Gepstein L (2004) Electromechanical integration of cardiomyocytes derived from human embryonic stem cells. Nat Biotechnol 22:1282–1289

Kelly RG, Buckingham ME (2002) The anterior heart-forming field: voyage to the arterial pole of the heart. Trends Genet 18:210–216

Klug MG, Soonpaa MH, Koh GY, Field LJ (1996) Genetically selected cardiomyocytes from differentiating embryonic stem cells form stable intracardiac grafts. J Clin Invest 98:216–224

Kolossov E, Fleischmann BK, Liu Q, Bloch W, Viatchenko-Karpinski S, Manzke O, Ji GJ, Bohlen H, Addicks K, Hescheler J (1998) Functional characteristics of ES cell-derived cardiac precursor cells identified by tissue-specific expression of the green fluorescent protein. J Cell Biol 143:2045–2056

Krishnan P, King MW, Neff AW, Sandusky GE, Bierman KL, Grinnell B, Smith RC (2001) Human truncated Smad 6 (Smad 6s) inhibits the BMP pathway in Xenopus laevis. Dev Growth Differ 43:115–132

Lints TJ, Parsons LM, Hartley L, Lyons I, Harvey RP (1993) Nkx-2.5: a novel murine homeobox gene expressed in early heart progenitor cells and their myogenic descendants. Development 119:969

Loebel DA, Watson CM, De Young RA, Tam PP (2003) Lineage choice and differentiation in mouse embryos and embryonic stem cells. Dev Biol 264:1–14

Lough J, Barron M, Brogley M, Sugi Y, Bolender DL, Zhu X (1996) Combined BMP-2 and FGF-4, but neither factor alone, induces cardiogenesis in non-precardiac embryonic mesoderm. Dev Biol 178:198–202

Makino S, Fukuda K, Miyoshi S, Konishi F, Kodama H, Pan J, Sano M, Takahashi T, Hori S, Abe H, Hata J, Umezawa A, Ogawa S (1999) Cardiomyocytes can be generated from marrow stromal cells in vitro. J Clin Invest 103:697–705

Maltsev VA, Ji GJ, Wobus AM, Fleischmann BK, Hescheler J (1999) Establishment of beta-adrenergic modulation of L-type Ca^{2+} current in the early stages of cardiomyocyte development. Circ Res 84:136–145

Martin GR (1981) Isolation of a pluripotent cell line from early mouse embryos cultured in medium conditioned by teratocarcinoma stem cells. Proc Natl Acad Sci U S A 78:7634–7638

McBurney MW, Jones-Villeneuve EM, Edwards MK, Anderson PJ (1982) Control of muscle and neuronal differentiation in a cultured embryonal carcinoma cell line. Nature 299:165–167

Menasche P (2004) Skeletal myoblast transplantation for cardiac repair. Expert Rev Cardiovasc Ther 2:21–28

Meyer N, Jaconi M, Landopoulou A, Fort P, Puceat M (2000) A fluorescent reporter gene as a marker for ventricular specification in ES-derived cardiac cells. FEBS Lett 478:151–158

Molkentin JD, Lin Q, Duncan SA, Olson EN (1997) Requirement of the transcription factor GATA4 for heart tube formation and ventral morphogenesis. Genes Dev 11:1061–1072

Muller M, Fleischmann BK, Selbert S, Ji GJ, Endl E, Middeler G, Muller OJ, Schlenke P, Frese S, Wobus AM, Hescheler J, Katus HA, Franz WM (2000) Selection of ventricular-like cardiomyocytes from ES cells in vitro. FASEB J 14:2540–2548

Mummery C, Ward D, van den Brink CE, Bird SD, Doevendans PA, Opthof T, Brutel de la Riviere A, Tertoolen L, van der Heyden M, Pera M (2002) Cardiomyocyte differentiation of mouse and human embryonic stem cells. J Anat 200:233–242

Mummery C, Ward-van Oostwaard D, Doevendans P, Spijker R, van den Brink S, Hassink R, van der Heyden M, Opthof T, Pera M, de la Riviere AB, Passier R, Tertoolen L (2003) Differentiation of human embryonic stem cells to cardiomyocytes: role of coculture with visceral endoderm-like cells. Circulation 107:2733–2740

Murry CE, Soonpaa MH, Reinecke H, Nakajima H, Nakajima HO, Rubart M, Pasumarthi KB, Virag JI, Bartelmez SH, Poppa V, Bradford G, Dowell JD, Williams DA, Field LJ (2004) Haematopoietic stem cells do not transdifferentiate into cardiac myocytes in myocardial infarcts. Nature 428:664–668

Nakamura T, Sano M, Songyang Z, Schneider MD (2003) A Wnt- and beta-catenin-dependent pathway for mammalian cardiac myogenesis. Proc Natl Acad Sci U S A 100:5834–5839

Nascone N, Mercola M (1995) An inductive role for the endoderm in Xenopus cardiogenesis. Development 121:515–523

Olson EN, Schneider MD (2003) Sizing up the heart: development redux in disease. Genes Dev 17:1937–1956

Pandur P, Lasche M, Eisenberg LM, Kuhl M (2002) Wnt-11 activation of a non-canonical Wnt signalling pathway is required for cardiogenesis. Nature 418:636–641

Paquin J, Danalache BA, Jankowski M, McCann SM, Gutkowska J (2002) Oxytocin induces differentiation of P19 embryonic stem cells to cardiomyocytes. Proc Natl Acad Sci U S A 99:9550–9555

Passier R, Mummery C (2003) Origin and use of embryonic and adult stem cells in differentiation and tissue repair. Cardiovasc Res 58:324–335

Passier R, Ward-van Oostwaard D, Snapper J, Kloots K, Hassink R, Kuijk E, Roelen B, Brutel de la Riviere A, Mummery C (2005) Increased cardiomyocyte differentiation from human embryonic stem cells in serum-free cultures. Stem Cells 23:772–780

Rathjen J, Rathjen PD (2001) Mouse ES cells: experimental exploitation of pluripotent differentiation potential. Curr Opin Genet Dev 11:587–594

Rathjen J, Lake JA, Bettess MD, Washington JM, Chapman G, Rathjen PD (1999) Formation of a primitive ectoderm like cell population, EPL cells, from ES cells in response to biologically derived factors. J Cell Sci 112:601–612

Reiter JF, Alexander J, Rodaway A, Yelon D, Patient R, Holder N, Stainier DY (1999) Gata5 is required for the development of the heart and endoderm in zebrafish. Genes Dev 13:2983–2995

Roebroek AJ, Umans L, Pauli IG, Robertson EJ, van Leuven F, Van de Ven WJ, Constam DB (1998) Failure of ventral closure and axial rotation in embryos lacking the proprotein convertase Furin. Development 125:4863–4876

Sachinidis A, Fleischmann BK, Kolossov E, Wartenberg M, Sauer H, Hescheler J (2003a) Cardiac specific differentiation of mouse embryonic stem cells. Cardiovasc Res 58:278–291

Sachinidis A, Gissel C, Nierhoff D, Hippler-Altenburg R, Sauer H, Wartenberg M, Hescheler J (2003b) Identification of plateled-derived growth factor-BB as cardiogenesis-inducing factor in mouse embryonic stem cells under serum-free conditions. Cell Physiol Biochem 13:423–429

Saga Y, Miyagawa-Tomita S, Takagi A, Kitajima S, Miyazaki J, Inoue T (1999) MesP1 is expressed in the heart precursor cells and required for the formation of a single heart tube. Development 126:3437–3447

Schneider MD, Gaussin V, Lyons KM (2003) Tempting fate: BMP signals for cardiac morphogenesis. Cytokine Growth Factor Rev 14:1–4

Schultheiss TM, Xydas S, Lassar AB (1995) Induction of avian cardiac myogenesis by anterior endoderm. Development 121:4203–4214

Schultheiss TM, Burch JB, Lassar AB (1997) A role for bone morphogenetic proteins in the induction of cardiac myogenesis. Genes Dev 11:451–462

Shi Y, Katsev S, Cai C, Evans S (2000) BMP signaling is required for heart formation in vertebrates. Dev Biol 224:226–237

Shin CH, Liu ZP, Passier R, Zhang CL, Wang DZ, Harris TM, Yamagishi H, Richardson JA, Childs G, Olson EN (2002) Modulation of cardiac growth and development by HOP, an unusual homeodomain protein. Cell 110:725–735

Snir M, Kehat I, Gepstein A, Coleman R, Itskovitz-Eldor J, Livne E, Gepstein L (2003) Assessment of the ultrastructural and proliferative properties of human embryonic stem cell-derived cardiomyocytes. Am J Physiol Heart Circ Physiol 285: H2355–H2363

Thomson JA, Itskovitz-Eldor J, Shapiro SS, Waknitz MA, Swiergiel JJ, Marshall VS, Jones JM (1998) Embryonic stem cell lines derived from human blastocysts. Science 282:1145–1147

Van den Eijnden-van Raaij AJ, van Achterberg TA, van der Kruijssen CM, Piersma AH, Huylebroeck D, de Laat SW, Mummery CL (1991) Differentiation of aggregated murine P19 embryonal carcinoma cells is induced by a novel visceral endoderm-specific FGF-like factor and inhibited by activin A. Mech Dev 33:157–165

Van der Heyden MA, Defize LH (2003) Twenty-one years of P19 cells: what an embryonal carcinoma cell line taught us about cardiomyocyte differentiation. Cardiovasc Res 58:292–302

Ventura C, Maioli M (2000) Opioid peptide gene expression primes cardiogenesis in embryonal pluripotent stem cells. Circ Res 87:189–194

Wang D, Chang PS, Wang Z, Sutherland L, Richardson JA, Small E, Krieg PA, Olson EN (2001) Activation of cardiac gene expression by myocardin, a transcriptional cofactor for serum response factor. Cell 105:851–862

Wang D, Passier R, Liu ZP, Shin CH, Wang Z, Li S, Sutherland LB, Small E, Krieg PA, Olson EN (2002) Regulation of cardiac growth and development by SRF and its cofactors. Cold Spring Harb Symp Quant Biol 67:97–105

Wobus AM, Wallukat G, Hescheler J (1991) Pluripotent mouse embryonic stem cells are able to differentiate into cardiomyocytes expressing chronotropic responses to adrenergic and cholinergic agents and Ca^{2+} channel blockers. Differentiation 48:173–182

Wobus AM, Kaomei G, Shan J, Wellner MC, Rohwedel J, Ji G, Fleischmann B, Katus HA, Hescheler J, Franz WM (1997) Retinoic acid accelerates embryonic stem cell-derived cardiac differentiation and enhances development of ventricular cardiomyocytes. J Mol Cell Cardiol 29:1525–1539

Xu C, Police S, Rao N, Carpenter MK (2002) Characterization and enrichment of cardiomyocytes derived from human embryonic stem cells. Circ Res 91:501–508

Yamagishi H, Yamagishi C, Nakagawa O, Harvey RP, Olson EN, Srivastava D (2001) The combinatorial activities of Nkx2.5 and dHAND are essential for cardiac ventricle formation. Dev Biol 239:190–203

Zaffran S, Frasch M (2002) Early signals in cardiac development. Circ Res 91:457–469

Zandstra PW, Bauwens C, Yin T, Liu Q, Schiller H, Zweigerdt R, Pasumarthi KB, Field LJ (2003) Scalable production of embryonic stem cell-derived cardiomyocytes. Tissue Eng 9:767–778

Zeng X, Miura T, Luo Y, Bhattacharya B, Condie B, Chen J, Ginis I, Lyons I, Mejido J, Puri RK, Rao MS, Freed WJ (2004) Properties of pluripotent human embryonic stem cells BG01 and BG02. Stem Cells 22:292–312

HEP (2006) 174:123–146
© Springer-Verlag Berlin Heidelberg 2006

Autocrine and Intracrine Signaling for Cardiogenesis in Embryonic Stem Cells: A Clue for the Development of Novel Differentiating Agents

C. Ventura[1,2] ($\boxtimes$) · A. Branzi[1,2]

[1]Laboratory of Molecular Biology and Stem Cell Engineering,
National Institute of Biostructures and Biosystems, University of Bologna, Bologna, Italy
cvent@libero.it

[2]S. Orsola-Malpighi Hospital, Institute of Cardiology, Pavilion 21, Via Massarenti 9,
40138 Bologna, Italy

Abstract Cardiogenesis, one of the earliest and most complex morphogenetic events in the embryo, is not fully understood at the molecular level and is typically a low-yield process. Affording a high throughput of cardiogenesis from a suitable population of pluripotent cells is therefore a major assignment in the perspective of a stem cell therapy for heart failure. Analysis of cardiac lineage commitment in mouse embryonic stem cells and in vivo models of cardiac differentiation revealed that a number of crucial growth factors are released from precursor cells, acting in an autocrine fashion on specific plasma membrane receptors to prime a cardiogenic decision. Nevertheless, it is increasingly becoming evident that cell nuclei harbor the potential for intrinsic signal transduction pathways. The term "intracrine" has been proposed for growth regulatory peptides that have been shown to act within their cell of synthesis at the level of the nuclear envelope, chromatin, or other sub-nuclear components. Considerable evidence links known intracrines with transcriptional responses and self-sustaining loops that behave as long-lived signals and impart features characteristic of differentiation, growth regulation and cell memory. This review focuses on a number of autocrine and intracrine systems within the context of cardiac differentiation and emphasizes the identification of cardiogenic mechanisms as a clue for the development of unprecedented differentiating strategies. In this regard, recently synthesized mixed esters of hyaluronan with butyric and retinoic acid primed the expression of cardiogenic genes and elicited a remarkable increase in cardiomyocyte yield in mouse embryonic stem cells. This demonstrates the potential for chemically modifying the gene program of cardiac differentiation without the aid of gene transfer technologies and sets the basis for the design of a novel generation of chemicals suited for the organization of targeted lineage patterning in stem cells.

Keywords Embryonic stem cells · Cardiogenesis · Gene transcription · Differentiating agents

1
Introduction

Mouse embryonic stem (ES) cells have been shown to behave as pluripotent, self-renewable elements that can be committed to multiple lineages, including cardiac myocytes. Due to these features, ES cells proved to be an invaluable model to take a glimpse of the molecular events underlying the specification of a myocardial fate. In this regard, a selected number of lineage-restricted transcription factors, including the zinc finger-containing GATA-4 and the homeodomain Nkx-2.5, has been found to be essential for cardiogenesis in different animal species (Biben and Harvey 1997; Grepin et al. 1995; Heikinheimo et al. 1994; Jiang and Evans 1996; Lints et al. 1993), including humans (Benson et al. 1999; Schott et al. 1998). However, the identification of genes and signaling patterning recruited for the expression of cardiogenic transcription factors is only partially exploited. So far, different cardiogenic growth factors recognized by specific cell-surface receptors have been identified and the signaling mechanisms coupled with receptor activation have been increasingly dissected. A common feature in a number of these growth factors is their potential of being released by a pluripotent cell in the extracellular space, acting in an autocrine fashion onto targeted plasma membrane receptors to elicit a biological effect (Fig. 1). However, there is also increasing evidence to support intracellular sites of growth factor action and a large body of data indicating that such action is not rare (Cook et al. 2001; Re 2000, 2002, 2003). Within this context, the term "intracrine" has been proposed for the action of a peptide hormone either within its cell of synthesis or after internalization (Fig. 1). It is now agreed that an intracrine must retain the potential of being found in the extracellular space producing a response after binding to a membrane receptor such as a traditional endocrine, paracrine, or autocrine. In addition, a putative intracrine factor must be found in association with one or more intracellular organelles not associated with secretory or degratory structures (these may arguably be viewed as extensions of the extracellular space).

The present review will focus on a number of autocrine/intracrine systems involved in a cardiogenic decision in pluripotent ES cells, and will discuss the

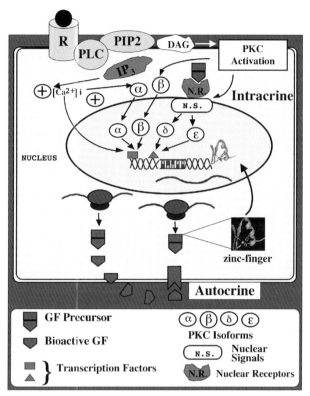

Fig. 1 Autocrine/intracrine signaling in ES cell cardiogenesis. Selected growth factors may trigger complex subcellular redistribution patterning of PKC isoforms, encompassing both nuclear translocation (PKC-α, -β_1, and -β_2) and/or the activation of nuclear-embedded isozymes (PKC-δ, and -ϵ). Nuclear PKCs play a major role in the activation of lineage-restricted transcription factors (i.e., GATA-4 and Nkx-2.5), which have been found to be essential for cardiogenesis in different animal species including humans. A common feature in a number of growth factors (LIF, dynorphin peptides, Wnts) is their potential of being released by a pluripotent cell in the extracellular space, acting in an autocrine fashion onto a targeted plasma membrane receptor to elicit a differentiating response. There is also increasing evidence to support intracellular sites of growth factor action. The term intracrine has been proposed for the action of a peptide hormone either within its cell of synthesis or after internalization. Binding sites for intracrines have been detected in the nuclear envelope, chromatin, or both, as well as in other nuclear components. Nuclear endorphin receptors have been identified in pluripotent mouse ES cells and their stimulation with dynorphin B in nuclei isolated from undifferentiated cells has been shown to trigger nuclear PKC activity as well as GATA-4 and Nkx-2.5 gene transcription. Preprodynorphin itself possesses structural similarity to helix-loop-helix DNA binding proteins and exhibits cysteine-rich regions characteristic of zinc-finger domains. This raises the possibility that opioid peptide precursors may act as intracrines mimicking transcription factor dynamics

discovery of related signaling patterning as a potential clue for the development of novel differentiating agents.

2
Leukemia Inhibitory Factor

Leukemia inhibitory factor (LIF), a member of the interleukin (IL)-6 family of cytokines, is a pleiotropic growth factor that exists in two isoforms, a diffusible molecule (D-LIF) and an extracellular matrix-bound isoform (M-LIF) (Conquet et al. 1992; Rathjen et al. 1990). LIF is recognized by a receptor complex, a LIF-specific receptor (LIFR) and the signal transducer gp130 (Gearing et al. 1992; Godard et al. 1992), encompassing multiple downstream signaling, including the Janus kinase/signal transducers and activators of transcription (JAK/STAT), and the mitogen-activated protein (MAP) kinase pathways (Kunisada et al. 1998). Besides acting as a growth factor in hematopoiesis, bone, and neuroectodermal tissue, LIF also acts as an inhibitor of differentiation on ES cells (Taupin et al. 1998) and seems to affect developmental stages in different cells of the cardiovascular system in an opposite manner (Kirby et al. 1993; Paradis et al. 1998; Pepper et al. 1995; Towle et al. 1998). M-LIF has been found to act as an inhibitor of mesodermal differentiation during gastrulation (Conquet et al. 1992), while before gastrulation, LIF is downregulated to undetectable low levels, likely to allow commitment to the mesodermal lineage. These observations and the finding that M-LIF expression increases in the neonatal myocardium and elicits an antiapoptotic effect or hypertrophic response via the STAT3 pathway in primary cultures of embryonic or neonatal cardiomyocytes (Kunisada et al. 1998; Sheng et al. 1996) corroborate the hypothesis that LIF may finely tune cardiogenesis in a developmental stage-dependent fashion.

As shown by Bader et al. (2000), D-LIF is secreted at very low rates by STO fibroblasts and at significantly increased rates by SNL76/7 fibroblasts used as feeder cells to keep ES cells in an undifferentiated state (Bader et al. 2000). While D-LIF did not appear to be involved in early cardiogenic commitment in ES-derived embryoid bodies, the addition of D-LIF after mesodermal precursors had become committed to the cardiac lineage dose-dependently attenuated differentiation of cardiomyocytes, even at subpicomolar concentrations (Bader et al. 2000). Although these data may only suggest a paracrine role of D-LIF secreted by co-cultured fibroblast in in vitro models of ES cell cardiogenesis, a major role for autocrine D- and/or M-LIF, secreted by the ES cell itself within committed embryoid bodies, is inferred from a number of experimental observations in the study of Bader et al. (2000). First, in $lif^{-/-}$ embryoid bodies timely differentiation of cardiomyocytes was remarkably hampered and delayed, as compared to wild type cells. Secondly, the cardiac phenotype could be partially rescued by adding pM D-LIF to $lif^{-/-}$ embryoid bodies, indicating that autocrine LIF, which includes M-LIF in murine cells, is essential for initiation of differentiation of cardiomyocytes from embryoid bodies. Within this context, the complexity of the LIF action is highlighted by the fact that with increasing concentrations of D-LIF, differentiation of cardiomyocytes in $lif^{-/-}$ embryoid bodies was attenuated in a dose-dependent manner, indicating that, after the inductive event, autocrine LIF may attenuate cardiac differentiation. Akin to these findings is the observation that in ES cells lacking the LIF receptor gene cardiomyogenesis was also severely hampered and delayed (Bader et al. 2000).

In their study, Bader et al. (2000) also provided evidence that despite its effects on cardiomyogenesis, D-LIF added in nanomolar concentrations promoted proliferation and longevity of fully differentiated cardiomyocytes, acting as a renewal factor contributing to the maintenance of the acquired cardiac phenotype in embryoid bodies. It is noteworthy that LIF-neutralizing antibodies blocked the antiapoptotic effect observed in the presence of D-LIF and SNL76/7 fibroblasts, and reduced longevity of cardiomyocytes well below the value observed in the absence of any fibroblasts, indicating that autocrine secretion of LIF by embryoid bodies contributes to the longevity of cardiomyocytes.

Understanding the maintenance of the differentiated state of cardiomyocytes is now a major area of inquiry. Compelling evidence indicates that each developmental stage of cardiogenesis is subtly handled by a hierarchy of regulators. Once cardiomyocytes are fully differentiated, feedback mechanisms may be required to maintain their stable state and sustain a threshold level of critical regulators of the cardiac phenotype. A role in maintenance of the cardiac phenotype has been demonstrated for the muscle-specific intermediate filament protein desmin (Li et al. 1996; Milner et al. 1996). At the stage of a fully differentiated state of cardiomyocytes, M- and D-LIF exert this type of maintaining role at very low concentrations, presumably together with a plethora of other factors, owing to the shared usage of gp130.

3
The Wnt Pathway

The Wnt (mouse Int-1 and *Drosophila* wingless) genes encode a large family of secreted proteins that constitute key signaling molecules involved in the regulation of embryonic patterning, cell proliferation, and the definition of cell fates and organ architecture (Brown and Moon 1998; Wodarz and Nusse 1998). So far, at least 24 vertebrate Wnts have been identified and have been shown to bind members of the Frizzled family of receptors. To date, 11 members of the Frizzled family of Wnt receptors have been identified in mice, all displaying a seven-serpentine transmembrane motif. Wnt signaling has first been believed to proceed through a pathway controlled by β-catenin (Brown and Moon 1998; Wodarz and Nusse 1998). In this scheme, Wnt binding to

Frizzled receptors activates the intracellular transducer Dishevelled (Rattner et al. 1997), resulting in inhibition of glycogen synthase kinase-3β (GSK-3β), and stabilization of β-catenin (Nusse 1999). Free β-catenin forms nuclear complexes with members of the TCF/LEF family of transcription factors, regulating the expression of numerous genes. In the absence of a Wnt/receptor complex, β-catenin is associated with a complex including GSK-3β, Axin and the adenomatous polyposis coli tumor suppressor protein (ACP) (Wodarz and Nusse 1998). In the absence of Wnt signaling, phosphorylation of β-catenin by GSK-3β results in its ubiquitination and subsequent degradation by proteosomes (Aberle et al. 1997). Low Wnt signaling also involves the association of TCF/LEF with Groucho, a transcriptional inhibitor (Nusse 1999).

The first evidence suggesting that some Wnt and Frizzled homologs may signal through a β-catenin-independent pathway came from a number of observations in zebrafish and *Xenopus*. The phenotype resulting from the overexpression of the 5HT1c serotonin receptor in *Xenopus* embryos resembled that elicited by overexpressing Wnt-5A (Ault et al. 1996; Slusarski et al. 1997a; Yang-Snyder et al. 1996). Since 5HT1c is a serpentine receptor that modulates intracellular Ca^{2+} handling in a G-protein-coupled fashion, this finding led to the hypothesis that Wnt-5A signaling may proceed through a similar pathway. Additionally, Wnt-5A but not the axis-inducing Wnt-8 was found to stimulate intracellular Ca^{2+} release (Slusarski et al. 1997a). A similar patterning of gene expression was also observed upon ectopic expression of both Wnt-5A and 5HT1c (Slusarski et al. 1997a). In this regard, the observation that Wnt-5A signaling was able to block a gene program expressed in response to Wnt-8 signaling suggests that distinct Wnt pathways may converge in an antagonistic manner through signal transduction mechanisms that still remain to be fully elucidated (Slusarski et al. 1997b).

Concerning the process of cardiogenesis, proteins have been found to act both through β-catenin-related pathways and noncanonical signaling. In *Xenopus laevis*, among the *Xenopus* Wnt genes, Wnt-11 was found to exhibit a spatiotemporal pattern of expression correlating with specification of the cardiac lineage. In pluripotent animal cap cells, overexpression of Wnt-11 resulted in sufficiently inducing the early cardiac genes GATA-4, GATA-6, and XNkx-2.5, as well as α-myosin heavy chain (MHC) and TnIc (Pandur et al. 2002), which are characteristic of and specific for terminally differentiated cardiomyocytes. In these experiments, absence of the panmesodermal marker Xbra and the panendodermal marker Sox17b suggested that cardiac induction by XWnt-11 is direct and independent of germ-layer specification. Loss- and gain-of-function experiments provided evidence that Wnt-11 is required for heart formation in *Xenopus* embryos and is sufficient to induce a contractile phenotype in embryonic explants (Pandur et al. 2002). In the same study, experiments designed to assess whether Wnt/β-catenin signaling may mimic Wnt-11 activity in animal caps revealed that overexpression of β-catenin failed to induce the expression of GATA-4, GATA-6, and cardiac actin, MHC or TnIc. In Xenopus explants from the dorsal marginal zone (DMZ), Pandur et al. (2002) found that a protein kinase C (PKC) inhibitor was able to phenocopy the downregulatory effect exerted by dnWnt-11 on cardiac gene transcription, while specific inhibition of CamKII was ineffective, implicating the involvement of PKC but not CamKII in Wnt-11-induced cardiogenesis. Akin to these findings, is the observation that the expression of cardiac genes in DMZ explants could be rescued from dnWnt-11-mediated inhibition by the PKC activator PMA (Pandur et al. 2002). This negative effect could also be compensated by JNK overexpression. Consonant with these findings is the observation that Wnt-11 overexpression by itself elicited JNK1 phosphorylation. Requirement for PKC patterning in JNK activation was inferred from the capability of PKC inhibitors to prevent JNK activation by Wnt-11.

Differently from the results obtained in *Xenopus* embryos, in the pluripotent mouse cell line P19CL6, which recapitulates early steps for cardiac specification, a β-catenin-dependent pathway was found to be responsible for the cardiogenic action of Wnt proteins. In this system, early and late cardiac genes are upregulated by 1% DMSO, and spontaneous beating occurs. Wnt3A and Wnt8A were induced days before even the earliest cardiogenic transcription factors (Nakamura et al. 2003). Such an induction was combined with increased levels of β-catenin and led to the onset of cardiogenic transcription factors, cardiogenic growth factors, and sarcomeric myosin heavy chains (Nakamura et al. 2003). Differentiation was blocked by constitutively active glycogen synthase kinase-3β, an intracellular inhibitor of the Wnt-β-catenin pathway; conversely, lithium chloride, which inhibits GSK-3β, and Wnt3A-conditioned medium upregulated early cardiac markers and the proportion of differentiated cells (Nakamura et al. 2003). Consonant with these findings is the requirement of β-catenin-Tcf/Lef pathway for the myogenic signaling evoked by lithium in rat H9c2 cardiomyoblasts (Kashour et al. 2003).

It is now evident that autocrine/paracrine mechanisms are a major context for Wnt patterning in different animal species. Secretion of Wnt proteins is a priming step in the autocrine loop associated with Wnt signaling. Secreted Wnts share a signature WNT motif (C-K-C-HG-[LIVMT]-S-G-x-C), 22 conserved cysteines, many highly charged amino acid residues, and several potential glycosylation sites. Based on their amino acid sequences, Wnt proteins should be soluble, secreted glycoproteins. Nevertheless, Wnts do not exhibit the properties expected of soluble hydrophilic proteins. Analysis of *Drosophila* Wnt-1 expression in transgenic S2 cells revealed that only about 20% of the secreted protein is present in soluble conditioned medium; the majority of the extracellular Wnt-1 is associated with the cell surface and extracellular matrix (Reichsman et al. 1996). Recent work by Willert et al. (2003) has shown that murine Wnt-3a is palmitoylated at a conserved cysteine residue (Cys 77). Their discovery suggests for the first time that lipid modifications may account for the unusual behavior of Wnt ligands. *Drosophila* Wnt-1 also undergoes a lipid modification. Lipidation occurs in the ER and is dependent on porcupine, a putative O-acyltransferase. Porcupine is required for Wnt-1 activity, and porcupine homologs have been identified in *Xenopus*, mouse, human, and *Candida elegans* (Caricasole et al. 2002; Tanaka et al. 2000; Thorpe et al. 1997). How lipidation affects Wnt signaling is a question now under investigation. Many types of proteins, including cytosolic, transmembrane, and secreted proteins, are known to undergo S-palmitoylation, the reversible addition of palmitate to a cysteine via a thioester bond (Linder and Deschenes 2003). Such a modification can affect both protein localization and function. Palmitoylation increases protein hydrophobicity, and promotes membrane association; it also affects intracellular trafficking (Linder and Deschenes 2003). Palmitoylated proteins are frequently targeted to specific intracellular organelles, as well as to detergent-resistant microdomains (DRMs) located at the plasma membrane (Ikonen and Simons 1998; Patterson 2002). These DRMs, commonly referred to as lipid rafts, are rich in cholesterol and glycosphingolipids and exist in a separate liquid-ordered phase within the plasma membrane (Simons and Ikonen 1997), forming signal transduction centers.

Although Wnt-dependent autocrine/paracrine mechanisms have been demonstrated in a wide variety of nonmyocardial developmental models in vitro and in vivo (Rawadi et al. 2003; Shea et al. 2003; Shimizu et al. 1997), the molecular dissection of these mechanisms within the process of cardiomyogenesis has been only partially exploited. In this regard, the possibility that Wnt proteins may act in an autocrine fashion during cardiac differentiation is strongly suggested by the finding that DMSO-induced cardiogenesis in P19CL6 cells was mediated by the increase in the expression of endogenous Wnt proteins and could be executed without adding exogenous Wnts (Nakamura et al. 2003). Such a view is further inferred from the observation that the DMSO effect was suppressed by Frizzled-8Fc, a soluble Wnt antagonist that inhibited the transcription of both cardiogenic and cardiac-specific genes, as well as the appearance of spontaneously beating colonies (Nakamura et al. 2003). The involvement of autocrine/paracrine mechanisms in the cardiogenesis primed by Wnt signaling is also supported by studies in avian morphogenesis showing that Wnt-11 is expressed in early mesoderm in a pattern that overlaps with the precardiac regions (Eisenberg and Eisenberg 1999). Further dissection of Wnt-related dynamics in cardiac differentiation reveals that autocrine/paracrine interplay(s) may be more complex than expected. It has long been observed that repressive signals from the neural tube block cardiogenesis in vertebrates. It has been shown that a signal from the neural tube that blocks cardiogenesis in the adjacent anterior paraxial mesoderm of stage 8–9 chick embryos can be mimicked by ectopic expression of either Wnt-3a or Wnt-1, both of which are expressed in the dorsal neural tube (Tzahor and Lassar 2001). Hence, while mesodermal-expressed Wnt proteins are important orchestrators of cardiac differentiation, different Wnt proteins and their related signals from the neural tube normally act to block cardiogenesis in the adjacent anterior paraxial mesendoderm. Interestingly, repression of cardiogenesis by the neural tube can be overcome by ectopic expression of a secreted Wnt antagonist (Tzahor and Lassar 2001). Within this context, a number of secreted Frizzled-like proteins (sFRP) with a conserved N-terminal frizzled motif have been identified (Finch et al. 1997; Melkonyan et al. 1997; Rattner et al. 1997). sFRP are now regarded as major conductors of a negative autocrine feedback loop toward Wnt signaling. FrzA, the bovine counterpart of the murine sFRP-1 (93% identity) is involved in vascular cell growth control and antagonizes Xwnt-8 and hWnt-2 signaling in *Xenopus* embryos (Duplaa et al. 1999; Xu et al. 1998). sFRP-1 was found to be expressed in the heart and in the visceral yolk sac during mouse development, and displayed overlapping expression patterns with mWnt-8 during heart morphogenesis (Jaspard et al. 2000). From 8.5 to 12.5 d.p.c., sFRP-1 is expressed in cardiomyocytes together with mWnt-8 but neither in the pericardium nor in the endocardium; at 17.5 d.p.c., they are no longer present in the heart (Jaspard et al. 2000). In their study, Jaspard et al. (2000) also found that in mouse adult tissues, sFRP-1 is highly detected in the aortic endothelium and media and in cardiomyocytes, while mWnt-8 is not detected in these areas. sFRP-1 is also strongly expressed during early phases of the vascularization process in embryonic vasculature where it is thought to negatively interfere with Wnt signaling (Dufourcq et al. 2002). Hence, downregulatory signals by sFRP may provide a spatial and timely patterning for the action of Wnt proteins and may affect the interplay of adjacent morphogenetic areas in the developmental embryo. This view is further supported by the finding that sizzled, a secreted Frizzled-related protein expressed ventrally during and after gastrulation, functions in a negative feedback loop that limits allocation of mesodermal cells to the extreme ventral fate, with direct consequences for morphogenesis (Collavin and Kirschner 2003). Although the biochemical activity of sizzled is apparently very different from that of other secreted Frizzled-related proteins, and does not involve inhibition of Wnt8, these data are consistent with the hypothesis that different sFRP may be part of self-organizing regulatory circuits controlling cell behavior and differentiation at a distance from the organizer.

4
Endorphins and Autocrine Regulation of Protein Kinase C Signaling in Cardiogenesis

Opioid peptides govern important physiological responses, including pain (Matthes et al. 1996), behavior (Konig et al. 1996), learning, and memory (Jiang et al. 1989; Rigter 1978), and have also been shown to affect cell growth in a wide variety of normal and malignant tissues (Maneckjee and Minna 1992; Zagon et al. 1985). We previously provided evidence that endorphin peptides and their related receptors are tightly coupled with PKC signaling and regulate major functional features in adult myocardial cells. Dynorphin B, a biologically active end-product of the prodynorphin gene acting as a natural agonist of κ opioid receptors, was initially found to be expressed in myocardial cells (Ventura et al. 1994, 1995) and to act at cell surface opioid receptors priming phosphoinositide turnover (Ventura et al. 1991b, 1992) and remarkable changes in cytosolic Ca^{2+} and pH homeostasis (Ventura et al. 1991a, 1992). Moreover, prodynorphin gene and dynorphin B expression, as well as PKC signaling, were upregulated in cardiac myocytes isolated from Syrian cardiomyopathic hamsters (Ventura and Pintus 1997; Ventura et al. 1997a, 1997b), suggesting that opioid peptide gene expression may be involved in the modulation of myocardial growth and differentiation. The possibility that the adult myocardial cell may have retained a "memory" of a system involved in cardiac lineage specification during the embryonic stage is supported by the finding that P19 embryonal pluripotent cells express the prodynorphin gene and are able to synthesize and secrete bioactive dynorphin B (Ventura and Maioli 2000). In this study, exposure of P19 cells to dynorphin B primed the expression of the cardiac lineage restricted GATA-4 and Nkx-2.5 genes, followed by the transcription of the cardiac-specific genes MHC and myosin light chain-2V (MLC-2V). These changes in the expression of cardiogenic and cardiac-specific genes ultimately ensued in the appearance of beating colonies of cardiac myocytes. Within this context, we have recently investigated whether PKC activation may be a major requirement for ES cell cardiogenesis and whether this activation may be coupled with an autocrine circuit involving both endorphin gene expression and the synthesis and secretion of endorphin peptides (Ventura et al. 2003a). These issues were addressed in GTR1 cells, a derivative of R1 mouse ES cells that contain a transgene encoding the cardiomyocyte-specific MHC promoter driving the puromycin-resistance gene, and afford genetic selection of a virtually pure population of ES-derived cardiomyocytes. Similar to P19 cells, GTR1 ES cells expressed the prodynorphin gene and were able to synthesize and secrete dynorphin B. Moreover, following LIF removal their cardiac differentiation was associated with a remarkable increase in prodynorphin gene and dynorphin B expression. Our experimental data revealed the presence of κ opioid receptors in a plasma membrane-enriched fraction obtained from undifferentiated ES cells, with specific binding ranging between 75% and 85% of the total bound and a single dissociation constant (K_d) in the low nM range (Ventura et. al 2003a). A marked increase in the maximal binding capacity (B_{max}) for a radiolabeled ligand of κ opioid receptors was evident in plasma membranes that had been isolated from puromycin-selected cardiac myocytes. Coupling of cell surface opioid receptors and secreted dynorphin B to PKC signaling during the process of cardiogenesis was inferred by the analysis of subcellular patterning of targeted isozymes (Ventura et al. 2003a). In this study, PKC-α, -β$_1$, -β$_2$, -δ and -ε were all increased in the nucleus of ES-derived cardiac myocytes (Fig. 1), as compared with nuclei from undifferentiated cells. In both groups of cells, PKC-δ and -ε were mainly expressed at nuclear level. PKC-α was only slightly expressed in the nucleus of undifferentiated cells and its increase in the cardiomyocyte nucleus depended on a translocation from the cytosolic compartment. On the contrary, the increase of both PKC-δ and PKC-ε in the nucleus of ES-derived cardiomyocytes occurred independently of enzyme translocation and appeared to reflect the overexpression of these isozymes detected in total cellular extracts from myocardial cells. Differently from PKC-δ and -ε, the nuclear increase in both PKC-β$_1$ and -β$_2$ observed in ES-derived cardiac myocytes was associated with enhanced isozyme expression in the cytosolic fraction of these cells, suggesting a complex interplay between selected PKC mRNA expression and isozyme redistribution within the cytosolic and nuclear compartments. Interestingly, exposure of GTR1 ES cells to different opioid receptor antagonists markedly reduced the number of cells committed to the cardiac lineage and prevented the nuclear increase of PKC-α, PKC-β$_1$, and PKC-β$_2$. Failure of opioid receptor antagonism to affect the amount of PKC-δ and -ε detectable in the nucleus excluded an involvement of cell surface opioid receptors in enhancing the expression of these isozymes during cardiac differentiation. A causal role for PKC signaling in the activation of a cardiogenic program of differentiation was substantiated by the finding that the two PKC inhibitors chelerythrine and calphostin C prevented the overexpression of the prodynorphin gene, as well as the onset of GATA-4 and Nkx-2.5 transcripts observed following LIF withdrawal (Ventura et al. 2003a). Requirement for PKC activation in cardiogenesis was further inferred by the fact that ES cell treatment with specific PKC inhibitors counteracted the expression of the cardiac-specific genes MHC and MLC-2V and suppressed ES cell differentiation into beating cardiomyocytes. On the whole, downregulation of prodynorphin gene and dynorphin B expression by PKC inhibitors prompts the hypothesis that changes in subcellular profiling of PKC isozymes may orchestrate an autocrine circuit of cardiogenesis involving a feed-forward stimulation of opioid gene expression sustained by coupling of secreted dynorphin B with plasma membrane opioid receptors (Fig. 1).

5
Intracrine Regulation of Cell Growth and Differentiation: Role for a Nuclear Endorphinergic System in Stem Cell Cardiogenesis

Consonant with the definition of intracrine provided in this review, a large number of heterogeneous peptides may be deemed as intracrines and many of them have been demonstrated in the nucleus. Binding sites for intracrines have been detected in the nuclear envelope, chromatin, or both, as well as in other nuclear components. An exhaustive list of different intracrines and their related intracellular sites has been recently reviewed (Re 2003). Considerable evidence links known intracrines with crucial transcriptional and developmental pathways. The renin-angiotensin system (RAS), one of the most widely investigated cardiovascular regulators, has also been found to operate as an intracrine. Labeled angiotensin has long been reported to traffic from the circulation to the nucleus of cardiomyocytes (Cook et al. 2001; Erdmann et al. 1996; Re 1989). Nuclear angiotensin receptors have been found in association with chromatin in different cell types and their stimulation has been shown to trigger transcriptional responses (Re 2000). Strikingly, exposure of isolated nuclei to angiotensin ensued in increased transcription of renin, angiotensinogen and platelet-derived growth factor (PDGF) (Cook et al. 2001; Eggena et al. 1996). The intracrine PTHrP (Aarts et al. 1999; Moroianu and Riordan 1994) induces keratinocyte differentiation (Aarts et al. 1999, 2001). CSF-1 acts in the development of both hematopoietic cells and skeletal muscle (Borycki et al. 1995; Tang et al. 2001). Nuclear binding sites have been detected for LIF (Gardiner et al. 2002; Gouin et al. 1999; Oka et al. 2002). Besides LIF, other peptides including VEGF, FGF-2, BDNF, and PDGF-BB exhibit nuclear binding (Re 2003) and have been shown to regulate the growth and/or differentiation of pluripotent mesenchymal stem cells. VEGF has been reported to maintain hematopoietic stem cell survival by an intracrine mechanism (Gerber et al. 2002).

Functional implications of the nuclear binding of intracrines are substantiated by compelling evidence that cell nuclei harbor the potential for intrinsic signal transduction pathways (Fig. 1). This is indicated by the presence of nuclear enzymes and substrates associated with the synthesis of diacylglycerol and inositol phospholipids. In isolated rat liver nuclei, the nuclear envelope was first found to synthesize in vitro phosphatidic acid, PtdIns(4)P and PtdIns(4,5)P2 (Cocco et al. 1987; Smith and Wells 1983). Moreover, nuclear inositol phospholipids have been consistently shown to serve as regulators of chromatin structure (Sylvia et al. 1986; Yu et al. 1998) and nuclear phosphoinositide-related signaling has been reported to operate in conjunction with the activation of nuclear PKC isozymes affording gene transcription regulation (Ventura et al. 1995, 1997a). Consonant with these findings is our recent observation that PKC-δ and -ε were constitutively expressed in the nucleus of undifferentiated ES cells and that their expression was remarkably enhanced in nuclei isolated from ES-derived cardiac myocytes (Ventura et al. 2003a). These data raise the question of whether cardiogenesis may also involve the intervention of intracrines coupling nuclear-embedded signaling kinases to the activation of a gene program of cardiac differentiation.

In this regard, confocal microscopy analysis of immunoreactive dynorphin B in GTR1 ES cells revealed that immunoreactive dynorphin B-like material was consistently detectable within undifferentiated cells and was remarkably enhanced in puromycin-selected cardiomyocytes (Ventura et al. 2003b). In this study, binding experiments performed in the presence of [^{3}H]U-69,593, a selective radiolabeled κ opioid receptor ligand, demonstrated the presence of highly specific κ opioid-binding sites in nuclei isolated from undifferentiated GTR1 cells. The Scatchard plots of ligand binding were linear with a single dissociation constant (K_d) in the low nanomolar range. It should be noted that B_{max} values were highly enhanced in nuclei of ES-derived cardiac myocytes, suggesting that the availability of nuclear opioid-binding sites for intracellular endorphins may be a developmentally regulated process and that nuclear opioid receptors may be part of the molecular machinery coaxing ES cells to a cardiac lineage.

Nuclear run-off experiments revealed that a direct exposure of nuclei isolated from undifferentiated ES cells to dynorphin B dose-dependently increased the transcription rate of the two cardiac lineage-promoting genes GATA-4 and Nkx-2.5 (Ventura et al. 2003b). Similar transcriptional responses were elicited by nuclear exposure to U-50,488H (U-50), a selective synthetic κ opioid receptor agonist. Endorphin-primed gene transcription was suppressed in a stereospecific fashion by selective opioid receptor antagonists. Failure of both dynorphin B and U-50 to affect transcription of genes promoting skeletal muscle or neuronal specification seems to exclude a generalized activation of repressed genes and suggests that coupling of nuclear opioid receptors to GATA-4 and Nkx-2.5 gene transcription may represent a mechanism pertaining to ES cell cardiogenesis. The finding that exposure of ES cell nuclei to dynorphin B enhanced prodynorphin gene transcription (Ventura et al. 2003b) indicates that dynorphin B-mediated induction of cardiogenic genes may involve a tonic feed-forward stimulation elicited at nuclear level by the opioid peptide on its coding gene. This is consonant with other observations indicating that several intracrines appear to directly upregulate their own synthesis and/or the expression of other components associated with their signaling patterning through intracellular actions (i.e., nuclear binding of dynorphin B triggers prodynorphin gene transcription as well as GATA-4 and Nkx-2.5 transcription in ES cell cardiogenesis). This ensues in the formation of multiple intracellular loops where both feed-forward or feed-back mechanisms have been detected, like those described for the pairs angiotensin/renin, angiotensin/angiotensinogen, angiotensin/PDGF, CSF-1/CSF-1, insulin/nuclear insulin receptor (for a review, see Re 2003). Within this scenario, it has also been found that intracellular actions of intracrines may both be similar or contrary to the action of those same intracrines at the cell-surface level. In this regard, PTHrP may both enhance or suppress cell proliferation according to its nuclear or plasma membrane binding, respectively (Re 1999), while angiotensin has been found to upregulate angiotensinogen expression by acting either extra- or intracellularly (Re 1999; Eggena et al. 1996).

There is now increasing agreement that self-sustaining intracrine-related loops may behave as long-lived signals and impart features characteristic of differentiation, growth regulation and cell memory. Concerning ES cell cardiogenesis, the possibility that the activation of nuclear-embedded signaling may represent a major component in an endorphin-sustained intracrine loop is prompted by the observation that undifferentiated ES nuclei harbored both PKC-δ and -ε (Ventura et al. 2003a) and that chelerythrine and calphostin C abrogated the transcription of cardiogenic genes primed by nuclear exposure to dynorphin B (Ventura et al. 2003b). Akin to these results, in the same study we provided evidence that nuclei isolated from undifferentiated cells were able to phosphorylate the high-affinity fluorescent PKC substrate acrylodan-labeled MARCKS peptide. Such an activity could be suppressed by the same PKC inhibitors that abolished the transcription evoked by the activation of nuclear opioid receptors (Ventura et al. 2003b) and were previously found to abrogate the cardiac differentiation in ES cells (Ventura et al. 2003a). Moreover, nuclear exposure to dynorphin B induced a significant, time-dependent increase in nuclear PKC activity that was antagonized by selective κ opioid receptor antagonists. Hence, in ES cells intracrine signals for myocardial differentiation may be fashioned by a nuclear endorphinergic system encompassing dynorphin B-mediated stimulation of nuclear opioid receptors, the activation of nuclear PKC signaling, and the onset of a cardiogenic program of gene expression (Fig. 1). In actual fact, the opioid peptide precursor preprodynorphin has been found to display structure similarity with the helix-loop-helix motif of multiple DNA binding proteins and to exhibit cysteine-rich regions characteristic of zinc-finger domains (Bakalkin et al. 1991). This raises the possibility that the processing of prodynorphin peptides may prime intracrine interactions, recapitulating homeodomain protein feed-back loops (Fig. 1).

Among the endorphinergic systems, the peptide products of the preproenkephalin gene are also worthy of consideration as growth factors affecting cell growth and differentiation. In nonmyocardial cells, preproenkephalin has been shown to behave as a nuclear protein responsive to growth arrest and differentiation signals (Bottger and Spruce 1995), suggesting that enkephalins may also be deemed as intracrines. Concerning the cardiovascular system, both methionine enkephalin and other peptide products of the proenkephalin gene have been detected in the rat heart (Dumont et al. 1990; Tang et al. 1983), as well as in guinea pig, hamster, and dog myocardium (Barron et al. 1992; Weihe et al. 1983). Proenkephalin mRNA was found to be more abundant in rat heart than in either the brain or the adrenal medulla, two tissues that have long been known to express high concentrations of opioid peptides (Howells et al. 1986). In addition, the detection of comparable amounts of proenkephalin mRNA in both ventricles and in myocyte cultures suggested that proenkephalin gene expression could be primarily associated with the myocardial cell. An opioid growth factor (OGF), the pentapeptide [Met^5]enkephalin, has been identified in both eukaryotes and prokaryotes and has been shown to act as a potent inhibitor of cell replication (Zagon and McLaughlin 1991, 1992; Zagon et al. 1985). OGF is also thought to be important in cellular maturation and survival (Meriney et al. 1991), and in the outgrowths of rabbit corneal epithelium it has been found to inhibit cell proliferation and to alter cell migration and the orchestration of cells into a specific architecture (Zagon et al. 1995). In the developing rat heart, OGF has been shown to regulate DNA synthesis at the level of both myocardial and epicardial cells, suggesting a role for OGF as a tonic modulator of cardiac morphogenesis (McLaughlin 1996). Whether the observed changes in DNA synthesis may be related to hyperplasia and/or hypertrophy and whether the proenkephalin gene and its related end-products may also be involved in ES cell cardiogenesis remain to be established.

6
Molecular Dissection of Embryonic Stem Cell Cardiogenesis: A Clue for the Development of Novel Differentiating Agents

Cell lineage specification is fashioned at multiple interconnected levels and is controlled by a complex interplay between cell signaling, nucleosomal assembly, the establishment of multifaceted transcriptional motifs, and the temporal and spatial organization of chromatin in loops and domains. Recent developments in the area of stem cell research have been boosted by an increasing understanding of transcriptional regulation and epigenetic modifications, including histone acetylation, DNA methylation, and chromatin remodeling. This is a crucial issue in ES cell cardiogenesis, since the rescuing potential of ES cells is limited by the fact that ES-derived cardiomyocytes withdraw early from the cell cycle (Klug et al. 1995, 1996). The development of strategies affording high-throughput of cardiogenesis from pluripotent cells would have obvious therapeutic potential. However, overexpression of cardiogenic genes by vector-mediated gene transfer is a cumbersome approach that may perturb normal homeostasis in both ES cells and recipient tissues, and cannot be readily envisioned in humans.

We have recently developed hyaluronan (HA) mixed esters with retinoic acid (RA) and butyric (BU) acid (Fig. 2), and provided evidence that these compounds (HBR) act as novel differentiating agents eliciting a remarkable increase in the yield of cardiomyocytes derived from mouse ES cells (Ventura et al. 2004). A rationale for the synthesis of these novel glycoconjugates is prompted by a number of interrelated observations. The HA receptor CD44 is highly expressed by cardiogenic cells and by the fused endothelial tubes and surrounding muscular epimyocardium within the early embryonic mouse heart (Wheatley et al. 1993). Normal cardiac morphogenesis and HA-mediated transformation of mouse epithelium into mesenchyme are abrogated by disruption of HA synthase-2 (Camenisch et al. 2000). HA can be translocated into various cell types via a receptor-mediated endocytosis, being consistently detected in close association with nuclear heterochromatin (Collis et al. 1998; Tammi et al. 2001). Intracellular HA-binding molecules (hyaladherins) translocate to the nucleus upon mitogenic stimulation (Majumdar et al. 2002), serving as substrates or activators for MAP kinases (Zhang et al. 1998), or acting as vertebrate homologues of proteins involved in splicing or cell cycle regulation (Deb and Datta 1996; Grammatikakis et al. 1995). An interference of RA signaling with cardiac differentiation is supported by the finding that inactivation of the RXRα gene and vitamin A deficiency caused embryonal death due to cardiac hypoplasia and ventricular chamber defects (Sucov et al. 1994). In this regard, abnormal heart development is observed by combining mouse strains with mutant RAR and RXR subtypes (Kastner et al. 1994; Mendelsohn et al. 1994). Moreover, in vitro studies demonstrated that all-*trans* RA increased the efficiency of cardiogenic differentiation in ES cells (Wobus et al. 1997). Concerning BU, its histone deacetylase inhibitory action alters chromatin structure, increasing transcription factor accessibility to target *cis*-acting regulatory sites (Wolffe and Pruss 1996). Recent developments concerning epigenetic modifications reveal that histone acetylation, DNA methylation, and chromatin remodeling are intimately connected to afford modulation of targeted gene transcription (Fig. 2). Accordingly, basic helix-loop-helix transcription factors interact with transcriptional coactivators possessing histone acetyltransferase activity (Ogryzko et al. 1996) and histone deacetylase inhibitors have been reported to enhance RXR/RAR heterodimer action (Fig. 2), promoting crucial developmental pathways in pluripotent cells (Dilworth et al. 2000; McCue et al. 1984). In general, histone acetylation, through the action of histone acetylases, correlates with gene activation, while histone deacetylation through histone deacetylases is linked with gene silencing.

On the whole, these considerations suggest that HA that is taken up may regulate cellular events from within subcellular compartments and may also act as a carrier for internalization of HA-grafting synthetic compounds. Within this context, the newly developed glycoconjugate HBR was found to remarkably increase the expression of the two cardiac lineage-promoting genes GATA-4 and Nkx-2.5 (Ventura et al. 2004). In these studies, HBR also enhanced prodynorphin gene expression, and the synthesis and secretion of dynorphin B. Nuclear run-off transcription analyses indicated that these effects occurred at the transcriptional level. The activation of such a cardiogenic program of gene transcription was associated with an increase in the expression of the cardiac-specific genes MHC and MLC-2V. Akin with the recruitment of PKC patterning in ES cell cardiogenesis, the transcriptional responses elicited by HBR, as well as the expression of cardiac-specific genes were suppressed by specific PKC inhibitors. ES cell exposure to HBR elicited a remarkable and dose-dependent increase in the number of spontaneously beating colonies, as compared to untreated controls (Ventura et al. 2004). Treatment with an ester of HA with RA (HR) or exposure to RA, HA, or BU alone induced a significantly lower increase in the number of beating colonies, as compared with HBR. The possibility that each of the HA-grafted moieties in HBR may additively act in a cardiogenic response was inferred by the observation that a combined treatment with HA and RA, or with HA and BU, resulted in increased cardiomyocyte yield, and mimicked the increase in the number of beating colonies observed in the presence of the corresponding HA monoesters HR or HB. Accordingly, cell treatment with an association of HB and HR led to a further increase in the yield of ES-derived cardiomyocytes. Nevertheless, in the presence of HB + HR the cardiomyocyte yield was still significantly lower than in HBR-treated cells (Ventura et al. 2004). This finding suggests that a competition for the

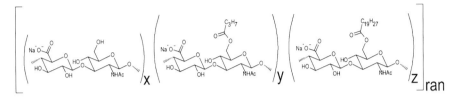

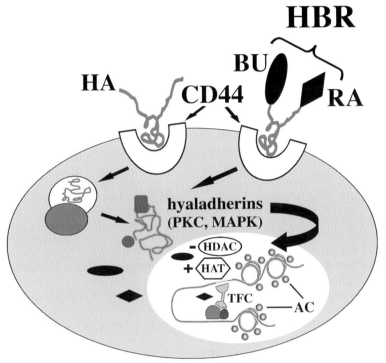

Fig. 2 Butyric and retinoic acid mixed esters of hyaluronan: toward the synthesis of novel differentiating agents. Hyaluronan mixed esters with butyric and retinoic acid (*HBR*) act as novel differentiating agents remarkably increasing the yield of ES-derived cardiomyocytes. The general formula of hyaluronan esters represent a random copolymer (*ran*) of three distinct dimeric repeating units, among which x are nonsubstituted, y are butyrylated, and z are retinoylated. The hyaluronan receptor CD44 is highly expressed by cardiogenic cells and by the fused endothelial tubes and surrounding muscular epimyocardium within the early embryonic mouse heart. Hyaluronan that is taken up may regulate cellular events from within subcellular compartments and may also act as a carrier for hyaluronan-grafting synthetic compounds. Intracellular hyaluronan-binding molecules (hyaladherins) translocate to the nucleus upon mitogenic stimulation, serving as substrates or activators for crucial signaling kinases or acting as vertebrate homologs of proteins involved in splicing or cell cycle regulation. Butyrate (*BU*) inhibits histone deacetylase activity (*HDAC*), an effect that alters chromatin structure, increasing transcription factor accessibility to target *cis*-acting regulatory sites (*AC*, acetyl groups). Retinoic acid (*RA*), HDAC inhibitors and coactivators possessing histone acetyltransferase activity (*HAT*) interact with transcription factor complexes (*TFC*), priming chromatin remodeling and targeted developmental fates

same uptake system of the two monoesters may have altered an optimal intracellular BU/RA ratio and/or their timely sequence of action and indicates that a maximal differentiating response is achieved when both BU and RA are concomitantly internalized by the mixed ester. Whether an intracellular release of RA and BU may represent a major requirement for the biological activity of HBR, or whether it may also act as a bioconjugate remains to be established.

It is noteworthy that HBR failed to affect the transcription rate of MyoD and neurogenin1, two genes involved in skeletal myogenesis and neuronal determination, respectively, indicating that a novel generation of mixed esters of hyaluronan may be proposed to organize lineage patterning in ES cells.

On the whole, these results demonstrate the potential for chemically modifying the gene program of cardiac differentiation in ES cells without the aid of gene transfer technologies, which may pave the way for novel approaches in tissue engineering and myocardial regeneration.

References

Aarts MM, Levy D, He B, Stregger S, Chen T, Richard S, Henderson JE (1999) Parathyroid hormone-related protein interacts with RNA. J Biol Chem 274:4832–4838

Aarts MM, Davidson D, Corlukja A, Petroulakis E, Guo J, Bringhurst FR, Galipeau J, Henderson JE (2001) PTHrP promotes quiescence and survival of serum deprived chondrocytes by inhibiting rRNA synthesis. J Biol Chem 276:37934–37943

Aberle H, Bauer A, Stappert J, Kispert A, Kemler R (1997) β-catenin is a target for the ubiquitin-proteasome pathway. EMBO J 16:3797–3804

Ault KT, Durmowicz G, Galione A, Harger PL, Busa WB (1996) Modulation of Xenopus embryo mesoderm-specific gene expression and dorsoanterior patterning by receptors that activate the phosphatidylinositol cycle signal transduction pathway. Development 122:2033–2041

Bader A, Al-Dubai H, Weitzer G (2000) Leukemia inhibitory factor modulates cardiogenesis in embryoid bodies in opposite fashions. Circ Res 86:787–794

Bakalkin GY, Ponomariev D, Sarkysian RA, Terenius L (1991) Sequence similarity between opioid peptide precursors and DNA binding proteins. FEBS Lett 282:175–177

Barron BA, Gaugl JF, Gu H, Caffrey JL (1992) Screening for opioids in the dog heart. J Mol Cell Cardiol 24:67–77

Benson DW, Silberbach GM, Kavanaugh-McHugh A, Cottrill C, Zhang Y, Riggs S, Smalls O, Johnson MC, Watson MS, Seidman JG, Seidman CE, Plowden J, Kugler JD (1999) Mutations in the cardiac transcription factor Nkx-2.5 affect diverse cardiac developmental pathways. J Clin Invest 104:1567–1573

Biben C, Harvey RP (1997) Homeodomain factor Nkx-2.5 controls left/right asymmetric expression of bHLH gene eHand during heart development. Genes Dev 11:1357–1369

Borycki AG, Smadja F, Stanley R, Leibovitch SA (1995) Colony-stimulating factor 1 (CSF-1) is involved in an autocrine growth control of rat myogenic cells. Exp Cell Res 218:213–222

Bottger A, Spruce BA (1995) Proenkephalin is a nuclear protein responsive to growth arrest and differentiation signals. J Cell Biol 130:1251–1262

Brown JD, Moon RT (1998) Wnt signaling: why is everything so negative? Curr Opin Cell Biol 10:182–187

Camenisch TD, Spicer AP, Brehm-Gibson T, Biesterfeldt J, Augustine ML, Calabro A Jr, Kubalak S, Klewer SE, McDonald JA (2000) Disruption of hyaluronan synthase-2 abrogates normal cardiac morphogenesis and hyaluronan-mediated transformation of epithelium to mesenchyme. J Clin Invest 106:349–360

Caricasole A, Ferraro T, Rimland JM, Terstappen GC (2002) Molecular cloning and initial characterization of the MG61/PORC gene, the human homologue of the Drosophila segment polarity gene Porcupine. Gene 288:147–157

Cocco L, Gilmour RS, Ognibene A, Letcher AJ, Manzoli FA, Irvine RF (1987) Synthesis of polyphosphoinositides in nuclei of Friend cells. Evidence for polyphosphoinositide metabolism inside the nucleus which changes with cell differentiation. Biochem J 248:765–770

Collavin L, Kirschner MW (2003) The secreted Frizzled-related protein Sizzled functions as a negative feedback regulator of extreme ventral mesoderm. Development 130:805–816

Collis L, Hall C, Lange L, Ziebell M, Prestwich R, Turley EA (1998) Rapid hyaluronan uptake is associated with enhanced motility: implications for an intracellular mode of action. FEBS Lett 440:444–449

Conquet F, Peyrieras N, Tiret L, Brulet P (1992) Inhibited gastrulation in mouse embryos overexpressing the leukemia inhibitory factor. Proc Natl Acad Sci U S A 89:8195–8199

Cook JL, Zhang Z, Re RN (2001) In vitro evidence for an intracellular site of angiotensin action. Circ Res 89:1138–1146

Deb TB, Datta K (1996) Molecular cloning of human fibroblast hyaluronic acid-binding protein confirms its identity with P-32, a protein copurified with splicing factor SF2. J Biol Chem 271:2206–2212

Dilworth FJ, Fromental-Ramain C, Yamamoto K, Chambon P (2000) ATP-driven chromatin remodeling activity and histone acetyltransferases act sequentially during transactivation by RAR/RXR in vitro. Mol Cell 6:1049–1058

Dufourcq P, Couffinhal T, Ezan J, Barandon L, Moreau C, Daret D, Duplaa C (2002) FrzA, a secreted frizzled related protein, induced angiogenic response. Circulation 106:3097–3103

Dumont M, Sabourin L, Lemaire S (1990) Alterations of heart dynorphin-A in the development of spontaneously hypertensive rats. Neuropeptides 15:43–48

Duplaa C, Jaspard B, Moreau C, D'Amore PA (1999) Identification and cloning of a secreted protein related to the cysteine-rich domain of frizzled. Evidence for a role in endothelial cell growth control. Circ Res 84:1433–1445

Eggena P, Zhu JH, Sereevinyayut S, Giordani M, Clegg K, Andersen PC, Hyun P, Barrett JD (1996) Hepatic angiotensin II nuclear receptors and transcription of growth-related factors. J Hypertens 14:961–968

Eisenberg CA, Eisenberg LM (1999) WNT11 promotes cardiac tissue formation of early mesoderm. Dev Dyn 216:45–58

Erdmann B, Fuxe K, Ganten D (1996) Subcellular localization of angiotensin II immunoreactivity in the rat cerebellar cortex. Hypertension 28:818–824

Finch PW, He X, Kelley MJ, Uren A, Schaudies RP, Popescu NC, Rudikoff S, Aaronson SA, Varmus HE, Rubin JS (1997) Purification and molecular cloning of a secreted, Frizzledrelated antagonist of Wnt action. Proc Natl Acad Sci U S A 94:6770–6775

Gardiner NJ, Cafferty WB, Slack SE, Thompson SW (2002) Expression of gp130 and leukaemia inhibitory factor receptor subunits in adult rat sensory neurones: regulation by nerve injury. J Neurochem 83:100–109

Gearing DP, Comeau MR, Friend DJ, Gimpel SD, Thut CJ, McGourty J, Brasher KK, King JA, Gillis S, Mosley B, Ziegler SF, Cosman D (1992) The IL-6 signal transducer, gp130: an oncostatin M receptor and affinity converter for the LIF receptor. Science 255:1434–1437

Gerber HP, Malik AK, Solar GP, Sherman D, Liang XH, Meng G, Hong K, Marsters JC, Ferrara N (2002) VEGF regulates haematopoietic stem cell survival by an internal autocrine loop mechanism. Nature 417:954–958

Godard A, Heymann D, Raher S, Anegon I, Peyrat MA, Le Mauff B, Mouray E, Gregoire M, Virdee K, Soulillou JP, Moreau JF, Jaques Y (1992) High and low affinity receptors for human interleukin for DA cells/leukemia inhibitory factor on human cells: molecular characterization and cellular distribution. J Biol Chem 267:3214–3222

Gouin F, Couillaud S, Cottrel M, Godard A, Passuti N, Heymann D (1999) Presence of leukaemia inhibitory factor (LIF) and LIF-receptor chain (gp190) in osteoclast-like cells cultured from human giant cell tumour of bone. Ultrastructural distribution. Cytokine 11:282–289

Grammatikakis N, Grammatikakis A, Yoneda M, Yu Q, Banerjee SD, Toole BP (1995) A novel glycosaminoglycan-binding protein is the vertebrate homologue of the cell cycle control protein, Cdc37. J Biol Chem 270:16198–16205

Grepin C, Robitaille L, Antakly T, Nemer M (1995) Inhibition of transcription factor GATA-4 expression blocks in vitro cardiac muscle differentiation. Mol Cell Biol 15:4095–4102

Heikinheimo M, Scandrett JM, Wilson DB (1994) Localization of transcription factor GATA-4 to regions of the mouse embryo involved in cardiac development. Dev Biol 164:361–373

Howells RD, Kilpatrick DL, Bailey LC, Noe M, Udenfriend S (1986) Proenkephalin mRNA in rat heart. Proc Natl Acad Sci U S A 83:1960–1963

Ikonen E, Simons K (1998) Protein and lipid sorting from the trans-Golgi network to the plasma membrane in polarized cells. Semin Cell Dev Biol 9:503–509

Jaspard B, Couffinhal T, Dufourcq P, Moreau C, Duplaa C (2000) Expression pattern of mouse sFRP-1 and mWnt-8 gene during heart morphogenesis. Mech Dev 90:263–267

Jiang HK, Owyang VV, Hong JS, Gallagher M (1989) Elevated dynorphin in the hippocampal formation of aged rats: relation to cognitive impairment on a spatial learning task. Proc Natl Acad Sci U S A 86:2948–2951

Jiang Y, Evans T (1996) The Xenopus GATA-4/5/6 genes are associated with cardiac specification and can regulate cardiac-specific transcription during embryogenesis. Dev Biol 174:258–270

Kashour T, Burton T, Dibrov A, Amara F (2003) Myogenic signaling by lithium in cardiomyoblasts is Akt independent but requires activation of the beta-catenin-Tcf/Lef pathway. J Mol Cell Cardiol 35:937–951

Kastner P, Grondona JM, Mark M, Gansmuller A, LeMeur M, Decimo D, Vonesch JL, Dolle P, Chambon P (1994) Genetic analysis of RXRα developmental function: convergence of RXR and RAR signaling pathways in heart and eye morphogenesis. Cell 78:987–1003

Kirby ML, Kumiski DH, Myers T, Cerjan C, Mishima N (1993) Backtransplantation of chick cardiac neural crest cells cultured in LIF rescues heart development. Dev Dyn 198:296–311

Klug MG, Soonpaa MH, Field LJ (1995) DNA synthesis and multinucleation in embryonic stem cell-derived cardiomyocytes. Am J Physiol 268:H1913–H1921

Klug MG, Soonpaa MH, Koh GY, Field LJ (1996) Genetically selected cardiomyocytes from differentiating embryonic stem cells form stable intracardiac grafts. J Clin Invest 98:216–224

Konig M, Zimmer AM, Steiner H, Holmes PV, Crawley JN, Brownstein MJ, Zimmer A (1996) Pain responses, anxiety and aggression in mice deficient in pre-proenkephalin. Nature 383:535–538

Kunisada K, Tone E, Fujio Y, Matsui H, Yamauchi-Takihara K, Kishimoto T (1998) Activation of gp130 transduces hypertrophic signals via STAT3 in cardiac myocytes. Circulation 98:346–352

Li Z, Colucci-Guyon E, Pincon-Raymond M, Mericskay M, Pournin S, Paulin D, Babinet C (1996) Cardiovascular lesions and skeletal myopathy in mice lacking desmin. Dev Biol 175:362–366

Linder ME, Deschenes RJ (2003) New insights into the mechanisms of protein palmitoylation. Biochemistry 42:4311–4320

Lints TJ, Parsons LM, Hartley L, Lyons I, Harvey RP (1993) Nkx-2.5: a novel murine homeobox gene expressed in early heart progenitor cells and their myogenic descendants. Development 119:419–431

Majumdar M, Meenakshi J, Goswami SK, Datta K (2002) Hyaluronan binding protein 1 (HABP1)/C1QBP/p32 is an endogenous substrate for MAP kinase and is translocated to the nucleus upon mitogenic stimulation. Biochem Biophys Res Commun 291:829–837

Maneckjee R, Minna JD (1992) Nonconventional opioid binding sites mediate growth inhibitory effects of methadone on human lung cancer cells. Proc Natl Acad Sci U S A 89:1169–1173

Matthes HW, Maldonado R, Simonin F, Valverde O, Slowe S, Kitchen I, Befort K, Dierich A, Le Meur M, Dolle P, Tzavara E, Hanoune J, Roques BP, Kieffer BL (1996) Loss of morphine-induced analgesia, reward effect and withdrawal symptoms in mice lacking the mu-opioid-receptor gene. Nature 383:819–823

McCue PA, Gubler ML, Sherman MI, Cohen BN (1984) Sodium butyrate induces histone hyperacetylation and differentiation of murine embryonal carcinoma cells. J Cell Biol 98:602–608

McLaughlin PJ (1996) Regulation of DNA synthesis of myocardial and epicardial cells in developing rat heart by [Met^5]enkephalin. Am J Physiol 271:R122–R129

Melkonyan HS, Chang WC, Shapiro JP, Mahadevappa M, Fitzpatrick PA, Kiefer MC, Tomei LD, Umansky SR (1997) SARPs: a family of secreted apoptosis-related proteins. Proc Natl Acad Sci U S A 94:13636–13641

Mendelsohn C, Lohnes D, Decimo D, Lufkin T, LeMeur M, Chambon P, Mark M (1994) Function of the retinoic acid receptors (RARs) during development (II). Multiple abnormalities at various stages of organogenesis in RAR double mutants. Development 120:2749–2771

Meriney SD, Ford MJ, Oliva D, Pilar G (1991) Endogenous opioids modulate neuronal survival in the developing avian ciliary ganglion. J Neurosci 11:3705–3717

Milner DJ, Weitzer G, Tran D, Bradley A, Capetanaki Y (1996) Disruption of muscle architecture and myocardial degeneration in mice lacking desmin. J Cell Biol 134:1255–1270

Moroianu J, Riordan JF (1994) Nuclear translocation of angiogenic proteins in endothelial cells: an essential step in angiogenesis. Biochemistry 33:12535–12539

Nakamura T, Sano M, Songyang Z, Schneider MD (2003) A Wnt- and beta-catenin-dependent pathway for mammalian cardiac myogenesis. Proc Natl Acad Sci U S A 100:5834–5839

Nusse R (1999) WNT targets. Repression and activation. Trends Genet 15:1–3

Ogryzko VV, Schiltz RL, Russanova V, Howard BH, Nakatani Y (1996) The transcriptional coactivators p300 and CBP are histone acetyltransferases. Cell 87:953–959

Oka M, Tagoku K, Russell TL, Nakano Y, Hamazaki T, Meyer EM, Yokota T, Terada N (2002) CD9 is associated with leukemia inhibitory factor-mediated maintenance of embryonic stem cells. Mol Biol Cell 13:1274–1281

Pandur P, Läsche M, Eisenberg LM, Kühl M (2002) Wnt-11 activation of a non-canonical Wnt signalling pathway is required for cardiogenesis. Nature 418:636–641

Paradis H, Arceci RJ, Adams LC, Gendron RL (1998) Differentiation responses of embryonic endothelium to leukemia inhibitory factor. Exp Cell Res 240:7–15

Patterson SI (2002) Posttranslational protein S-palmitoylation and the compartmentalization of signaling molecules in neurons. Biol Res 35:139–150

Pepper MS, Ferrara N, Orci L, Montesano R (1995) Leukemia inhibitory factor (LIF) inhibits angiogenesis in vitro. J Cell Sci 108:73–83

Rathjen PD, Toth S, Willis A, Heath JK, Smith AG (1990) Differentiation inhibiting activity is produced in matrix-associated and diffusible forms that are generated by alternate promoter usage. Cell 62:1105–1114

Rattner A, Hsieh JC, Smallwood PM, Gilbert DJ, Copeland NG, Jenkins NA, Nathans J (1997) A family of secreted proteins contains homology to the cysteine-rich ligand-binding domain of frizzled receptors. Proc Natl Acad Sci U S A 94:2859–2863

Rawadi G, Vayssiere B, Dunn F, Baron R, Roman-Roman S (2003) BMP-2 controls alkaline phosphatase expression and osteoblast mineralization by a Wnt autocrine loop. J Bone Miner Res 18:1842–1853

Re RN (1989) The cellular biology of angiotensin: paracrine, autocrine and intracrine actions in cardiovascular tissues. J Mol Cell Cardiol 21:63–69

Re RN (1999) The nature of intracrine peptide hormone action. Hypertension 34:534–538

Re RN (2000) On the biological actions of intracellular angiotensin. Hypertension 35:1189–1190

Re RN (2002) The origins of intracrine hormone action. Am J Med Sci 323:43–48

Re RN (2003) The intracrine hypothesis and intracellular peptide hormone action. Bioessays 25:401–409

Reichsman F, Smith L, Cumberledge S (1996) Glycosaminoglycans can modulate extracellular localization of the wingless protein and promote signal transduction. J Cell Biol 135:819–827

Rigter H (1978) Attenuation of amnesia in rats by systemically administered enkephalins. Science 200:83–85

Schott JJ, Benson DW, Basson CT, Pease W, Silberbach GM, Moak JP, Maron BJ, Seidman CE, Seidman JG (1998) Congenital heart disease caused by mutations in the transcription factor Nkx-2.5. Science 281:108–111

Shea CM, Edgar CM, Einhorn TA, Gerstenfeld LC (2003) BMP treatment of C3H10T1/2 mesenchymal stem cells induces both chondrogenesis and osteogenesis. J Cell Biochem 90:1112–1127

Sheng Z, Pennica D, Wood WI, Chien KR (1996) Cardiotrophin-1 displays early expression in the murine heart tube and promotes cardiac myocyte survival. Development 122:419–428

Shimizu H, Julius MA, Giarre M, Zheng Z, Brown AM, Kitajewski J (1997) Transformation by Wnt family proteins correlates with regulation of beta-catenin. Cell Growth Differ 8:1349–1358

Simons K, Ikonen E (1997) Functional rafts in cell membranes. Nature 387:569–572

Slusarski DC, Corces VG, Moon RT (1997a) Interaction of Wnt and Frizzled homologue triggers G-protein-linked phosphatidylinositol signaling. Nature 390:410–413

Slusarski DC, Yang-Snyder J, Busa WB, Moon RT (1997b) Modulation of embryonic intracellular Ca^{2+} signaling by Wnt-5A. Dev Biol 182:114–120

Smith CD, Wells WW (1983) Phosphorylation of rat liver nuclear envelopes. II. Characterization of in vitro lipid phosphorylation. J Biol Chem 258:9368–9373

Sucov HM, Dyson E, Gumeringer CL, Price J, Chien KR, Evans RM (1994) RXRa mutant mice establish a genetic basis for vitamin A signaling in heart morphogenesis. Genes Dev 8:1007–1018

Sylvia VL, Joe CO, Norman JO, Curtin GM, Busbee DL (1986) Phosphatidylinositol-dependent activation of DNA polymerase alpha. Biochem Biophys Res Commun 135:880–885

Tammi R, Rilla K, Pienimaki JP, MacCallum DK, Hogg M, Luukkonen M, Hascall VC, Tammi M (2001) Hyaluronan enters keratinocytes by a novel endocytic route for catabolism. J Biol Chem 276:35111–35122

Tanaka K, Okabayashi K, Asashima M, Perrimon N, Kadowaki T (2000) The evolutionarily conserved porcupine gene family is involved in the processing of the Wnt family. Eur J Biochem 267:4300–4311

Tang F, Costa E, Schwartz JP (1983) Increase of proenkephalin mRNA, and enkephalin content of rat striatum after daily injection of haloperidol for 2 to 3 weeks. Proc Natl Acad Sci U S A 80:3841–3844

Tang SS, Zheng GG, Wu KF, Chen GB, Liu HZ, Rao O (2001) Autocrine and possible intracrine regulation of HL-60 cell proliferation by macrophage colony-stimulating factor. Leuk Res 25:1107–1114

Taupin JL, Pitard V, Dechanet J, Miossec V, Gualde N, Moreau JF (1998) Leukemia inhibitory factor: part of a large ingathering family. Int Rev Immunol 16:397–426

Thorpe CJ, Schlesinger A, Carter JC, Bowerman B (1997) Wnt signaling polarizes an early C. elegans blastomere to distinguish endoderm from mesoderm. Cell 90:695–705

Towle MF, Mondragon-Escorpizo M, Norin A, Fukada K (1998) Deprivation of leukemia inhibitory factor by its function-blocking antibodies augments T cell activation. J Interferon Cytokine Res 18:387–392

Tzahor E, Lassar AB (2001) Wnt signals from the neural tube block ectopic cardiogenesis. Genes Dev 15:255–260

Ventura C, Pintus G (1997) Opioid peptide gene expression in the primary hereditary cardiomyopathy of the Syrian hamster. Part III. Autocrine stimulation of prodynorphin gene expression by dynorphin B. J Biol Chem 272:6699–6705

Ventura C, Maioli M (2000) Opioid peptide gene expression primes cardiogenesis in embryonal pluripotent stem cells. Circ Res 87:189–194

Ventura C, Capogrossi MC, Spurgeon HA, Lakatta EG (1991a) κ-opioid peptide receptor stimulation increases cytosolic pH and myofilament responsiveness to Ca^{2+} in cardiac myocytes. Am J Physiol 261:H1671–H1674

Ventura C, Guarnieri C, Stefanelli C, Cirielli C, Lakatta EG, Capogrossi MC (1991b) Comparison between alpha-adrenergic and κ-opioidergic mediated inositol(1,4,5)P3/inositol(1,3,4,5)P4 formation in adult cultured rat ventricular cardiomyocytes. Biochem Biophys Res Commun 179:972–978

Ventura C, Spurgeon HA, Lakatta EG, Guarnieri C, Capogrossi MC (1992) κ and δ opioid receptor stimulation affects cardiac myocyte function and Ca^{2+} release from an intracellular pool in myocytes and neurons. Circ Res 70:66–81

Ventura C, Guarnieri C, Vaona I, Campana G, Pintus G, Spampinato S (1994) Dynorphin gene expression and release in the myocardial cell. J Biol Chem 269:5384–5386

Ventura C, Pintus G, Vaona I, Bennardini F, Pinna G, Tadolini B (1995) Phorbol ester regulation of opioid peptide gene expression in myocardial cells. J Biol Chem 270:30115–30120

Ventura C, Pintus G, Fiori MG, Bennardini F, Pinna G, Gaspa L (1997a) Opioid peptide gene expression in the primary hereditary cardiomyopathy of the Syrian hamster. Part I. Regulation of prodynorphin gene expression by nuclear protein kinase C. J Biol Chem 272:6685–6692

Ventura C, Pintus G, Tadolini, B (1997b) Opioid peptide gene expression in the primary hereditary cardiomyopathy of the Syrian hamster. Part II. Role of intracellular calcium loading. J Biol Chem 272:6693–6698

Ventura C, Zinellu E, Maninchedda E, Fadda M, Maioli M (2003a) Protein kinase C signaling transduces endorphin-primed cardiogenesis in GTR1 embryonic stem cells. Circ Res 92:617–622

Ventura C, Zinellu E, Maninchedda E, Maioli M (2003b) Dynorphin B is an agonist of nuclear opioid receptors coupling nuclear protein kinase C activation to the transcription of cardiogenic genes in GTR1 embryonic stem cells. Circ Res 92:623–629

Ventura C, Maioli M, Asara Y, Santoni D, Scarlata I, Cantoni S, Perbellini A (2004) Butyric and retinoic mixed ester of hyaluronan: a novel differentiating glycoconjugate affording a high-throughput of cardiogenesis in embryonic stem cells. J Biol Chem 279:23574–23579

Weihe E, McKnight AT, Corbett AD, Kosterlitz HW (1985) Proenkephalin- and prodynorphin-derived opioid peptides in guinea pig heart. Neuropeptides 5:453–456

Wheatley SC, Isacke CM, Crossley PH (1993) Restricted expression of the hyaluronan receptor, CD44, during postimplantation mouse embryogenesis suggests key roles in tissue formation and patterning. Development 119:295–306

Willert K, Brown JD, Danenberg E, Duncan AW, Weissman IL, Reya T, Yates JR 3rd, Nusse R (2003) Wnt proteins are lipid-modified and can act as stem cell growth factors. Nature 423:448–452

Wobus AM, Kaomei G, Shan J, Wellner MC, Rohwedel J, Ji G, Fleischmann B, Katus HA, Hescheler J, Franz WM (1997) Retinoic acid accelerates embryonic stem cell-derived cardiac differentiation and enhances development of ventricular cardiomyocytes. J Mol Cell Cardiol 29:1525–1539

Wodarz A, Nusse R (1998) Mechanisms of Wnt signaling in development. Annu Rev Cell Dev Biol 14:59–88

Wolffe AP, Pruss D (1996) Targeting chromatin disruption: transcription regulators that acetylate histones. Cell 84:817–819

Xu Q, D'Amore PA, Sokol SY (1998) Functional and biochemical interactions of Wnts with FrzA, a secreted Wnt antagonist. Development 125:4767–4776

Yang-Snyder J, Miller JR, Brown JD, Lai CJ, Moon RT (1996) A frizzled homolog functions in a vertebrate Wnt signaling pathway. Curr Biol 6:1302–1306

Yu H, Fukami K, Watanabe Y, Ozaki C, Takenawa T (1998) Phosphatidylinositol 4,5-bisphosphate reverses the inhibition of RNA transcription caused by histone H1. Eur J Biochem 251:281–287

Zagon IS, Rhodes RE, McLaughlin PJ (1985) Distribution of enkephalin immunoreactivity in germinative cells of developing rat cerebellum. Science 227:1049–1051

Zagon IS, McLaughlin PJ (1991) Identification of opioid peptides regulating proliferation of neurons and glia in the developing nervous system. Brain Res 542:318–323

7

Zagon IS, McLaughlin PJ (1992) An opioid growth factor regulates the replication of microorganisms. Life Sci 50:1179–1187

Zagon IS, Sassani JW, McLaughlin PJ (1995) Opioid growth factor modulates corneal epithelial outgrowth in tissue culture. Am J Physiol 268:R942–R9450

Zhai L, Chaturvedi D, Cumberledge S (2004) Drosophila Wnt-1 undergoes a hydrophobic modification and is targeted to lipid rafts, a process that requires Porcupine. J Biol Chem 279:33220–33227

Zhang S, Chang MC, Zylka D, Turley S, Harrison R, Turley EA (1998) The hyaluronan receptor RHAMM regulates extracellular-regulated kinase. J Biol Chem 273:11342–11348

HEP (2006) 174:147–167
© Springer-Verlag Berlin Heidelberg 2006

Therapeutic Potential of Stem Cells in Diabetes

E. Roche · R. Enseñat-Waser · J. A. Reig · J. Jones · T. León-Quinto · B. Soria (✉)

Instituto de Bioingenieria, Universidad Miguel Hernandez, 03550 San Juan, Spain
bsoria@upos.es

Abstract Stem cells possess the ability to self-renew by symmetric divisions and, under certain circumstances, differentiate to a committed lineage by asymmetric cell divisions. Depending on the origin, stem cells are classified as either embryonic or adult. Embryonic stem cells are obtained from the inner cell mass of the blastocyst, a structure that appears during embryonic development at day 6 in humans and day 3.5 in mice. Adult stem cells are present within tissues of adult organisms and are responsible for cell turnover or repopulation of tissues under normal or exceptional circumstances. Taken together, stem cells might represent a potential source of tissues for cell therapy protocols, and diabetes is a candidate disease that may benefit from cell replacement protocols. The pathology of type 1 diabetes is caused by the autoimmune destruction or malfunction of pancreatic β cells, and consequently, a lack of insulin. The absence of insulin is life-threatening, thus requiring diabetic patients to take daily hormone injections from exogenous sources; however, insulin injections do not adequately mimic β cell function. This results in the development of diabetic complications such as neuropathy, nephropathy, retinopathy and diverse cardiovascular disorders. This chapter intends to summarize the possibilities opened by embryonic and adult stem cells in regenerative medicine for the cure of diabetes.

Keywords Diabetes · Insulin · Stem cells · Cell therapy · β cells

Abbreviations

AFP	α-Fetoprotein
ASCs	Adult stem cells

bFGF	Basic fibroblast growth factor
CHIBs	Cultivated human islet buds
CMV	Cytomegalovirus promoter
EBs	Embryoid bodies
EGF	Epidermal growth factor
EGFP	Enhanced green fluorescent protein
ESCs	Embryonic stem cells
GFAP	Glial fibrillary acidic protein
HGF	Hepatic growth factor
IGFs	Insulin-like growth factors
IL-3	Interleukin-3
IPSCs	Islet pluripotent stem cells
ITSFn	Insulin + transferring + selenium + fibronectin
KGF	Keratinocyte growth factor
LIF	Leukaemia inhibitory factor
MAPCs	Multipotent adult progenitor cells
MBP	Myelin basic protein
NF-200	Neurofilament-200
M-CSF	Macrophage colony stimulating factor
NIPs	Nestin-positive islet-derived progenitors
Pax4	Paired homeobox 4
Pax6	Paired homeobox 6
Pdx1	Pancreatic duodenal homeobox 1
PGCs	Primordial germ cells
STZ	Streptozotocin
TH	Tyrosine hydroxylase

1
Introduction

1.1
Diabetes

Diabetes is characterized by a default in insulin secretion (low secretion or even total absence of the hormone) that impairs adequate control of glycaemia, leading to a general metabolic dysfunction and death. The main cause of the disease is the specific destruction of insulin-producing cells (β cells), located within the endocrine pancreas inside typical cell structures called islets of Langerhans. Diabetes is classified as type 1 and type 2 (DeFronzo et al. 2004).

In type 1 diabetes, β cells are destroyed by the immune system of the individual. There are other rare forms of type 1 diabetes of idiopathic origin, although in the majority of the cases it is an autoimmune disease. Antibodies against proteins located at the surface of the β cell (anti-islet), and against intracellular proteins (anti-glutamate dehydrogenase, anti-tyrosin phosphatase) have been described (Benoist et al. 1997; Mathis et al. 2001). The disease affects mainly, but not exclusively, children and young people. In fact, recent findings indicate that 5%–15% of adults initially diagnosed with type 2 diabetes can suffer a less severe and slow progressing form of type 1 diabetes called latent autoimmune diabetes (LADA) (Zimmet et al. 2001).

Type 2 diabetes represents a more complex pathological entity in which environmental factors and genetic predisposition co-participate to different degrees (Saltiel 2001; Bell and Polonsky 2001). Either insulin secretion defects or insulin resistance appears first, and this is initially compensated by an increased secretion of the hormone (hyperinsulinaemia) (Polonsky et al. 1996; Zierath et al. 2000). However, insulin resistance cannot cause severe diabetes, as has been demonstrated in transgenic models (Bruning et al. 1998). The dysfunction of pancreatic β cells seems to be the key event to culminate in overt type 2 diabetes (Poitout and Robertson 1996). This is related to an excess of circulating nutrients (mainly glucose and fatty acids) that can affect β cell function, impairing insulin secretion and gene expression profiles (glucolipotoxicity) (Prentki et al. 2000; Roche 2003). Therefore, there is a strong correlation between type 2 diabetes and hyperlipidaemia, hypercholesterolaemia, excess weight and obesity (DeFronzo et al. 2004). This disease affects mainly people of industrialized countries, with a prevalence of 10%. In addition, this incidence is increasing dramatically, and it is estimated that in 20 years' time, this value will double. The activation of cell suicide programs (apoptosis) culminates, long-term, with β cell loss, such that chronically type 2 diabetes becomes similar to type 1 (Prentki et al. 2000; Maechler and Wollheim 2001). Therefore, both pathologies would benefit from cell replacement protocols.

1.2
Islet Transplantation and the Need for Alternative Sources of Cells

At the present time, there is no definitive cure for diabetes. Insulin injection does not mimic the precise regulation that β cells exert on glucose homeostasis, leading long term to the development of complications in diabetic patients (Brownlee 2001). Replacement of the damaged organ (i.e. islets) seems to be a logical strategy to treat diabetes, and recently, a transplantation protocol of islets of Langerhans isolated from cadaveric donors has been established by the group of Dr. Shapiro in Edmonton, Alberta, Canada (Shapiro et al. 2000).

This strategy has several advantages with respect to surgical interventions that involve the double transplantation of kidney and pancreas. First, only islets of Langerhans (the structures containing insulin), and not the whole pancreas, are transplanted. Islets comprise the endocrine portion (1%) of the pancreas, while the exocrine part (99%) is devoted to food digestion. In one sense, islets can be considered as densely microvascularized and innervated micro-organs that contain a heterogeneous population of cells specialized in hormone production (i.e. α cells/glucagon, β cells/insulin, δ cells/somatostatin and PP cells/pancreatic polypeptide). Adult pancreas contains 1 million islets and each islet contains around 2,000 cells 60% of which are β cells. Therefore, the transplantation of islets vs whole pancreas has obvious advantages with respect to the amount of the organ that must be manipulated during isolation and surgery. However, semiautomatic islet isolation from the pancreas is time-consuming and of low yield (50%), thus requiring the use of two pancreata per recipient. Second, the Edmonton protocol employs a combination of immune suppressors, such as sirolimus, tacrolimus and daczimulab, to permit long-term islet survival (Shapiro et al. 2000). Nevertheless, this immune-suppression protocol, which has limited adverse side effects, would be expected to affect normal immunological responses (Oluwole et al. 2004). Third, the main improvement of the Edmonton protocol resides in the isolation method itself. This method utilizes a special device called a Ricordi chamber that combines mechanical disruption with enzymatic digestion by liberase (a highly purified blend of collagenase) or recombinant collagenase (Gray et al. 2004; Barshes et al. 2004; Georges et al. 2002; Brandhorst et al. 2003), the combination of which has improved the purity, yield, and survival of islets from donor pancreas. Fourth, islet transplantation is less invasive and economically more viable than organ transplantation. Pancreas transplantation, often performed as a double transplant with kidney, requires major surgery with general anaesthesia, prolonged hospital stays and considerable financial costs for insurance companies. Islet transplantation, in contrast, only requires minor surgery (intraperitoneal injection into the portal vein) and local anaesthesia, thus facilitating rapid patient recovery with substantially reduced economic costs.

During the past 4 or more years, over 400 patients worldwide have benefited from this therapeutic intervention. In addition to avoiding daily insulin injections, major complications have been circumvented, and a reduction in diabetic complications generally has been observed during the follow-up of these patients (Ryan et al. 2002). However, due to the scarcity of cadaveric pancreata and the low yield of islets obtained by this procedure (50%), not all people have access to this surgical intervention. New cell sources, therefore, are necessary for an efficient replacement protocol, and in this sense stem cells offer a promising possibility that deserves to be explored.

2
Embryonic Stem Cells

Embryonic stem cells (ESCs) are obtained from the inner cell mass of the blastocyst, a structure that appears during embryonic development at day 6 in humans and day 3.5 in mice (Smith 2001). The main properties of these cells include a robust capacity for self-renewal and the potential to differentiate into specific cell lineages (Wobus and Boheler 2005). Due to this plasticity, ESCs are generally considered pluripotent, and because of the recent success in generating insulin-producing cells from ESCs, the therapeutic potential will be considered in more detail.

2.1
Spontaneous Differentiation

Cultured mouse ESCs form characteristic adherent colonies in the presence of leukaemia inhibitory factor (LIF), a cytokine that maintains the cells in an undifferentiated state. Alternatively, the undifferentiated phenotype is maintained by growing ESCs on feeder layers of mitotically inactivated fibroblasts. Under these conditions, cells express a characteristic gene pattern of pluripotentiality, including Oct3/4; Nanog, ESG-1 genes, SSEA-1 surface antigen and alkaline phosphatase activity (Smith 2001; Mitsui et al. 2003; Tanaka et al. 2002). In contrast, human ESCs do not respond to human LIF and when cultured on fibroblast feeder layers, they still initiate differentiation processes (Smith 1991), which effectively renders these cells more difficult to cultivate in vitro than mouse ESCs.

During continuous culture and after several passages, we have observed that undifferentiated mouse ES cell lines (R1 and D3) yield heterogeneous cell populations. According to the pattern of gene expression, these cells correspond to ectodermal lineages that express specific markers after several passages, such as glial fibrillary acidic protein (GFAP) and neurofilament-200 (NF-200). A likely explanation pointed out by others is that ESCs do not require complex extracellular signals to differentiate to ectoderm, supporting a default model for in vitro differentiation (Ying et al. 2003). This may explain why ectoderm derivatives are easily obtained in bioengineering protocols. Clonal selection could circumvent this problem, although it is recommended to check the pattern of gene expression in ESC cultures after several passages, even in the presence of LIF (Fig. 1).

The transfer from adherent culture conditions to suspension cultures and LIF withdrawal are key manipulations that activate in vitro differentiation programs. Under these conditions, cells form aggregates called embryoid bodies (EBs), in which markers from different lineages are evident (Smith 1991). The molecular determinants that modulate differentiation in EBs are still unknown, but it has been suggested that gradients in oxygen, nutrients and growth factors, as well as cell connections, interactions and paracrine factors are instrumental (Roche et al. 2003).

Taking into account the gene expression profile, different cell lineages form within EBs, including ectoderm, mesoderm and endoderm. Cell precursors present in EBs could theoretically yield specific cell types present in the adult organism or in intermediate stages of embryonic development. Ectoderm markers, such as NF-200 and GFAP, are detected from day 1 in EBs; however, mesoderm markers, such as brachyury, α- and β-myosin heavy chain as well as atrial natriuretic peptide present a delayed expression (3–10 days) in EBs. Endoderm markers, such as α-fetoprotein (AFP) and glucagon (Soria et al. 2001), are observed much later in 10- to 20-day EBs. The determinants that regulate the evolution of all these cell precursors in EBs are still unknown. On

a   b

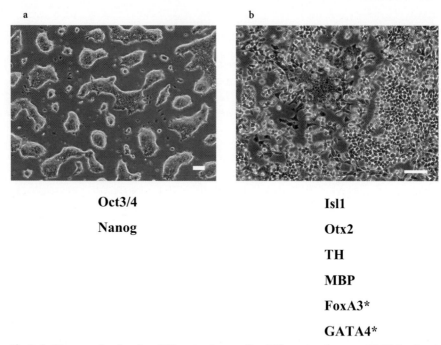

Oct3/4   Isl1

Nanog   Otx2

                                            TH

                                            MBP

                                            FoxA3*

                                            GATA4*

Fig. 1a,b Micrographs showing different cultures of undifferentiated mouse R1-ESCs after 8 (**a**) and 26 (**b**) passages in the presence of LIF. Gene markers characteristic of each passage are listed. Markers of pluripotency are expressed in **a**. Genes characteristics of ectoderm are expressed in **b**. Markers of primitive endoderm (*) are expressed also in **b** when cells are seed highly confluent. Bar, 100 μm

one hand and as mentioned before, ectoderm precursors seem to respond to a default mechanism (Ying et al. 2003), although alternative pathways cannot be discarded. In addition, determinants effective in derivation of mesoderm and endoderm lineages are also unknown, although some data demonstrate the participation of mesendoderm precursors (Kubo et al. 2004). On the other hand, the exact identity in vitro for endoderm (primitive or definitive) is not clear due to the number of markers shared by both lineages (Ku et al. 2004; Milne et al. 2005) (Fig. 2).

In addition, expression of Oct3/4 (marker of pluripotency) suggests the presence of residual undifferentiated cells at the level of EBs in standard protocols of differentiation in the absence of LIF. Oct3/4 is downregulated when cells initiate a differentiation process (Niwa et al. 2000). In vivo, Oct3/4 is reduced during gastrulation, when cells differentiate into the three germ layers. In vitro, this occurs approximately after day 6 of culture in EBs, although a residual population of positive cells remains for long periods of incubation. This population has been observed and purified following transfection of R1 mouse ESCs with a genetic construction containing the Oct3/4 gene promoter

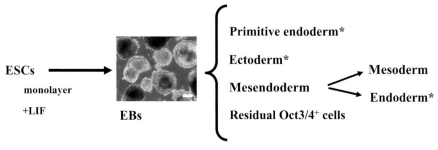

Fig. 2 Proposed pattern of lineage differentiation in EBs (micrograph) cultured in vitro. Ectoderm appears quickly and requires no complex signals. Primitive endoderm and residual undifferentiated cells Oct3/4+ are also present, and the existence of a mesendoderm lineage that forms meso- and endoderm can be envisioned. All of the proposed pathways require additional detailed studies. *Lineages that can derive insulin-positive cells. Bar, 100 μm

driving the expression of the enhanced green fluorescent protein (EGFP). Derived EBs displayed a characteristic fluorescence during the first 24 h in culture. According to the fluorescence intensity, the population of positive cells expressing Oct3/4 was maintained at over 95% for 5 days. However, there was an evident reduction of the EGFP expression after day 6 of culture. At day 8, the fluorescence and the population of EGFP-positive cells were dramatically decreased as the differentiation of most cells into the EBs progressed. Finally, a small proportion of residual green fluorescent cells was still present in the EBs, even after 30 days of culture (Fig. 3).

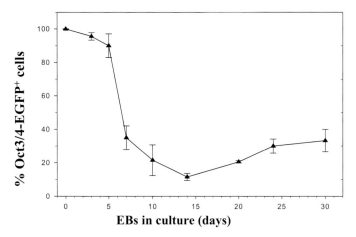

Fig. 3 Time course of fluorescent cells (%) in EBs obtained from mouse R1-ESCs transfected with a DNA construct in which Oct3/4 promoter drives the expression of EGFP. Fluorescence cell sorting analysis shows the presence of a residual undifferentiated population (20%) Oct3/4+

At this time (30 days), EGFP-positive cells were isolated from EBs by cell sorting and further cultured. Two possibilities were considered in order to better characterize these Oct3/4-positive cells: presence of residual undifferentiated cells or in vitro generation of primordial germ cells (PGCs) that also are positive for Oct3/4 (Pesce et al. 1998). To discriminate between these two alternatives, we determined by quantitative PCR the expression of VASA (Mvh), a marker for PGCs (Toyooka et al. 2000). VASA expression in sorted cells was very low, similar to values determined in undifferentiated R1 ESCs. This result reinforces the alternative idea that these Oct3/4-positive cells could be residual undifferentiated cells. To test this possibility, we studied the development of these cells after subcutaneous injection into immunodeficient mice. Some weeks after injection, we observed the presence of tumours displaying different cell types. Altogether, this result supports pluripotence latency in vitro in these cells, which is somehow switched on in an in vivo environment. The factors and mechanisms participating in these processes are still unknown.

Gating selection strategies could eliminate these cells from culture in bioengineering protocols; however, the presence of tumors reported after transplantation in several reports indicates apparently that these residual cells cannot totally be extinguished under standard culture conditions (Lumelsky et al. 2001). These results demonstrate that a small fraction of residual undifferentiated cells remains in EBs in conditions that support the differentiation of the rest of cells. Due to their potential to form tumours, in vitro extinction protocols or in vivo biosafety mechanisms should be considered in future research when using ESCs.

Insulin together with other pancreatic hormones has been observed during spontaneous differentiation in EBs as early as 10–23 days (Soria et al. 2001). However, the parental lineage leading to insulin-positive cells has not been properly characterized. In this vein, ectoderm, extraembryonic endoderm as well as definitive endoderm are all candidate lineages capable of expressing this hormone (Melloul et al. 2002). These considerations are instrumental in bioengineering protocols in which the final cell product has to mimic as much as possible β cell function. Little is known about the differentiation and function of insulin-positive cells derived from lineages outside of definitive endoderm. In the case of ectoderm, recent reports suggested that pro-insulin is working as a growth factor, controlling apoptotic processes during neuronal development in stages in which insulin-like growth factors (IGFs) are absent (Vicario-Abejón et al. 2003). Rodents have two insulin genes, known as insulin I and II. The insulin I gene is exclusively expressed in pancreatic tissue, while insulin II is expressed in islets, yolk sac and certain neurons (Melloul et al. 2002). The consideration of the differences observed in terms of gene regulation, hormone processing and production could be instrumental in order to design reproducible protocols for obtaining insulin-secreting cells suitable for replacement trials (Hernández-Sánchez et al. 2003) (Table 1).

Table 1 Key differences (1–5) and similarities (6–9) displayed by insulin-positive cells derived from ectoderm and definitive endoderm that could be instrumental in bioengineering protocols

Component	Ectoderm	Endoderm
1. Processing	Prepronsulin→proinsulin	Prepronsulin→proinsulin →insulin
2. Gene regulation	During development	By nutrients
3. Genes	Insulin II (mouse)	Insulin I (mouse)
4. Amount	1×	1,000×
5. Function	Growth factor	Anabolic hormone
	Tissue remodelling	Nutrient homeostasis
6. Components of excitatory machinery		
7. Proteins of the secretory pathway		
8. Glucose-sensing machinery		
9. Transcription factors		

2.2
Directed Differentiation

A well-detailed and definitive in vitro protocol to obtain insulin-secreting cells for replacement trials does not exist at present. However, different approaches have been developed by several laboratories for mouse and human ESCs. These may be classified into three categories, even though the working protocols are in fact a combination of each. The strategies are:

1. Gating selection protocols

2. Coaxial methods

3. Directional strategies.

2.2.1
Gating Selection Protocols

Gating technology or cell trapping systems confer an advantage to certain groups of cells, based on the expression of specific genes, like those that confer resistance to antibiotics or express fluorescence proteins (i.e. EGFP). This strategy is a relatively simple genetic approach that produces essentially pure cultures of precursors or differentiated cells from ESCs.

In this method, ESCs are transfected with two DNA selection cassettes (i.e. transgenes) that are often incorporated into a common DNA vector. The first cassette makes use of a constitutively active promoter to drive expression of a gene (usually drug resistance protein), which can be used to select cells that have incorporated the DNA-construct (clonal selection). The second DNA cassette utilizes a promoter to drive the expression of the second transgene (i.e. drug-resistance protein, EGFP, cell-surface marker) exclusively in one cell type, to facilitate the purification of the desired cell type (Klug et al. 1996; Li et al. 1998; Müller et al. 2000; Soria et al. 2000).

The strategy used to obtain insulin-secreting cells from ESCs (Soria et al. 2000) consists of a selection protocol based on resistance to two antibiotics: hygromycin, under the control of the constitutive promoter of the phosphoglycerate kinase gene, and neomycin, under the control of the regulatory regions of the insulin gene promoter. A key point to consider with this strategy, particularly in lineages other than definitive endoderm, is the possibility that insulin expression may differ from that seen in β cells. Ideally, the expression of the gene driving the selection cassettes must be specific and unique for the final cell type. If the promoter-gene construct is expressed in other cell types, then cell selection with gating technology will be sub-optimal.

Gating technology could also be used to enrich lineage precursors that expression selection transgenes under the control of promoters expressed at intermediate stages of development. Based on this idea, we have recently developed a new gating protocol designed to isolate islet precursor cells through the use of a construct containing the Nkx6.1 gene promoter and neomycin resistance cassette (León-Quinto et al. 2004). Nkx6.1 is a transcription factor functionally active during intermediate stages of embryonic development of islet cell precursors and in the final differentiated stage of β cells (Chakrabarti and Mirmira 2003). The selection with neomycin, together with specific culture conditions, including addition of nicotinamide, anti-sonic hedgehog and conditioned media from pancreatic buds, produced a pure population of cells co-expressing insulin, Pdx1, Nkx6.1, glucokinase, GLUT-2 and Sur-1. In vitro, the selected cells responded to increasing concentrations of extracellular glucose, and when cell grafts were transplated under the kidney capsule of streptozotocin-treated diabetic mice for 3 weeks, resting glucose levels were restored to normal. When the graft was removed, the mice once again became hyperglycaemic (Fig. 4). Although insulin content was still very low, these cells generated reproducible amounts of intracellular hormone that may be increased in future protocols (León-Quinto et al. 2004).

The use of gating technology to obtain precursor cells has an important advantage, because progenitor cells are capable of proliferating and generating large cell numbers. However, the cells will need to undergo further maturation protocols in order to develop fully functional insulin-releasing cells suitable for cell replacement trials. In conclusion, gating selection protocols are being used in combination with directed differentiation protocols to increase the

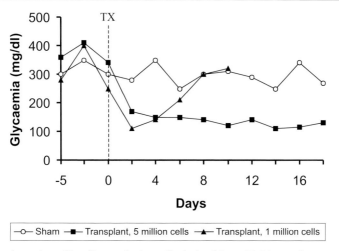

Fig. 4 Transplantation of insulin-producing cells derived from Nkx6.1-neo[r] expressing ESCs under the kidney capsule of STZ-diabetic animals normalize blood glucose (León-Quinto et al. 2004). This effect is dependent on the cell mass transplanted. *TX*, day of transplantation

proportion of islet progenitors and differentiated cells that can be obtained for possible therapeutic purposes (León-Quinto et al. 2004).

2.2.2
Coaxial Methods

Coaxial methods employ differentiation strategies based on the addition of specific growth factors to the culture medium to drive ESCs to generate insulin-positive cells. Good examples of this methodology involve protocols developed to isolate nestin-positive cells as precursors of endocrine pancreatic cells. The principle protocol using this methodology comprises five steps (Lumelsky et al. 2001):

1. Expansion of ESCs in the presence of LIF

2. EB formation in the absence of LIF

3. Selection of nestin-positive cells in the outgrowth phase by plating the EBs in serum-free ITSFn medium (DMEM/F12 containing insulin, transferrin, selenium and fibronectin)

4. Expansion of nestin-positive cells in serum-free N2 medium (DMEM/F12 containing B27 supplement, insulin, transferrin, selenium, progesterone and putrescine supplemented with bFGF [basic fibroblast growth factor])

5. Expression of insulin, performed by incubation of the cells in N2 medium as clusters (as previously described by Soria et al. 2000), but in the absence of bFGF and in the presence of nicotinamide (proposed also by Soria et al. 2000)

Due to the low insulin content obtained through this protocol, additional modifications proved necessary. These include the addition of the phospho-inositide-3-kinase inhibitors LY294002 or wortmannin in step 5 (Hori et al. 2002), the introduction of growth factors, such as KGF and EGF (keratinocyte and epidermal growth factors, respectively), and in step 4, the use of gating selection strategies (Moritoh et al. 2003; Miyazaki et al. 2004). All of these modifications have led to modest increases of insulin content insufficient to be considered useful in transplantation trials. Furthermore, comparison of different protocols based on nestin-positive cell selection suggests that ISTFn and bFGF selected cells are committed to neuroectoderm before pancreatic differentiation is induced (Kania et al. 2004).

Nestin, which is usually considered a marker of neuronal lineages, is abundantly expressed in rat and human pancreatic islets (Zulewski et al. 2001); however, the role of nestin progenitors of islet cells remains controversial. Some authors have suggested that nestin-positive cells could play a role in the formation of the microvasculature of the islet (Treutelaar et al. 2003; Piper et al. 2002); consequently, bioengineered cells that express nestin and that are isolated by coaxial protocols, may not correspond to differentiated β cells. Instead, these cells may only have an ability to mimic some aspects of β cell function. Interestingly, some groups have been able to obtain insulin-positive cells from human ESCs based on the selection of nestin precursors developed in mice (Segev et al. 2004). This method was improved by lowering the glucose concentration in step 5, as previously described (Soria et al. 2000). The authors of this publication claimed that the final cells were immature islet-like aggregates, because of the low cell responsiveness to glucose and co-expression of insulin with other pancreatic endocrine hormones, such as glucagon and somatostatin (Polak et al. 2000). Although improvements in this protocol are necessary, this demonstrates that human ESCs can be bioengineered in vitro to produce insulin-secreting cells, opening exciting possibilities in diabetes treatment.

2.2.3
Directional Strategies

The aim of directional strategies is to achieve constitutive overexpression of key transcription factors implicated in β cell function or development through transfection of constructs containing the corresponding cDNAs and regulated by strong constitutive promoters (i.e. CMV). These strategies are generally used to complement coaxial protocols. For example, one group used ESCs stably transfected with Pdx1 or Pax4 to promote insulin-positive cells together with the nestin selection strategy (Blyszczuk et al. 2003). PDX1 and PAX4 proteins are both master regulators of β cell differentiation and function (Chakrabarti and Mirmira 2003); however, Pax4 overexpressing cells demonstrated better yields of insulin production than Pdx1 overexpressing cells in the background of nestin positive-cell selection. Insulin-producing cells also can be obtained using the same differentiation protocol without nestin selection (Blyszczuk et al. 2004), indicating that nestin may not be the best candidate gene for pancreatic selection.

It is currently difficult to judge the efficacy of the different protocols from various laboratories. In order to compare results, all approaches from mouse ESCs or human ESCs need to optimize characterization criteria. For instance, insulin immunostaining and radioimmunodetection techniques are currently inadequate, because the hormone can be taken up by apoptotic cells from the culture medium (Rajagopal et al. 2003). Indeed, insulin is added to the culture medium in many protocols, and this hormone is present in variable amounts among lots of serum used for cell culture experiments. Analysis of C-peptide and mRNA levels of insulin, therefore, may represent better markers of endogenous insulin biosynthesis.

3
Adult Stem Cells and Somatic Cells

Adult stem cells (ASCs), present within tissues of adult organisms, are responsible for cell turnover or repopulation of tissues in normal and under exceptional circumstances (Fuchs et al. 2004). Relative to ESCs, the proliferation potential of ASCs seems to be limited. ASCs, which may be committed to specific cell fates, also exhibit less plasticity in terms of differentiation potential; however, several laboratories have reported that ASCs could transdifferentiate to other cell types. This latter finding has led to expectations for autotransplantation protocols (Wagers and Weissman 2004), but the capacity of ASCs to fuse with differentiated cells, and thus acquire the recipient phenotype in the new niche, has led to questions concerning the true plasticity of these cells (Wagers and Weissman 2004). Nevertheless, autologous ASCs have a major advantage with respect to ESCs in terms of immune compatibility i.e. ASCs will not undergo immune attack once transplanted to the recipient. The possibilities offered by both cell types to generate insulin-producing cells will be discussed in more detail.

3.1
From Endoderm-Derived Tissues

In addition to pancreas, liver is derived from embryonic endoderm, and it may represent an interesting source of ASCs capable of generating insulin-producing cells. Gene therapy protocols have already shown that insulin can be properly expressed in liver cells (Efrat 1998). This is likely due to the fact that hepatocytes share many phenotypic characteristics with β cells, including the glucose transporter GLUT-2 and glucokinase. Hepatic cells are, therefore, candidates for ectopic insulin production that may be achieved through the expression of insulin under the control of liver-specific promoters (i.e. phosphoenolpyruvate carboxykinase) (Efrat 1998) or by overexpression of certain transcription factors essential for β cell function such as Pdx1 or NeuroD combined with betacellulin (Ferber et al. 2000; Kojima et al. 2003).

Alternatively, liver stem cells, such as oval hepatic cells, can be thought of as another possible source for insulin-producing cells. Isolated oval cells in vitro are maintained in an undifferentiated state through the use of specific culture conditions that utilize serum withdrawal, 5 mM glucose and the presence of LIF. Differentiation to insulin-positive structures can be performed by adding 10% serum and increasing glucose concentration up to 23 mM in the absence of LIF. The resulting cells express islet markers such as Pdx1, Pax4, Pax6, Nkx2.2, Nkx6.1, insulin I and II, glucagon, pancreatic polypeptide and GLUT-2. Transplantation of these cells in the renal capsule of streptozotocin-diabetic NOD-SCID mice resulted in the recovery of normoglycaemia (Yang et al. 2002).

In addition, a recent report described the use of progenitor cells, obtained from human fetal liver, transfected with a construct coding for the catalytic subunit of the human telomerase gene. Subsequent transfection of these cells with Pdx1 resulted in differentiation to insulin-positive cells, and transplantation of this cell population to diabetic animals ($n = 4$) produced normoglycaemia (Zalzman et al. 2003). Importantly, the sham controls did not die and remained hyperglycaemic throughout the experiment.

Altogether, these studies suggest the potential use of autologous liver biopsies as a source of ASCs to generate functional islet-like structures for cell replacement in diabetes. Because many of these cells co-express a variety of pancreatic hormones, improvements will be required to increase the functional maturation of these cells, prior to any therapeutic application (Polak et al. 2000).

3.2
From Mesoderm-Derived Tissues

Mesoderm-derived bone marrow is an important reservoir of ASCs in the adult organism, and it may represent an alternative source of ASCs that can circumvent many of the problems associated with hepatic cells. A side population of cells from this niche has already been isolated that displays a degree plasticity that goes beyond normal blood and bone turnover. These cells, called MAPCs (multipotent adult progenitor cells), can be expanded in vitro and differentiated to cells positive for ectodermal, mesodermal and endodermal lineage markers (Jiang et al. 2002). Nevertheless the isolation of insulin-containing cells from MAPCs has not been reported.

Alternatively, one report showed the possibility of using highly purified bone marrow stem cells for pancreas repopulation (Ianus et al. 2003); however, this observation has not been confirmed by other laboratories (Choi et al. 2003;

Lechner et al. 2004). The possibility of generating new blood vessels from bone marrow stem cells could explain these divergent results. Since signals derived from the vasculature play an instrumental role in early pancreas development (Lammert et al. 2001; Kim and Hebrok 2001), pancreatic repopulation could be due to new blood vessel formation that favours islet regeneration (Hess et al. 2003). Nevertheless, the existence of a pancreatic pluripotent stem cell population that responds to a variety of extracellular factors cannot be excluded.

Monocytes from peripheral blood also may represent an alternative source. Monocytes appear not to be committed to becoming a terminally differentiated cells of the myeloid lineage, but can be reprogrammed in vitro by exposure to cytokines (IL-3 and M-CSF). Further exposure to EGF, HGF and nicotinamide differentiates human progenitor cells of monocyte origin to insulin-containing cells (Ruhnke et al. 2005). Transplantation of 2–3 million insulin-secreting cells under the kidney capsule of STZ-diabetic mice also led to correction of hyperglycaemia within 2 days.

4
Pancreas Regeneration

Endocrine pancreas, together with the nervous system and heart, is included in the group of organs that do not display obvious proliferation capacity in vivo (Potten and Loeffler 1990; Podolsky 1993; Yoo et al. 1998; Thorgeirsson 1996; Gage et al. 1995). Nevertheless, progenitor stem cells have been isolated from those nonproliferative tissues, suggesting the possibility of developing strategies to isolate, expand and differentiate these quiescent cells both in vitro and in vivo (Wagers and Weissman 2004; Fuchs et al. 2004).

In this sense, it has been proposed that exocrine pancreatic cells could transdifferentiate to insulin-producing cells; however, the exact identity of the parental cell as well as additional phenotypic and functional studies of the final cell product are necessary in order to identify novel sources of cells for transplantation (Baeyens et al. 2005). Several studies have documented the potential of pancreatic duct epithelium to differentiate in vitro into islet-like structures, suggesting that this is a candidate location for islet progenitors in adult pancreas (Bonner-Weir et al. 2000; Ramiya et al. 2000). Indeed, duct epithelium can be easily purified from cadaveric pancreata free from other cell types, due to its exceptional adherent capacity to cell culture surfaces. Conditions for expansion, differentiation and maturation used DMEM/F12 serum-free medium containing ITS (insulin + transferrin + selenium), keratinocyte growth factor (specific for duct expansion), nicotinamide and 8 mM glucose. Finally, Matrigel (commercial analogues of extracellular matrix) was added to allow the formation of cell aggregates called CHIBs (cultivated human islet buds) (Bonner-Weir et al. 2000) that were positive for insulin (evidenced by immune detection, dithizone staining and RT-PCR), glucagon and other islet markers, such as Pdx1. In vitro incubation of CHIBs in the presence of 20 mM glucose resulted in a 2.5-fold increase in insulin release with respect to 5 mM glucose after 24 h of incubation (Bonner-Weir et al. 2000).

Another study reported the identification of isolated IPSCs (islet pluripotent stem cells) budding from pancreatic ducts isolated from prediabetic NOD mice. These IPSCs showed enhanced insulin secretion in response to stimulating glucose concentrations and other secretagogues. Furthermore, IPSCs partially reversed hyperglycaemia when transplanted to the kidney capsule of diabetic NOD mice (Ramiya et al. 2000). Nevertheless, the observation reported with IPSCs, which contain low amounts of insulin in vitro, suggests additional mechanisms operating in vivo, even though a nephrectomy has not been performed to test this possibility.

Both CHIBs and IPSCs seem to arise from pluripotent cells present in duct epithelium, the identity of which remains unknown. Certain laboratories claim that these cells are positive for nestin, a protein present in neurofilaments, and negative for cytokeratin 19, an intermediate filament that is present in the rest of the cells of ductal epithelium. The presence of nestin-positive cells has been associated with islet structures, and these cells have been named NIPs (nestin-positive islet-derived progenitors). Cultured NIPs isolated from rat and human islets displayed the capacity to express hepatic markers as well as endo-and exocrine pancreatic genes (Zulewski et al. 2001); however, the proposal of NIPs as candidates for islet precursors has been questioned after recent findings showing participation of nestin-expressing cells in islet microvasculature of transgenic animals (Treutelaar et al. 2003).

In any case, all these reports strongly demonstrate the plasticity of duct epithelium to differentiate in vitro to islet-like structures in response to specific mitogenic signals (Bonner-Weir et al. 2000; Ramiya et al. 2000; Jamal et al. 2003). The presence of β cell precursors outside the ducts (i.e. NIPs) represents an interesting alternative, but strong evidence is still missing. Furthermore, data from other laboratories suggest that new β cells are coming from the replication of pre-existing β cells, questioning the existence of a stem cell population in pancreatic tissue (Dor et al. 2004). However, the experimental design to address this key question was based on genetic lineage tracing for insulin gene expression. The data of the study do not exclude the participation of islet precursors from ducts or even the presence of progenitors located inside islets, provided that these candidates are only committed to form β cells and are capable of expressing insulin in early stages of differentiation. The low turnover of pancreatic tissue suggests that cell replication may occur in response to specific insults, some of which can be characterized in animal models, such as pancreatectomy or streptozotocin injection. Nevertheless, certain points need to be clarified in more detail. For example, it is presently unknown whether putative endocrine pancreatic stem cells respond equally to different mitogenic signals and insults or what role β cell heterogeneity plays in regenerative processes. Altogether the data indicate that additional work will help answer these and other questions to ultimately identify the best potential endocrine-pancreatic stem cell population.

At the present time, the plasticity of duct epithelium to form insulin-positive cells seems promising, but this system needs to be improved to increase insulin content or adjust the secretory response to acute nutrient demands. On the other hand, both the identification of islet precursors and the design of protocols to stimulate in vivo differentiation represent key challenges in this field. Assuming some degree of success in the generation of islet tissue from ducts or from pre-existing islet-precursors, new perspectives for regenerative medicine in diabetes treatment by either autotransplantation or from exploitation of cadaveric pancreata can be realistically envisioned.

References

Baeyens L, De Breuck S, Lardon J, Mfopou JK, Rooman I, Bouwens L (2005) In vitro generation of insulin-producing beta cells from adult exocrine pancreatic cells. Diabetologia 48:49–57

Barshes NR, Lee T, Goodpasture S, Brunicardi FC, Alejandro R, Ricordi C, Soltes G, Barth M, Hamilton D, Goss JA (2004) Achievement of insulin independence via pancreatic islet transplantation using a remote isolation center: a first-year review. Transplant Proc 36:1127–1129

Bell GI, Polonsky KS (2001) Diabetes mellitus and genetically programmed defects in β-cell function. Nature 414:788–791

Benoist C, Mathis D (1997) Cell death mediators in autoimmune diabetes. No shortage of suspects. Cell 89:1–3

Blyszczuk P, Czyz J, Kania G, Wagner M, Roll U, St-Onge L, Wobus A (2003) Expression of Pax4 in embryonic stem cells promotes differentiation of nestin-positive progenitor and insulin-producing cells. Proc Natl Acad Sci U S A 100:998–1003

Blyszczuk P, Asbrand C, Rozzo A, Kania G, St-Onge L, Rupnik M, Wobus AM (2004) Embryonic stem cells differentiate into insulin-producing cells without selection of nestin-expressing cells. Int J Dev Biol 48:1095–1104

Bonner-Weir S, Taneja M, Weir GC, Tatarkiewicz K, Song K-H, Sharma A, O'Neil JJ (2000) In vitro cultivation of human islets from expanded ductal tissue. Proc Natl Acad Sci U S A 97:7999–8004

Brandhorst H, Brandhorst D, Hess F, Ambrosius D, Brendel M, Kawakami Y, Bretzel RG (2003) Successful human islet isolation utilizing recombinant collagenase. Diabetes 52:1143–1146

Brownlee M (2001) Biochemistry and molecular cell biology of diabetic complications. Nature 414:813–820

Bruning JC, Michael MD, Winnay JN, Hayashi T, Horsch D, Accili D, Goodyear LJ, Kahn CR (1998) A muscle-specific insulin receptor knockout exhibits features of the metabolic syndrome of NIDDM without altering glucose tolerance. Mol Cell 2:559–569

Chakrabarti SK, Mirmira RG (2003) Transcription factors direct the development and function of pancreatic β cells. Trends Endocrinol Metab 14:78–84

Choi JB, Uchino H, Azuma K, Iwashita N, Tanaka Y, Mochizuki H, Migita M, Shimada T, Kawamori R, Watada H (2003) Little evidence of transdifferentiation of bone marrow-derived cells into pancreatic beta cells. Diabetologia 46:1366–1374

DeFronzo RA, Ferrannini E, Keen H, Zimmet P (2004) International textbook of diabetes mellitus, 3rd edn. John Wiley, Chichester, UK

Dor Y, Brown J, Martínez OI, Melton DA (2004) Adult pancreatic β-cells are formed by self-duplication rather than stem-cell differentiation. Nature 429:41–46

Efrat S (1998) Prospects for gene therapy of insulin-dependent diabetes mellitus. Diabetologia 41:1401–1409

Ferber S, Halkin A, Cohen H, Ber I, Einav Y, Goldberg I, Barshack I, Seijffers R, Kopolovic J, Kaiser N, Karasik A (2000) Pancreatic and duodenal homeobox gene 1 induces expression of insulin genes in liver and ameliorates streptozotocin-induced hyperglycemia. Nat Med 6:568–572

Fuchs E, Tumbar T, Guasch G (2004) Socializing with the neighbors: stem cells and their niche. Cell 116:769–778

Gage FH, Ray J, Fisher LJ (1995) Isolation, characterization, and use of stem cells from CNS. Annu Rev Neurosci 18:159–192

Georges P, Muirhead RP, Williams L, Holman S, Tabiin MT, Dean SK, Tuch BE (2002) Comparison of size, viability, and function of fetal pig islet-like cell clusters after digestion using collagenase or liberase. Cell Transplant 11:539–545

Gray DW, Sudhakaran N, Titus TT, McShane P, Johnson P (2004) Development of a novel digestion chamber for human and porcine islet isolation. Transplant Proc 36:1135–1138

Hernández-Sánchez C, Mansilla A, de la Rosa EJ, Pollerberg GE, Martínez-Salas E, de Pablo F (2003) Upstream AUGs in embryonic proinsulin mRNA control its low translation level. EMBO J 22:5582–5592

Hess D, Li L, Martin M, Sakano S, Hill D, Strutt B, Thyssen S, Gray DA, Bhatia M (2003) Bone marrow-derived stem cells initiate pancreatic regeneration. Nat Biotech 21:763–770

Hori Y, Rulifson IC, Tsai BC, Heit JJ, Cahoy JD, Kim SK (2002) Growth inhibitors promote differentiation of insulin-producing tissue from embryonic stem cells. Proc Natl Acad Sci U S A 99:16105–16110

Ianus A, Holz GG, Theise ND, Hussain MA (2003) In vivo derivation of glucose-competent pancreatic endocrine cells from bone marrow without evidence of cell fusion. J Clin Invest 111:843–850

Jamal A-M, Lipstt M, Hazrati A, Paraskevas S, Agapitos D, Maysinger D, Rosenberg L (2003) Signals for death and differentiation: a two-step mechanism for in vitro transformation of adult islets of Langerhans to duct epithelial structures. Cell Death Diff 10:987–996

Jiang Y, Jahagirdar BN, Reinhardt RL, Schwartz RE, Keene CD, Ortiz-González XR, Reyes M, Lenvik T, Lund T, Blackstad M, Du J, Aldrich S, Lisberg A, Lew WC, Largaespada DA, Verfaillie CM (2002) Pluripotency of mesenchymal stem cells derived from adult marrow. Nature 418:41–49

Kania G, Blyszczuk P, Wobus AM (2004) The generation of insulin-producing cells from embryonic stem cells– a discussion of controversial findings. J Dev Biol 48:1061–1064

Kim SK, Hebrok M (2001) Intercellular signals regulating pancreas development and function. Genes Dev 15:111–127

Klug MG, Soonpa MH, Koh GY, Field LJ (1996) Genetically selected cardiomyocytes from differentiating embryonic stem cells form stable intracardiac grafts. J Clin Invest 98:216–224

Kojima H, Fujimiya M, Matsumura K, Younan P, Imaeda, H, Maeda M, Chan L (2003) NeuroD-betacellulin gene therapy induces islet neogenesis in the liver and reverses diabetes in mice. Nat Med 9:596–603

Ku HT, Zhang N, Kubo A, O'Connor R, Mao M, Keller G, Bromberg JS (2004) Committing embryonic stem cells to early endocrine pancreas in vitro. Stem Cells 22:1205–1217

Kubo A, Shinozaki K, Shannon JM, Kouskoff V, Kennedy M, Woo S, Fehling HJ, Keller G (2004) Development of definitive endoderm from embryonic stem cells in culture. Development 131:1651–1662

Lammert E, Cleaver O, Melton D (2001) Induction of pancreatic differentiation by signals from blood vessels. Science 294:564–567

Lechner A, Yang Y-G, Blacken RA, Wang L, Nolan AL, Habener JF (2004) No evidence for significant transdifferentiation of bone marrow into pancreatic β-cells in vivo. Diabetes 53:616–623

León-Quinto T, Jones J, Skoudy A, Burcin M, Soria B (2004) In vitro directed differentiation of mouse embryonic stem cells into insulin-producing cells. Diabetologia 47:1442–1451

Li M, Pevny L, Lovell-Badge R, Smith A (1998) Generation of purified neural precursors from embryonic stem cells by lineage selection. Curr Biol 8:971–974

Lumelsky N, Blondel O, Laeng P, Velasco I, Ravin R, McKay R (2001) Differentiation of embryonic stem cells to insulin-secreting structures similar to pancreatic islets. Science 292:1389–1394

Maechler P, Wollheim CB (2001) Mitochondrial function in normal and diabetic β-cells. Nature 414:807–812

Mathis D, Vence L, Benoist C (2001) β-Cell death during progression to diabetes. Nature 414:792–798

Melloul D, Marshak S, Cerasi E (2002) Regulation of insulin gene transcription. Diabetologia 45:309–326

Milne HM, Burns CJ, Kitsou-Mylona IK, Luther MJ, Minger SL, Persaud SJ, Jones PM (2005) Generation of insulin-expressing cells from mouse embryonic stem cells. Biochem Biophys Res Commun 328:399–403

Mitsui K, Tokuzawa Y, Itoh H, Segawa K, Murakami M, Takahashi K, Maruyama M, Maeda M, Yamanaka S (2003) The homeoprotein Nanog is required for maintenance of pluripotency in mouse epiblast and ES cells. Cell 113:631–642

Miyazaki S, Yamato E, Miyazaki J (2004) Regulated expression of Pdx1 promotes in vitro differentiation of insulin-producing cells from embryonic stem cells. Diabetes 53:1030–1037

Moritoh Y, Yamato E, Yasui Y, Miyazaki S, Miyazaki J (2003) Analysis of insulin-producing cells during in vitro differentiation from feeder-free embryonic stem cells. Diabetes 52:1163–1168

Müller M, Fleischmann BK, Selbert S, Ji GJ, Endl E, Middeler G, Müller OJ, Schlenke P, Frese S, Wobus AM, Hescheler J, Katus HA, Franz WM (2000) Selection of ventricular-like cardiomyocytes from ES cells in vitro. FASEB J 14:2540–2548

Niwa H, Miyazaki J, Smith AG (2000) Quantitative expression of Oct3/4 defines differentiation, dedifferentiation or self-renewal of ES cells. Nat Genet 24:372–376

Oluwole SF, Oluwole OO, Adeyeri AO, DePaz HA (2004) New strategies in immune tolerance induction. Cell Biochem Biophys Suppl 40:27–48

Pesce M, Gross MK, Scholer HR (1998) In line with our ancestors: Oct4 and the mammalian germ. Bioessays 20:722–732

Piper K, Ball SG, Turnpenny LW, Brickwod S, Wilson DI, Hanley NA (2002) Beta-cell differentiation during human development does not rely on nestin-positive precursors: implications for stem cell-derived replacement therapy. Diabetologia 45:1045–1047

Podolsky DK (1993) Regulation of intestinal epithelial proliferation: a few answers, many questions. Am J Physiol 264:G179–G186

Poitout V, Robertson RP (1996) An integrated view of β-cell dysfunction in type 2 diabetes. Annu Rev Med 47:69–83

Polak M, Bouchareb-Banaei L, Scharfmann R, Czernichow P (2000) Early pattern of differentiation in the human pancreas. Diabetes 49:225–232

Polonsky KS, Sturis J, Bell GI (1996) Non-insulin dependent diabetes mellitus. A genetically programmed failure of the β-cell to compensate for insulin resistance. N Engl J Med 334:777–783

Potten CS, Loeffler M (1990) Stem cells: attributes, cycles, spirals, pitfalls and uncertainties. Lessons for and from the crypt. Development 110:1001–1020

Prentki M, Roduit R, Lameloise N, Corkey BE Assimacopoulos-Jeannet F (2000) Glucotoxicity, lipotoxicity and pancreatic β-cell failure: a role for malonyl-CoA, PPARα and altered lipid partitioning? Can J Diabetes Care 25:36–46

Rajagopal J, Anderson WJ, Kume S, Martínez OI, Melton DA (2003) Insulin staining of ES cell progeny from insulin uptake. Science 299:363

Ramiya VK, Maraist M, Arfors KE, Schatz DA, Peck AB, Cornelius JG (2000) Reversal of insulin-dependent diabetes using islets generated in vitro from pancreatic stem cells. Nat Med 6:278–282

Roche E (2003) Type 2 diabetes: gluco-lipo-toxicity and pancreatic β-cell dysfunction. Ars Pharmaceutica 44:313–332

Roche E, Sepulcre MP, Enseñat-Waser R, Maestre I, Reig JA, Soria B (2003) Bio-engineering insulin-secreting cells from embryonic stem cells: a review of progress. Med Biol Eng Comp 41:384–391

Ruhnke M, Ungefroren H, Nussler A, Martin F, Brulport M, Schorman W, Hengstler JG, Klapper W, Ulrichs K, Hutchinson JA, Soria B, Parwaresch RM, Heeckt P, Kremer B, Fändrich F (2005) Differentiation of in-vitro modified human peripheral monocytes into hepatocyte-like and pancreatic islet-like cells. Gastroenterology 128:174–1786

Ryan EA, Lakey JRT, Paty BW, Imes S, Korbutt GS, Kneteman NM, Bigam D, Rajotte RV, Shapiro AMJ (2002) Successful islet transplantation. Continued insulin reserve provides long-term glycemic control. Diabetes 51:2148–2157

Saltiel AR (2001) New perspectives into the molecular pathogenesis and treatment of type 2 diabetes. Cell 104:517–529

Segev H, Fishman B, Ziskind A, Shulman M, Itskovitz-Eldor J (2004) Differentiation of human embryonic stem cells into insulin-producing clusters. Stem Cells 22:265–274

Shapiro AMJ, Lakey JRT, Ryan EA, Korbutt GS, Toth E, Warnock GL, Kneteman NM, Rajotte RV (2000) Islet transplantation in seven patients with type 1 diabetes mellitus using a corticoid-free immunosuppressive regime. N Eng J Med 343:230–238

Smith AG (1991) Culture and differentiation of embryonic stem cells. J Tissue Culture Methods 13:89–94

Smith AG (2001) Embryo-derived stem cells: of mice and men. Annu Rev Cell Dev Biol 17:435–462

Soria B, Roche E, Berná G, León-Quinto T, Reig JA, Martín F (2000) Insulin-secreting cells derived from embryonic stem cells normalize glycemia in streptozotocin-induced diabetic mice. Diabetes 49:157–162

Soria B, Skoudy A, Martín F (2001) From stem cells to beta cells: new strategies in cell therapy of diabetes mellitus. Diabetologia 44:407–415

Tanaka TS, Kunath T, Kimber WL, Jaradat SA, Stagg CA, Usuda M, Yokota T, Niwa H, Rossant J, Ko MS (2002) Gene expression profiling of embryo-derived stem cells reveals candidate genes associated with pluripotency and lineage specificity. Genome Res 12:1921–1928

Thorgeirsson SS (1996) Hepatic stem cells in liver regeneration. FASEB J 10:1249–1256

Toyooka Y, Tsunekawa N, Takahashi Y, Matsui Y, Satoh M, Noce T (2000) Expression and intracellular localization of mouse Vasa-homologue protein during germ cell development. Mech Dev 93:139–149

Treutelaar MK, Skidmore JM, Dias-Leme CL, Hara M, Zhang L, Simeone D, Martin DM, Burant CF (2003) Nestin-lineage cells contribute to the microvasculature but not endocrine cells of the islet. Diabetes 52:2503–2512

Vicario-Abejón C, Yusta-Boyo MJ, Fernández-Moreno C, de Pablo F (2003) Locally born olfactory bulb stem cells proliferate in response to insulin-related factors and require endogenous insulin-like growth factor-I for differentiation into neurons and glia. J Neurosci 23:895–906

Wagers AJ, Weissman IL (2004) Plasticity of adult stem cells. Cell 116:639–648

Wobus AM, Boheler KR (2005) Embryonic stem cells: prospects for developmental biology and cell therapy. Physiol Rev 85:636–678

Yang L, Li S, Hatch H, Ahrens K, Cornelius JG, Petersen BE, Peck AB (2002) In vitro transdifferentiation of adult hepatic stem cells into pancreatic endocrine hormone-producing cells. Proc Natl Acad Sci U S A 99:8078–8083

Ying Q-L, Stavridis M, Griffiths D, Li M, Smith A (2003) Conversion of embryonic stem cells into neuroectodermal precursors in adherent monoculture. Nat Biotechnol 21:183–186

Yoo JU, Barthel TS, Nishimura K, Solchaga L, Caplan AI, Goldberg VM, Johnstone B (1998) The chondrogenic potential of human bone-marrow-derived mesenchymal progenitor cells. J Bone Joint Surg 80:1745–1757

Zalzman M, Gupta S, Giri RK, Berkovich I, Sappal BS, Karnieli O, Zern MA, Fleischer N, Efrat S (2003) Reversal of hyperglycemia in mice by using human expandable insulinproducing cells differentiated from fetal liver progenitor cells. Proc Natl Acad Sci U S A 100:7253–7258

Zierath JR, Krook A, Wallberg-Henriksson H (2000) Insulin action and insulin resistance in human skeletal muscle. Diabetologia 43:821–835

Zimmet P, Alberti KGMM, Shaw J (2001) Global and societal implications of the diabetes epidemic. Nature 414:782–787

Zulewski H, Abraham EJ, Gerlach MJ, Daniel PB, Moritzs W, Müller B, Vallejo M, Thomas MK, Habener JF (2001) Multipotential nestin-positive stem cells isolated from adult pancreatic islets differentiate ex vivo into pancreatic endocrine, exocrine and hepatic phenotypes. Diabetes 50:521–533

HEP (2006) 174:169–183
© Springer-Verlag Berlin Heidelberg 2006

The Stem Cell Continuum:
A New Model of Stem Cell Regulation

P. J. Quesenberry (✉) · G. A. Colvin · M. S. Dooner

Research Department, Roger Williams Medical Center, 825 Chalkstone Avenue,
Providence RI, 02908, USA
pquesenberry@rwmc.org

Abstract Most models of hematopoiesis have been hierarchical in nature. This is based on a large volume of correlative data. Recent work has indicated that, at least at the stem/progenitor level, hematopoiesis may, in fact, be a continuum of transcriptional opportunity. The most primitive hematopoietic stem cells are either continually cycling at a slow rate or entering and exiting cell cycle. Associated with this cycle passage are changes in functional phenotype including reversible alterations in engraftment, adhesion protein expression, cytokine receptor expression, homing to marrow, and progenitor cell numbers. Global gene expression, as measured in one point in cycle, is also markedly altered. The differentiation potential of the marrow as it transits cell cycle in response to a set differentiation stimulus also shows marked variations. This cycle-related plasticity has been clearly established for hematopoiesis. It also holds for the ability of murine marrow stem cells to home to lung and to convert to pulmonary cells. These data indicate that bone marrow stem cells can probably not be defined as discrete entities but must rather be studied on a population basis. They also indicate that mathematical modeling will become progressively more important in this field.

Keywords Stem cell · Continuum · Hierarchy · Progenitor · Differentiation

1
Introduction

One of the strongest tenets of experimental hematology has been that the system is intrinsically hierarchical in nature. Models have included an early multipotent stem cell with tremendous proliferative and differentiative potential that gives rise to a progressively more differentiated series of progenitors which lose proliferative renewal potential as they gain differentiated characteristics. Finally, these progenitors result in the development of specific lineages of morphologically defined hematopoietic cell lines including NK cells, T cells, B cells, granulocytes, megakaryocytes/platelets, erythrocytes, and monocyte/macrophages. Data has been evolving over the years to suggest alternative models with less order and with a great deal more flexibility. Below we present the evolution of these models.

2
The Hierarchy

Marrow stem cell/progenitor regulation has been presumed to be hierarchical in nature based upon impressive correlative studies (Cronkite 1975). The recovery of granulopoiesis and erythropoiesis after different myeloablative treatments to rodents virtually established a hierarchy at the levels of morphologically recognizable differentiated myeloid cells. It was clear in these studies that myeloblasts gave rise to promyelocytes, which then gave rise to myelocytes and metamyelocytes, band forms, and polymorphonuclear granulocytes then sequentially followed. Similarly in the erythroid lineage, erythroblasts gave rise to pronormoblasts, which then produced basophilic erythroblasts followed by polychromatophilic normoblasts, orthochromatic normoblasts and then reticulocytes and mature erythrocytes. Thymidine labeling studies showed that there were both proliferating and maturing compartments in these lineages. Bradley and Metcalf (1966) and Pluznik and Sachs (1965) introduced the in vitro clonal assays for granulocytes and macrophages, which appeared to identify progenitors committed to the production of these cells. Earlier, the colony-forming unit spleen had been described by Till and McCulloch (1961) as a pluripotent myeloid stem cell, which gave rise to erythroid, granulocytic, and megakaryocytic lineages. It was thus natural to assume that the CFUs gave rise to the granulocyte-macrophage colony-forming unit culture (GM-CFU-C), which, in turn, gave rise to mature granulocytes and macrophages. When megakaryocyte and erythroid colony assays were introduced, similar lineage hierarchies were assumed (McLeod et al. 1976; 1974; Iscove and Sieber

1975; Nakeff et al. 1975; Metcalf et al. 1975). The description of progenitors requiring multiple cytokines and which gave rise to larger proliferative units, the high-proliferative colony-forming cell (HPP-CFC) (Bradley and Hodgson 1979; McNiece et al. 1988a, 1988b), the burst-forming unit erythroid (BFU-e) (Heath et al. 1976; Gregory 1976), and the burst-forming unit megakaryocyte (BFU-mega) (Long et al. 1985; Briddell et al. 1989) simply suggested a more complex hierarchy within the progenitor compartment. Eventually, progenitors with virtually every possible lineage combination have been described and these have been placed in a more and more complex hierarchical tree. In a similar fashion, engraftable stem cells have been subsetted by the degree of retention of the supravital dye rhodamine into short-term and long-term repopulation cells (Bertoncello et al. 1989). A very complex but still orderly hierarchy could be constructed from these observations. There were perhaps some indications that things might not be this simple. In general, progenitors could not be cleanly separated from one another and engraftable stem cells, but this was assumed to be due to a lack of cell surface or metabolic cell characteristics, which could facilitate such separations. However, there were some observations, which did not support this overall hierarchical model. Dr. Makio Ogawa and colleagues carried out a series of elegant experiments in which they isolated cells from primitive hematopoietic blast colonies in vitro, and then, when these cells divided under permissive cytokine conditions, separated daughter cells and determined the differentiated progeny of these cells (Ogawa et al. 1985; Nakahata and Ogawa 1982; Suda et al. 1983, 1984; Quesenberry 1991). In these experiments, any change in the differentiation phenotype would have had to occur through one cell cycle transit of the daughter cells. I quote from an editorial in *Experimental Hematology* titled "The Blueness of Stem Cells" (Quesenberry 1991), in which I commented on these studies.

"Then, Dr. Ogawa came along and messed everything up. He described a bewildering array of different colony types with from one to five lineages arising from single cells. Anyone who carries out particularly elegant experiments and derives important new insights can be very irritating, especially to those of us who would like to be the ones reporting the work. Dr. Ogawa continues to be an irritant, but perhaps the most devastating Ogawian data are the daughter cell experiments, which indicate that within one cell cycle transit totally different lineages may be pursued by two daughter cells derived from a blast colony cell. This discovery was akin to exploding a bomb in the center of the hierarchical models, although most of us keep presenting such models because it is simply too messy to incorporate Ogawa's cell cycle data." The sister cell cloning experiments indicated that within one cell cycle transit quite different differentiation outcomes could be seen. In about 20% of the cases, clones from daughter cells derived from the original blast colony cell, showed different lineages—one colony might be erythroid-megakaryocyte, while the sister clone might give rise to macrophages and granulocytes. This certainly did not fit with a hierarchical scheme of differentiation; in fact, it was strong

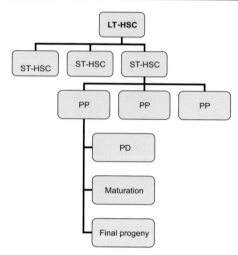

Fig. 1 A classical hierarchical model of hematopoiesis. LT-HSC represents the long-term engraftable marrow stem cell and ST-HSC the short-term engraftable marrow stem cell. *HSC* stands for hematopoietic stem cell. *PP* represents a primitive progenitor cell and *PD* a more differentiated progenitor cell. *Maturation* represents the differentiated maturing marrow compartment, and *final progeny* represents the end cell of a particular lineage

evidence against such a scheme, although the implications of these data were not vigorously pursued at the time.

Thus, the hierarchy of the hematopoietic stem progenitor system has become a strongly held tenet of most workers in this field, such that challenges to this concept can provoke quite strong comments from grant or manuscript reviewers. I speak from painful personal experience. I think that the hierarchical concept may have attained the status of an idol of the mind, as so lucidly described by Francis Bacon in 1620 (*Novum Organum*). The concepts of a hierarchical and a continuum model of hematopoiesis are presented in Figs. 1 and 2.

3
The Continuum

A series of investigations, to be detailed below, has shown that critical features of the phenotype of the classically defined marrow stem cell are, in fact, not stable but fluctuate dramatically over time and, most importantly, these fluctuations are reversible, i.e., they do not represent differentiation. Furthermore, we have found striking correlations with cell cycle state and changes in the stem cell phenotype. These observations would not be of particular consequence if the normal primitive marrow stem cells were a quiescent noncycling population, as has been standard dogma for years. However, it turns out that

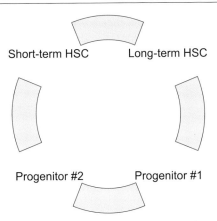

Short-term HSC   Long-term HSC

Progenitor #2   Progenitor #1

Fig. 2 A continuum model of hematopoiesis. *HSC* represents hematopoietic stem cell as assayed by either short- or long-term engraftment. The continuum circle could represent cell cycle or other as yet unknown cellular attributes

the marrow stem cell department as defined by many workers is a cycling population of cells. They represent cells, which are either cycling continuously, but slowly, or, alternatively, cycling intermittently, at a more rapid rate. The quiescent dogma is puzzling because a look at studies characterizing stem cells with regard to cycle status reveals that they have always shown a small percentage of cells to be in S phase. These studies, of course, just give a transient window on cycle status, and these data would indicate that most stem cells are probably cycling, but simply at a lower rate than some other populations. This was definitively shown by Bradford and colleagues (Bradford et al. 1997). These investigators fed BALB/c mice BrdU in their drinking water over time and then determined, at different points in the feeding schedule, the percentage of LRH stem cells which took up the label. Labeling would indicate that the cells had synthesized DNA and passed through S-phase, since BrdU is incorporated into DNA when DNA is synthesized. By week 4, 60±14% of LRH had labeled, and the estimated T1/2 for labeling was 19 days. These studies were confirmed by Chesire et al. (1999) using a different stem cell separation and mouse strain and with faster kinetics. Recently, our group (Pang et al. 2003), in studies trying to address whether DNA damage–repair might be involved in the observed BrdU labeling, confirmed the Bradford studies.

The concept that stem cells are a cycling cell population is further supported by studies showing rapid cycle induction of long-term renewal cells when cells are cultured in cytokines (Reddy et al. 1997) or when they are engrafted into normal or irradiated hosts (Nilsson et al. 1997). When cells transit the cell cycle, the chromatin coverage continuously changes. This would lead to continuous shifts in regions of the chromosome, which would be available for interactions with transcription factors. This, in turn, suggests that the ability to respond to a specific differentiation inductive stimulus would also be continually changing, certain outcomes being favored at certain points in cell cycle (Cerny and Quesenberry 2004). Experiments addressing this point will be presented below. This, of course, immediately suggests a continuum model of hematopoiesis rather than a hierarchical one.

We will begin with the studies on engraftment.

4
Engraftment

In the attempts to increase engraftment of murine marrow stem cells into non-myeloablated host mice, we were surprised to observe a marked decrease in engraftment when marrow cells had been incubated in the cytokines interleukin-3 (IL-3), IL-6, IL-11, and steel factor. These cytokines had been chosen because at the time we were also attempting to obtain engraftment of retroviral trans-duced stem cells into nonmyeloablated mice, and this was the cytokine cocktail used to cycle marrow cells in order to obtain retroviral integration into stem cell DNA. In these studies, we were attempting to transfer the MDR-1 gene, and we obtained very high rates of in vitro transduction, reasonable rates of long-term engraftment, but only marginal levels of gene transfer (Kittler et al. 1997). A conclusion from these studies is that cytokines cycled the stem cells giving us very good in vitro transduction, but that these particular cells en-grafted very poorly. When we carried out studies on normal murine marrow cells incubated with IL-3, IL-6, IL-11, and steel factor (cytokine cocktail 1), we found that at 48 h of culture there was a profound decrease in engraftment, and this was seen whether marrow was transplanted into nonmyeloablated hosts (Peters et al. 1995) or evaluated in a competitive setting in lethally irradiated host mice (Peters et al. 1996). This could, of course, simply represent loss of engraftability with differentiation into progenitors.

Critical experiments followed showing that loss of engraftability at either 8 weeks or 6 months after cell infusion was not a permanent state, but was, in fact, reversible (Habibian et al. 1998). These studies were carried out on unseparated marrow, but when highly purified lineage-negative rhodamine 123 low and Hoechst 33342 low (LRH) stem cells were cultured under the same cytokine conditions, it was found that there was a highly predictable transit through cell cycle with the first cycle ending at about 36–38 h and with subsequent cycles lasting 12 h out to at least five additional cycle transits (Reddy et al. 1997). In these studies, marked and reversible alterations in engraftment capacity were seen over 2-h intervals, and a prominent loss of engraftment was seen in the late S/early G_2 period of cycle (Habibian et al. 1998). Further studies showed that there was little effect on short-term engraftment (Peters et al. 1999), but that the further analysis was carried out after cell infusion, the more profound the cytokine/cycle induced engraftment defect. We also established that these results were not due to differential in vitro adherence to

Table 1 Engraftment results with cytokine stimulated stem cell cycle transit

Long-term engraftment is reversibly lost in late S/early G_2, but in the same population short-term engraftment is preserved.

Shifts of the engraftment phenotype can occur within 2-h time intervals.

The same results are obtained whether engraftment is in nonmyeloablated or myeloablated hosts.

Purified marrow stem cells and unseparated marrow give the same engraftment results.

The engraftment results are not due to in vitro adherence.

Similar results are obtained with a different cytokine cocktail (thrombopoietin, Flt3, and steel factor, cocktail 2) with a loss of engraftment in the same cell cycle phases, although the kinetics of cycle transit are different with this cytokine combination.

---

plastic and, with more recent studies, this variable has been removed by the use of nonadherent Teflon bottle cultures (Peters et al. 2002). More recently, these results have been duplicated studying purified LRH cells cultured in IL-3, IL-6, IL11, and steel factor and, again, showing a reversible defect in late S/early G_2 (Lambert et al. 2003). These engraftment results are summarized in Table 1.

5
Homing

We addressed whether this loss of engraftment capacity could be due to alterations in homing efficiency. We established a homing assay in nonmyeloablated mice using 5-(and 6)-carboxyflyorescein diacetate succinimidyl ester (CFSE) labeled lineage-negative Sca-1[+] (Lin-Sca-1[+]) marrow stem cells (Cerny et al. 2002). These cells were injected by tail vein into untreated mice and marrow harvested at varying times and then analyzed on a high-speed MoFlo cell sorter for fluorescent positive events using a large event analysis with at least 16 million events analyzed. These studies showed that homing of Lin-Sca-1[+] cells plateaued by 1 h and, at 3 h after infusion was linear between 50,000 and 1,000,000 infused cells. The plateau persisted out to 16 h, the longest time analyzed. Previous work had shown that engrafting stem cells entered S-phase within 12 h of in vivo infusion (Nilsson et al. 1997) and, thus, we established a homing assay in which the homed cells would not have proliferated and on the plateau of the homing curve. This assay utilized 250,000 infused CFSE labeled Lin-Sca-1[+] marrow cells and then recovered cells 3 h later for a large event MoFlo sorter analysis. In this setting, there were between 40–50 positive events per 1 million cells analyzed, and from 7.45% to 9.32% of infused cells homed.

We also established an in vitro stem cell homing assay. Here we analyzed adherence to pre-established Dexter culture stromal cells of engraftable stem cells from whole marrow suspensions (Frimberger et al. 2001). Using a competitive transplant assay into lethally irradiated mice, we found that the number of hematopoietic stem cells adhering to stroma was substantial at 20 min, increased in the 1st hour, and then remained constant at 1, 6, and 24 h of adherence. By 1 h of adherence in vitro, 70.7% of the predicted engraftment from equivalent numbers of unmanipulated marrow cells was observed to be adherent to the stromal cells.

These data from an in vivo infusion assay and an in vitro adherence assay gave remarkably similar results, with very rapid "homing" plateauing within 1 h after infusion or cell addition. Using the in vivo assay, we determined that homing of stem cells cultured for 48 h in IL-3, IL-6, IL-11, and steel factor was defective when compared to noncultured cells (Cerny et al. 2002). This is a time point in these cytokine stimulated cultures when engraftment is markedly and reproducibly decreased, suggesting that changes in homing may underlie the observed changes in engraftment.

As homing is probably mediated, at least in part, by stem cell adhesion receptors, we evaluated these in the above models (Berrios et al. 2001; Becker et al. 1999). We first investigated receptor expression and modulation on Lin-Sca-1$^+$ marrow stem cells using Northern blot, quantitative PCR, and flow analysis. Normal Lin-Sca-1$^+$ cells expressed a number of adhesion receptors including integrins α_L, α_1, α_3, α_4, α_5, α_6, β_1, L-selectin, CD44, and PECAM. Adhesion of Lin-Sca-1$^+$ cells to Dexter stroma was blocked by about 90% with antibodies to PECAM-1, α_4, and β_4 and partially blocked by antibodies to CD44, L-selectin, and α_4. When these stem cells were incubated in IL-3, IL-6, IL-11, and steel factor for 24 or 48 h, the proportion of cells expressing α_4 and β_1 were decreased. Other receptors were variably modulated with α_2, showing a decrease at 24 h with an increase at 48 h, and L-selectin showing an increase at 24 h with a subsequent decrease at 48 h. Adhesion of these cells to fibronectin after cytokine incubation correlated with the expression of α_4.

In more recent unpublished studies using real-time PCR, we have shown expression of CXCR4 and SDF-1 in these cells and modulation with cycle transit.

Adhesion receptor expression was also examined in LRH cells under the same cytokine culture conditions, but at 0, 16, and 48 h of culture. Here too, variable alterations in adhesion protein levels were noted with transit through cell cycle. Purified LRH stem cells studied with immunofluorescence showed variable expression of α_L, α_4, α_5, α_6, β_1, L-selectin and PECAM. Once again, expression of α_4 and β_1 were decreased at 48 h of culture. A variable modulation of the other adhesion receptors was also seen at 16 and 48 h with reversible alterations seen with L-selectin, PECAM, α_5 and α_L.

These studies indicated that adhesion proteins showed a cell cycle-associated modulation, that many of the changes were reversible, and that the changes in homing and engraftment might be secondary to changes in adhesion pro-

Table 2 Homing and adhesion protein expression with cell cycle transit

Stem cell homing in vivo to marrow or in vitro on Dexter culture stroma is very rapid and plateaus by 1 h.

Homing in vivo by Lin-Sca-1$^+$ marrow stem cells is defective at a time point when engraftment is defective.

Both Lin-Sca-1$^+$ and LRH purified murine marrow stem cells express a wide variety of adhesion receptors.

These receptors show variable and reversible changes in expression at different time points in a cytokine-stimulated cell cycle transit.

A consistent finding is that integrin α_4 is markedly decreased at 48 h of cytokine culture, a time point when both homing and engraftment is depressed.

tein expression. The homing and adhesion protein results are summarized in Table 2.

We recently utilized in vivo phage display biopanning and discovered that CD84 may be an important homing peptide. The role of CD84 in the above biology remains to be determined (Nowakowski et al. 2004).

6
Switch to a Progenitor Phenotype: The Progenitor/Stem Cell Inversion

Progenitors have been felt to differentiate from more primitive marrow stem cells such as LRH or Lin-Sca-1$^+$ cells. This is part of the traditional stem cell hierarchy. However, we have generated data indicating that the progenitor phenotype is quite labile as a cell progresses through cell cycle and, that as progenitor numbers increase, the number of engraftable stem cells decrease and, most importantly, that these shifts in phenotype are reversible (Colvin et al. 2004). We utilized two different systems in these studies; in one marrow cells were studied in conventional liquid culture with cytokines, while in the other cells were cultured with cytokines in rotating wall vessel cultures, which simulate microgravity. The cytokines for these experiments were thrombopoietin, Flt3, and steel factor. Cells under these conditions were also highly synchronized as to cell cycle, with up to 98% of cells labeling with propidium during the first cell cycle passage. Synchrony was determined using both propidium labeling and ^{3}HtdR labeling, and while the kinetics of cell cycle transit were slower, stem cells were still found to have an engraftment defect at lateS/earlyG$_2$. In these studies, HPP-CFC and CFU-c were assayed at different points in cycle and found to show marked fluctuation in numbers through one cell cycle transit. Perhaps most impressive was the reciprocal relationship between progenitor and engraftable stem cell numbers. When progenitors were increased frequently over twofold, engraftable stem cells were decreased by a similar magnitude, and these changes were reversible within one cycle transit. We termed these stem cell/progenitor inversions. These data suggested that the progenitor and the engraftable stem cell might be the same cell, simply changing phenotype on a continuum.

7
Differentiation Hotspots in Cell Cycle Transit

The concept of a changing phenotype as a stem cell progressed through cell cycle with associated changes in chromatin coverage and transcriptional opportunity would suggest that the potential of a cell to respond to a specific differentiation inductive signal would change as it passed through different cell cycle phases. We tested this hypothesis by culturing LRH cells in thrombopoietin, Flt3, and steel factor and then at different points in cell cycle transit, the cells were subcultured in liquid culture in a differentiation cytokine cocktail consisting of G-CSF, GM-CSF, and steel factor; differentiation was determined 14 days later. In these unpublished but relatively definitive experiments, we found a differentiation hotspot in mid-S phase for megakaryocytes. A large production of megakaryocytes was seen at this point, which was reversible within one cell cycle transit, i.e., before the next population doubling. This further supported our concept of a continuum (Colvin et al. 2004).

8
Global Gene Expression and Other Stem Cell-Specific Gene Expression

We studied the genetic phenotype of purified LRH marrow stem cells in IL-3, IL-6, IL-11, and steel factor stimulated cell culture at 0 and 48 h of culture (Lambert et al. 2003). Gene expression of quiescent (0 h) and cycling (48 h) stem cells was compared with lineage-positive cells by 3' end PCR differential display analysis. Individual PCR bands were quantified using a 0–9 scale, and results were visualized using color-coded matrices. We defined a set of 637 transcripts expressed in stem cells and not expressed in lineage-positive cells. Gene expression analyzed at 0 and 48 h showed a major shift from stem cell genes being highly expressed at 0 h (at isolation), and turned off at 48 h of culture, while cell division genes were turned on at 48 h.

In other studies, we have also shown fluctuations through cell cycle transit in cytokine receptor expression (Pang et al. 2003) and, utilizing real-time PCR, seen fluctuations in the expression of different stem cell markers such as Sca-1 and c-kit, in differentiation markers such as Mac-1 and CD4, and in various transcription factors, which have been invoked as stem cell regulators.

9
Plasticity and Plasticity: Plasticity Squared

We have entered the era of stem cell plasticity. The above discussion could be described as "in-tissue" plasticity. However, what most consider as stem cell plasticity is the ability of marrow stem cells to produce cells of nonhematopoietic tissues in nonhematopoietic organs. We, and others, have extensively commented on the capacity of adult marrow cells to produce cells in multiple different lineages, and on the rather mindless debate, which has grown up around this field. We have termed this "Ignoratio Elenchi," the use of red herrings to divert attention. I will make just a few points before getting back to the continuum concept. First, the capacity of marrow stem cells, including highly purified marrow stem cells, to make nonmarrow cells has been repeatedly demonstrated. Second, it is clearly highly functional in at least one well-studied model of liver disease, the FAH-negative ($^-$) mouse (Lagassee et al. 2000). Third, it is quite significant, or if you will, robust, in liver, lung, and skeletal muscle (Lagassee et al. 2000; Krause et al. 2001; Abedi et al. 2004). The phenomena of cell fusion occurs in some models and not others and, in fact, was present in the FAH$^-$ model in which some mice were cured of this otherwise fatal liver disease.

We have studied the conversion of marrow cells to lung cells using a green-fluorescent protein transgenic marrow source engrafted after irradiation into a wild type C57BL/6J host mouse. We then employed cardiotoxin injection into the anterior tibialis muscle or intratracheal bleomycin as lung injuries, and evaluated lung at varying times after cardiotoxin injury. In these studies, we routinely see conversion of marrow cells to CD45-GFP$^+$ lung cells, about half of which mark as either type 1 or type 2 pneumocytes. Of interest with regard to the continuum concept, we have found that if we engraft mid-S-phase marrow cells from thrombopoietin, Flt3, and steel factor-stimulated cultures, the number of conversions is increased up to threefold and, at times, we see that over 30% of lung cells have derived from marrow (Dooner et al. 2004). Thus, we see one form of plasticity on top of another form of plasticity. This increase in conversion events also reverses within one cell cycle transit. We term this plasticity squared or P^2.

10
A Continuum Model of Hematopoiesis

The above discussion outlines a series of studies which show that under defined experimental conditions, the phenotype of what we have referred to as the primitive marrow engrafting stem cell is quite labile over time and that the changes seen are not permanent differentiation steps.

Table 3 Marrow stem cell lability over time

Cytokine culture
Engraftment
Homing
Adhesion protein expression
Progenitor number
Differentiation in response to a set stimulus
Cytokine receptor expression
Stem cell surface marker
Stem cell transcription factors
Global gene expression
Conversion to lung cells
Circadian rhythm
Engraftment
Progenitor numbers

This is, of course, not consistent with a hierarchical model of hematopoiesis. A continuum concept is not as neat and orderly as a hierarchical concept, but offers an attractively flexible system with a tremendous amount of potential, which can be selectively expressed given a particular set of circumstances, such as tissue injury or exposure to a specific mix of inductive cytokines. Many questions remain to be answered. Are the changes due to the cytokines separate from cycle phase, only the cycle phase without the cytokines, or a combination of the two? We have demonstrated dramatic fluctuations in the progenitor and engraftment phenotype with circadian rhythm (D'Hondt et al. 2004), and these fluctuations seem to change in different seasons. Could our observations relate to circadian cycle, or could the circadian cycle and cell cycle phase together determine the phenotypic changes? However, whatever the specific underlying mechanism, the lability of the phenotype over time appears to be established, as is the fact that changes seen can be reversible; thus, the continuum concept. A summary of stem cell lability over time is presented in Table 3.

The continuum concept indicates that the stem cell as a discrete entity defined by cell surface markers, metabolic characteristics, or other functional features, probably cannot be defined, but rather must be defined on a population basis. This, in turn, suggests that we have arrived at a point where reductionist studies alone will be less and less informative; rather, studies of patterns over time will be necessary in order to begin to understand the marrow stem cell system. Mathematical modeling will become an increasingly important and necessary part of this research.

Acknowledgements Supported by: NIH, 1 P20 RR018757; NHLBI, R01 HL073749; NIDDK, R01 DK60084; NIDDK, R01 DK60090; HLB, HL-02–017.

References

Abedi M, Greer D, Colvin G, Demers D, Dooner M, Harpel J, Heinz-Ulrich W, Lambert JF, Quesenberry PJ (2004) Robust conversion of marrow cells to skeletal muscle with formation of marrow-derived muscle cell colonies: a multifactorial process. Exp Hematol 32:426–434

Becker PS, Nilsson SK, Li Z, Berrios VM, Dooner MS, Cooper CJ, Hsieh CC, Quesenberry PJ (1999) Adhesion receptor expression by hematopoietic cell lines and murine progenitors: modulation by cytokines and cell cycle status. Exp Hematol 27:533–541

Berrios VM, Dooner GJ, Nowakowski G, Frimberger A, Valinski H, Quesenberry PJ, Becker PS (2001) The molecular basis for the cytokine-induced defect in homing and engraftment of hematopoietic stem cells. Exp Hematol 29:1326–1335

Bertoncello I, Bradley TR, Dunlop JM, Hodgson GS (1989) The concentration and resolution of primitive hemopoietic cells from normal mouse bone marrow by negative selection using monoclonal antibodies and Dynabead monodisperse magnetic microspheres. Exp Hematol 17:484a

Bradley TR, Metcalf D (1966) The growth of mouse bone marrow cells in vitro. Aust J Exp Biol Med Sci 44:287–299

Bradford GB, Williams B, Rossi R, Bertoncello I (1997) Quiescence, cycling, and turnover in the primitive hematopoietic stem cell compartment. Exp Hematol 25:445–453

Briddell RA, Brandt JE, Straneva JE, Srour EF, Hoffman R (1989) Characterization of the human burst-forming unit-megakaryocyte. Blood 74:145–151

Cerny J, Quesenberry PJ (2004) Chromatin remodeling and stem cell theory of relativity. J Cell Physiol 201:1–16

Cerny J, Dooner MS, McAuliffe CI, Habibian H, Stencil K, Berrios V, Reilly J, Carlson JE, Cerny AM, D'Hondt L, Benoit B, Lambert JF, Colvin GA, Nilsson S, Becker P, Quesenberry P (2002) Homing of purified murine lymphohematopoietic stem cells: a cytokine-induced defect. J Hematother Stem Cell Res 11:913–922

Cheshier SH, Morrison SJ, Liao X, Weissman IL (1999) In vivo proliferation and cell cycle kinetics of long-term self-renewing hematopoietic stem cells. Proc Natl Acad Sci U S A, 96:3120–3125

Colvin GA, Lambert JF, Moore BE, Carlson JE, Dooner MS, Abedi M, Cerny J, Quesenberry PJ (2004) Intrinsic hematopoietic stem cell/progenitor plasticity: inversions. J Cell Physiol 199:20–31

Colvin GA, Dooner MS, Abedi M, Demers D, Lambert JF, Ramanathan M, Bitar I, Huerta F, Aliotta J, Quesenberry PJ (2004) Hotspots of differentiation found in clonally derived purified murine marrow stem cells (abstract). Exp Hematol 32:48

Cronkite EP (1975) Hemopoietic stem cells. An analytic review of hemopoiesis. Pathobiol Annu 5:35–69

D'Hondt L, McAuliffe C, Damon J, Reilly J, Carlson J, Dooner M, Colvin G, Lambert JF, Habibian H, Hsieh C, Stencel K, Quesenberry PJ (2004) Circadian variations of bone marrow engraftability. J Cell Physiol 200:63–70

Dooner MS, Pimentel J, Colvin GA, Abedi M, Aliotta J, Demers D, Greer D, Cerny J, Dooner G, Quesenberry PJ (2004) Engraftment and homing of whole bone marrow and stem cells to lung (abstract). Exp Hematol 32:91

Frimberger AE, Stering AI, Quesenberry PJ (2001) An in vitro model of hematopoietic stem cell homing and maintenance of engraftable stem cells. Blood 98:1012–1018

Gregory CJ (1976) Erythropoietin sensitivity as a differentiation marker in the hemopoietic system: studies of three erythropoietic colony responses in culture. J Cell Physiol 89:289–301

Habibian HK, Peters SO, Hsieh CC, Wuu J, Vergilis K, Grimaldi CI, Reilly J, Carlson JE, Frimberger AE, Stewart FM, Quesenberry PJ (1998) The fluctuating phenotype of the lymphohematopoietic stem cell with cell cycle transit. J Exp Med 188:393–398

Heath DS, Axelrad AA, McLeod DL, Shreeve MM (1976) Separation of the erythropoietin-responsive progenitors BFU-E and CFU-E in mouse bone marrow by unit gravity sedimentation. Blood 47:777–792

Iscove NN, Sieber F (1975) Erythroid progenitors in mouse bone marrow detected my macroscopic colony formation in culture. Exp Hematol 3:32–43

Kittler EL, Peters SO, Crittenden RB, Debatis ME, Ramshaw HS, Stewart FM, Quesenberry PJ (1997) Cytokine-facilitated transduction leads to low-level engraftment in nonablated hosts. Blood 90:865–872

Krause DS, Theise ND, Collector MI, Henegariu O, Hwang S, Gardner R, Neutzel S, Sharkis SJ (2001) Multi-organ, multi-lineage engraftment by a single bone marrow-derived stem cell. Cell 105:369–377

Lagassee E, Connors H, Al-Dhalimy M, Reitsma M, Dohse M, Osborne L, Wang X, Finegold M, Weissman IL, Grompe M (2000) Purified hematopoietic stem cells can differentiate into hepatocytes in vivo. Nat Med 6:1229–1234

Lambert JF, Liu M, Colvin GA, Dooner M, McAuliffe CI, Becker PS, Forget BG, Weissman SM, Quesenberry PJ (2003) Marrow stem cells shift gene expression and engraftment phenotype with cell cycle transit. J Exp Med 197:1563–1572

Long MW, Gragowski LL, Heffner CH, Boxer LA (1985) Phorbol diesters stimulate the development of an early murine progenitor cell. The burst-forming unit-megakaryocyte. J Clin Invest 76:431–438

McLeod DL, Shreeve MM, Axelrad AA (1974) Improved plasma culture system for production of erythrocytic colonies in vitro: quantitative assay method for CFU-E. Blood 44:517–534

McLeod DL, Shreve MM, Axelrad AA (1976) Induction of megakaryocytes colonies with platelet formation in vitro. Nature 261:492–494

McNiece IK, Stewart FM, Deacon DM, Quesenberry PJ (1988a) Synergistic interactions between hematopoietic growth factors as detected by in vitro mouse bone marrow colony formation. Exp Hematol 16:383–388

McNiece IK, Robinson BE, Quesenberry PJ (1988b) Stimulation of murine colony-forming cells with high proliferative potential by the combination of GM-CSF and CSF-1. Blood 72:191–195

McNiece IK, Kriegler AB, Quesenberry PJ (1989a) Studies on the myeloid synergistic factor from 5637: comparison with interleukin-1 alpha. Blood 73:919–923

McNiece IK, Stewart FM, Deacon DM, Temeles DS, Zsebo KM, Clark SC, Quesenberry PJ (1989b) Detection of a human CSF with a high proliferative potential. Blood 74:609–612

McNiece IK, Andrews R, Stewart FM, Clark S, Boone T, Quesenberry PJ (1989c) Action of IL-3, G-CSF, and GM-CSF on highly enriched human hematopoietic progenitor cells: Synergistic interaction of GM-CSF plus G-CSF. Blood 74:110–114

Metcalf D, MacDonald HR, Odartchenko N, Sordat B (1975) Growth of mouse megakaryocyte colonies in vitro. Proc Natl Acad Sci U S A 72:1744–1748

Nakahata T, Ogawa M (1982) Hemopoietic colony-forming cells in umbilical cord blood with extensive capability to generate mono- and multipotential hemopoietic progenitors. J Clin Invest 70:1324–1328

Nakeff A, Dicke KA, Noord van MJ (1975) Megakarocytes in agar cultures of mouse bone marrow. Ser Haematol 8:4–21

Nilsson SK, Dooner MS, Quesenberry PJ (1997) Synchronized cell-cycle induction of engrafting long-term repopulating stem cells. Blood 90:4646–4650

Nowakowski GS, Dooner MS, Valinski HM, Mihaliak AM, Quesenberry PJ, Becker PS (2004) A specific heptapeptide from phage display peptide library homes to bone marrow and binds to primitive hematopoietic stem cells. Stem Cells 22:1030–1038

Ogawa M, Pharr PN, Suda T (1985) Stochastic nature of stem cell functions in culture. Alan R. Liss, New York, pp 11–19

Pang L, Reddy PV, McAuliffe CI, Colvin GA, Quesenberry PJ (2003) Studies on BrdU labeling of hematopoietic cells: stem cells and cell lines. J Cell Physiol 197:251–260

Peters SO, Kittler EL, Ramshaw HS, Quesenberry PJ (1995) Murine marrow cells expanded in culture with IL-3, IL-6, IL-11, and SCF acquire an engraftment defect in normal hosts. Exp Hematol 23:461–469

Peters SO, Kittler EL, Ramshaw HS, Quesenberry PJ (1996) Ex vivo expansion of murine marrow cells with interleukin-3 (IL-3), IL-6, IL-11, and stem cell factor leads to impaired engraftment in irradiated hosts. Blood 87:30–37

Peters SO, Habibian HK, Vergilis K, Quesenberry PJ (1999) Effects on cytokines on stem cell engraftment depends on time of evaluation post-marrow infusion. Int J Hematol 70:112–118

Peters SO, Habibian H, Quesenberry PJ (2002) Cytokine modulation of murine stem cell engraftment: the role of adherence of plastic surfaces. Intl J Hematol 76:84–90

Pluznik DH, Sachs L (1965) The cloning of normal "mast" cells in tissue culture. J Cell Physol 66:319–324

Quesenberry PJ (1991) The blueness of stem cells. Exp Hematol 19:725–728

Reddy GP, Tiarks CY, Pang L, Wuu J, Hsieh CC, Quesenberry PJ (1997) Cell cycle analysis and synchronization of pluripotent hematopoietic progenitor stem cells. Blood 90:2293–2299

Suda T, Suda J, Ogawa M (1983) Single-cell origin of mouse hemopoietic colonies expressing multiple lineages in variable combinations. Proc Natl Acad Sci U S A 80:6689–6693

Suda T, Suda J, Ogawa M (1984) Disparate differentiation in mouse hemopoietic colonies derived from paired progenitors. Proc Natl Acad Sci U S A 81:2520–2524

Till JE, McCulloch EA (1961) A direct measurement of the radiation sensitivity of normal mouse bone marrow cells. Radiat Res 14:213–222

HEP (2006) 174:185–227
© Springer-Verlag Berlin Heidelberg 2006

Markers of Adult Tissue-Based Stem Cells

M. R. Alison[1] (✉) · M. Brittan[1] · M. J. Lovell[2] · N. A. Wright[2]

[1]Centre for Diabetes and Metabolic Medicine, Queen Mary's School of Medicine
and Dentistry, Institute of Cell and Molecolar Science, Whitechapel, London E1 2AT, UK
m.alison@qmul.ac.uk

[2]Histopathology Unit, Cancer Research UK,
44 Lincoln's Inn Fields, London WC2A 3PX, UK

Abstract The expectation generated by the pluripotentiality of embryonic stem (ES) cells
has initiated a renaissance in stem cell biology. While ES cells can be harvested in abundance
and appear to be the most versatile of cells for regenerative medicine, adult stem cells also
hold promise, but the identity and subsequent isolation of these comparatively rare cells
remains problematic in most tissues, perhaps with the notable exception of the bone marrow.
Identifying surface molecules (markers) that would aid in stem cell isolation is thus a major
goal for stem cell biologists. Moreover, the characterization of normal stem cells in specific
tissues may provide a dividend for the treatment of cancer. There is a growing belief that the
successful treatment of neoplastic disease will require specific targeting of the cancer stem
cells, cells that may well have many of the characteristics of their normal counterparts.

Keywords Stem cells · Side population cells · ABC membrane transporters · Telomerase ·
Integrins · Bromodeoxyuridine · ^{3}H-thymidine · Label retaining cells · Ki-67 · CD34 ·
CD133 · Musashi-1 · Nestin · p63

1
Introduction

The identification of molecular markers that best facilitate the isolation and
characterization of stem cell populations has long been a worthwhile challenge.
In studies of the haematopoietic system, both experimental and clinical, the expression of the sialomucin CD34 has traditionally been exploited to enrich cells
with long-term marrow repopulation capacity, though not all haematopoietic
stem cells (HSCs) express this marker (Bonnet 2002). Moreover, it was in the
bone marrow that cells with the key properties of adult stem cells, namely
self-renewal and multilineage potential, were first recognized. In fact, such
cells were first described operationally back in 1961 by Till and McCulloch
as cells that gave rise to multilineage haematopoietic colonies in the spleen
(colony forming units-spleen [CFU-S]). Indeed, the ability of a single cell to
give rise to a large family of descendants (clonogenicity), containing all the
lineages normally found in that cell's tissue of origin is considered a reasonably
robust proof of 'stemness' (Fig. 1). For example, the recently proposed stem
cells of the human heart and brain have met these criteria (Beltrami et al.
2003; Sanai et al. 2004); the former producing monoclonally-derived colonies
containing cells expressing proteins consistent with either cardiomyocyte, endothelia or smooth muscle differentiation, the latter colonies demonstrating
neuronal, oligodendrocytic and astrocytic differentiation. Some have argued
that stem cell markers are like the spots on a Dalmatian dog, useful for iden-

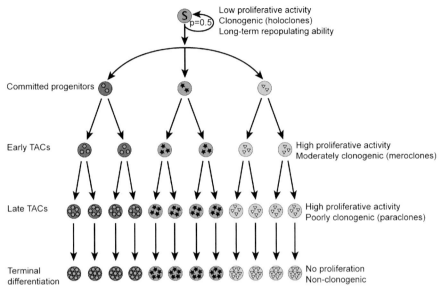

Fig. 1 In most renewing systems, a cell hierarchy can be recognized in which a few self-renewing stem cells (p = probability of self-renewal) give rise to a limited number of committed progenitors, also called transit amplifying cells (*TACs*). TACs have limited proliferation potential and eventually give rise to reproductively sterile terminally differentiated cells. In vitro, stem cells, early TACs and late TACs are thought to generate holoclones, meroclones and paraclones, respectively

tification, but which do not appear to play an essential role in dog (stem cell) function (Fig. 2). This assertion seems counterintuitive from an evolutionary standpoint, and, for example, many so-called markers have a function consistent with the protection of these valuable cells e.g. ABC transporters to efflux potential toxins and high expression of extracellular matrix (ECM) receptors such as integrins to anchor cells to the underlying basement membrane. In this chapter, we describe some general markers that may serve in stem cell identification, along with more tissue-restricted markers, but noting that in each case these markers are not generally specific to any one tissue. We should also add that some markers may represent 'a moving target' in that their expression may vary without loss of stem cell function (Dorrell et al. 2000; Deschaseaux et al. 2003), at least in vitro.

2
Common Attributes of Stem Cells

Stem cells appear to be located in all organs of the body, though in ageing organs such as the heart their regenerative powers seem muted (Sussman

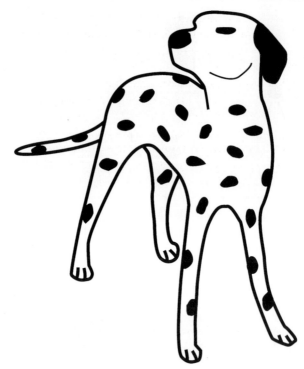

Fig. 2 Are markers of stem cells merely good for recognition (like spots on a dog) or do they serve a function?

and Anversa 2004). With regard to their attributes, we can make some broad descriptions that might aid in identification.

2.1
Strategic Placement

When cell migration occurs in a tissue, stem cells are at the beginning of the flux. Particularly where cell flux is unidirectional, e.g. epidermis, stem cells are at one end of the cell escalator in the basal layer, with cells being shed at the surface. This makes sense if the stem cell population is to be preserved; a niche may achieve the same goal (see below).

2.2
Self-Renewal

Stem cells in any tissue are a self-renewing population, achieving this if, on average, each stem cell division gives rise to one replacement stem cell and one transit amplifying cell (TAC) by asymmetric cell division. Equally well, stem cell numbers would remain constant if only symmetrical divisions occurred provided that each time a stem cell gave rise to two daughter TACs, another stem cell gave rise to two daughter stem cells (Fig. 3). Stem cells are normally located in a restrictive environment called a niche (French, recess), and in a tissue such as the small intestine, the niche is found close to the crypt base at the origin of a bidirectional flux (Fig. 7B). Interactions within the stem cell niche, a specialized environment composed of mesenchymal cells and extracellular matrix, are crucial to the self-renewal process and the controlling factors are rapidly becoming elucidated. In the *Drosophila* ovariole, a stem cell niche known as the germarium has been defined, and here the germline stem cell (GSC) number is maintained by the close apposition of GSCs with cap cells; Armadillo

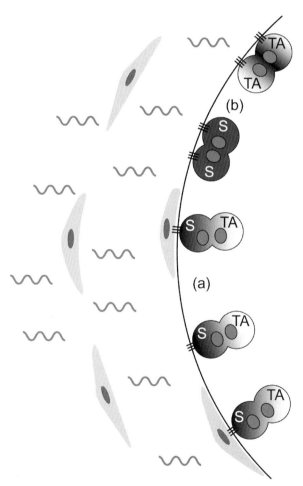

Fig. 3 The stem cell niche. (*a*) Stem cell self-renewal can be achieved if all stem cells divide asymmetrically with the mitotic cleavage plane parallel to the basement membrane. Alternatively (*b*) symmetrical divisions can achieve the same end-result: population asymmetry

(fly β-catenin) and decapentaplegic (DPP) (a homologue of mammalian bone morphogenetic proteins [BMPs]) signalling are involved (Gonalez-Reyes 2003). Likewise, in the *Drosophila* testis, GSC number is strictly controlled by the interaction with so-called hub cells (Yamashita et al. 2003); in both the ovariole and testis, disruption of DPP signalling and/or Armadillo/APC interactions can result in supernumerary GSCs due to alterations in the orientation of the mitotic axes (see Fig. 3). In mammals, cadherin/catenins and BMP signalling are also involved in the maintenance of haematopoietic stem cell number through interactions with osteoblasts (Zhang et al. 2003).

2.3
Small in Number

Stem cells are a small percentage of the total cellularity. In the mouse small intestine, there are perhaps four to five stem cells near the bottom of the crypt out of a total crypt population of about 250 cells (Marshman et al. 2002). Likewise, in skeletal muscle, satellite cells comprise about 5% of all nuclei. In the bone marrow, the multipotential haematopoietic stem cell is even rarer, with a frequency of 1 in 10,000 or more amongst all bone marrow cells.

2.4
Undifferentiated

Stem cells are relatively undifferentiated. In most tissues, the stem cells do not have the functional specializations of the progeny that they give rise to.

2.5
Slowly Cycling

Stem cells are slowly cycling but highly clonogenic. Teleologically it would seem prudent to restrict stem cell division because DNA synthesis can be error-prone. Thus, in many tissues we see that stem cells divide less frequently than TACs. In the intestine, the stem cells cycle less frequently than the more luminally located TACs (Marshman et al. 2002), and in the human epidermis the integrin-bright cells have a lower level of proliferation than the other basal cells (see Sect. 3.6.1). In hair follicles, the hair shaft and its surrounding sheaths are derived from TACs in the hair bulb that is itself replenished by the bulge stem cells. As befits true stem cells, the bulge cells divide less frequently but are more clonogenic than the TACs of the hair bulb.

2.6
Side Populations

In 1996, Goodell et al. reported on a new method for the isolation of HSCs based on the ability of the HSCs to efflux a fluorescent dye. Like the activity of the P-glycoprotein (encoded by the *mdr1* gene), this activity was verapamil-sensitive. Cells subjected to Hoechst 33342 dye staining and fluorescence activated cell sorting (FACS) analysis can give a fluorescent profile, as illustrated in Fig. 4. Those that actively efflux the Hoechst dye appear as a distinct population of cells on the side of the profile; hence the name the side population (SP) has been given to these cells. Numerous studies now point to the fact that the SP phenotype of HSCs in mice and humans is largely determined by the expression of a protein known as the ABCG2 transporter (ATP-binding cassette [ABC] subfamily G member 2, also known as BCRP1) (Scharenberg et al. 2002; Kim et al. 2002; Zhou et al. 2002; Guo et al. 2003). Additionally, a diverse range of adult tissues (e.g. skeletal muscle, brain, liver and spleen) contain $CD34^+$ SP cells capable of forming haematopoietic colonies in vitro, indicating that the bone marrow is not the sole provenance of adult haematopoiesis (Asakura and Rudnicki 2002). Moreover, tissues such as brain and skeletal muscle not only have a much higher proportion of $CD34^-$ compared to $CD34^+$ SP cells, but these cells do not express nestin or satellite cell markers, respectively, suggesting that SP cells represent a distinct class of tissue-specific stem cells, perhaps present in all tissues (Asakura and Rudnicki 2002; Zhou et al. 2001)? The ABC superfamily of membrane transporters is one of the largest protein classes known, characterized by expression of an ATP-binding cassette region functioning to hydrolyse ATP to support energy-dependent substrate exportation against steep concentration gradients across membranes, principally from the intracellular cytoplasm to the extracellular space (Klein et al. 1999; Borst and Elferink 2002; Schinkel and Jonker 2003). The ATP-binding cassette is a 200- to 250-amino acid mini-protein harbouring two short conserved peptide motifs (Walker A and Walker B), involved in ATP binding, with a third conserved sequence (the ABC signature) interposed between the Walker A and B sequences (Klein et al. 1999). A highly informative website compiled by Michael Muller's group at Wageningen University, The Netherlands (http://www.nutrigene.4 t.com/humanabc.htm) currently lists 48 human ABC transporters organized into seven families (Table 1).

Table 1 Families of ABC transporter proteins

Family	Number of members	Symbols
ABC1 (subfamily A)	12	ABCA1-ABCA12
MDR/TAP (subfamily B)	11	ABCB1-ABCB11
CFTR/MRP (subfamily C)	12	ABCC1-ABCC12
ALD (subfamily D)	4	ABCD1-ABCD4
OABP (subfamily E)	1	ABCE1
GCN20 (subfamily F)	3	ABCF1-ABCF3
White (subfamily G)	5	ABCG1-ABCG5

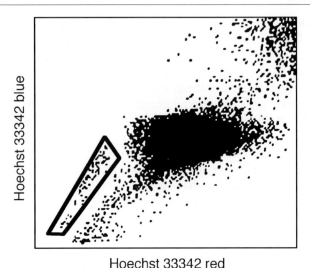

Hoechst 33342 red

Fig. 4 Hypothetical SP profile for bone marrow. *Vertical axis* shows blue Hoechst fluorescence, *horizontal axis* shows red Hoechst fluorescence. SP cells indicated within the trapezoid gate have a low uptake of dye and a high blue:red ratio. Typically, SP cells comprise about 0.05% of the total bone marrow cells and are highly enriched for long-term repopulating activity

ABC transporters play a role in the transport of drugs (xenobiotics) and drug conjugates. Their role is exemplified by MDR1 (ABCB1 or P-glycoprotein), MRP1 (the multidrug resistance protein 1, ABCC1) and BCRP1 (breast cancer resistance protein 1, ABCG2) whose expression is associated with multidrug resistance (MDR) in cancer cells (Litman et al 2000); BCRP1 is a half-transporter that functions as a homo- or heterodimer, and is unique amongst half-transporters in that it is localized to the plasma membrane (Rocchi et al. 2000). Drug resistance results from the ability of the transporters to extrude several classes of anticancer drugs, lowering effective concentrations within the cell. For example, MDR1 is able to cause the greatest resistance to bulky amphipathic drugs such as paclitaxel (taxol) anthracyclines and *Vinca* alkaloids. SP cells can be isolated from human tumours, and probably contribute significantly to tumour drug resistance (Hirschmann-Jax et al. 2005).

ABC transporters have emerged as an important new field of investigation in the regulation of stem cell biology (Bunting 2002), and manipulation of the system can result in stem cell amplification (Bunting et al. 2000). Furthermore, in skeletal muscle, CD34$^+$/CD45$^-$ cells expressing ABCG2 mRNA can give rise to endothelial and skeletal muscle cells (Tamaki et al. 2002), and it has been claimed that marrow-derived SP cells in skeletal muscle specifically engraft into endothelium during injury-induced vascular regeneration while non-SP cells from the same source engraft into smooth muscle (Majka et al. 2003). In the pancreas too, multipotential progenitors can express the neural stem cell marker nestin along with ABCG2 and MDR1 (Lechner et al. 2002), and MDR1 expression is a feature of the recipient cells that engraft the myocardium of transplanted female hearts in male recipients (Quaini et al. 2002). SP cells have also been isolated from human and mouse breast tissue, and murine SP cells can give rise to both myoepithelial and luminal breast epithelial cell lineages when transplanted into cleared fat pads (Alvi et al. 2003). ABC transporters are not the only cytoprotective molecules present in adult stem cells; aldehyde dehydrogenase (ALDH) is a detoxifying enzyme expressed at high levels in HSCs (see Sect. 3.1.1), while some liver and pulmonary airway stem cells may be resistant to potential toxins through low expression of drug-metabolizing cytochrome P450 enzymes (see Sects. 3.4 and 3.11, respectively).

2.7
Maintenance of Genome Integrity

In addition to an infrequently dividing nature, stem cells would also appear to have devised a strategy for maintaining genome integrity. Termed the 'immortal strand' hypothesis by John Cairns (Cairns 1975), stem cells can apparently designate one of the two strands of DNA in each chromosome as a template strand, such that in each round of DNA synthesis while both strands of DNA are copied, only the template strand and its copy is allocated to the daughter cell that remains a stem cell (Fig. 5). Thus, any errors in replication would be readily transferred (within one generation) to TACs that are soon lost from the population. Such a mechanism probably accounts for the ability of putative stem cells to be label-retaining cells (LRCs) after injection of DNA labels when stem cells are being formed. However, as we shall see, most investigators have attributed the presence of LRCs to the infrequent cycling of stem cells in vivo, without testing for the ability of LRCs to further synthesize DNA and divide, yet still segregating the immortal DNA strands from sister chromatids into the daughter cell that remains a stem cell; there have been notable exceptions to this omission (Potten et al. 2002; Merok et al. 2002; see Sect. 3.3.3).

2.8
Generic Stem Cell Markers

A number of molecules are expressed by a variety of putative organ-specific stem cells and these are listed in Table 2. Collectively these molecules appear to be involved in maintaining 'stemness', ensuring longevity, adhesion to a niche and a slow cycling habitus. The transcription factor Oct-4, important for the maintenance of pluripotency in embryonic stem cells, has been claimed to be expressed in a variety of adult stem cells, but the identity of the cells illustrated is unclear (Tai et al. 2005).

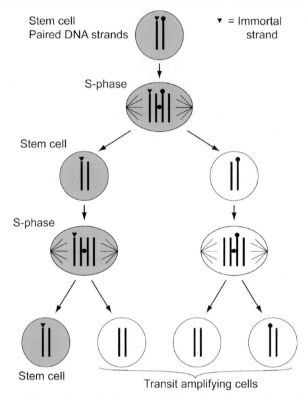

Fig. 5 The immortal strand hypothesis. Genomic integrity of stem cells can be preserved if newly synthesized strands of DNA are always allocated to TACs, and stem cells retain the immortal (template) strand. The template strand of each chromosome is established when stem cells are being created

Table 2 Examples of generic stem cell markers

Marker	Function (known or proposed)
CD34, CD133, integrins	Cell adhesion to substratum
Bcl-2, telomerase, ABC transporters	Cell survival
c-kit	Receptor for stem cell factor (SCF)
Musashi 1	Asymmetrical cell division, stem cell renewal
Nestin	Embryonic intermediate filament
p27^{Kip1}	Inhibition of cyclin-dependent kinases
p63	p53 homologue

3
Organ-Specific Stem Cells

3.1
Bone Marrow

Leaving aside the potential of bone marrow cells to generate the likes of cardiomyocytes, hepatocytes and neurons – so-called transdifferentiation or plasticity (Alison et al. 2003), the adult marrow contains, not one, but at least three ostensibly discrete stem cell populations; haematopoietic stem cells (HSCs), mesenchymal stem cells (MSCs) and endothelial precursor cells (EPCs).

3.1.1
Haematopoietic Stem Cells

HSCs are rare cells, with a frequency of 1 in 10^4 to 1 in 10^5 amongst bone marrow cells. The expression of the cell surface sialomucin CD34 has, for a long time, been the basis for the selection of HSCs, and the mainstay of HSC transplantation is currently still the selection of CD34$^+$ cells. However, repopulating cell assays in the likes of fetal preimmune sheep and immunodeficient mice suggest that HSCs can be either CD34$^+$ or CD34$^-$, and that selection of CD34$^+$ cells may exclude more primitive cells (Bonnet 2002). Such cells might express ABCG2, a common determinant of the SP phenotype (Zhou et al. 2001), and it seems that ABCG2 expression is greatest in CD34-negative cells and is downregulated in CD34$^+$ and, of course, with specific lineage differentiation. Another alternative to CD34 may be the expression of CD133 (AC133) (Bhatia 2001), a 120-kDa glycosylated protein containing five transmembrane domains, though whether this marker is superior to CD34 in selecting for HSCs is unclear. Nevertheless, the initiation of human acute myeloid leukaemia (AML) in NOD/SCID mice by AML cell transplantation appears to be the provenance of the CD34$^+$ CD38$^-$ fraction (Bonnet and Dick 1997).

The expression of CD34 probably depends on the degree of activation; CD34$^-$ negative cells being quiescent while CD34$^+$ cells are activated self-renewing cells – likened to a flexible continuum rather than a hierarchy. Differences in gene expression between quiescent and activated HSCs have been explored (Venezia et al. 2004). Because the expression of CD34 is rather a 'moving target', purification on the basis of a more robust marker might seem desirable. Thus, Storms et al. (1999) have exploited the fact that HSCs have high levels of aldehyde dehydrogenase (ALDH), a detoxifying enzyme that confers resistance to alkylating agents such as cyclophosphamide. They describe a substrate that can be used to isolate cells with high ALDH activity by flow cytometry since the fluorescent reaction product is retained within viable cells. This so-called Aldefluor reagent system has been recommended because of its simplicity (Armstrong et al. 2004). Hess et al. (2004) have purified HSCs from human cord blood on the basis of high ALDH. They comprised 23% of the Lin- fraction and highly co-expressed markers such as $CD34^+$ $CD38^-$ and $CD34^-$ $CD133^+$; the $ALDH^{high}$ Lin^- cells were clonogenic in vitro and able to repopulate immune-deficient mice with committed progenitors and primitive repopulating cells. VEGFR2 (KDR in humans) expression alone or in combination with the likes of CD133 or CD34 has also been suggested as a good marker of HSCs (Ziegler et al.1999).

Sca-1 (stem cell antigen 1, Ly-6A/E) is an 18-kDa phosphatidylinositol-anchored protein expressed on murine multipotent HSCs, frequently used in combination with negative selection for a number of cell surface markers characteristic of commitment toward haematolymphoid lineages (Lin^-) to select for murine HSCs. In the mouse, usually a panel of surface markers, in the absence of all lineage markers (Lin^-) is employed to identify HSCs, commonly isolated as c-Kit^+ Thy 1.1^{lo} Lin^- Sca-1^+ (KTLS). Recent advances in HSC biology have been reviewed by Bonde et al. (2004).

3.1.2
Mesenchymal Stem Cells

In comparison to HSCs, MSCs, also known as marrow stromal cells, are not well antigenically characterized. In vitro, single cell suspensions of bone marrow generate colonies of adherent stromal cells that can readily differentiate into either bone, cartilage or fat, but can also be coaxed in to many other cell types. Each colony is derived from a single cell called a colony-forming unit fibroblast (CFU-F). MSCs are rare, declining in frequency with age, being present in bone marrow aspirates at a frequency of $0.1–5/10^5$ cells in rodents and $1–20/10^5$ in humans (Short et al. 2003). STRO-1 is an antibody that positively identifies MSCs, and the frequency of CFU-F is enriched 100-fold in the STRO-1^+/Glycophorin A^- population compared to the STRO-1^+/Glycophorin A^+ population. In the mouse, the Sca-1^+ Lin^- $CD31^-$ $CD45^-$ fraction has a plating efficiency of approximately 30% for CFU-F. In human bone marrow, the combined use of the STRO-1 and VECAM-1 (CD106) antibodies results in a fraction with a plating efficiency of almost 50% for CFU-F (Gronthos et al. 2003). MSCs can be partly defined by a huge range of both positive and negative phenotypic staining characteristics, but none of these traits are specific to MSCs (reviewed in Pittenger and Martin 2004; Tropel et al. 2004; Otto and Rao 2004). Apart from bone marrow, MSCs can also be found in connective tissue, adipose tissue and muscle.

3.1.3
Endothelial Progenitor Cells

EPCs constitute a unique population of peripheral blood mononuclear cells derived from bone marrow that are involved in postnatal angiogenesis during wound healing, limb ischaemia, postmyocardial infarction, atherosclerosis and tumour vascularization. HSCs and EPCs are seemingly derived from a common precursor called a haemangioblast, so in the bone marrow these cells share many antigenic determinants, including CD34, CD133, Sca-1, c-Kit, Tie-2 and Flk-1 (Iwami et al. 2004; Hristov and Weber 2004; Khakoo and Finkel 2005). However, once in the circulation, these cells express markers of endothelial commitment, including von Willebrand factor (vWF) and VE-cadherin (Hristov and Weber 2004). The primitive EPC is probably best defined as $CD133^+$ $CD34^+$ $Flk-1^+$.

3.2
Musculoskeletal Stem Cells

Sources of stem cells for musculoskeletal repair include bone marrow, peritrabecular tissues in cancellous bone, cartilage, muscle, fat and pericytes: collectively known as connective tissue stem cells, most of which seem multipotent.

3.2.1
Cartilage

Articular cartilage is a unique avascular load-bearing live tissue that does not normally self-repair. In the bovine, Dowthwaite et al. (2004) have suggested that appositional cartilage growth is achieved by stem/progenitor cells on the articular surfaces; these cells expressed the $\alpha5\beta1$ integrin, the classical fibronectin receptor and expression of Notch 1 appeared to identify the most clonogenic cells.

3.2.2
Bone

Osteoblastic progenitors can be recognized in vitro as cells that make colonies that express alkaline phosphatase (CFU-APs), and in humans there are on average 55 CFU-APs/10^6 nucleated bone marrow cells (Muschler et al. 2001); in both sexes there is a decline in frequency with age. The exact nature of osteogenic stem cells is unclear, Muschler et al. (2003) advocates the term 'connective tissue progenitors' (CTPs) to encompass a heterogeneous group of multipotential stem cells responsible for musculoskeletal renewal and repair. This would include pericytes, present outside the basement membrane of small blood vessels and fibroblastic cells in the bone marrow known as Westin-Bainton cells; it is uncertain whether these cells are true stem cells or transit amplifying cells, but progenitors eventually give rise to secretory osteoblasts with limited self-renewal capacity (short-lived, $\sim$40 days) that produce bone matrix, and finally long-lived osteocytes are produced.

3.2.3
Skeletal Muscle

It is generally accepted that unipotential satellite cells, comprising 5% of the nuclei present within muscle fibres, located outside the myofibre but beneath the basement membrane, are the major source of myogenic cells for growth and repair of postnatal skeletal muscle (Fig. 6). Such cells are highly expressive of M-cadherin (Goldring et al. 2002). Though the role of the bone marrow in providing cells for muscle regeneration has been much vaunted (Camargo et al. 2003), the indigenous satellite cell has been reaffirmed as the major player (Sherwood et al. 2004; Partridge 2004). Preactivated satellite cells are CD34[+] Sca1[−] (Zammit and Beauchamp 2001); other markers include the transcription factor Pax7, but once activated by injury the myogenic genes *Myf-5* and *MyoD* are switched on (reviewed in Chen and Goldhammer 2003). A population of muscle-derived stem cells, distinct from satellite cells, that are CD34[+] Sca1[+] has also been described (Huard et al. 2003).

3.3
Gastrointestinal Tract

The gastrointestinal tract (GIT) is lined by region-specific epithelial coverings, beginning with stratified squamous epithelia lining the oral cavity and oesophagus, progressing to the gastric glands of the stomach, moving distally to the small intestine where the simple epithelial lining is thrown into invaginations (crypts) and finger-like projections (villi), and finally to the colorectum where crypts are still present but villi are absent.

3.3.1
Oesophagus

The surface of the human oesophagus is relatively flat, but invaginations of the basement membrane produce tall papillary structures within the stratified epithelium. Cell proliferation is confined to the basal and immediately epibasal

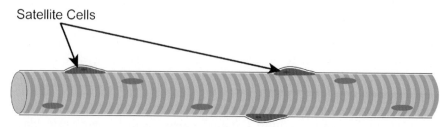

Fig. 6 Satellite cells are located between the multinucleated myotube and the underlying basement membrane, proliferating after damage with cell progeny becoming incorporated into the myotube

layers, with cell division more common in the papillary basal layer (PBL) than in the flat interpapillary basal layer (IBL) (Seery 2002). In the PBL, the mitotic axes tend to be parallel to the basement membrane, so both daughter cells remain in the basal layer, whereas in the IBL, the mitotic axes tend to be at right angles to the basement membrane; thus, one daughter cell remains a stem cell and the other daughter cell becomes a transit amplifying cell in the more proliferatively active epibasal layers (see Fig. 3). Unlike the cells of the PBL and epibasal cells, oesophageal stem cells are thought to be relatively undifferentiated, not expressing CKs 13, 14 and 15. Okumura et al. (2003) also isolated a fraction of human oesophageal cells that expressed a relatively low level of both CK13 and involucrin, and observed that these cells were additionally characterized by high expression of the low-affinity neurotrophin receptor p75^{NTR} but low β1 integrin expression; such cells behaved as stem cells in vitro. The expression of p75^{NTR} may also characterize unipotent stem cells of other squamous epithelia such as uterine cervix.

3.3.2
Stomach

In the stomach, the epithelial lining is folded to form structures called gastric glands; the gastric stem cells are located and maintained within a mesenchymal niche situated towards the centre of the gland (Fig. 7a). Thus, cell flux in the glands is bidirectional, cells descending downwards toward the gland base and upwards toward the surface via the gastric pit (Wright and Alison 1984). In the mouse, RT-PCR analysis of cells retrieved from the niche by laser capture microdissection has indicated that gene expression closely matches that found in HSCs (Mills et al. 2002). Surprisingly, there are very few 'markers' described for gastric stem cells; however, Bjerknes and Cheng (2002) have established that multipotential progenitor cells exist in the mouse stomach. Using a mutagenicity strategy with ethylnitrosourea, they created mutant clones in adult hemizygous ROSA26 mice in vivo that did *not* express β-galactosidase, and all cell lineages could be found in a single clone – persuasive evidence for the existence of multipotential cells. From ultrastructural observations in the isthmic region of human stomach, Karam et al. (2003) have suggested that perhaps the stem cells are so-called mini-granule cells, cells with minute, dense or cored secretory granules, somewhat akin to the granule-free cells found in the mouse. An RNA-binding protein of 39 kDa, known as Musashi1 (Msi-1) was first identified in *Drosophila* and thought responsible for the asymmetric divisions of sensory organ precursor cells (Sakakibara et al. 1996); it may also be a marker for gut stem cells. The location of Msi-1-expressing cells coincides with the zone of active proliferation, at least in *Xenopus laevis* (Ishizuya-Oka et al. 2003).

3.3.3
Small and Large Intestine

In the small intestine, the stem cells are located in a postulated stem cell niche in the crypt base, just superior to the Paneth cells, although some intermingling with Paneth cells may occur (Fig. 7b). In the large intestine, in the absence of Paneth cells, stem cells occupy the crypt bottom. The mesenchymal intestinal sub-epithelial myofibroblasts and their secreted basement membrane factors (in particular Wnts) are believed to form and maintain the stem cell niche, and thereby regulate epithelial cell function. The stem cells give rise to transit amplifying cells, which proliferate and differentiate as they migrate upward in the crypt towards the intestinal lumen. The neural stem cell marker, Msi-1, believed to suppress neural cell differentiation, positively regulates the transcriptional repressor molecule, Hes-1. In the mouse small intestine, Msi-1 and Hes-1 are co-expressed in the cells just above the Paneth cell zone, thus these markers may denote the stem cell zone, though Hes-1 expression additionally extends to proliferative cells higher up the crypt (Kayahara et al. 2003). Musashi-1 mRNA and protein expression has been confirmed in the murine intestinal stem cell zone (Potten et al. 2003), though after crypt damage, Msi-1 expression appeared to be expressed by many proliferative cells above the stem cell zone – possibly as a consequence of the long half-life of the protein in conjunction with rapidly cycling regenerating cells. In human colonic crypts, expression of Msi-1 in scattered cells between cell positions 1–10 supports

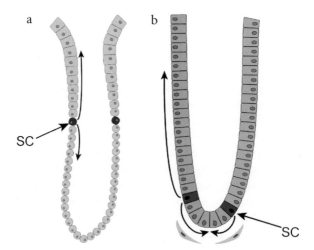

Fig. 7 a In the gastric glands, stem cells are located in the isthmic region just beneath the foveolus (gastric pit), and TACs are located above and below this region. **b** In the small intestine, stem cells are in a ring at about cell position 4–5 (counting from the base), and migration is mostly upwards towards the crypt orifice, though there is also migration of Paneth cells towards the crypt base

the notion that Msi-1 is a marker of stem cells, and probably also some TACs (Nishimura et al. 2003). A *reduced* expression of E-cadherin has been reported in the putative stem cell zone of the human small bowel crypt (Escaffit et al. 2005).

Since the discovery that the absence of Tcf-4 results in mice failing to maintain a stem cell compartment in the intestine (Korinek et al. 1998), it has become very clear that β-catenin/Tcf-4 signalling is a major determinant of proliferation vs differentiation in the crypt. Wnt glycoproteins secreted by the sub-epithelial myofibroblasts, through binding to Frizzled receptors on epithelial cells, are responsible for disabling the intracellular machinery (APC, axin, GSK-3β) that normally functions to phosphorylate excess β-catenin and target it for ubiquitination and proteasomal destruction. Thus, nuclear β-catenin itself may mark stem cells (van de Wetering et al. 2002), and the proteins encoded by β-catenin target genes (e.g. CD44 and c-Myc) do appear to be expressed in stem cells as well as some other proliferative cells. Likewise, receptor tyrosine kinases of the Eph subfamily, particularly EphB2 and EphB3, are targets of β-catenin/Tcf-4 signalling, thus are expressed in the stem cell zone, but again it appears, also in other proliferative cells in superior cell positions (Batlle et al. 2002; Sancho et al. 2003, 2004).

In common with many other tissues, the location of the intestinal stem cell zone has been inferred by the presence of label-retaining cells (LRCs). Potten et al. (2002), first labelled intestinal epithelial cells by a course of ^{3}H-thymidine injections at a time of stem cell expansion that occurred either during early postnatal life or after severe mucosal injury, noting several weeks later that the heavily ^{3}H-thymidine-labelled cells (LRCs) were predominantly in cell positions 4 and 5, though some LRCs were observed higher up the crypt, notably cell positions 6–9. In theory, LRCs (putative stem cells) exist either because of their infrequent cycling (thus label is not so diluted by division in comparison to other proliferatively competent cells), or because these cells have a mechanism for selectively retaining the so-called template DNA strand during the duplication and segregation of sister chromatids—the immortal strand hypothesis (Cairns 2002) (Fig. 5). To demonstrate that the latter mechanism was operative in the generation of small intestinal LRCs, Potten et al. further labelled the ^{3}H-thymidine-labelled mice with a course of bromodeoxyuridine (BrdU) injections, observing that the LRCs soon became both ^{3}H-thymidine- and BrdU-positive, but then they rapidly lost the BrdU label, indicating that ^{3}H-thymidine label retention was not due to the cells remaining out of cycle.

3.4
Liver

The liver is normally proliferatively quiescent, but hepatocyte loss uncomplicated by virus infection or inflammation invokes a rapid regenerative response from all cell types in the liver to restore the organ to its pristine state. More-over, hepatocyte transplants in animals have shown that a certain proportion of hepatocytes in foetal and adult liver can clonally expand, suggesting that hepa-toblasts/hepatocytes are themselves the functional stem cells of the liver. More severe liver injury can activate a facultative stem cell compartment located within the intrahepatic biliary tree, giving rise to cords of bipotential tran-sit amplifying cells (oval cells/hepatic progenitor cells), that can ultimately differentiate into hepatocytes and biliary epithelial cells (Fig. 8; Alison et al. 2004).

If all surviving hepatocytes can regenerate in response to a large hepatocyte loss, are there any markers that identify a particular subset that may be more clonogenic? If rats are treated with retrorsine, a compound metabolized by the hepatocyte's cytochrome P450 mixed function oxidase system to a metabolite that forms DNA adducts, blocking the cell's ability to proliferate, then in response to a two-thirds partial hepatectomy, regeneration is accomplished by the activation, expansion and differentiation of so-called small hepatocyte-like progenitors (SHPCs) (Gordon et al. 2000). These cell clusters lacked CYP enzymes that are usually readily induced by retrorsine, and this probably accounts for their resistance to the anti-proliferative effects of retrorsine. Ferry and colleagues have provided persuasive evidence that these SHPCs are clonally derived, seemingly at random from amongst all hepatocytes (Avril et al. 2004), but we have no further clues as to the identity of these seemingly relatively undifferentiated hepatocytes.

The clonogenic potential of transplanted adult hepatocytes has been very impressively shown in the fumarylacetoacetate hydrolase (Fah) null mouse,

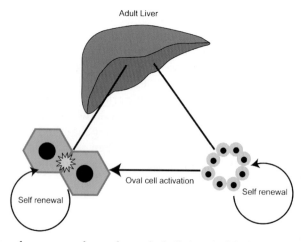

Fig. 8 In the liver, hepatocytes that make up the bulk (90%) of the liver are the regenerative cells after most injuries, but when hepatocyte regeneration is impeded some bile duct cells give rise to oval cells (TACs) that can differentiate into hepatocytes

a model of hereditary type 1 tyrosinaemia, where a profoundly strong positive selection pressure is exerted on the transplanted wild type cells due to liver failure (Overturf et al. 1997), but here again we have no idea if a subset of hepatocytes is responsible. Fujikawa et al. (2003) have, like Suzuki and colleagues in foetal liver (Suzuki et al. 2000, 2002), identified a population of CD49f$^+$, CD29$^+$, c-kit$^-$, CD45$^-$ and Ter119$^-$ cells in adult mouse liver, that were bipotential and clonogenic in vitro.

When either massive damage is inflicted upon the liver or regeneration after damage is compromised, a *potential* stem cell compartment located within the smallest branches of the intrahepatic biliary tree is activated. This so-called oval cell or ductular reaction, comprising TACs, expands this biliary-derived population before they differentiate into either hepatocytes or cholangiocytes (Alison et al. 1996, 1997, 1998, 2004). In rats, oval cells are predominantly derived from the canal of Hering, and thus this is the location of a stem cell niche (Paku et al. 2001). However, there does not appear to be any specific marker that identifies a subset of biliary cells that are in any way different from the bulk of the cholangiocyte population. Thus, perhaps all biliary cells, or at least those in the smallest ducts, have stem cell potential, and they can be recognized by expression of typical cholangiocyte proteins such as CK7 and 19, GGT and glutathione-S-transferase (GST-P) along with a host of monoclonal antibodies raised against cytoskeletal proteins and unknown surface antigens (Alison 2003). Moreover, antigens traditionally associated with haematopoietic cells can also be expressed by oval cells, including c-kit, flt-3, Thy-1 and CD34 (Baumann et al. 1999; Petersen et al. 1998; Lemmer et al. 1998; Omori et al. 1997). Several ABC transporter proteins are expressed by regenerating ductules in damaged human liver (Ros et al. 2003), and the ABCG2/BCRP1 protein marks rat oval cells (Shimano et al. 2003), adding support to the proposal that ABC transporter proteins are intimately involved in the biology of stem/progenitor cells in many tissues. However, is the expression of these ABC transporters in liver ductules a genuine marker of stem cells/progenitors or merely a reflection of the protective role these proteins undoubtedly perform within the biliary tree against toxic bile constituents (Scheffer et al. 2002)? The correct answer is probably the latter since it is highly unlikely that all the reactive ductular cells are stem cells or even progenitors, and many are imminently going to differentiate into hepatocytes and cholangiocytes. Nevertheless, the expression of ABC transporters adds incrementally to the battery of already established markers for this stem cell-initiated response.

3.5
Pancreas

The pancreas is essentially two different tissues (Fig. 9): the exocrine pancreas, organized into acini and a branching duct system that produces digestive enzymes, and the endocrine tissue, the islets of Langerhans, that produce the

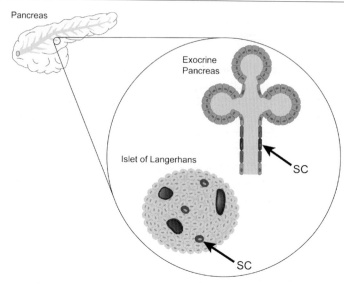

Fig. 9 Pancreas has both exocrine (ducted gland) and endocrine (islets of Langerhan) components. Both ducts and islets appear able to generate new endocrine tissue, particularly new insulin-producing β cells

hormones glucagon, insulin, somatostatin and pancreatic polypeptide from four separate cell types, α, β, δ and PP cells, respectively. There are about 1 million islets in a human pancreas, each composed of roughly 3,000 cells of which 75% are insulin-producing β cells. It is the renewal of β cells that is of primary interest for the treatment of diabetes, a disease that currently afflicts 200 million people worldwide. There is no doubt that insulin-producing β cells can, and do divide throughout life, but there is as yet no clearly identifiable adult pancreatic stem cell (Bonner-Weir and Sharma 2002). There are a number of studies reporting that β cells can be generated from islet tissue in culture: equally well, ductal tissue can be cultured to produce β cells, and pancreatic ducts have been proposed as the location of β cell and islet neogenesis in many models of pancreatic damage.

In pancreatic ontogeny, a coordinated cascade of transcription factors is required for β cell development (Wang et al. 2004). Ngn3 specifies endocrine fate and induces Pax4, that along with Nkx2.2 and Nkx6.1 rapidly induces Pax6 and Islet1. The program of β cell differentiation is complete once Pdx1 increases, HB9 is induced and insulin synthesis begins. These transcription factors may be useful markers of β cell progenitors in the adult. Indeed, such factors are expressed in ducts that appear to be responsible for the rapid islet neogenesis that occurs after a 90% partial pancreatectomy (Px) in the rat (Bonner Weir and Sharma 2002). Of course, such gene expression undoubtedly reflects a differentiation program in TACs rather than in stem cells (Zhang and Sarvetnick 2003; Holland et al. 2004). Numerous other studies point to the fact that ductal cells from mouse (Peck et al. 2002), rat (Kim et al. 2004) and human pancreas (Bonner-Weir et al. 2000) can generate all the pancreatic endocrine cell types under controlled in vitro conditions, but the identity of any multipotential stem cell is still lacking. However, Ramiya et al. (2000) do describe small round epithelioid cells that arise in cultures of ducts from prediabetic NOD mice that give rise to all pancreatic endocrine cell types.

Seaberg et al. (2004) have described clonal colonies derived with equal frequency ($\sim$2 colonies/10^4 cells) from both ducts and islets of mouse pancreas, and from both the nestin-positive and -negative fractions of these cell types. Occasional primary cells were nestin$^+$/Pdx1$^+$, but neither the primary cells nor the cultured cells expressed markers of pluripotency such as Oct-4 or Nanog. These cells were called pancreas-derived multipotent precursors (PMPs); clonal colonies expressed markers of the three neural lineages and all pancreatic lineages. The islets have been suggested as a location of stem cells for β cell replacement in many species. Following a course of BrdU labelling in the 1st week of postnatal life, Pdx1-positive LRCs were found within and on the periphery of rat pancreatic islets (Duvillie et al. 2003). Zulewski et al. (2001) describe the long-term culture of undifferentiated hormone-negative, nestin-positive cells (nestin-positive islet-derived progenitor [NIP] cells) from human and rat pancreatic islet cell cultures: upon altering culture conditions, these cells expressed Pdx1 and became hormone-positive. Nestin-positive cells were also found in ducts, but the utility of nestin as a marker is controversial since nestin can also be expressed by fibroblast-like cells in pancreatic stroma (Bonner-Weir and Sharma 2002). Other markers of these NIP cells include the GLP-1 receptor (Abraham et al. 2002), while up to 2% of cultured human NIP cells have an SP phenotype based upon ABCG2 and ABCB1 (MDR1) activity (Lechner et al. 2002). In mice treated with the β cell poison, streptozotocin, where blood glucose was normalized by insulin treatment, Guz et al. (2001) believe that regeneration was accomplished by two progenitor populations, one being positive for the glucose 2 transporter (GLUT-2) and the other co-expressing Pdx1 and somatostatin. In human and canine pancreas, small cells (7–10 μm in diameter), organized into clusters and restricted to small islets, positive for numerous markers (Pdx1, synaptophysin, insulin, glucagons, pancreatic polypeptide, somatostatin, α-FP and Bcl-2) could be progenitors (Petropavlovskaia and Rosenberg 2002). Finally, we should note studies that suggest that there are no stem cells in the mouse pancreatic islets (Dor et al. 2004). Using a genetic labelling strategy, it was suggested that no β cells arose from undifferentiated (insulin-negative) stem cells, despite an almost doubling of β cell mass during the 1st year of life, instead proposing that β cells arose from self-duplication. Of course, this does not close the door on the possibility that there are stem cells for β cell replacement in the mouse: they may in fact be insulin-positive?

3.6
Stratified Squamous Epithelia

3.6.1
Epidermis

The skin is lined by a stratified keratinizing squamous epithelium, the inter-follicular epidermis (IFE) (Fig. 10). Normally, cell proliferation is confined to the basal layer of cells that make contact with the underlying basement membrane. The basal layer is contiguous with cells of the outer root sheath that form the outermost layer of hair follicles. There are also attendant eccrine and

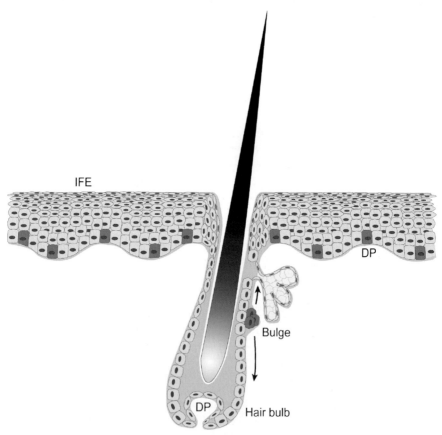

Fig. 10 In the epidermis, stem cells are present in the interfollicular epidermis (*IFE*) and bulge region. In human skin, stem cells may be located over dermal papillae at most sites, but other studies suggest a more random localization. The bulge is the location of multipotential stem cells that produce progeny that migrate upwards toward the IFE and downwards toward the hair bulb. The hair bulb is the location of rapidly dividing TACs that are nourished by the blood vessels in the dermal papilla (*DP*)

apocrine sweat glands that vary in frequency according to site, and sebaceous glands usually, but not exclusively associated with hair follicles. Until relatively recently, epidermal stem cell identity was inferred either by their ability to retain DNA labels that had been administered in the immediate postnatal period (LRCs) or by their growth potential in vitro (Barrandon and Green 1987). When human keratinocytes were cultured at clonal density, three different types of cell were recognized based on the size of clones generated in a single plating: the largest clones were called holoclones, consisting of small undifferentiated cells, most of which were capable of forming proliferative colonies on passaging – it is assumed that holoclone-generating cells in vitro are the stem cells in vivo. Meroclones (early TACs, see Fig. 1) had intermediate growth potential and paraclones (late TACs) abort and differentiate after very few passages.

Of course, neither label retention nor in vitro clonogenicity allow easy isolation of epidermal stem cells, but a number of studies have highlighted that selection of basal keratinocytes with the highest expression of the β1 integrin (integrin[bri] cells) enriches for cells with a high colony forming efficiency (Jones and Watt 1993; Jones et al. 1995). However, integrin[bri] cells make up 40% of basal cells in human epidermis, but probably only 10% of basal cells are stem cells (Jensen et al. 1999). These integrin[bri] cells tended to be clustered over the tips of dermal papillae in most skin sites, with the notable exception of the plantar and palmar surfaces (Owens and Watt 2003), had a low level of cell proliferation, and it was suggested that TACs migrated laterally away from the stem cell clusters. This notion was supported by the fact that integrin[dull] cells were more mobile on type IV collagen than integrin[bri] cells. However, a recent study following the fate of genetically marked cells in human epidermis (Ghazizadeh and Taichman 2005), while confirming that integrin[bri] cells, were concentrated over dermal papillae, suggested instead that stem cells are scattered all along the basal layer, giving rise to cells that migrate solely upwards forming columns of cells reminiscent of EPU-like structures. In mouse epidermis, where there is a relatively flat interface with the underlying dermis, it is well established that individual stem cells give rise to TACs and their differentiated progeny within spatial units called epidermal proliferative units (EPUs) that stretch from the basal layer to the surface. A LRC occupies a central position in the basal layer of each EPU along with up to a dozen other cells, most of which are TACs (Wu and Morris 2005). Melanoma chondroitin sulphate proteoglycan (MCSP) is another potential stem cell marker, co-localizing with the β1 integrin (Legg et al. 2003); most Ki-67 positive cells are found outside the patches of β1 integrin/MCSP[+] cells. Another marker used in combination with β1 integrin has been the low expression of desmosomal proteins such as desmoplakin and desmoglein3 (Dsg3) (Wan et al. 2003); the selection of β1[bri]Dsg3[dull] enriched for cells with high clonogenicity.

Rather than selecting for β1 integrin-expressing cells, Kaur and colleagues (Kaur and Li 2000; Webb and Kaur 2004; Li and Kaur 2005) have noted superior colony-forming ability from cells selected on the basis of expression of the hemidesmosomal integrin α6, which partners β4 to attach cells to the basement membrane component, laminin V. Combined with low expression of the transferrin receptor (CD71), such $α6^{bri}CD71^{dim}$ cells comprised about 2%–5% of $CK14^+$ basal cells in human epidermis, being blast-like in morphology, highly clonogenic and lacking CK10, a differentiation marker. Furthermore, such cells could regenerate a full thickness epidermis in organotypic culture.

In the hair follicle, the bulge region is clearly the stem cell niche (Alonso and Fuchs 2003; Fuchs et al. 2004; Tumbar et al. 2004) (Fig. 10). Very elegant transplantation studies have demonstrated that the progeny of bulge stem cells can regenerate the whole follicle, and furthermore the bulge can also contribute to cells of the IFE (Oshima et al. 2001). Bulge cells have many of the attributes expected of stem cells, they divide infrequently in vivo, but can form large colonies in vitro (Oshima et al. 2001). By comparison, TACs in the hair bulb divide frequently in vivo but are poorly clonogenic in vitro. LRCs are generally found below the sebaceous glands in the bulge region of mouse hair follicles (Braun et al. 2003), and CK15 expression combined with a high expression of the α6β4 integrin characterizes most, but not all LRCs. Transcriptional profiling of bulge cells has shown that they express many mRNAs typical of stem cells including SCF, Eph receptors, CD34 and tenascin (Tumbar et al. 2004), while Morris et al. (2004) have also noted that bulge cells have a gene expression profile consistent with maintaining proliferative quiescence and an undifferentiated state.

3.6.2
Cervix

Surprisingly little is known about the identity of the stem cells proposed to maintain the lining of the female genital tract such as that of the vagina and uterus. The uterus is lined principally by the endometrium, an epithelial lining thrown into deep folds that vary in depth dependent on the menstrual cycle. This gives way to the endocervical canal of the uterine cervix, lined by a simple columnar epithelium, again with contiguous glands: the endocervical crypts. At the neck of the uterus, the simple columnar epithelium gives way, at the so-called transformation zone, to the stratified squamous epithelium of the ectocervix. The acidic vaginal environment results in squamous metaplasia of the transformation zone, preceded by the appearance of sub-columnar reserve cells that undergo hyperplasia before forming metaplastic squamous epithelium indistinguishable from the squamous epithelia of the ectocervix. Like the basal cells of the original squamous epithelium, these reserve cells have round nuclei and little cytoplasm. p63, a homologue of p53, appears to be particularly important to the development of the female genital tract (Ince et al. 2002) and is expressed by reserve cells, reserve cell hyperplasia and the basal cells of the ectocervix (Martens et al. 2004). p63-expressing cells are also found in basal endometrial glands as well as in mouse epidermal basal cells (O'Connell et al. 2001). Witkiewicz et al. (2005) propose that basal cells derive from columnar cells in the endocervix, and like other studies, found that p63 was a good cellular marker; additionally these cells co-expressed high levels of Bcl-2 and CK5. However, p63 expression marks all basal cells; thus, it is unclear if p63 is an authentic stem cell marker.

3.7
Mammary Glands

As in many tissues, the identity of stem cells in the mammalian breast is the subject of controversy. The collective wisdom is that they reside in the terminal ductal lobuloalveolar units (TDLUs) (see Fig. 11) as small undifferentiated cells in the luminal cell layer that do not make contact with the lumen. These cells are bipotential, giving rise to luminal and myoepithelial cells (reviewed in Smalley and Ashworth 2003; Clarke et al. 2003). Most studies have been carried out on the mouse, and in murine mammary glands, the SP fraction is enriched for stem cells, determined by the proportion of LRCs and the ability to repopulate cleared (indigenous epithelial cells removed to allow engraftment of transplanted cells) mammary fat pads in vivo with both myoepithelial and luminal lineages (Welm et al. 2003; Alvi et al. 2003). Most of the SP cells express Sca-1 (Welm et al. 2002). Based on a number of studies in humans, three specific phenotypes appear to be emerging; myoepithelial cells are CALLA$^+$ (common acute lymphoblastic leukaemia antigen) CK14$^+$ αSMA$^+$ vimentin$^+$, luminal cells are MUC1$^+$ CK18$^+$ ESA$^+$ (epithelial surface antigen), while stem

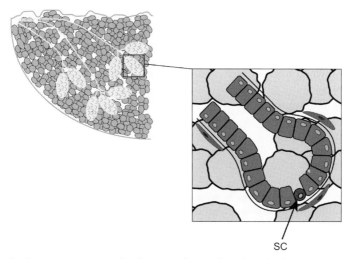

SC

Fig. 11 In the human mammary gland, stem cells are thought to be located in the terminal ductule lobuloalveolar units (TDLUs, *boxed area*) as small cells that do not make contact with the luminal surface

cells have an $\alpha6^+$ CK19$^+$ ESA$^+$ MUC1$^-$ CALLA$^-$ phenotype (Stingl et al. 2001; Gudjonsson et al. 2002; Clarke et al. 2003). Using DNA radiolabelling of human breast tissue implanted into nude mice, LRCs can be found that often express oestrogen and progesterone receptors. Moreover, in common with many other putative stem cells, these cells were enriched for the expression of p21^{CIP1} and Musashi-1 (Clarke et al. 2005). The relationship of the normal stem cell phenotype to that of the ESA$^+$ CD44$^+$ CD24$^{-/low}$ human breast cancer cells, able to propagate breast cancer in NOD/SCID mice with as few as 100 cells, is still to be fully determined (Al-Hajj et al. 2003).

3.8
Male Gonadal and Accessory Sex Tissue

3.8.1
Testis

In the mammalian testis, the mitotic divisions occur amongst the various generations of so-called type A spermatogonia that are located on the basement membrane of the seminiferous tubule (Fig. 12); the meiotic reduction divisions and further differentiation towards terminally differentiated spermatozoa occurs centripetally. Spermatogonia that are relatively devoid of heterochromatin are called A_{pale}, and those occurring as single cells (incidence of ~2 in 10^4 testicular cells) are probably the stem cells. Their distribution is not random in mouse and rat; rather they are located in those areas of seminiferous tubules

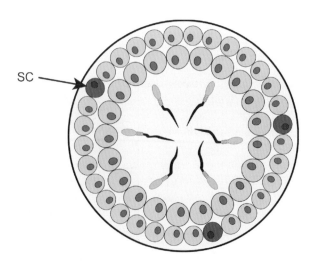

Fig. 12 In the seminiferous epithelium, stem cells and TACs all reside on the basement membrane as various generations of spermatogonia; the meiotic reduction divisions occur in spermatocytes that have moved to a more luminal position and further maturation towards spermatozoa occurs in yet more luminally positioned cells

that border on interstitial (niche?) tissue (Chiarni-Garcia et al. 2003). The mouse testis has been widely studied. Shinohara et al. (1999) selected stem cells on the basis of expression of c-Kit and the $\beta1$ and $\alpha6$ integrins (laminin receptor). The expression of the transcription factors Oct-4 and Plfz has also been used to define murine testicular stem cells (Buaas et al. 2004), while Kubota et al. (2003) have described spermatogonial stem cells as being MHC-1$^+$ Thy-1$^+$ c-Kit$^-$ CD24$^+$ $\alpha6^+$ αv^- Sca-1$^-$ CD34$^-$, but interestingly found that the SP fraction contained no cells capable of in vivo testis repopulation. By contrast, Lassalle et al. (2004) found that the SP population (dependent on ABCG2 activity) was highly enriched for in vivo cell repopulation ability, these cells expressing the $\alpha6$ integrin and Stra8, a premeiotic germ cell-specific cytoplasmic protein.

3.8.2
Prostate

Anatomically the prostate gland varies greatly between species, but can essentially be described as an exocrine gland enveloping the urethra at the base of the bladder, composed of blind-ending tubules that open into the urethra. In the mouse, based on the location of LRCs, prostatic epithelial stem cells are thought to be in the proximal regions of prostatic ducts, close to the urethra (Tsujimura et al. 2002). Human prostatic stem cells are thought to be multipotential (Huss et al. 2004), able to generate secretory, basal and neuroendocrine cells, located amongst basal cells that form a continuous layer between the luminal secretory cells and the basement membrane (Hudson 2004). Based on colony growth in vitro, Hudson (2004) has proposed a cytokeratin-based differentiation pathway in which stem cells are CK5/CK14-positive, giving rise to TACs that lose expression of CK14, but gain CK17 and 19. CD44, Bcl-2, p63 and p27^{Kip1} are further markers of basal cells, but not necessarily stem cells. Richardson et al. (2004) has identified the expression of CD133 in 1% of human prostate basal cells; these cells uniquely co-expressed $\alpha2\beta1$ integrins and possessed two important attributes of putative stem cells: a high level of in vitro proliferation coupled with the ability to reconstitute acini in immunocompromised mice. p63 is a reliable marker of prostatic basal cells and is certainly required for the maintenance of basal cells, but curiously, p63 and basal cells are not required for the differentiation of urogenital sinus into neuroendocrine and luminal epithelial cells (Kurita et al. 2004).

3.9
Heart

Cardiovascular disease is one of the major causes of morbidity and mortality in the developed world, and encouragingly, the use of autologous bone marrow as a cell therapy appears a realistic option (Kajstura et al. 2005). Only relatively recently has the proliferative potential of cardiomyocytes been acknowledged (Beltrami et al. 2001), with up to 4% of myocyte nuclei adjacent to infarcts found to express Ki-67. Anversa and Nadal-Ginard (2002) identified cells in the myocardium expressing antigens commonly found in stem cells, c-Kit, Sca-1 and MDR1. In aged rats, Beltrami et al. (2003) observed Lin$^-$ c-Kit$^+$ cells at a frequency of 1 in 10^4 myocytes (Fig. 13); these cells were negative for the pan leucocyte marker CD45 and the endothelial/haematopoietic marker CD34, though the possibility that these cells were circulating cells, presumably bone marrow-derived, could not be discounted. These freshly sorted c-Kit$^+$ cells did not express markers for cardiomyocytes (cardiac myosin), endothelia (von Willebrand factor, CD31), nor smooth muscle cells (α-SMA), but a small proportion (7%–10%) did express the transcription factors Nkx2.5 and GATA4, suggestive of early cardiomyocyte commitment. These cells were clonogenic in vitro, able to produce cardiomyocytes, endothelia and smooth muscle cells from single cells; they could also contribute to all these three lineages following intracardiac injection in a model of infarction. Putative stem cells have also been isolated from human heart (Messina et al. 2004), these cells expressed CD34, c-Kit, Flk-1 (KDR) and CD31, formed large colonies (cardiospheres) in vitro and could differentiate into cardiomyocytes, endothelia and smooth muscle cells after orthotopic transplantation into SCID/beige mice with myocardial infarction. Very recently, Laugwitz et al. (2005) have isolated what appear to be cardiac progenitors (cardioblasts) from rodent and human hearts based on the expression of the LIM-homeodomain transcription factor islet-1 (isl1). These cells decreased in frequency postnatally, but they could be expanded and differentiated in vitro into seemingly functional cardiomyocytes.

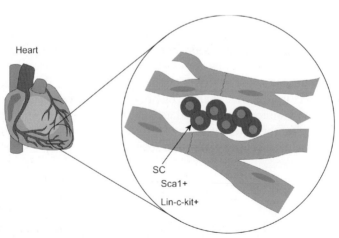

Fig. 13 Putative cardiac stem cells are found in clusters between cardiomyocytes, particularly in areas of least mechanical stress

3.10
Kidney

The kidney has a low rate of cell turnover under steady state conditions, but can regenerate tubular epithelium after injury. The identity of any renal stem cells has not been readily forthcoming. Since the kidney develops centrifugally, the medulla is the oldest region and thus could be the location of a stem cell niche (Al-Awqati and Oliver 2002). The renal papilla has also been proposed, based on the distribution of BrdU-labelled cells after a period of postnatal labelling, but the frequency of LRCs (40%) was far too high for them all to be stem cells (Oliver et al. 2004): nevertheless they disappeared after ischaemic injury and displayed clonal growth in vitro. An SP population has been isolated from rat kidney, but these cells did not contribute to renal repair when injected into recipient rats (Iwatani et al. 2004). A putative kidney stem cell has been isolated from the cortical interstitium of human kidney, making up 0.8% of all cortical cells; these cells expressed Pax-2 and CD133 along with mesenchymal markers such as CD73, CD29 and CD44 (Bussolati et al. 2005). These cells were capable of in vitro expansion and differentiation into epithelia and endothelia, and formed tubular structures and endothelia in the damaged kidneys of SCID mice.

3.11
Lung

The lung is a complex three-dimensional structure composed of a branching system of airways that serve to conduct the inspired air to the distal alveolar-capillary units (air sacs). Progress in identifying lung stem cells has been impeded by the slow turnover of airway and alveolar epithelium, but the consensus view is that there is no single multipotential stem cell for the lung, but rather there are regiospecific stem cell zones in the proximal and distal lung (Fig. 14). In the mouse trachea, cells scattered in the ducts of submucosal glands expressing high levels of CK5, that were LRCs after a period of BrdU labelling during tracheal injury, are likely stem/progenitor cells for this pseudostratified epithelium (Borthwick et al. 2001). Tracheal basal cells are also present, and expression of p63 appears important for their self-maintenance (Daniely et al. 2004). The mouse bronchial tree is lined by a number of cell types including basal cells, ciliated cells and nonciliated cells (serous, goblet and Clara cell secretory protein [CCSP]-expressing CE cells). Here, both CE cells and basal cells appear to be able to act as multipotential stem cells, for when CE cells are selectively ablated, a major subset of basal cells (basal cells identified by the binding of the lectin *Griffonia simplicifolia isolectin B_4* [GSI-B_4]) upregulate CK14 and are able to regenerate the entire epithelium (Hong et al. 2004). In the bronchiolar epithelium, stem cell function appears to be the property of rare pollutant-resistant CE cells, co-localized with pulmonary neuroendocrine cells (PNECs), normally located in cell clusters termed neu-

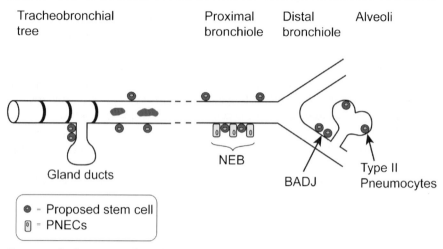

Fig. 14 In the lung, a number of candidate stem cells have been proposed. In the proximal airways, scattered basal cells and cells located in the ducts of submucosal glands are likely stem cells. More proximally, pollutant-resistant Clara cells either amongst pulmonary neuroendocrine cells (*PNECs*) in neuroepithelial bodies (*NEBs*) or close to bronchoalveolar duct junctions (*BADJ*) appear to have a stem cell function. In the alveoli, proliferative type II pneumocytes replenish lost type I cells

roepithelial bodies (NEBs); PNECs can only act as progenitors for more PNECs (Reynolds et al. 2000). Pollutant resistance of CE cells appears to be related to a deficiency in the phase I drug metabolizing enzyme CYP450 2F2. At the bronchoalveolar duct junction (BADJ), Giangreco et al. (2002) have identified other pollutant-resistant CE cells, not associated with NEBs, that probably serve a stem cell function in the terminal bronchioles; CE cells that were also LRCs were located within three cell diameters of the BADJ. A nonhaematopoietic (CD45⁻) SP population has been isolated from murine lung, and, like NEB-associated variant CE cells, these cells showed expression of CCSP and absence of CYP450 2F2; a frequency of less than 0.9% amongst intrapulmonary conducting airway epithelia is consistent with a low abundance of stem cells (Giangreco et al. 2004). In the alveoli, type II pneumocytes are widely believed to be the stem/progenitor cells, undergoing hyperplasia in response to the loss of the squamous type I pneumocytes, giving rise to type I cells as well as self-renewing. Type II cells are characteristically recognized by the presence of intracellular lamellar bodies and the production of surfactant proteins.

3.12
Brain

During development, the neuroepithelial cells in the embryonic ventricular layer generate most of the neurons and glia (astrocytes and oligodendrocytes);

in the adult human brain, the consensus view is that oligodendrocytes are the stem cells (Doetsch 2003). In the mouse, Johansson et al. (1999) believe that the ventricle-lining cells, the ciliated ependymal cells are the stem cells (Fig. 15). After their labelling in vivo, these cells could differentiate into olfactory bulb neurons, while in vitro these cells produced clones (neurospheres) that showed trilineage potential (neurons – βlll-tubulin; astrocytes – GFAP; 04 – oligodendrocytes). The ependymal cells commonly expressed nestin and the Notch 1 receptor; their proliferation rate speeded up after injury and in most mitotic cells the cleavage plane was parallel to the luminal surface (see Fig. 3). Nestin is an embryonic intermediate filament expressed by the neuroepithelial stem cells of the neural tube (Lendahl et al. 1990), and nestin is downregulated when

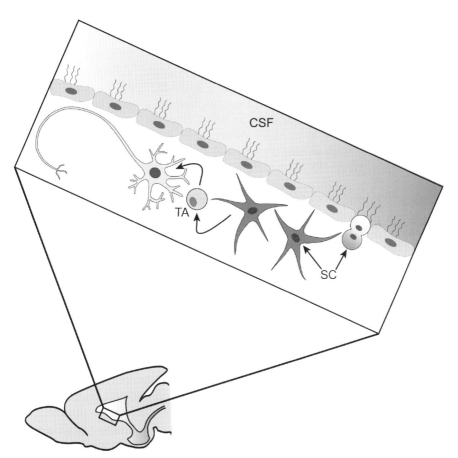

Fig. 15 In the brain, a major site of neurogenesis in adulthood appears to be close to the ventricles that convey the cerebrospinal fluid (*CSF*). In mice, the ciliated ependymal cells may serve as stem cells (*SC*), but in humans, astrocytes located in the subventricular zone (*SVZ*) have been proposed as stem cells

neural stem cells differentiate (Liu et al. 2004). Despite claims for the ependymal cells as having stem cell credentials, the consensus view is that in the mouse, the subventricular zone (SVZ) of the lateral ventricles and the dentate gyrus of the hippocampus are the main sites of adult neurogenesis. The SVZ is separated from the lateral ventricle by a single layer of multiciliated ependymal cells; the stem cells are GFAP$^+$ astrocytes, sometimes extending a single cilium between the overlying ependymal cells (Doetsch 2003). In the hippocampus, these astrocytes are located in the subgranular zone (SGZ). Using electron microscopy, characteristic astrocyte features include glycogen granules, thick bundles of intermediate filaments and gap junctions. They may also express SSEA-1 (stage specific embryonic antigen-1, a cell surface carbohydrate found on ES cells) and Musashi1. Musashi1 is a highly conserved neural RNA binding protein highly enriched in neural stem cells, having a role in stem cell self-renewal by repressing translation of the Notch inhibitor m-Numb (Okano et al. 2002); activating Notch leads to transactivation of the *HES1* gene, so maintaining the immature proliferative status of Musashi1-expressing cells.

In human brain, Sunai et al. (2004) have identified ribbons of astrocytes in the SVZ lining the lateral ventricles; a Ki-67 labelling index of 0.7% was observed in these cells *in* vivo and neurospheres displaying trilineage differentiation could be derived from single cells. Cells with similar in vitro potential have been isolated from human subcortical white matter using an antibody, A2B5 that recognizes an immature neural ganglioside (Nunes et al. 2003). How these putative stem cells relate to the CD133$^+$ cells isolated from human medulloblastoma that can form colonies in vitro (Singh et al. 2003) and propagate the tumour in NOD/SCID mice (Singh et al. 2004) is unclear at present. In the rat brain, Sox-2, a transcription factor expressed in neuroepithelial progenitors, is expressed by proliferating cells in the SVZ and SGZ, including GFAP$^+$ astroglia (Komitova and Eriksson 2004). After spinal cord injury in the rat, gray and white matter astrocytes upregulate nestin expression, are able to clonally expand and show trilineage differentiation in vitro (Lang et al. 2004).

3.13
Eye

The limbus is a narrow ring of tissue between the cornea and conjunctiva (Fig. 16). Limbal stem cells give rise to the complex multilayered structure of the cornea that functions in protection, refraction and transparency. These stem cells are LRCs, form holoclones in vitro, are relatively undifferentiated, and lack CK3 and CK12 unlike the suprabasal cells of the limbus and all layers of the cornea (Boulton and Albon 2004). At the corneal margin, basal cells express vimentin and CKs 3 and 12, they also cycle more rapidly than those cells away from the margin. In the human limbus, a side population based on ABCG2 activity has been identified that appeared to be highly clonogenic in vitro, these cells also expressed high levels of p63 and the α9 integrin (Chen et al.

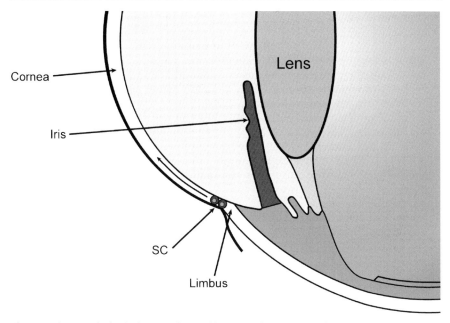

Fig. 16 In the eye, the limbal region, located between the cornea and conjunctiva, is the likely stem cell zone

2004; De Paiva et al. 2005). In the retina, about 0.2% of pigmented cells in the ciliary margin have stem/progenitor cell properties, expressing transcription factors such as Pax6 and Hes1, nestin and $p27^{kip1}$, are able to clonally proliferate and show multipotential differentiation (Boulton and Albon 2004).

4
Conclusions

Stem cells in different tissues have common attributes that enable their self-maintenance, survival and maintenance of genomic integrity. In tissues with a continual cell turnover, stem cells are located in niches at the beginning of any flux to avoid getting swept away in the cell escalator: high expression of cell adhesion molecules by such cells is a common trait. As we have observed, stem cell location is often inferred by the presence of LRCs, commonly taken as indicative of a slowly cycling habitus; whether all stem cells additionally operate a mechanism to preserve immortal DNA strands remains to be proven. More recently, transcriptional profiling has been employed to enable a signature of 'stemness' to be defined; pluripotential embryonic stem cells have been an abundant source of analysable cells, and in due course will lead to the discovery of more markers of adult stem cells.

References

Abraham EJ, Leech CA, Lin JC, Zulewski H, Habener JF (2002) Insulinotropic hormone glucagon-like peptide-1 differentiation of human pancreatic islet-derived progenitor cells into insulin-producing cells. Endocrinology 143:3152–3161

Al-Awqati Q, Oliver JA (2002) Stem cells in the kidney. Kidney Int 61:387–395

Al-Hajj M, Wicha MS, Benito-Hernandez A, Morrison SJ, Clarke MF (2003) Prospective identification of tumorigenic breast cancer cells. Proc Natl Acad Sci U S A 100:3983–3988

Alison MR (2003) Characterization of the differentiation capacity of rat-derived hepatic stem cells. Semin Liver Dis 23:325–336

Alison MR, Golding M, Sarraf CE, Edwards RJ, Lalani EN (1996) Liver damage in the rat induces hepatocyte stem cells from biliary epithelial cells. Gastroenterology 110:1182–1190

Alison MR, Golding M, Lalani E-N, Nagy P, Thorgeirsson S, Sarraf C (1997) Wholesale hepatocytic differentiation in the rat from ductular oval cells, the progeny of biliary stem cells. J Hepatol 26:343–352

Alison MR, Golding M, Lalani E-N, Sarraf CE (1998) Wound healing in the liver with particular reference to stem cells. Phil Trans R Soc Lond B 353:1–18

Alison MR, Poulsom R, Otto WR, Vig P, Brittan M, Direkze NC, Preston SL, Wright NA (2003) Plastic adult stem cells: will they graduate from the school of hard knocks? J Cell Sci 116:599–603

Alison MR, Vig P, Russo F, Bigger BW, Amofah E, Themis M, Forbes S (2004) Hepatic stem cells: from inside and outside the liver? Cell Prolif 37:1–21

Alonso L, Fuchs E (2003) Stem cells of the skin epithelium. Proc Natl Acad Sci U S A 100 [Suppl 1]:11830–11835

Alvi AJ, Clayton H, Joshi C, Enver T, Ashworth A, Vivanco MM, Dale TC, Smalley MJ (2003) Functional and molecular characterisation of mammary side population cells. Breast Cancer Res 5:R1–R8

Anversa P, Nadal-Ginard B (2002) Myocyte renewal and ventricular remodelling. Nature 415:240–243

Armstrong L, Stojkovic M, Dimmick I, Ahmad S, Stojkovic P, Hole N, Lako M (2004) Phenotypic characterization of murine primitive hematopoietic progenitor cells isolated on basis of aldehyde dehydrogenase activity. Stem Cells 22:1142–1151

Asakura A, Rudnicki MA (2002) Side population cells from diverse adult tissues are capable of in vitro hematopoietic differentiation. Exp Hematol 30:1339–1345

Avril A, Pichard V, Bralet MP, Ferry N (2004) Mature hepatocytes are the source of small hepatocyte-like progenitor cells in the retrorsine model of liver injury. J Hepatol 41:737–743

Barrandon Y, Green H (1987) Three clonal types of keratinocyte with different capacities for multiplication. Proc Natl Acad Sci U S A 84:2302–2306

Batlle E, Henderson JT, Beghtel H, van den Born MM, Sancho E, Huls G, Meeldijk J, Robertson J, van de Wetering M, Pawson T, Clevers H (2002) Beta-catenin and TCF mediate cell positioning in the intestinal epithelium by controlling the expression of EphB/ephrinB. Cell 111:251–263

Baumann U, Crosby HA, Ramani P, Kelly DA, Strain AJ (1999) Expression of the stem cell factor receptor c-kit in normal and diseased pediatric liver: identification of a human hepatic progenitor cell? Hepatology 30:112–117

Beltrami AP, Urbanek K, Kajstura J, Yan SM, Finato N, Bussani R, Nadal-Ginard B, Silvestri F, Leri A, Beltrami CA, Anversa P (2001) Evidence that human cardiac myocytes divide after myocardial infarction. N Engl J Med 344:1750–1757

Beltrami AP, Barlucchi L, Torella D et al (2003) Adult cardiac stem cells are multipotent and support myocardial regeneration. Cell 114:763–776

Bhatia M (2003) AC133 expression in human stem cells. Leukemia 15:1685–1688

Bjerknes M, Cheng H (2002) Multipotential stem cells in adult mouse gastric epithelium. Am J Physiol Gastrointest Liver Physiol 283:G767–G777

Bonde J, Hess DA, Nolta JA (2004) Recent advances in hematopoietic stem cell biology. Curr Opin Hematol 11:392–398

Bonner-Weir S, Sharma A (2002) Pancreatic stem cells. J Pathol 197:519–526

Bonner-Weir S, Taneja M, Weir GC, Tatarkiewicz K, Song KH, Sharma A, O'Neil JJ (2000) In vitro cultivation of human islets from expanded ductal tissue. Proc Natl Acad Sci U S A 97:7999–8004

Bonnet D (2002) Haematopoietic stem cells. J Pathol 197:430–440

Bonnet D, Dick JE (1997) Human acute myeloid leukemia is organized as a hierarchy that originates from a primitive hematopoietic cell. Nat Med 3:730–737

Borst P, Elferink RO (2002) Mammalian ABC transporters in health and disease. Annu Rev Biochem 71:537–592

Borthwick DW, Shahbazian M, Krantz QT, Dorin JR, Randell SH (2001) Evidence for stem-cell niches in the tracheal epithelium. Am J Respir Cell Mol Biol 24:662–670

Boulton M, Albon J (2004) Stem cells in the eye. Int J Biochem Cell Biol 36:643–657

Braun KM, Niemann C, Jensen UB, Sundberg JP, Silva-Vargas V, Watt FM (2003) Manipulation of stem cell proliferation and lineage commitment: visualisation of label-retaining cells in wholemounts of mouse epidermis. Development 130:5241–5255

Buaas FW, Kirsh AL, Sharma M, McLean DJ, Morris JL, Griswold MD, de Rooij DG, Braun RE (2004) Plzf is required in adult male germ cells for stem cell self-renewal. Nat Genet 36:647–652

Bunting KD (2002) ABC transporters as phenotypic markers and functional regulators of stem cells. Stem Cells 20:11–20

Bunting KD, Zhou S, Lu T, Sorrentino BP (2000) Enforced P-glycoprotein pump function in murine bone marrow cells results in expansion of side population stem cells in vitro and repopulating cells in vivo. Blood 96:902–909

Bussolati B, Bruno S, Grange C, Buttiglieri S, Deregibus MC, Cantino D, Camussi G (2005) Isolation of renal progenitor cells from adult human kidney. Am J Pathol 166:545–555

Cairns J (1975) Mutation selection and the natural history of cancer. Nature 255:197–200

Cairns J (2002) Somatic stem cells and the kinetics of mutagenesis and carcinogenesis. Proc Natl Acad Sci U S A 99:10567–10570

Camargo FD, Green R, Capetanaki Y, Jackson KA, Goodell MA (2003) Single hematopoietic stem cells generate skeletal muscle through myeloid intermediates. Nat Med 9:1520–1527

Chen JC, Goldhamer DJ (2003) Skeletal muscle stem cells. Reprod Biol Endocrinol 1:101

Chen Z, de Paiva CS, Luo L, Kretzer FL, Pflugfelder SC, Li DQ (2004) Characterization of putative stem cell phenotype in human limbal epithelia. Stem Cells 22:355–366

Chiarini-Garcia H, Raymer AM, Russell LD (2003) Non-random distribution of spermatogonia in rats: evidence of niches in the seminiferous tubules. Reproduction 126:669–680

Clarke RB, Anderson E, Howell A, Potten CS (2003) Regulation of human breast epithelial stem cells. Cell Prolif 36 [Suppl 1]:45–58

Clarke RB, Spence K, Anderson E, Howell A, Okano H, Potten CS (2005) A putative human breast stem cell population is enriched for steroid receptor-positive cells. Dev Biol 277:443–456

Daniely Y, Liao G, Dixon D, Linnoila RI, Lori A, Randell SH, Oren M, Jetten AM (2004) Critical role of p63 in the development of a normal esophageal and tracheobronchial epithelium. Am J Physiol Cell Physiol 287:C171–C181

De Paiva CS, Chen Z, Corrales RM, Pflugfelder SC, Li DQ (2005) ABCG2 transporter identifies a population of clonogenic human limbal epithelial cells. Stem Cells 23:63–73

Deschaseaux F, Gindraux F, Saadi R, Obert L, Chalmers D, Herve P (2003) Direct selection of human bone marrow mesenchymal stem cells using an anti-CD49a antibody reveals their CD45med, low phenotype. Br J Haematol 122:506–517

Doetsch F (2003) The glial identity of neural stem cells. Nat Neurosci 6:1127–1134

Dor Y, Brown J, Martinez OI, Melton DA (2004) Adult pancreatic beta-cells are formed by self-duplication rather than stem-cell differentiation. Nature 429:41–46

Dorrell C, Gan OI, Pereira DS, Hawley RG, Dick JE (2000) Expansion of human cord blood CD34(+)CD38(-) cells in ex vivo culture during retroviral transduction without a corresponding increase in SCID repopulating cell (SRC) frequency: dissociation of SRC phenotype and function. Blood 95:102–110

Dowthwaite GP, Bishop JC, Redman SN, Khan IM, Rooney P, Evans DJ, Haughton L, Bayram Z, Boyer S, Thomson B, Wolfe MS, Archer CW (2004) The surface of articular cartilage contains a progenitor cell population. J Cell Sci 117:889–897

Duvillie B, Attali M, Aiello V, Quemeneur E, Scharfmann R (2003) Label-retaining cells in the rat pancreas: location and differentiation potential in vitro. Diabetes 52:2035–2042

Escaffit F, Perreault N, Jean D, Francoeur C, Herring E, Rancourt C, Rivard N, Vachon PH, Pare F, Boucher MP, Auclair J, Beaulieu JF (2005) Repressed E-cadherin expression in the lower crypt of human small intestine: a cell marker of functional relevance. Exp Cell Res 302:206–220

Fuchs E, Tumbar T, Guasch G (2004) Socializing with the neighbors: stem cells and their niche. Cell 116:769–778

Fujikawa T, Hirose T, Fujii H, Oe S, Yasuchika K, Azuma H, Yamaoka Y (2003) Purification of adult hepatic progenitor cells using green fluorescent protein (GFP)-transgenic mice and fluorescence-activated cell sorting. J Hepatol 39:162–170

Ghazizadeh S, Taichman LB (2005) Organization of stem cells and their progeny in human epidermis. J Invest Dermatol 124:367–372

Giangreco A, Reynolds SD, Stripp BR (2002) Terminal bronchioles harbor a unique airway stem cell population that localizes to the bronchoalveolar duct junction. Am J Pathol 161:173–182

Giangreco A, Shen H, Reynolds SD, Stripp BR (2004) Molecular phenotype of airway side population cells. Am J Physiol Lung Cell Mol Physiol 286:L624–L630

Goldring K, Partridge T, Watt D (2002) Muscle stem cells. J Pathol 197:457–467

Gonzalez-Reyes A (2003) Stem cells, niches and cadherins: a view from Drosophila. J Cell Sci 116:949–954

Goodell MA, Brose K, Paradis G, Conner A, Mulligan R (1996) Isolation and functional properties of murine hematopoietic stem cells that are replicating in vivo. J Exp Med 183:1797–1806

Gordon GJ, Coleman WB, Hixson DC, Grisham JW (2000) Liver regeneration in rats with retrorsine-induced hepatocellular injury proceeds through a novel cellular response. Am J Pathol 156:607–619

Gronthos S, Zannettino AC, Hay SJ, Shi S, Graves SE, Kortesidis A, Simmons PJ (2003) Molecular and cellular characterisation of highly purified stromal stem cells derived from human bone marrow. Cell Sci 116:1827–1835

Gudjonsson T, Villadsen R, Nielsen HL, Ronnov-Jessen L, Bissell MJ, Petersen OW (2002) Isolation, immortalization, and characterization of a human breast epithelial cell line with stem cell properties. Genes Dev 16:693–706

Guo Y, Lubbert M, Engelhardt M (2003) CD34(-) Hematopoietic stem cells: current concepts and controversies. Stem Cells 21:15–20

Guz Y, Nasir I, Teitelman G (2001) Regeneration of pancreatic beta cells from intra-islet precursor cells in an experimental model of diabetes. Endocrinology 142:4956–4968

Hess DA, Meyerrose TE, Wirthlin L, Craft TP, Herrbrich PE, Creer MH, Nolta JA (2004) Functional characterization of highly purified human hematopoietic repopulating cells isolated according to aldehyde dehydrogenase activity. Blood 104:1648–1655

Hirschmann-Jax C, Foster AE, Wulf GG, Goodell MA, Brenner MK (2005) A distinct "side population" of cells in human tumor cells: implications for tumor biology and therapy. Cell Cycle 4203–205

Holland AM, Gonez LJ, Harrison LC (2004) Progenitor cells in the adult pancreas. Diabetes Metab Res Rev 20:13–27

Hong KU, Reynolds SD, Watkins S, Fuchs E, Stripp BR (2004) Basal cells are a multipotent progenitor capable of renewing the bronchial epithelium. Am J Pathol 164:577–588

Hristov M, Weber C (2004) Endothelial progenitor cells: characterization, pathophysiology, and possible clinical relevance. J Cell Mol Med 8:498–508

Huard J, Cao B, Qu-Petersen Z (2003) Muscle-derived stem cells: potential for muscle regeneration. Birth Defects Res C Embryo Today 69:230–237

Hudson DL (2004) Epithelial stem cells in human prostate growth and disease. Prostate Cancer Prostatic Dis 7:188–194

Huss WJ, Gray DR, Werdin ES, Funkhouser WK Jr, Smith GJ (2004) Evidence of pluripotent human prostate stem cells in a human prostate primary xenograft model. Prostate 60:77–90

Ince TA, Cviko AP, Quade BJ, Yang A, McKeon FD, Mutter GL, Crum CP (2002) p63 Coordinates anogenital modeling and epithelial cell differentiation in the developing female urogenital tract. Am J Pathol 161:1111–1117

Ishizuya-Oka A, Shimizu K, Sakakibara S, Okano H, Ueda S (2003) Thyroid hormone-upregulated expression of Musashi-1 is specific for progenitor cells of the adult epithelium during amphibian gastrointestinal remodeling. J Cell Sci 116:3157–3164

Iwami Y, Masuda H, Asahara T (2004) Endothelial progenitor cells: past, state of the art, and future. J Cell Mol Med 8:488–497

Iwatani H, Ito T, Imai E, Matsuzaki Y, Suzuki A, Yamato M, Okabe M, Hori M (2004) Hematopoietic and nonhematopoietic potentials of Hoechst(low)/side population cells isolated from adult rat kidney. Kidney Int 65:1604–1614

Jensen UB, Lowell S, Watt FM (1999) The spatial relationship between stem cells and their progeny in the basal layer of human epidermis: a new view based on whole-mount labelling and lineage analysis. Development 126:2409–2418

Johansson CB, Momma S, Clarke DL, Risling M, Lendahl U, Frisen J (1999) Identification of a neural stem cell in the adult mammalian central nervous system. Cell 96:25–34

Jones PH, Harper S, Watt FM (1995) Stem cell patterning and fate in human epidermis. Cell 80:83–93

Jones PH, Watt FM (1993) Separation of human epidermal stem cells from transit amplifying cells on the basis of differences in integrin function and expression. Cell 73:713–724

Kajstura J, Rota M, Whang B, Cascapera S, Hosoda T, Bearzi C, Nurzynska D, Kasahara H, Zias E, Bonafe M, Nadal-Ginard B, Torella D, Nascimbene A, Quaini F, Urbanek K, Leri A, Anversa P (2005) Bone marrow cells differentiate in cardiac cell lineages after infarction independently of cell fusion. Circ Res 96:127–137

Karam SM, Straiton T, Hassan WM, Leblond CP (2003) Defining epithelial cell progenitors in the human oxyntic mucosa. Stem Cells 21:322–336

Kaur P, Li A (2000) Adhesive properties of human basal epidermal cells: an analysis of keratinocyte stem cells, transit amplifying cells, and postmitotic differentiating cells. J Invest Dermatol 114:413–420

Kayahara T, Sawada M, Takaishi S, Fukui H, Seno H, Fukuzawa H, Suzuki K, Hiai H, Kageyama R, Okano H, Chiba T (2003) Candidate markers for stem and early progenitor cells, Musashi-1 and Hes1, are expressed in crypt base columnar cells of mouse small intestine. FEBS Lett 535:131–135

Khakoo AY, Finkel T (2005) Endothelial progenitor cells. Annu Rev Med 56:79–101

Kim M, Turnquist H, Jackson J et al (2002) The multidrug resistance transporter ABCG2 (breast cancer resistance protein 1) effluxes Hoechst 33342 and is overexpressed in hematopoietic stem cells. Clin Cancer Res 8:22–28

Kim SY, Lee SH, Kim BM, Kim EH, Min BH, Bendayan M, Park IS (2004) Activation of nestin-positive duct stem (NPDS) cells in pancreas upon neogenic motivation and possible cytodifferentiation into insulin-secreting cells from NPDS cells. Dev Dyn 230:1–11

Klein I, Sarkadi B, Varadi A (1999) An inventory of the human ABC proteins. Biochim Biophys Acta 1461:237–262

Komitova M, Eriksson PS (2004) Sox-2 is expressed by neural progenitors and astroglia in the adult rat brain. Neurosci Lett 369:24–27

Korinek V, Barker N, Moerer P et al (1998) Depletion of epithelial stem-cell compartments in the small intestine of mice lacking Tcf-4. Nat Genet 19:379–383

Kubota H, Avarbock MR, Brinster RL (2003) Spermatogonial stem cells share some, but not all, phenotypic and functional characteristics with other stem cells. Proc Natl Acad Sci U S A 100:6487–6492

Kurita T, Medina RT, Mills AA, Cunha GR (2004) Role of p63 and basal cells in the prostate. Development 131:4955–4964

Lang B, Liu HL, Liu R, Feng GD, Jiao XY, Ju G (2004) Astrocytes in injured adult rat spinal cord may acquire the potential of neural stem cells. Neuroscience 128:775–783

Lassalle B, Bastos H, Louis JP, Riou L, Testart J, Dutrillaux B, Fouchet P, Allemand I (2004) 'Side population' cells in adult mouse testis express Bcrp1 gene and are enriched in spermatogonia and germinal stem cells. Development 131:479–487

Laugwitz KL, Moretti A, Lam J, Gruber P, Chen Y, Woodard S, Lin LZ, Cai CL, Lu MM, Reth M, Platoshyn O, Yuan JX, Evans S, Chien KR (2005) Postnatal isl1+ cardioblasts enter fully differentiated cardiomyocyte lineages. Nature 433:647–653

Lechner A, Leech CA, Abraham EJ, Nolan AL, Habener JF (2002) Nestin-positive progenitor cells derived from adult human pancreatic islets of Langerhans contain side population (SP) cells defined by expression of the ABCG2 (BCRP1) ATP-binding cassette transporter. Biochem Biophys Res Commun 293:670–674

Legg J, Jensen UB, Broad S, Leigh I, Watt FM (2003) Role of melanoma chondroitin sulphate proteoglycan in patterning stem cells in human interfollicular epidermis. Development 130:6049–6063

Lemmer ER, Shepard EG, Blakolmer K, Kirsch RE, Robson SC (1998) Isolation from human fetal liver of cells co-expressing CD34 haematopoietic stem cell and CAM 5.2 pancytokeratin markers. J Hepatol 29:450–454

Lendahl U, Zimmerman LB, McKay RD (1990) CNS stem cells express a new class of intermediate filament protein. Cell 60:585–595

Li A, Kaur P (2005) FACS enrichment of human keratinocyte stem cells. Methods Mol Biol 289:87–96

Litman T, Brangi M, Hudson E et al (2000) The multidrug-resistant phenotype associated with overexpression of the new ABC half-transporter, MXR (ABCG2). J Cell Sci 113:2011–2021

Liu SY, Zhang ZY, Song YC, Qiu KJ, Zhang KC, An N, Zhou Z, Cai WQ, Yang H (2004) SVZa neural stem cells differentiate into distinct lineages in response to BMP4. Exp Neurol 190:109–121

Majka SM, Jackson KA, Kienstra KA, Majesky MW, Goodell MA, Hirschi KK (2003) Distinct progenitor populations in skeletal muscle are bone marrow derived and exhibit different cell fates during vascular regeneration. J Clin Invest 111:71–79

Marshman E, Booth C, Potten CS (2002) The intestinal epithelial stem cell. Bioessays 24:91–98

Martens JE, Arends J, Van der Linden PJ, De Boer BA, Helmerhorst TJ (2004) Cytokeratin 17 and p63 are markers of the HPV target cell, the cervical stem cell. Anticancer Res 24:771–775

Merok JR, Lansita JA, Tunstead JR, Sherley JL (2002) Cosegregation of chromosomes containing immortal DNA strands in cells that cycle with asymmetric stem cell kinetics. Cancer Res 62:6791–6795

Messina E, De Angelis L, Frati G, Morrone S, Chimenti S, Fiordaliso F, Salio M, Battaglia M, Latronico MV, Coletta M, Vivarelli E, Frati L, Cossu G, Giacomello A (2004) Isolation and expansion of adult cardiac stem cells from human and murine heart. Circ Res 95:911–921

Mills JC, Andersson N, Hong CV, Stappenbeck TS, Gordon JI (2002) Molecular characterization of mouse gastric epithelial progenitor cells. Proc Natl Acad Sci U S A 99:14819–14824

Morris RJ, Liu Y, Marles L, Yang Z, Trempus C, Li S, Lin JS, Sawicki JA, Cotsarelis G (2004) Capturing and profiling adult hair follicle stem cells. Nat Biotechnol 22:411–417

Muschler GF, Nitto H, Boehm CA, Easley KA (2001) Age- and gender-related changes in the cellularity of human bone marrow and the prevalence of osteoblastic progenitors. J Orthop Res 19:117–125

Muschler GF, Midura RJ, Nakamoto C (2003) Practical modeling concepts for connective tissue stem cell and progenitor compartment kinetics. J Biomed Biotechnol 3:170–193

Nishimura S, Wakabayashi N, Toyoda K, Kashima K, Mitsufuji S (2003) Expression of musashi-1 in human colon crypt cells. Dig Dis Sci 48:1523–1529

Nunes MC, Roy NS, Keyoung HM, Goodman RR, McKhann G 2nd, Jiang L, Kang J, Nedergaard M, Goldman SA (2003) Identification and isolation of multipotential neural progenitor cells from the subcortical white matter of the adult human brain. Nat Med 9:439–447

O'Connell JT, Mutter GL, Cviko A, Nucci M, Quade BJ, Kozakewich HP, Neffen E, Sun D, Yang A, McKeon FD, Crum CP (2001) Identification of a basal/reserve cell immunophenotype in benign and neoplastic endometrium: a study with the p53 homologue p63. Gynecol Oncol 80:30–36

Okano H, Imai T, Okabe M (2002) Musashi: a translational regulator of cell fate. J Cell Sci 115:1355–1359

Okumura T, Shimada Y, Imamura M, Yasumoto S (2003) Neurotrophin receptor p75(NTR) characterizes human esophageal keratinocyte stem cells in vitro. Oncogene 22:4017–4026

Oliver JA, Maarouf O, Cheema FH, Martens TP, Al-Awqati Q (2004) The renal papilla is a niche for adult kidney stem cells. J Clin Invest 114:795–804

Omori N, Omori M, Evarts RP et al (1997) Partial cloning of rat CD34 cDNA and expression during stem cell-dependent liver regeneration in the adult rat. Hepatology 26:720–727

Oshima H, Rochat A, Kedzia C, Kobayashi K, Barrandon Y (2001) Morphogenesis and renewal of hair follicles from adult multipotent stem cells. Cell 104:233–245

Otto WR, Rao J (2004) Tomorrow's skeleton staff: mesenchymal stem cells and the repair of bone and cartilage. Cell Prolif 37:97–110

Overturf K, al-Dhalimy M, Ou CN, Finegold M, Grompe M (1997) Serial transplantation reveals the stem-cell-like regenerative potential of adult mouse hepatocytes. Am J Pathol 151:1273–1280

Owens DM, Watt FM (2003) Contribution of stem cells and differentiated cells to epidermal tumours. Nat Rev Cancer 3:444–451

Paku S, Schnur J, Nagy P, Thorgeirsson SS (2001) Origin and structural evolution of the early proliferating oval cells in rat liver. Am J Pathol 158:1313–1323

Partridge T (2004) Reenthronement of the muscle satellite cell. Cell 119:447–448

Peck AB, Cornelius JG, Chaudhari M, Shatz D, Ramiya VK (2002) Use of in vitro-generated, stem cell-derived islets to cure type 1 diabetes: how close are we? Ann N Y Acad Sci 958:59–68

Petersen BE, Goff JP, Greenberger JS, Michalopoulos GK (1998) Hepatic oval cells express the hematopoietic stem cell marker Thy-1 in the rat. Hepatology 27:433–445

Petropavlovskaia M, Rosenberg L (2002) Identification and characterization of small cells in the adult pancreas: potential progenitor cells? Cell Tissue Res 31:51–58

Pittenger MF, Martin BJ (2004) Mesenchymal stem cells and their potential as cardiac therapeutics. Circ Res 95:9–20

Potten CS, Owen G, Booth D (2002) Intestinal stem cells protect their genome by selective segregation of template DNA strands. J Cell Sci 115:2381–2388

Potten CS, Booth C, Tudor GL, Booth D, Brady G, Hurley P, Ashton G, Clarke R, Sakakibara S, Okano H (2003) Identification of a putative intestinal stem cell and early lineage marker; musashi-1. Differentiation 71:28–41

Quaini F, Urbanek K, Beltrami AP, Finato N, Beltrami CA, Nadal-Ginard B, Kajstura J, Leri A, Anversa P (2002) Chimerism of the transplanted heart. N Engl J Med 346:5–15

Ramiya VK, Maraist M, Arfors KE, Schatz DA, Peck AB, Cornelius JG (2000) Reversal of insulin-dependent diabetes using islets generated in vitro from pancreatic stem cells. Nat Med 6:278–282

Reynolds SD, Giangreco A, Power JHT, Stripp BR (2000) Neuroepithelial bodies of pulmonary airways serve as a reservoir of progenitor cells capable of epithelial regeneration. Am J Pathol 156:269–278

Richardson GD, Robson CN, Lang SH, Neal DE, Maitland NJ, Collins AT (2004) CD133, a novel marker for human prostatic epithelial stem cells. J Cell Sci 117:3539–3545

Rocchi E, Khodjakov A, Volk EL et al (2000) The product of the ABC half-transporter gene ABCG2 (BCRP/MXR/ABCP) is expressed in the plasma membrane. Biochem Biophys Res Commun 271:42–46

Ros JE, Libbrecht L, Geuken M, Jansen PL, Roskams TA (2003) High expression of MDR1, MRP1, and MRP3 in the hepatic progenitor cell compartment and hepatocytes in severe human liver disease. J Pathol 200:553–560

Sakakibara S, Imai T, Hamaguchi K, Okabe M, Aruga J, Nakajima K, Yasutomi D, Nagata T, Kurihara Y, Uesugi S, Miyata T, Ogawa M, Mikoshiba K, Okano H (1996) Mouse-Musashi-1, a neural RNA-binding protein highly enriched in the mammalian CNS stem cell. Dev Biol 176:230–242

Sanai N, Tramontin AD, Quinones-Hinojosa A et al (2004) Unique astrocyte ribbon in adult human brain contains neural stem cells but lacks chain migration. Nature 427:740–744

Sancho E, Batlle E, Clevers H (2003) Live and let die in the intestinal epithelium. Curr Opin Cell Biol 15:763–770

Sancho E, Batlle E, Clevers H (2004) Signaling pathways in intestinal development and cancer. Annu Rev Cell Dev Biol 20:695–723

Scharenberg CW, Harkey MA, Torok-Storb B (2002) The ABCG2 transporter is an efficient Hoechst 33342 efflux pump and is preferentially expressed by immature human
hematopoietic progenitors. Blood 99:507–512

Scheffer GL, Kool M, de Haas M et al (2002) Tissue distribution and induction of human
multidrug resistant protein 3. Lab Invest 82:193–201

Schinkel AH, Jonker JW (2003) Mammalian drug efflux transporters of the ATP binding
cassette (ABC) family: an overview. Adv Drug Deliv Rev 55:3–29

Seaberg RM, Smukler SR, Kieffer TJ, Enikolopov G, Asghar Z, Wheeler MB, Korbutt G, van
der Kooy D (2004) Clonal identification of multipotent precursors from adult mouse
pancreas that generate neural and pancreatic lineages. Nat Biotechnol 22:1115–1124

Seery JP (2002) Stem cells of the oesophageal epithelium. J Cell Sci 115:1783–1789

Sherwood RI, Christensen JL, Weissman IL, Wagers AJ (2004) Determinants of skeletal
muscle contributions from circulating cells, bone marrow cells, and hematopoietic stem
cells. Stem Cells 22:1292–1304

Shimano K, Satake M, Okaya A, Kitanaka J, Kitanaka N, Takemura M, Sakagami M, Terada N,
Tsujimura T (2003) Hepatic oval cells have the side population phenotype defined by
expression of ATP-binding cassette transporter ABCG2/BCRP1. Am J Pathol 163:3–9

Shinohara T, Avarbock MR, Brinster RL (1999) beta1- and alpha6-integrin are surface
markers on mouse spermatogonial stem cells. Proc Natl Acad Sci U S A 96:5504–5509

Short B, Brouard N, Occhiodoro-Scott T, Ramakrishnan A, Simmons PJ (2003) Mesenchymal
stem cells. Arch Med Res 34:565–571

Singh SK, Clarke ID, Terasaki M et al (2003) Identification of a cancer stem cell in human
brain tumors. Cancer Res 63:5821–5828

Singh SK, Hawkins C, Clarke ID, Squire JA, Bayani J, Hide T, Henkelman RM, Cusimano MD,
Dirks PB (2004) Identification of human brain tumour initiating cells. Nature 432:396–
401

Smalley M, Ashworth A (2003) Stem cells and breast cancer: a field in transit. Nat Rev Cancer
3:832–844

Stingl J, Eaves CJ, Zandieh I, Emerman JT (2001) Characterization of bipotent mammary
epithelial progenitor cells in normal adult human breast tissue. Breast Cancer Res Treat
67:93–109

Storms RW, Trujillo AP, Springer JB, Shah L, Colvin OM, Ludeman SM, Smith C (1999)
Isolation of primitive human hematopoietic progenitors on the basis of aldehyde dehydrogenase activity. Proc Natl Acad Sci U S A 96:9118–9123

Sussman MA, Anversa P (2004) Myocardial aging and senescence: where have the stem cells
gone? Annu Rev Physiol 66:29–48

Suzuki A, Zheng Y, Kondo R, Kusakabe M, Takada Y, Fukao K, Nakauchi H, Taniguchi H
(2000) Flow-cytometric separation and enrichment of hepatic progenitor cells in the
developing mouse liver. Hepatology 32:1230–1239

Suzuki A, Zheng Yw YW, Kaneko S, Onodera M, Fukao K, Nakauchi H, Taniguchi H (2002)
Clonal identification and characterization of self-renewing pluripotent stem cells in the
developing liver. J Cell Biol 156:173–184

Tai MH, Chang CC, Olson LK, Trosko JE (2005) Oct4 expression in adult human stem cells:
evidence in support of the stem cell theory of carcinogenesis. Carcinogenesis 26:495–502

Tamaki T, Akatsuka A, Ando K, Nakamura Y, Matsuzawa H, Hotta T, Roy RR, Edgerton VR
(2002) Identification of myogenic-endothelial progenitor cells in the interstitial spaces
of skeletal muscle. J Cell Biol 157:571–577

Till JE, McCulloch EA (1961) A direct measurement of the radiation sensitivity of normal
mouse bone marrow cells. Radiat Res14:213–222

Tropel P, Noel D, Platet N, Legrand P, Benabid AL, Berger F (2004) Isolation and characterisation of mesenchymal stem cells from adult mouse bone marrow. Exp Cell Res 295:395–406

Tsujimura A, Koikawa Y, Salm S, Takao T, Coetzee S, Moscatelli D, Shapiro E, Lepor H, Sun TT, Wilson EL (2002) Proximal location of mouse prostate epithelial stem cells: a model of prostatic homeostasis. J Cell Biol 157:1257–1265

Tumbar T, Guasch G, Greco V, Blanpain C, Lowry WE, Rendl M, Fuchs E (2004) Defining the epithelial stem cell niche in skin. Science 303:359–363

Van de Wetering M, Sancho E, Verweij C, de Lau W, Oving I, Hurlstone A, van der Horn K, Batlle E, Coudreuse D, Haramis AP, Tjon-Pon-Fong M, Moerer P, van den Born M, Soete G, Pals S, Eilers M, Medema R, Clevers H (2002) The beta-catenin/TCF-4 complex imposes a crypt progenitor phenotype on colorectal cancer cells. Cell 111:241–250

Venezia TA, Merchant AA, Ramos CA, Whitehouse NL, Young AS, Shaw CA, Goodell MA (2004) Molecular signatures of proliferation and quiescence in hematopoietic stem cells. PLoS Biol 2:e301

Wan H, Stone MG, Simpson C, Reynolds LE, Marshall JF, Hart IR, Hodivala-Dilke KM, Eady RA (2003) Desmosomal proteins, including desmoglein 3, serve as novel negative markers for epidermal stem cell-containing population of keratinocytes. J Cell Sci 116:4239–4248

Wang J, Elghazi L, Parker SE, Kizilocak H, Asano M, Sussel L, Sosa-Pineda B (2004) The concerted activities of Pax4 and Nkx2.2 are essential to initiate pancreatic beta-cell differentiation. Dev Biol 266:178–189

Webb A, Li A, Kaur P (2004) Location and phenotype of human adult keratinocyte stem cells of the skin. Differentiation 72:387–395

Welm BE, Tepera SB, Venezia T, Graubert TA, Rosen JM, Goodell MA (2002) Sca-1(pos) cells in the mouse mammary gland represent an enriched progenitor cell population. Dev Biol 245:42–56

Welm B, Behbod F, Goodell MA, Rosen JM (2003) Isolation and characterization of functional mammary gland stem cells. Cell Prolif 36 [Suppl 1]:17–32

Witkiewicz AK, Hecht JL, Cviko A, McKeon FD, Ince TA, Crum CP (2005) Microglandular hyperplasia: a model for the de novo emergence and evolution of endocervical reserve cells. Hum Pathol 36:154–161

Wright NA, Alison MR (1984) Biology of epithelial cell populations. Vol 2. Clarendon Press, Oxford

Wu WY, Morris RJ (2005) In vivo labeling and analysis of epidermal stem cells. Methods Mol Biol 289:73–78

Yamashita YM, Jones DL, Fuller MT (2003) Orientation of asymmetric stem cell division by the APC tumor suppressor and centrosome. Science 301:1547–1550

Zammit PS, Beauchamp JR (2001) The skeletal muscle satellite cell: stem cell or son of stem cell? Differentiation 68:193–204

Zhang J, Niu C, Ye L et al (2003) Identification of the haematopoietic stem cell niche and control of the niche size. Nature 425:836–841

Zhang YQ, Sarvetnick N (2003) Development of cell markers for the identification and expansion of islet progenitor cells. Diabetes Metab Res Rev 19:363–374

Zhou S, Schuetz JD, Bunting KD et al (2001) The ABC transporter Bcrp1/ABCG2 is expressed in a wide variety of stem cells and is a molecular determinant of the side-population phenotype. Nat Med 7:1028–1034

Zhou S, Morris JJ, Barnes Y, Lan L, Schuetz JD, Sorrentino BP (2002) Bcrp1 gene expression is required for normal numbers of side population stem cells in mice, and confers relative protection to mitoxantrone in hematopoietic cells in vivo. Proc Natl Acad Sci U S A 99:12339–12344

Ziegler BL, Valtieri M, Porada GA, De Maria R, Muller R, Masella B, Gabbianelli M, Casella I, Pelosi E, Bock T, Zanjani ED, Peschle C (1999) KDR receptor: a key marker defining hematopoietic stem cells. Science 285:1553–1558

Zulewski H, Abraham EJ, Gerlach MJ, Daniel PB, Moritz W, Muller B, Vallejo M, Thomas MK, Habener JF (2001) Multipotential nestin-positive stem cells isolated from adult pancreatic islets differentiate ex vivo into pancreatic endocrine, exocrine, and hepatic phenotypes. Diabetes 50:521–533

HEP (2006) 174:229–247
© Springer-Verlag Berlin Heidelberg 2006

Designer Cytokines for Human Haematopoietic Progenitor Cell Expansion: Impact for Tissue Regeneration

S. Rose-John

Department of Biochemistry, Christian-Albrechts-Universität zu Kiel,
Olshausenstrasse 40, 24098 Kiel, Germany
rosejohn@biochem.uni-kiel.de

Abstract Haematopoietic stem cells after bone marrow transplantation can expand 100-fold and thereby completely reconstitute the haematopoietic system. Such an expansion has so far not been achieved in vitro using cytokines and growth factors. An interesting parallel exists between haematopoietic stem cells and mouse embryonic stem cells. In both cell types, massive gp130 stimulation results in an inhibition of cellular differentiation. For both cell types, several intrinsic transcription factors are known which, when overexpressed, lead to massive self-renewal of the cells. It is currently unknown how in haematopoietic stem cells these intrinsic transcription factors, which include HOXB4 and Bmi-1, can be stimulated by extrinsic signals. Once such signals have been identified, they will be combined with the hyperstimulation of gp130 using designer cytokines. Additional strategies include a cell-permeable version of the HOXB4 protein and members of the WNT family of ligands. These strategies might eventually lead to an expansion of haematopoietic stem cells to a similar extent as that observed after bone marrow transplantation. Should haematopoietic stem cell expansion prove feasible and safe, there is great potential for the treatment of leukaemic disorders but also for the treatment of less severe diseases and non-malignant genetic disorders.

Keywords Haematopoietic stem cell · Expansion · Cytokine · Receptor · Transcription factor

Abbreviations

BMP	Bone morphogenetic protein
CNTF	Ciliary neurotrophic factor
CT-1	Cardiotrophin-1
G-CSF	Granulocyte colony stimulating factor
gp130	Glycoprotein 130 kDa
IL	Interleukin
JAK	Janus kinase
L	Ligand
LIF	Leukaemia inhibitory factor
R	Receptor
S	Soluble
SCF	Stem cell factor
SH2	Src homology 2
SHC	SH2 and collagen homology domain containing protein
STAT	Signal transducer and activator of transcription
TPO	Thrombopoietin

1
Introduction

A major milestone in progress in medical research in the past 20 years was the discovery of proteins that regulate the communication between cells of the body and those of the immune system. These proteins, called cytokines, are responsible for the preservation and restoration of homeostasis by coordination of lymphoid cells, inflammatory cells and haematopoietic cells. The involvement of these molecules in many diseases is underlined by marked changes in cytokine levels during pathologic states. Before using cytokines as therapeutic agents, a few important characteristics of cytokines need to be considered. One of them, termed pleiotropy, describes the fact that many cytokines exhibit different activities on a variety of cells. This implies the possibility of undesired side effects, especially during systemic administration. Many activities are shared between different cytokines, an attribute called redundancy. Blocking one cytokine pathway might, therefore, not be sufficient to inhibit a pathologic state. Moreover, cytokines often affect the synthesis of other cytokines. Blocking or enhancing one cytokine pathway may influence other cytokine pathways, leading to unpredictable effects. The stimulation of proliferation of haematopoietic stem cells largely depends on cytokines. Moreover, the differentiation response of such cells is controlled by cytokine pathways. Therefore, the molecular understanding of cytokine signalling pathways and cytokine receptor activation can be helpful to influence the expansion of haematopoietic stem cells in vivo as well as in vitro.

2
Cytokines and Haematopoietic Stem Cells

Haematopoietic stem cells are adult stem cells which are of great importance in the treatment of leukaemic disorders (Eaves et al. 1999) and autoimmune diseases (Radbruch and Thiel 2004) since after ablative chemotherapy, the entire haematopoietic system can be reconstituted from a few haematopoietic stem cells. In vivo, an expansion of more than 100-fold occurs following bone marrow transplantation (Pawliuk et al. 1996), whereas in vitro the expansion of haematopoietic cells is limited (see below).

Haematopoietic stem cells can be obtained from umbilical cord blood, from bone marrow and from peripheral blood after stem cells have been mobilized by treatment of the donor with the cytokine G-CSF (Conneally et al. 1997; Sorrentino 2004). Since the numbers of haematopoietic stem cells obtained from donors are often insufficient to reconstitute the entire haematopoietic system, the identification of conditions under which ex vivo expansion of haematopoietic stem cells occur are subject to intense research (Bruno et al. 2004; Sorrentino 2004).

The ex vivo expansion of haematopoietic stem cells has been studied by many groups and it has been found that the cultivation of these cells in the presence of various cytokines and growth factors leads to a significant proliferation response of the haematopoietic cells. Among these cytokines and growth factors, interleukin-6 (IL-6), IL-3 and stem cell factor (SCF) have been shown to be efficient mediators of cell expansion (Ikebuchi et al. 1987). However, although large cell numbers could be obtained, the increase in number of true haematopoietic stem cells after ex vivo expansion has only been in the range of up to three to five, indicating that differentiation was accompanied by depletion of primitive stem cells in cultures (Zandstra et al. 1997). Therefore strategies to define cytokines and growth factor cocktails that would help to inhibit the differentiation of haematopoietic stem cells during expansion have been followed by many groups. This chapter will first focus on the properties and the use of cytokines of the gp130 family for the expansion of haematopoietic stem cells, embryonic stem cells and tissue repair (Rose-John 2002). Furthermore, recent results which led to the definition of intrinsic factors needed for the massive expansion of haematopoietic stem cells will be evaluated.

2.1
The gp130 Family of Cytokines

The IL-6 family of cytokines acts via receptor complexes that contain at least one subunit of the ubiquitously expressed signal transducing protein gp130 (Taga and Kishimoto 1997). The family comprises IL-6, IL-11, ciliary neurotrophic factor (CNTF), cardiotrophin-1 (CT-1), cardiotrophin-like cytokine (CLC), leukaemia inhibitory factor (LIF), and oncostatin M (OSM) (Taga and

Kishimoto 1997), and the two newly characterized cytokines IL-27 and IL-31 (Dillon et al. 2004; Pflanz et al. 2004). IL-6, IL-11, and CNTF first bind to specific receptors, and these complexes associate with a homodimer of gp130 in the case of IL-6 and IL-11 or, alternatively, with a heterodimer of gp130 and the related protein LIF receptor (LIF-R) in the case of CNTF. OSM and LIF first bind directly to gp130 and LIF-R, respectively, and form heterodimers with LIF-R and gp130. In addition, a gp130-related protein was described that can heterodimerize with gp130 and acts as an alternative OSM receptor (Mosley et al. 1996). Recently, this OSM receptor was also shown to interact with an additional cognate receptor that provides specificity for IL-31 (Dillon et al. 2004). CT-1 binds directly to the LIF-R and induces gp130/LIF-R heterodimer formation (Pennica et al. 1996). In addition, the presence of a specific glyco-sylphosphatidylinositol (GPI)-anchored CT-1 receptor on neuronal cells was postulated (Pennica et al. 1996).

As mentioned before, IL-6 first binds to the IL-6 receptor (IL-6R). The complex of IL-6 and IL-6R associates with the signal transducing membrane protein gp130, thereby inducing its dimerization and initiation of signalling (Fig. 1a) (Rose-John 2001; Taga and Kishimoto 1997). The gp130 receptor is expressed by all cells in the body, whereas IL-6R is mainly expressed by hepatocytes, neutrophils, monocytes/macrophages and some lymphocytes. A naturally occurring soluble form of the IL-6R (sIL-6R), which has been found in various body fluids, is generated by two independent mechanisms: limited proteolysis of the membrane protein and translation from an alterna-tively spliced mRNA (Abel et al. 2004; Althoff et al. 2000, 2001; Hundhausen et al. 2003; Lust et al. 1992; Matthews et al. 2003; Müllberg et al. 2000; Rose-John and Heinrich 1994). Interestingly, the sIL-6R, together with IL-6, stimu-lates cells which only express gp130 (Jones and Rose-John 2002; Kallen 2002; Mackiewicz et al. 1992; Taga et al. 1989), a process which has been named trans-signalling (Fig. 1b) (Jones and Rose-John 2002; Kallen 2002; Müllberg et al. 2000; Peters et al. 1998; Rose-John and Heinrich 1994). Recently, it has been shown that the sIL-6R strongly sensitizes target cells of IL-6 (Peters et al. 1996).

Furthermore, embryonic stem cells (Humphrey et al. 2004; Rose-John 2002), early haematopoietic progenitor cells (Audet et al. 2001; Hacker et al. 2003; Peters et al. 1997, 1998), T cells (Atreya et al. 2000; Becker et al. 2004), many neural cells (März et al. 1998; März et al. 1999), smooth muscle cells (Klouche et al. 1999) and endothelial cells (Romano et al. 1997) are only responsive to IL-6 in the presence of sIL-6R (Jones and Rose-John 2002).

2.2
Signalling of gp130

The dimerization of two gp130 receptor subunits results in a juxtaposition of the cytoplasmic portions of gp130, leading to activation of the associated

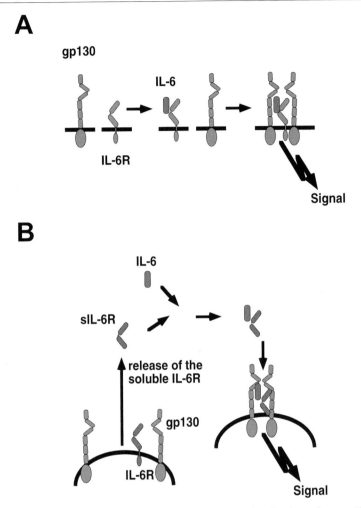

Fig. 1a, b IL-6 and IL-6R complex; Trans-signalling. **a** IL-6 first binds to the specific IL-6R forming the IL-6–IL-6R complex. This complex associates with gp130, induces gp130 dimerization and signal initiation. Note that neither IL-6 nor IL-6R alone exhibits a measurable affinity for gp130. **b** Trans-signalling of receptors for the IL-6 family of cytokines. The sIL-6R generated by shedding or alternative splicing binds its ligand with comparable affinity as the membrane-expressed IL-6R. The IL-6–sIL-6R complex initiates gp130 dimerization on a cell type lacking IL-6R expression and triggers cellular activation. Cells that only express gp130 but not the IL-6R are unable to respond to IL-6 itself. Activation of such cells in the presence of sIL-6R is called trans-signalling since the sIL-6R generated by one cell type enables a second cell type to elicit IL-6 responses

Janus kinase family (JAK) kinases. After tyrosine-phosphorylation of the cytoplasmic portions of gp130 by the JAKs, signal transducers and activators of transcription (STATs) are recruited via their SH2 domains, phosphorylated and thereby activated. The STATs translocate into the nucleus and act as transcription factors (Darnell 1997). Moreover, other substrates have been reported to become phosphorylated by JAKs, such as the adaptor protein Shc, leading to the activation of the ras-map-kinase pathway and the inositol trisphosphate (IP3) kinase, which activates pathways, which protect cells from apoptosis (Heinrich et al. 2003). STAT3 is the main STAT factor induced upon gp130 stimulation (Darnell 1997).

2.3
The Designer Cytokine Hyper-IL-6

The effective concentrations of IL-6 (50 ng/ml) and sIL-6R (1,000 ng/ml) (Sui et al. 1995) needed for the stimulation of human haematopoietic progenitor cells is high, considering a Kd of approximately 1 nmol/l (Rose-John et al. 1990; Yamasaki et al. 1988). Recently, it has been reported that the ligand–receptor

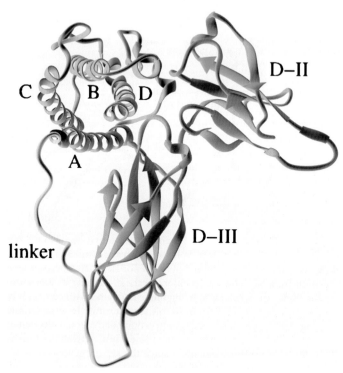

Fig. 2 Hyper-IL-6: a highly active designer cytokine consisting of IL-6 and soluble IL-6R. Molecular model of the fusion protein of IL-6 and sIL-6R (Hyper-IL-6) consisting of IL-6 and sIL-6R fused by a flexible peptide linker. *A–D* Denote the four helices of IL-6; D-II and D-III are the two cytokine-binding receptor domains of the sIL-6R which have been used for the construction of the Hyper-IL-6 fusion protein

interaction is mainly determined by the off-rate (Wells 1996), suggesting that the average half-life of the IL-6–sIL-6R complex might be shorter than the time needed to assemble the IL-6–sIL-6R/gp130 complex. Accordingly, to lower the effective dose needed for IL-6 bioactivity, IL-6 muteins with a lower off-rate have been generated that render the complexes with IL-6R more stable (Toniatti et al. 1996). As a novel approach, we postulated that the formation of the IL-6–IL-6R–gp130 complex could be enhanced by converting the IL-6–sIL-6R complex into a unimolecular protein by using a flexible polypeptide as a linker (Fig. 2). The distance between the C-terminus of IL-6R and the N-terminus of IL-6 was calculated from our three-dimensional model of the complex to be on the order of 40 Å (Grötzinger et al. 1997). Consequently, we used the 16 NH_2-terminal nonhelical and presumably flexible amino acid residues of IL-6 together with a 13-amino acid sequence rich in glycine and serine to connect IL-6 and the sIL-6R (Fischer et al. 1997). On gp130-expressing cells, this fusion protein that we called Hyper-IL-6 turned out to be fully active at 100- to 1,000-fold lower concentrations compared with the combination of unlinked IL-6 and sIL-6R (Fischer et al. 1997).

2.4
Gp130 Cytokines and Haematopoietic Stem Cells

In the mid-1990s, IL-6 and the soluble IL-6R were shown to play an important role in the regulation of expansion of haematopoietic stem cells. As outlined above, the soluble IL-6R can render cells which only express gp130 but no membrane-bound IL-6R responsive to the cytokine IL-6. Nakahata's group showed that IL-6 only in combination with the soluble IL-6R was very effective in stimulating the ex vivo expansion of haematopoietic stem cells (Heike and Nakahata 2002; Sui et al. 1995). The authors concluded that gp130 signalling in the presence of SCF dramatically stimulated the expansion of human primitive haematopoietic progenitor cells in vitro (Sui et al. 1995). Our group reported on the construction of transgenic mice, which overexpressed the human soluble IL-6R as well as human IL-6. These double transgenic mice, but not their single transgenic litter mates, showed massive extramedullary haematopoiesis in the liver and spleen, indicating that haematopoietic stem cells are responsive to IL-6 and the soluble IL-6R but not to IL-6 alone (Maione et al. 1998; Peters et al. 1997; Schirmacher et al. 1998). In subsequent studies, it was shown that the expression of the two transgenes led to the expression of genes in the liver which normally are only found in the foetal liver (Peters et al. 2001), raising the possibility that cellular differentiation is controlled by the gp130 cytokine receptor (Rose-John 2002).

The notion that early haematopoietic progenitor cells are only responsive to IL-6 and the soluble IL-6R but not to IL-6 alone was further supported by studies of Nakahata's team, who showed that during haematopoiesis the membrane-bound IL-6R is only expressed on haematopoietic progenitor cells when they started to undergo differentiation to the granulocyte/macrophage lineage (Tajima et al. 1996).

Given the important role of IL-6 and the soluble IL-6R in the regulation of expansion of haematopoietic stem cells, the fusion protein Hyper-IL-6 was tested for its ability to stimulate expansion of haematopoietic progenitor cells in vitro. It turned out that stimulation with Hyper-IL-6 was at least as effective as the separate proteins IL-6 and soluble IL-6R at 100–1,000 times lower concentrations than those used for the unlinked proteins (Audet et al. 2001; Chebath et al. 1997; Fischer et al. 1997; Hacker et al. 2003; Sui et al. 1995).

2.5
Gp130 and Tissue Regeneration

As outlined above, in IL-6/sIL-6R double transgenic mice, massive gp130 stimulation resulted in the expression of genes typically expressed only in foetal liver (Maione et al. 1998; Peters et al. 1997; Schirmacher et al. 1998). Since the promoter used to drive the expression of the human transgenic sIL-6R was only switched on after birth (Peters et al. 1996) and since the foetal gene expression in the liver only built up 8–16 weeks after birth, the most likely explanation was that massive gp130 stimulation reversed the differentiation status of adult hepatocytes to the status of foetal hepatocytes (Peters et al. 2001). Accordingly, we measured massive hepatocyte proliferation in the livers of 7-week-old IL-6/sIL-6R double transgenic mice but not in single transgenic animals (Maione et al. 1998; Schirmacher et al. 1998).

Since hepatocyte proliferation is not only typical for the foetal liver but also for liver regeneration, we hypothesized that massive gp130 stimulation via Hyper-IL-6 would also be beneficial in pathophysiological situations in which liver regeneration occurred. We first choose a mouse model in which liver regeneration was triggered by partial hepatectomy. After surgery, the animals were injected with IL-6 or Hyper-IL-6 and the time course of liver regeneration was followed. It turned out that treatment of the mice with recombinant Hyper-IL-6, but not with IL-6 alone, led to an earlier onset of hepatocellular proliferation, resulting in a marked acceleration of liver weight restoration. (Peters et al. 2000). In a different model, animals were treated with D-galactosamine, an agent that is known to induce liver damage. Seven hours after D-galactosamine administration, mice were treated with IL-6 or Hyper-IL-6 and the regeneration of the liver was followed. Hyper-IL-6 reversed the state of hepatotoxicity and enhanced the survival rates of rats suffering from fulminant hepatic failure after D-galactosamine administration (Galun et al. 2000). These results were further corroborated by experiments in which IL-6 or Hyper-IL-6 were administrated genetically. We constructed adenoviruses coding for IL-6 or Hyper-IL-6. These adenoviruses were injected into mice, which had received D-galactosamine. A single low dose of a Hyper-IL-6-encoding adenoviral vector, in contrast to an adeno-IL-6 vector, resulted in the maintenance of liver function, prevention of the progression of liver necrosis, induction of liver regeneration, and dramatically enhanced survival of the animals (Hecht et al. 2001).

The observation that massive gp130 stimulation can lead to tissue regeneration during acute liver failure led us to hypothesize that gp130 stimulation by Hyper-IL-6 might also be beneficial in animal models of acute renal failure. In initial experiments, Hyper-IL-6 turned out to be highly efficient in preventing the toxic effects of $HgCl_2$, which led to acute tubular necrosis (unpublished results).

3
Cytokines and Embryonic Stem Cells

In 1988, it was shown by Smith's group that the gp130 cytokine LIF completely blocked the differentiation of mouse embryonic stem cells (Smith et al. 1988; Williams et al. 1988). LIF acts via a heterodimeric receptor consisting of gp130 and the related protein LIF-R. Later it was demonstrated that gp130 stimulation of murine embryonic stem cells with IL-6 and soluble IL-6R (i.e. without stimulation of the LIF-R) also resulted in the maintenance if the pluripotential phenotype (Yoshida et al. 1994). Consequently, stimulation of mouse embryonic stem cells with Hyper-IL-6 also resulted in blockage of cellular differentiation (Viswanathan et al. 2002).

By using an engineered version of STAT3, which could be activated in a receptor independent fashion, Matsuda et al. showed that STAT3 activation and subsequent expression of the transcription factor Oct-4 is sufficient to support self-renewal of embryonic stem cells at high density in serum containing culture medium (Matsuda et al. 1999).

Interestingly, human embryonic stem cells do not require or respond to LIF (Reubinoff et al. 2000; Thomson et al. 1998). Since gp130 but not the LIF-R is ubiquitously expressed, one possible explanation was that human embryonic stem cells do not express the LIF-R but only the gp130 protein. Therefore the response of mouse and human embryonic stem cells to direct gp130 stimulation by Hyper-IL-6 (which only requires gp130) was directly compared. It turned out that both human and mouse embryonic stem cells express LIF-R mRNA and respond to both LIF and Hyper-IL-6 with an activation of STAT3. But in contrast to the situation in mouse cells, STAT3 activation was not sufficient to block cellular differentiation in human embryonic stem cells (Humphrey et al. 2004). These findings were recently confirmed by two independent reports (Daheron et al. 2004; Sumi et al. 2004). These results clearly established that the different behaviour of mouse and human embryonic stem cells is not due to differential receptor expression.

4
Expansion of Haematopoietic Stem Cells

Besides IL-3, IL-6 and SCF, other cytokines turned out to be effective in the ex vivo expansion of haematopoietic stem cells. The cytokine thrombopoietin (TPO), which had originally been identified and molecularly cloned as the cytokine responsible for the generation of platelets (de Sauvage et al. 1994; Lok et al. 1994), turned out to stimulate multilineage growth and progenitor cell expansion from primitive ($CD34^+$ $CD38^-$) human bone marrow progenitor cells (Goncalves et al. 1997; Ramsfjell et al. 1997). Flt-3 ligand (Flt-3L) is a cytokine which shares many features with the cytokine SCF. Both Flt-3L and SCF contain a transmembrane region and are therefore membrane-bound. It turned out that Flt-3L stimulated the self-renewal of primitive human haematopoietic cells (Petzer et al. 1996; Zandstra et al. 1997). Many other cytokines, morphogenic ligands and associated signalling components have in the meantime been shown to regulate self-renewal of haematopoietic stem cells in culture and in vivo (Sauvageau et al. 2004). Still, most strategies rely on the use of the cytokines SCF and Flt-3L with the addition of the cytokines IL-3, IL-6, Hyper-IL-6, IL-11and TPO (Hacker et al. 2003; Rose-John 2002; Sorrentino 2004).

4.1
The Provocative Role of gp130 Stimulation on Stem Cell Biology

As outlined above, gp130 stimulation on embryonic stem cells completely blocked differentiation of the cells (Smith et al. 1988; Williams et al. 1988). Of note, gp130 is the only receptor known which upon stimulation by its ligand has such a profound effect on the differentiation status of cells (Rose-John 2002; Smith 2001). Interestingly, a gene in *Drosophila* was found that encodes a cytokine receptor (Brown et al. 2001). Engagement of this cytokine receptor leads to the activation of the *Drosophila* JAK/STAT pathway (Harrison et al. 1988). The *Drosophila* genome encodes only one cytokine receptor and only one STAT protein (Brown et al. 2001). Moreover, the *Drosophila* cytokine receptor shows the highest homology to the mammalian gp130 receptor subunit. Therefore, there seems only one ancestor cytokine receptor, which mostly resembles the gp130 cytokine receptor. Importantly, two groups have published evidence that the JAK/STAT pathway is required for the control of self-renewal of germline stem cells in *Drosophila* (Kiger et al. 2001; Tulina and Matunis 2001). These data clearly demonstrate the pivotal role of the gp130/JAK/STAT signalling pathway for the prevention of cellular differentiation and for stem cell biology.

The role of the gp130 receptor during the expansion of haematopoietic stem cells therefore seems to be the suppression of cellular differentiation, whereas cytokines such as SCF and Flt-3L promote the concomitant proliferation of the cells (Eaves et al. 1999; Rose-John 2002). It should be noted, however, that even the massive stimulation of gp130 by the designer cytokine Hyper-IL-6 in combination with SCF and Flt-3L does not lead to unlimited expansion of haematopoietic stem cells. Audet et al. reported a more than tenfold expansion of competitive repopulation units of murine haematopoietic stem cells at an optimal Hyper-IL-6 concentration together with constant concentrations of SCF and Flt-3L (Audet et al. 2001).

4.2
HOXB4 Activation and Haematopoietic Stem Cell Expansion

Cytokine cocktail optimization did not result in unlimited expansion of hae-matopoietic stem cells (Conneally et al. 1997; Miller and Eaves 1997). In order to explore the intrinsic pathways leading to the expansion of haematopoietic stem cells, Humphries and colleagues has analyzed the role of members of the Hox family of transcription factors (Morgan et al. 2004). A dysregulation of these transcription factors has been shown to have effects on the proliferation, differentiation and self-renewal of haematopoietic stem cells. Remarkably, retroviral overexpression of the transcription factor HOXB4 has been shown to significantly enhance in vivo haematopoietic stem cell regeneration, with 1000-fold net increases of transduced haematopoietic stem cells (Sauvageau et al. 1995). The expanded murine stem cell population remained competitive in mouse repopulation assays and proved to be multipotent since B cells, T cells and myeloid cells were shown to be generated from these cells in primary and secondary recipient mice (Antonchuk et al. 2002).

To circumvent the need for retroviral transduction of haematopoietic stem cells, a recombinant human TAT-HOXB4 protein carrying the protein trans-duction domain of the HIV transactivating protein (TAT) fused to the human HOXB4 Protein was used as a potential growth factor for stem cells (Krosl et al. 2003). Such TAT fusion proteins are known to be efficiently taken up by cells via a mechanism that is not completely understood. The authors showed that exposure of haematopoietic stem cells to the fusion protein resulted in a significant expansion of stem cells, indicating that haematopoietic stem cell expansion induced by the TAT-HOXB4 protein was comparable to that induced by the HOXB4 gene carrying retrovirus during a similar period of observa-tion. The authors concluded that it was feasible to exploit the recombinant TAT-HOXB4 protein for rapid and significant ex vivo expansion of normal haematopoietic stem cells (Krosl et al. 2003).

4.3
The WNT Pathway and Haematopoietic Stem Cell Expansion

The WNT pathway, named after the *Drosophila* wingless and the oncogene int-1, has also been exploited to expand haematopoietic stem cells. WNT-mediated signalling controls numerous biological processes, including cell fate determination, cell migration and cell adhesion. Nineteen WNT genes are present in the genome of mammalian cells. These encode lipid modified signalling proteins, which are the ligands for the Frizzled family of receptors (Sauvageau et al. 2004; Sorrentino 2004). Without WNT-induced signalling, β-catenin is ubiquitylated and degraded by the proteasome. WNT signalling results in the inhibition of β-catenin degradation. The ectopic application of WNT proteins to haematopoietic stem cell cultures resulted in increased proliferation and expansion and self-renewal of these cells (Willert et al. 2003). Interestingly, WNT proteins are expressed by human stromal cells in foetal bone and Frizzled proteins have been detected on foetal liver haematopoietic stem cells (Sauvageau et al. 2004; Sorrentino 2004), indicating a possible role for this signalling pathway during normal haematopoiesis.

Of note, upregulation of the mRNA encoding HOXB4 was observed in haematopoietic stem cells that were transduced with a β-catenin-expressing retroviral vector, indicating that at least some of the effects of WNT might be mediated through HOXB4 (Reya et al. 2003).

Therefore, the use of WNT proteins for the in vitro expansion of haematopoietic stem cells will be examined in the future. Further research is required to determine which specific WNT molecules of this 19-member family are best suited for inducing the efficient expansion of haematopoietic stem cells (Sauvageau et al. 2004; Sorrentino 2004).

4.4
Bmi-1 and Self-Renewal of Haematopoietic Stem Cells

There has been evidence that the polycomb group gene Bmi-1 is centrally involved in the control of the cell cycle of haematopoietic stem cells (Sorrentino 2004). Intriguingly, although Bmi-1$^{-/-}$ mice show normal development of embryonic haematopoiesis, Bmi-1$^{-/-}$ haematopoietic stem cells exhibit a profound defect in self-renewal capacity (Park et al. 2003). This defect was mostly attributed to derepression of the Bmi-1 target proteins p16 and p19, since the deficiency of the genes coding for these proteins reverses the self-renewal defect in Bmi-1$^{-/-}$ haematopoietic stem cells (Park et al. 2003). Forced expression of Bmi-1 resulted in massive augmentation of haematopoietic stem cell activity (Iwama et al. 2004). Interestingly, the effect observed with forced expression of Bmi-1 can be qualitatively and quantitatively compared to the effect of a transduced HOXB4 gene into haematopoietic stem cells (Antonchuk et al. 2002). Although the molecular mechanism of the action of Bmi-1 and HOXB4 is not known, it can be speculated that early senescence of haematopoietic stem cells might be one reason for the depletion of haematopoietic stem cells in a Bmi-1$^{-/-}$ genetic background (Iwama et al. 2004). It can, however, not be excluded that Bmi-1 is also involved in the prevention of cellular differentiation during haematopoiesis. Such a notion is supported by recent data from C/EBPα$^{-/-}$

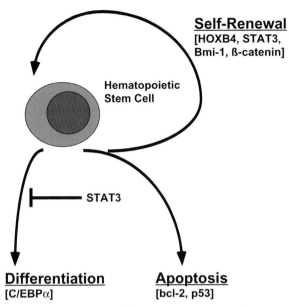

Fig. 3 Self-renewal and differentiation of haematopoietic stem cells. Haematopoietic stem cells can undergo self-renewal, differentiation and senescence/apoptosis. Several proteins have been recognized to be associated with these conditions. In the figure, the names of these proteins are given in *brackets*

mice. C/EBP is a transcription factor, which is needed for myeloid differentiation. C/EBP$\alpha^{-/-}$ haematopoietic stem cells show enhanced self-renewal capacity together with an increased Bmi-1 expression (Zhang et al. 2004).

These data collectively show that there are multiple checkpoints of haematopoietic stem cell proliferation, self-renewal and differentiation, and that there is possibly crosstalk between the pathways which are governed by gp130, WNT, HOXB4, C/EBP and Bmi-1 (Fig. 3) (Antonchuk et al. 2002; Iwama et al. 2004; Rose-John 2002; Willert et al. 2003; Zhang et al. 2004). Still, the molecular mechanism of such crosstalk between the different pathways remains to be elucidated.

5
Outlook

For mouse embryonic stem cells, it is known that self-renewal is dependent on signals from the cytokine LIF (Smith et al. 1988) and from either serum or bone morphogenetic proteins (BMP) (Ying et al. 2003). As in haematopoietic stem cells, several intrinsic transcription factors are known to be required for the maintenance of the undifferentiated state (Chambers and Smith 2004). These factors include the homeodomain proteins Oct4 and Nanog (Chambers et al.

2003). Overexpression of Nanog allowed self-renewal of murine embryonic stem cells even in the absence of LIF and BMP signals. Nanog was shown to act independent of the LIF-induced gp130 signal, although in the presence of gp130 signalling, self-renewal of embryonic stem cells was more efficient (Chambers et al. 2003). Nanog function required the presence of the transcription factor Oct4. It is, however, not known which extrinsic factors regulate the expression of Nanog. Human embryonic stem cells have been shown to lose the expression of Oct4 and Nanog whenever they undergo cellular differentiation (Humphrey et al. 2004).

In the case of haematopoietic stem cells, optimal extrinsic stimulation conditions which lead to profound expansion have yet to be defined. It can be hypothesized that the differentiation inhibiting signal exerted by massive gp130 stimulation will be a helpful component of an optimal cytokine cocktail (Rose-John 2002). Additional strategies might include a cell-permeable version of the HOXB4 protein and suited members of the WNT family of ligands. Since the forced expression of the transcription factors HOXB4 and Bmi-1 leads to the magnitude of haematopoietic stem cell expansion which is observed after bone marrow transplantation (Pawliuk et al. 1996), we at least know that such an expansion is possible in vitro. We can therefore be hopeful that such optimized extrinsic stimulation conditions will be worked out while we learn more about the complex biology of self-renewal of haematopoietic stem cells.

References

Abel S, Hundhausen C, Mentlein R, Berkhout TA, Broadway N, Siddall H, Dietrich S, Muetze B, Kallen KJ, Saftig P, Rose-John S, Ludwig A (2004) The transmembrane CXC-chemokine CXCL16 is expressed on vascular cells and shed by the activity of the disintegrin-like metalloproteinase ADAM10. J Immunol 172:6362–6372

Althoff K, Reddy P, Peschon J, Voltz N, Rose-John S, Müllberg J (2000) Contribution of the amino acid sequence at the cleavage site to the cleavage pattern of transmembrane proteins. Eur J Biochem 267:2624–2631

Althoff K, Müllberg J, Aasland D, Voltz N, Kallen K-J, Grötzinger J, Rose-John S (2001) Recognition sequences and structural elements contribute to shedding susceptibility of membrane proteins. Biochem J 353:663–672

Antonchuk J, Sauvageau G, Humphries RK (2002) HOXB4-induced expansion of adult hematopoietic stem cells ex vivo. Cell 109:39–45

Atreya R, Mudter J, Finotto S, Müllberg J, Jostock T, Wirtz S, Schütz M, Bartsch B, Holtmann M, Becker C, Strand D, Czaja J, Schlaak JF, Lehr HA, Autschbach F, Schürmann G, Nishimoto N, Yoshizaki K, Ito H, Kishimoto T, Galle PR, Rose-John S, Neurath MF (2000) Blockade of IL-6 transsignaling abrogates established experimental colitis in mice by suppression of the antiapoptotic resistance of lamina propria T cells. Nature Med 6: 583–588

Audet J, Miller CL, Rose-John S, Piret JM, Eaves CJ (2001) Distinct role of gp130 activation in promoting self-renewal divisions by mitogenically stimulated murine hematopoietic cells. Proc Natl Acad Sci U S A 98:1757–1762

Becker C, Fantini MC, Schramm C, Lehr HA, Wirtz S, Nikolaev A, Burg J, Strand S, Kiesslich R, Huber S, Ito H, Nishimoto N, Yoshizaki K, Kishimoto T, Galle PR, Blessing M, Rose-John S, Neurath MF (2004) TGF-beta suppresses tumor progression in colon cancer by inhibition of IL-6 trans-signaling. Immunity 21:491–501

Brown S, Hu N, Hombria JC (2001) Identification of the first invertebrate interleukin JAK/STAT receptor, the Drosophila gene domeless. Curr Biol 11:1700–1705

Bruno S, Gunetti M, Gammaitoni L, Perissinotto E, Caione L, Sanavio F, Fagioli F, Aglietta M, Piacibello W (2004) Fast but durable megakaryocyte repopulation and platelet production in NOD/SCID mice transplanted with ex-vivo expanded human cord blood CD34+ cells. Stem Cells 22:135–143

Chambers I, Smith A (2004) Self-renewal of teratocarcinoma and embryonic stem cells. Oncogene 23:7150–7160

Chambers I, Colby D, Robertson M, Nichols J, Lee S, Tweedie S, Smith A (2003) Functional expression cloning of Nanog, a pluripotency sustaining factor in embryonic stem cells. Cell 113:643–655

Chebath J, Fischer D, Kumar A, Oh JW, Kolett O, Lapidot T, Fischer M, Rose-John S, Nagler A, Slavin S, Revel M (1997) Interleukin-6 receptor-interleukin-6 fusion proteins with enhanced interleukin-6 type pleiotropic activities. Eur Cytokine Netw 8:359–365

Conneally E, Cashman J, Petzer A, Eaves CJ (1997) Expansion in vitro of transplantable human cord blood stem cells demonstrated using a quantitative assay of their lymphomyeloid repopulating activity in NOD/SCID mice. Proc Natl Acad Sci U S A 94:9836–9841

Daheron L, Opitz SL, Zaehres H, Lensch WM, Andrews PW, Itskovitz-Eldor J, Daley GQ (2004) LIF/STAT3 signaling fails to maintain self-renewal of human embryonic stem cells. Stem Cells 22:770–778

Darnell JE Jr (1997) STATs and gene regulation. Science 277:1630–1635

De Sauvage FJ, Hass PE, Spencer SD, Malloy BE, Gurney AL, Spencer SA, Darbonne WC, Henzel WJ, Wong SC, Kuang W-J, Oles KJ, Hultgren B, Solberg LA, Goeddel DV, Eaton DL (1994) Stimulation of megakaryocytopoiesis and thrombopoiesis by the c-Mpl ligand. Nature 369:533–538

Dillon SR, Sprecher C, Hammond A, Bilsborough J, Rosenfeld-Franklin M, Presnell SR, Haugen HS, Maurer M, Harder B, Johnston J, Bort S, Mudri S, Kuijper JL, Bukowski T, Shea P, Dong DL, Dasovich M, Grant FJ, Lockwood L, Levin SD, LeCiel C, Waggie K, Day H, Topouzis S, Kramer JB, Kuestner R, Chen Z, Foster D, Parrish-Novak J, Gross JA (2004) Interleukin 31, a cytokine produced by activated T cells, induces dermatitis in mice. Nat Immunol 5:752–760

Eaves C, Miller C, Conneally E, Audet J, Oostendorp R, Cashman J, Zandstra P, Rose-John S, Piret P, Eaves A (1999) Introduction to stem cell biology in vitro: threshold to the future. Ann N Y Acad Sci 872:1–8

Fischer M, Goldschmitt J, Peschel C, Kallen KJ, Brakenhoff JPJ, Wollmer A, Grötzinger J, Rose-John S (1997) A designer cytokine with high activity on human hematopoietic progenitor cells. Nature Biotech 15:142–145

Galun E, Zeira E, Shouval D, Pappo O, Peters M, Rose-John S (2000) Liver regeneration induced by a designed hIL-6/shIL-6R fusion protein reverses severe hepatocellular injury. FASEB J 14:1979–1987

Goncalves F, Lacout C, Villeval JL, Wendling F, Vainchenker W, Dumenil D (1997) Thrombopoietin does not induce lineage-restricted commitment of Mpl-R expressing pluripotent progenitors but permits their complete erythroid and megakaryocytic differentiation. Blood 89:3544–3553

Grötzinger J, Kurapkat G, Wollmer A, Kalai M, Rose-John S (1997) The family of the IL-6-type cytokines: specificity and promiscuity of the receptor complexes. Proteins: Structure, Function, Genetics 27:96–109

Hacker C, Kirsch RD, Ju X-S, Hieronymus T, Gust TC, Kuhl C, Jorgas T, Kurz SM, Rose-John S, Yokota Y, Zenke M (2003) Transcriptional profiling identifies Id2 function in dendritic cell development. Nat Immunol 4:380–386

Harrison DA, McCoon PE, Binari R, Gilman M, Perrimon N (1988) Drosophila unpaired encodes a secreted protein that activates the JAK signaling pathway. Genes Dev 12:3252–3263

Hecht N, Pappo O, Shouval D, Rose-John S, Galun E, Axelrod JH (2001) Hyper-IL-6 gene therapy reverses fulminant hepatic failure. Mol Therap 3:683–687

Heike T, Nakahata T (2002) Ex vivo expansion of hematopoietic stem cells by cytokines. Biochim Biophys Acta 1592:313–321

Heinrich PC, Behrmann I, Haan S, Hermanns HM, Muller-Newen G, Schaper F (2003) Principles of interleukin (IL)-6-type cytokine signalling and its regulation. Biochem J 374:1–20

Humphrey RK, Beattie GM, Lopez AD, Bucay N, King CC, Firpo M, Rose-John S, Hayek A (2004) Maintenance of pluripotency in human embryonic stem cells is Stat3 independent. Stem Cells 22:522–530

Hundhausen C, Misztela D, Berkhout TA, Broadway N, Saftig P, Hartmann D, Fahrenholz F, Postina R, Matthews V, Kallen K-J, Rose-John S, Ludwig A (2003) The disintegrin-like metalloproteinase ADAM 10 is involved in constitutive cleavage of CX3CL1 (fractalkine) and regulates CX3CL1-mediated cell-cell adhesion. Blood 102:1186–1195

Ikebuchi K, Wong GG, Clark SC, Ihle JN, Hirai Y, Ogawa M (1987) Interleukin 6 enhancement of interleukin 3-dependent proliferation of multipotential hemopoietic progenitors. Proc Natl Acad Sci U S A 84:9035–9039

Iwama A, Oguro H, Negishi M, Kato Y, Morita Y, Tsukui H, Ema H, Kamijo T, Katoh-Fukui Y, Koseki H, van Lohuizen M, Nakauchi H (2004) Enhanced self-renewal of hematopoietic stem cells mediated by the polycomb gene product Bmi-1. Immunity 21:843–851

Jones S, Rose-John S (2002) The role of soluble receptors in cytokine biology: the agonistic properties of the sIL-6R/IL-6 complex. Biochim Biophys Acta 1592:251–264

Kallen K-J (2002) The role of transsignalling via the agonistic soluble IL-6 receptor. Biochim Biophys Acta 1592:323–343

Kiger AA, Jones DL, Schulz C, Rogers MB, Fuller MT (2001) Stem cell self-renewal specified by JAK-STAT activation in response to a support cell cue. Science 294:2542–2545

Klouche M, Bhakdi S, Hemmes M, Rose-John S (1999) Novel path of activation of primary human smooth muscle cells: upregulation of gp130 creates an autocrine activation loop by IL-6 and its soluble receptor. J Immunol 163:4583–4589

Krosl J, Austin P, Beslu N, Kroon E, Humphries RK, Sauvageau G (2003) In vitro expansion of hematopoietic stem cells by recombinant TAT-HOXB4 protein. Nat Med 9:1428–1432

Lok S, Kaushansky K, Holly RD, Kuijper JL, Lofton-Day CE, Oort PJ, Grant FJ, Heipel MD, Burkhead SK, Kramer JM, Bell LA, Sprecher CA, Blumberg H, Johnson R, Prunkard D, Ching AFT, Mathewes SL, Bailey MC, Forstrom JW, Buddle MM, Osborn SG, Evans SJ, Sheppard PO, Presnell SR, O'Hara PJ, Hagen FS, Roth GJ, Foster DC (1994) Cloning and expression of murine thrombopoietin cDNA and stimulation of platelet production in vivo. Nature 369:565–568

Lust JA, Donovan KA, Kline MP, Greipp PR, Kyle RA, Maihle NJ (1992) Isolation of an mRNA encoding a soluble form of the human interleukin-6 receptor. Cytokine 4:96–100

Mackiewicz A, Schooltink H, Heinrich PC, Rose-John S (1992) Complex of soluble human IL-6-receptor/IL-6 up-regulates expression of acute-phase proteins. J Immunol 149:2021–2027

Maione D, Di Carlo E, Li W, Musiani P, Modesti A, Peters M, Rose-John S, Della Rocca C, Tripodi M, Lazzaro D, Taub R, Savino R, Ciliberto G (1998) Coexpression of IL-6 and soluble IL-6R causes nodular regenerative hyperplasia and adenomas of the liver. EMBO J 17:5588–5597

März P, Cheng J-C, Gadient RA, Patterson P, Stoyan T, Otten U, Rose-John S (1998) Sympathetic neurons can produce and respond to Interleukin-6. Proc Natl Acad Sci U S A 95:3251–3256

März P, Otten U, Rose-John S (1999) Neuronal activities of IL-6 type cytokines often depend on soluble cytokine receptors. Eur J Neurosci 11:2995–3004

Matsuda T, Nakamura T, Nakao K, Arai T, Katsuki M, Heike T, Yokota T (1999) STAT3 activation is sufficient to maintain an undifferentiated state of mouse embryonic stem cells. EMBO J 18:4261–4269

Matthews V, Schuster B, Schütze S, Bußmeyer I, Ludwig A, Hundhausen C, Sadowski T, Saftig P, Hartmann D, Kallen K-J, Rose-John S (2003) Cellular cholesterol depletion triggers shedding of the human interleukin-6 receptor by ADAM10 and ADAM17 (TACE). J Biol Chem 278:38829–38839

Miller CL, Eaves CJ (1997) Expansion in vitro of adult murine hematopoietic cells with transplantable lympho-myeloid reconstitution ability. Proc Natl Acad Sci U S A 94:13648–13653

Morgan R, Pettengell R, Sohal J (2004) The double life of HOXB4. FEBS Lett 578:1–4

Mosley B, De Imus C, Friend D, Boiani N, Thoma B, Park LS, Cosman D (1996) Dual oncostatin M (OSM) receptors. Cloning and characterization of an alternative signaling subunit conferring OSM-specific receptor activation. J Biol Chem 271:32635–32643

Müllberg J, Althoff K, Jostock T, Rose-John S (2000) The importance of shedding of membrane proteins for cytokine biology. Eur Cyt Netw 11: 27–38

Park IK, Qian D, Kiel M, Becker MW, Pihalja M, Weissman IL, Morrison SJ, Clarke MF (2003) Bmi-1 is required for maintenance of adult self-renewing haematopoietic stem cells. Nature 423:302–305

Pawliuk R, Eaves C, Humphries RK (1996) Evidence of both ontogeny and transplant dose-regulated expansion of hematopoietic stem cells in vivo. Blood 88:2852–2858

Pennica D, Arce V, Swanson TA, Vejsada R, Pollock RA, Armanini M, Dudley K, Phillips HS, Rosenthal A, Kato AC, Henderson CE (1996) Cardiotrophin-1, a cytokine present in embryonic muscle, supports long-term survival of spinal motoneurons. Neuron 17:63–74

Peters M, Jacobs S, Ehlers M, Vollmer P, Müllberg J, Wolf E, Brem G, Meyer zum Büschenfelde KH, Rose-John S (1996) The function of the soluble interleukin 6 (IL-6) receptor in vivo: sensitization of human soluble IL-6 receptor transgenic mice towards IL-6 and prolongation of the plasma half-life of IL-6. J Exp Med 183:1399–1406

Peters M, Schirmacher P, Goldschmitt J, Odenthal M, Peschel C, Dienes HP, Fattori E, Ciliberto G, Meyer zum Büschenfelde KH, Rose-John S (1997) Extramedullary expansion of hematopoietic progenitor cells in IL-6/sIL-6R double transgenic mice. J Exp Med 185: 755–766

Peters M, Müller A, Rose-John S (1998) Interleukin-6 and soluble interleukin-6 receptor: direct stimulation of gp130 and hematopoiesis. Blood 92:3495–3504

Peters M, Blinn G, Jostock T, Schirmacher P, Meyer zum Büschenfelde KH, Galle PR, Rose-John S (2000) Combined Interleukin-6 and soluble interleukin-6 receptor accelerates murine liver regeneration. Gastroenterology 119:1663–1671

Peters M, Solem F, Schirmacher P, Rose-John S (2001) IL-6 and soluble IL-6R induce stem cell factor (SCF) and Flt-3 ligand expression in vivo and in vitro. Exp Hematol 29:146–155

Petzer AL, Zandstra PW, Piret JM, Eaves CJ (1996) Differential cytokine effects on primitive (CD34+CD38–) human hematopoietic cells: novel responses to Flt3-ligand and thrombopoietin. J Exp Med 183:2551–2558

Pflanz S, Hibbert L, Mattson JD, Rosales R, Vaisberg E, Bazan JF, Phillips JH, McClanahan TK, de Waal Malefyt R, Kastelein RA (2004) WSX-1 and glycoprotein 130 constitute a signal-transducing receptor for IL-27. J Immunol 172:2225–2231

Radbruch A, Thiel A (2004) Cell therapy for autoimmune diseases: does it have a future? Ann Rheum Dis 63 [Suppl 2]:ii96–ii101

Ramsfjell V, Borge O, Cui L, Jacobsen SE (1997) Thrombopoietin directly and potently stimulates multilineage growth and progenitor cell expansion from primitive (CD34+ CD38–) human bone marrow progenitor cells: distinct and key interactions with the ligands for c-kit and flt3, and inhibitory effects of TGF-beta and TNF-alpha. J Immunol 158:5169–5177

Reubinoff BE, Pera MF, Fong CY, Trounson A, Bongso A (2000) Embryonic stem cell lines from human blastocysts: somatic differentiation in vitro. Nat Biotechnol 18:399–404

Reya T, Duncan AW, Ailles L, Domen J, Scherer DC, Willert K, Hintz L, Nusse R, Weissman IL (2003) A role for Wnt signalling in self-renewal of haematopoietic stem cells. Nature 423:409–414

Romano M, Sironi M, Toniatti C, Polentarutti N, Fruscella P, Ghezzi P, Faggioni R, Luini W, van Hinsbergh V, Sozzani S, Bussolino F, Poli V, Ciliberto G, Mantovani A (1997) Role of IL-6 and its soluble receptor in induction of chemokines and leukocyte recruitment. Immunity 6:315–325

Rose-John S (2001) Coordination of interleukin-6 biology by membrane bound and soluble receptors. Adv Exp Med Biol 495:145–151

Rose-John S (2002) GP130 stimulation and the maintenance of stem cells. Trends Biotechnol 20:417–419

Rose-John S, Heinrich PC (1994) Soluble receptors for cytokines and growth factors: generation and biological function. Biochem J 300:281–290

Rose-John S, Schooltink H, Lenz D, Hipp E, Dufhues G, Schmitz H, Schiel X, Hirano T, Kishimoto T, Heinrich PC (1990) Studies on the structure and regulation of the human hepatic interleukin-6 receptor. Eur J Biochem 190:79–83

Sauvageau G, Thorsteinsdottir U, Eaves CJ, Lawrence HJ, Largman C, Lansdorp PM, Humphries RK (1995) Overexpression of HOXB4 in hematopoietic cells causes the selective expansion of more primitive populations in vitro and in vivo. Genes Dev 9:1753–1765

Sauvageau G, Iscove NN, Humphries RK (2004) In vitro and in vivo expansion of hematopoietic stem cells. Oncogene 23:7223–7232

Schirmacher P, Peters M, Ciliberto G, Fattori E, Lotz J, Meyer zum Büschenfelde KH, Rose-John S (1998) Hepatocellular hyperplasia, plasmacytoma formation, extracellular hematopoiesis in interleukin (IL)-6/Soluble IL-6 receptor double-transgenic mice. Am J Pathol 153:639–648

Smith AG (2001) Embryo-derived stem cells: of mice and men. Annu Rev Cell Dev Biol 17:435–462

Smith AG, Heath JK, Donaldson DD, Wong GG, Moreau J, Stahl M, Rogers D (1988) Inhibition of pluripotential embryonic stem cell differentiation by purified polypeptides. Nature 336:688–690

Sorrentino BP (2004) Clinical strategies for expansion of haematopoietic stem cells. Nat Rev Immunol 4:878–888

Sui X, Tsuji K, Tanaka R, Tajima S, Muraoka K, Ebihara Y, Ikebuchi K, Yasukawa K, Taga T, Kishimoto T, Nakahata T (1995) gp130 and c-Kit signalings synergize for ex vivo expansion of human primitive hemopoietic progenitor cells. Proc Natl Acad Sci U S A 92:2859–2863

Sumi T, Fujimoto Y, Nakatsuji N, Suemori H (2004) STAT3 is dispensable for maintenance of self-renewal in nonhuman primate embryonic stem cells. Stem Cells 22:861–872

Taga T, Kishimoto T (1997) gp130 and the interleukin-6 family of cytokines. Annu Rev Immunol 15:797–819

Taga T, Hibi M, Hirata Y, Yamasaki K, Yasukawa K, Matsuda T, Hirano T, Kishimoto T (1989) Interleukin-6 triggers the association of its receptor with a possible signal transducer, gp130. Cell 58:573–581

Tajima S, Tsuji K, Ebihara Y, Sui X, Tanaka R, Muraoka K, Yoshida M, Yamada K, Yasukawa K, Taga T, Kishimoto T, Nakahata T (1996) Analysis of interleukin-6 receptor and gp130 expressions and proliferative capability of human CD34+ cells. J Exp Med 184:1357–1364

Thomson JA, Itskovitz-Eldor J, Shapiro SS, Waknitz MA, Swiergiel JJ, Marshall VS, Jones JM (1998) Embryonic stem cell lines derived from human blastocysts. Science 282:1145–1147

Toniatti C, Cabibbo A, Sporena E, Salvati AL, Cerretani M, Serafini S, Lahm A, Cortese R, Ciliberto G (1996) Engineering human interleukin-6 to obtain variants with strongly enhanced bioactivity. EMBO J 15:2726–2737

Tulina N, Matunis E (2001) Control of stem cell self-renewal in Drosophila spermatogenesis by JAK-STAT signaling. Science 294:2546–2549

Viswanathan S, Benatar T, Rose-John S, Lauffenburger D, Zandstra P (2002) Maintenance of ES cell pluripotentiality is regulated by the number and types of gp130-mediated signaling complexes. Stem Cells 20:119–138

Wang XP, Schunck M, Kallen KJ, Trautwein C, Rose-John S, Proksch E (2004) The interleukin-6 cytokine system regulates epidermal permeability barrier repair in wild-type and IL-6-deficient mice. J Invest Dermatol 123:124–131

Wells JA (1996) Binding in the growth hormone receptor complex. Proc Natl Acad Sci U S A 93:1–6

Willert K, Brown JD, Danenberg E, Duncan AW, Weissman IL, Reya T, Yates JR, Nusse R (2003) Wnt proteins are lipid-modified and can act as stem cell growth factors. Nature 423:448–452

Williams RL, Hilton DJ, Pease S, Willson TA, Stewart CL, Gearing DP, Wagner EF, Metcalf D, Nicola NA, Gough NM (1988) Myeloid leukaemia inhibitory factor maintains the developmental potential of embryonic stem cells. Nature 336:684–687

Yamasaki K, Taga T, Hirata Y, Yawata H, Kawanishi Y, Seed B, Taniguchi T, Hirano T, Kishimoto T (1988) Cloning and expression of the human interleukin-6 (BSF-2/IFN beta 2) receptor. Science 241:825–828

Ying QL, Nichols J, Chambers I, Smith A (2003) BMP induction of Id proteins suppresses differentiation and sustains embryonic stem cell self-renewal in collaboration with STAT3. Cell 115:281–292

Yoshida K, Chambers I, Nichols J, Smith A, Saito M, Yasukawa K, Shoyab M, Taga T, Kishimoto T (1994) Maintenance of the pluripotential phenotype of embryonic stem cells through direct activation of gp130 signalling pathways. Mech Dev 45:163–171

Zandstra PW, Conneally E, Petzer AL, Piret JM, Eaves CJ (1997) Cytokine manipulation of primitive human hematopoietic cell self-renewal. Proc Natl Acad Sci U S A 94:4698–4703

Zhang P, Iwasaki-Arai J, Iwasaki H, Fenyus ML, Dayaram T, Owens BM, Shigematsu H, Levantini E, Huettner CS, Lekstrom-Himes JA, Akashi K, Tenen DG (2004) Enhancement of hematopoietic stem cell repopulating capacity and self-renewal in the absence of the transcription factor C/EBP alpha. Immunity 21:853–863

HEP (2006) 174:249–282

Mesenchymal Stem Cells: Isolation, In Vitro Expansion and Characterization

N. Beyer Nardi (✉) · L. da Silva Meirelles

Genetics Department, Universidade Federal do Rio Grande do Sul, Av Bento Gonçalves 9500, Porto Alegre RS, CEP 91540–000, Brazil
nardi@ufrgs.br

Abstract Mesenchymal stem cells (MSC), one type of adult stem cell, are easy to isolate, culture, and manipulate in ex vivo culture. These cells have great plasticity and the potential for therapeutic applications, but their properties are poorly understood. MSCs can be found in bone marrow and in many other tissues, and these cells are generally identified through a combination of poorly defined physical, phenotypic, and functional properties; consequently, multiple names have been given to these cell populations. Murine MSCs have been directly applied to a wide range of murine models of diseases, where they can act as therapeutic agents per se, or as vehicles for the delivery of therapeutic genes. In addition to their systemic engraftment capabilities, MSCs show great potential for the replacement of damaged tissues such as bone, cartilage, tendon, and ligament. Their pharmacological importance is related to four points: MSCs secrete biologically important molecules, express specific receptors, can be genetically manipulated, and are susceptible to molecules that modify their natural behavior. Due to their low frequency and the lack of knowledge on cell surface markers and their location of origin, most information concerning MSCs is derived from in vitro studies. The search for the identity of the mesenchymal stem cell has depended mainly on three culture systems: the CFU-F assay, the analysis of bone marrow stroma, and the cultivation of mesenchymal stem cell lines. Other cell populations, more or less related to the MSC, have also been described. Isolation and culture conditions used to expand these cells rely on the ability of MSCs, although variable, to adhere to plastic surfaces. Whether these conditions selectively favor the expansion of different bone marrow precursors or cause similar cell populations to acquire different phenotypes is not clear. The cell populations could also represent different points of a hierarchy or a continuum of differentiation. These issues reinforce the urgent need for a more comprehensive view of the mesenchymal stem cell identity and characteristics.

Keywords Mesenchymal stem cell · Bone marrow stroma · Differentiation · Stem cell niche · Cell therapy · Genetic therapy

1
Introduction

Stem cells present in early embryonic stages are pluripotent and can generate all of the cell types found in adult organisms, whereas, adult stem cells exhibit a continuum of plasticity or multipotency. In adult humans, the first and one of the best-known stem cells to be described is the hematopoietic stem cell (HSC). A great variety of other stem/precursor cell types have also been described, but much less is known about their origin and maintenance in vivo as organ-specific stem cell pools (Nardi 2005).

The mesenchymal stem cell (MSC) is one of the most interesting of the adult stem cell types. These cells are easily isolated, cultured, and manipulated ex vivo. MSCs exhibit great plasticity and harbor the potential for therapeutic applications, but these cells are poorly defined. This has led to a heterogeneity of names and phenotypes ascribed by different groups to this cell population. MSCs are present in the bone marrow and in many other tissues, and these cells are presently identified through a combination of poorly defined physical, phenotypic, and functional properties. A number of recent reviews have adequately described the nature of MSCs (Short et al. 2003; Zipori 2004; Barry and Murphy 2004; Kassem et al. 2004; Baksh et al. 2004; Javazon et al. 2004), and the focus of this review will be to describe experimental approaches for their isolation, in vitro expansion, and characterization. We will also discuss the cellular therapeutic potentials of MSCs and place a special emphasis on the pharmacological prospects of these cells in vitro and in vivo.

2
The Identity of the Mesenchymal Stem Cell

For most cells present in adult organisms, mitosis is accompanied by differentiation. Stem cells are defined as those cells with the ability to proliferate without differentiating. At the moment, the very existence of a mesenchymal stem cell in vivo is not completely understood, since it is based on indirect evidence derived mainly from the in vitro cultivation of bone marrow and other tissues. This is true, but only to a point, because most types of adult stem cells can only be identified after isolation, which can then be examined through in vitro or in vivo assays to determine if they have the two main characteristics of stem cells: the ability to proliferate and to differentiate into mature cell types. Most of the information for MSCs, which are present at a low frequency, are derived from in vitro studies, due to a lack of information with respect to specific surface markers and their location in vivo. In vitro studies, by their very nature, may, however, introduce experimental artifacts (Javazon et al. 2004). This possibility is clearly described in several studies, including one reported by Rombouts and Ploemacher (2003), who compared the homing abilities of primary and culture-expanded MSCs in a syngeneic mouse model. Uncultured MSCs demonstrated highly efficient homing to bone marrow, but the infusion of immortalized multipotent syngeneic stromal cells, or even primary MSCs that had been cultured for only 24 h, were rarely if ever seen in the lymphohematopoietic organs. Murine MSCs were also reported to have a deficient capacity to home to bone marrow by Anjos-Afonso et al. (2004).

The identification of the mesenchymal stem cell has thus far depended on in vitro culture systems, which have provided very heterogeneous information and made the characterization of MSCs even more difficult. Three in vitro systems are generally employed to examine these cells: the CFU-F assay, the analysis of the bone marrow stroma, and the cultivation of mesenchymal stem cell lines. Other cell populations, more or less related to the MSC, have also been described.

2.1
The Colony-Forming Unit-Fibroblast

The first direct evidence that nonhematopoietic, mesenchymal precursor cells were present in the bone marrow originated from the work conducted in

Moscow during the 1960s and 1970s of Friedenstein and colleagues (reviewed in Phinney 2002). These pioneering experiments involved the incubation of bone marrow samples in tissue culture flasks. The presence of an adherent fraction could be seen within a few days, which proved highly heterogeneous. Around the 3rd–5th days, individual foci of two to four fibroblasts were observed among the histiocytes and mononuclear cells, which could differentiate into cells that could form small deposits of bone or cartilage (Friedenstein et al. 1976). These cells were termed colony forming unit-fibroblasts or CFU-F.

During the 1980s, several studies showed that cells isolated by the Friedenstein method were multipotent and could differentiate into osteoblasts, chondroblasts, adipocytes, and even myoblasts (reviewed in Prockop 1997). The frequency of CFU-F in bone marrow suspensions is very different among species, and the results are influenced by the culture conditions (reviewed in Short et al. 2003). Growth factors stimulating the proliferation of CFU-F include platelet-derived growth factor (PDGF), epidermal growth factor (EGF), basic fibroblast growth factor, transforming growth factor-β, and insulin-like growth factor-1 (Gronthos and Simmons 1995; Kuznetsov et al. 1997a; Baddoo et al. 2003; Bianchi et al. 2003). In contrast, cytokines such as interleukin 4 (IL-4) and interferon-alpha can inhibit the establishment of CFU-F (Wang et al. 1990; Gronthos and Simmons 1995). The formation of CFU-F has been considered indicative of mesenchymal stem cells, but a direct relationship between the two has not been clearly established, probably because of the great heterogeneity in morphology, cell size and differentiation potential observed among species and between colonies (Javazon et al. 2004).

2.2
The Bone Marrow Stroma

Stromal cells, along with extracellular matrix (ECM) components and soluble regulatory factors, have until recently been thought of as secondary components of a microenvironment required for sustained hematopoiesis (Nardi and Alfonso 1999). The stroma, studied both in vitro and in vivo, is composed of a very heterogeneous population of cells, which includes macrophages, fibroblasts, adipocytes, and endothelial cells (Dexter et al. 1976; Ogawa 1993). Adventitial reticular cells branch through the medullary cavity and provide a reticular network that supports hematopoietic cells. Marrow adipocytes control hematopoietic volume, such that impaired hematopoiesis is associated with increased accumulation of fat inclusions, and accelerated hematopoiesis is associated with loss of fat vacuoles. These processes determine the space available for hematopoietic cells (Tavassoli 1984). Adipocytes may also act as a reservoir for lipids needed during proliferation. Macrophages are important in the clean-up of ineffective erythropoiesis and in the removal of the nuclear pole that is produced during this process.

Stromal cells produce ECM components and both soluble and membrane-associated growth factors to form a dynamic structure that plays an active role in hematopoiesis, i.e., the hematopoietic stem cell niche. Matrix proteins in this microenvironment include fibronectin, collagen, vitronectin, and tenascin, and some of the most relevant soluble factors include stem cell factor (SCF), granulocyte-macrophage colony-stimulating factor (GM-CSF) and the granulocyte colony-stimulating factor (G-CSF). Representative adhesion molecules include members of the integrin superfamily (VLA-1, VLA-2, VLA-3, VLA-4, VLA-5, VLA-6) (reviewed in Whetton and Grahan 1999). Physical contact among the stromal cells is important for the regulation of this microenvironment. Although it has been shown that contact is not fundamental for the hematopoietic process to occur (Verfaillie 1992), it seems to be related to the quality of the hematopoietic cells produced (Breems et al. 1998). The stromal compartment has implications for human health, since abnormalities in the stromal compartment may represent a possible mechanism implicated in aplastic anemia (Kojima 1998) and in the abnormal behavior of Ph^+ cells in chronic myeloid leukemia (Cordero et al. 2004).

Based on the well-established generation of multiple types of mesenchymal cell from bone marrow, stromal stem cells were additionally proposed to exist by Owen (1985). Analogous to the hematopoietic system, they proposed that stromal stem cells reside in the bone marrow in their own niche, where the cells were able to self-renew and generate mature conjunctive/stromal cell types. The identity of this stem cell—which is now almost universally termed mesenchymal stem cell—is still, as stated above, poorly understood.

2.3
The Mesenchymal Stem Cell

The lack of consensus about the proper nomenclature needed to describe these cells has resulted in an incorrect, but synonymous use of the terms "marrow stromal cell" and "mesenchymal stem cell." Actually, stromal cells encompass all cells present in the bone marrow that are not part of the hematopoietic system. MSCs, on the other hand, correspond to that rare cell population that can form other MSCs and generate mature cells of mesenchymal tissues. Protocols involving the isolation of bone marrow cells based on their adherence to plastic surfaces result in the immediate establishment of stromal cell cultures, and not of MSC cultures. A more adequate term for the large number of cell types with the potential to differentiate into mesenchymal tissues would be "mesenchymal progenitor cell" (MPC), which would include cell types from a hierarchy immediately above the pluripotent MSC but intermediate to that represented by mature mesenchymal cell types.

Another point of debate is the fact that the HSC is itself of mesodermic origin, hence a type of MSC. For this reason, some authors prefer the term "nonhematopoietic mesenchymal stem cell." The fact that these cells, which are described below, may have alternative differentiation pathways that go beyond the normal limits of mesoderm and ectoderm formation renders the term "mesenchymal" inadequate. Probably, the best nomenclature to define this cell type would be "adult nonhematopoietic stem cell," followed by "plastic-adherent, bone-marrow derived stem cells". All these concepts, however, are already included when the term "mesenchymal stem cell" is used, and there is a tendency to accept this terminology, even though it is inadequate.

2.4
Other Cell Populations Related to the Mesenchymal Stem Cell

In addition to the heterogeneity, which characterizes MSC cultures established from various species or in different laboratories, some groups have described cell populations that are very similar to MSCs, but which have a different nomenclature. Bone marrow stromal (stem) cells (BMSSCs), stromal precursor cells (SPCs), and recycling stem cells (RS-1, RS-2) are some of these variations (Baksh et al. 2004 and references therein). More recently, D'Ippolito et al. (2004) described the marrow-isolated adult multilineage inducible (MIAMI) cells which, although isolated from humans, can proliferate extensively without showing signs of senescence or loss of differentiation potential (which, as described below, is not usual for human cells). These cells may represent a more primitive subset of bone marrow stem cells. Higher proliferative and differentiation potential has also been reported for the multipotential adult progenitor cell (MAPC) described by Catherine Verfaillie's group (Reyes et al. 2001; Reyes and Verfaillie 2001). Young et al. (2001) described human reserve pluripotent mesenchymal stem cells, present in the connective tissues of skeletal muscle and dermis.

Isolation and culture conditions used by the different groups are also variable, and probably represent the main factor responsible for the phenotype and function of the resulting cell populations. Whether these conditions selectively favor the expansion of different bone marrow precursors or cause similar cell populations to acquire different phenotypes is not clear. The cell populations could also represent different points in a hierarchy (Caplan 1994), and some studies suggest that this second alternative might be more realistic. Lodie et al. (2002), for instance, systematically compared different protocols used to isolate/expand human bone marrow adherent cells and concluded that the cell populations isolated by these various techniques are virtually indistinguishable. We have recently observed that the maintenance of MSC lines generated according to established protocols (Meirelles and Nardi 2003) but grown under MAPC conditions for 4 weeks induced changes in the immunophenotypic profile of the cells to become more similar to that of MAPCs (N. Nardi and L. Meirelles, unpublished results). In either case and as reported for hematopoietic stem cells (Pranke et al. 2001), these results demonstrate that the mesenchymal stem cell compartment is heterogeneous and that cultivation conditions can alter some of their basic properties. These points reinforce the urgent need for a more comprehensive view of the mesenchymal stem cell identity and its characteristics.

3
Distribution of the Mesenchymal Stem Cell

Although very poorly understood, the interaction of MSCs with their niche is as essential for their existence and function as it is for any other of the adult stem cells (Watt and Hogan 2000; Fuchs et al. 2004). The primary source of MSCs in adult individuals is the bone marrow, where they are immersed in the stroma (Pittenger et al. 1999). They are present at a low frequency in bone marrow, and recent studies employing the CFU-F assay suggest that in humans there is one MSC per 34,000 nucleated cells (Wexler et al. 2003). In mice, the frequency was estimated to be one for 11,300–27,000 nucleated cells (Meirelles and Nardi 2003). Once again, the heterogeneity of this microenvironment hampers the unraveling of its components and their relationship, and basic questions remain unanswered. What is the niche for the MSC? Do hematopoietic and mesenchymal stem cells share the same niche and exchange signals to drive proliferation and differentiation?

MSCs have been found in several other tissues and in ontogeny (Table 1). In mice, they were isolated from the brain, thymus, liver, spleen, kidney, muscle, and lungs of adult mice (L. Meirelles and N. Nardi, unpublished results), and other MSC-related populations such as MAPCs have been observed in different organs as well (Jiang et al. 2002). This distribution could be explained by different scenarios: (a) adult tissues contain independent reservoirs of similar

Table 1 Distribution of MSCs in different organs/tissues and ontogeny stages

Site	Species	Ontogeny stage	Reference
Adipose tissue	Human	Post-natal	Zuk et al. 2001, 2002
Adipose tissue	Mouse	Post-natal	Safford et al. 2002
Pancreas	Human	Fetal	Hu et al. 2003
Bone marrow	Human	Fetal	Campagnoli et al. 2001
Liver	Human	Fetal	Campagnoli et al. 2001
Blood	Human	Fetal	Campagnoli et al. 2001
Tendon	Mouse	Postnatal	Salingcarnboriboon et al. 2003
Synovial membrane	Mouse	Postnatal	de Bari et al. 2003
Amniotic liquid	Human	Fetal	in't Anker et al. 2003
Peripheral blood	Human	Postnatal	Zvaifler et al. 2000; Kuwana et al. 2003
Umbilical cord blood	Human	Fetal/postnatal	Alfonso et al. 2000

stem cells, whose characteristic traits are determined by signals released by each niche; (b) MSCs exist as a reservoir in one specific location, from which they circulate through the organism to colonize different tissues/organs; or (c) MSCs originate from cell populations belonging to blood vessels, and are, as a consequence, present through the whole organism. Since Bianco and Cossu (1999) suggested that MSCs originate from marrow pericytes, this third possibility has received experimental support (reviewed in Short et al. 2003). The issue is, however, still unclear.

4
Isolation and Culture of Mesenchymal Stem Cells

Few adult stem cell populations can be unequivocally identified, and isolation of these cells requires in vitro or in vivo experimentation and characterization based on immunophenotypic or functional traits. Hematopoietic stem cells, for instance, can be enriched through the selection of cells expressing surface markers such as CD34 in humans and Sca-1 in mice, or by their ability to exclude the DNA-binding dye Hoechst 33342 (Goodell et al. 1996). Mesenchymal stem cells lack clearly defined surface markers, so that the most widely used approach to isolate them relies on their ability to adhere to plastic surfaces (Wakitani et al. 1995; MacKay et al. 1998; Makino et al. 1999; Muraglia et al. 2000).

For the selective isolation of bone marrow MSCs, total cells are washed, counted, resuspended in culture medium, and plated in six-well tissue culture dishes at approximately 1.94×10^6 cells/cm^2. Nonadherent cells are removed 24–72 h later by changing the medium. After 1 week, a heterogeneous culture develops, which is generally referred to as bone marrow stroma (Fig. 1a). Maintenance of the culture with a twice-weekly medium change and removal of nonadherent cells results, after 2 or 3 weeks, in a relatively homogeneous culture of morphologically and immunophenotypically similar mesenchymal stem cells (Fig. 1b,c). Our experience shows that the identification of MSCs depends on the availability of a good inverted microscope with phase contrast, since they are difficult to visualize otherwise.

Cultures can be maintained for variable periods, depending on the species and organ of origin, by passaging and subculturing the adherent cells which are detached by trypsinization. Although Dulbecco's modified Eagle's medium (DMEM) is frequently employed for the culture of MSCs, other media have also been shown to be appropriate (reviewed by Otto and Rao 2004). The presence of HEPES buffer is also important in our experience.

In an attempt to further enrich the frequency of MSCs in the initial cell population, other methods have been developed, such as the immunodepletion of hematopoietic contaminants identified, for instance, by the molecules CD34, CD45, and CD11b (Kopen et al. 1999; Badoo et al. 2003; Ortiz et al. 2003).

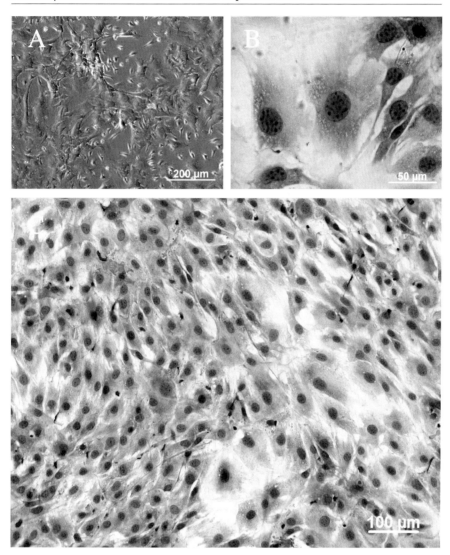

Fig. 1 a BALB/c bone marrow cells cultured for 1 week in DMEM with 10% FCS generate heterogeneous cell populations, referred to as bone marrow stromal cells (×100). Maintenance of the adherent cell population results in a homogeneous culture of mesenchymal stem cells of a flat-type morphology (**b**, ×400; **c**, ×100)

Other techniques involved cell size-based enrichment, involving the filtration of bone marrow cells through a 3-μm seive (Hung et al. 2002; Tuli et al. 2003), or changing plating densities (Colter et al. 2000; Sekiya et al. 2002). Since none of these approaches results in the establishment of homogeneous cell cultures, the development of efficient—and particularly reproducible—methods for the isolation and expansion of MSCs remains an important goal of this research field. It is possible that only when the true origin and nature of MSCs is better understood will we be able to confidently work with them in vitro.

Following removal of nonadherent cells 1–4 days after the establishment of the culture, cells are maintained with periodic passages until a relatively homogeneous population is established. Culture media may vary, but the most frequently used are Dulbecco's modified Eagle's medium (DMEM) and α-minimum essential medium (reviewed in Otto and Rao 2004). The batch of fetal calf serum employed to cultivate these cells may introduce phenotypic variations, which show that unknown factors influence the selection and expansion of these cells. The addition of specific growth factors is also important in defining the final characteristics of MSC cultures, and these are probably the main reasons for the heterogeneity observed in the mesenchymal stem cell types described in the literature. The growth of murine MAPCs, for instance, depends on the supplementation of leukemia inhibitory factor (LIF) and the use of fibronectin-coated surfaces (Jiang et al. 2002). The persistence of hematopoietic contaminants, shown by the presence of $CD45^+$ and $CD11b^+$ cells in the cultures, has also been reported (Phinney et al. 1999).

Ideal culture conditions would maintain mesenchymal stem cells with (a) phenotypic and functional characteristics similar to those exhibited in their original niche, (b) indefinite proliferation, and (c) a capacity to differentiate into multiple lineages. Since the in situ characteristics of MSCs are not known, efforts have concentrated in the last two objectives. The self-renewal potential of MSCs is not definitely established and can vary greatly according to the methodology used and the species (Bianco et al. 2001), but cells can be expected to expand for at least 40 population doublings (PDs) before their growth rate decreases significantly, as seen with human MSCs (Bruder et al. 1997). Supplementation of growth factors can also modify these results. Fibroblast growth factor-2 (FGF-2), for instance, was shown to increase the lifespan of human MSCs to more than 70 PDs (Bianchi et al. 2003). Murine MSCs, on the other hand, show apparently unlimited in vitro growth capacity (Meirelles and Nardi 2003 and unpublished observations). The high self-renewal capacity shown by murine MSCs without evidence of replicative senescence is probably related to that of rat oligodendrocyte precursor cells (Tang et al. 2001).

Cell seeding density may also influence the expansion capacity of mesenchymal stem cells. Human MSCs, for instance, expand to much higher PDs when plated at low density than at high density, with an increase of total cells from 60- to 2,000-fold (Colter et al. 2000). On the other hand, the establishment of long-term cultures of murine mesenchymal stem cells is dependent on a minimal cell density of 2×10^6 bone marrow cells/cm^2 (Meirelles and Nardi 2003). Long-term culture and high cell density are also determinants of loss of differentiation potential for human cells, another indication that the conditions for the in vitro maintenance of MSCs differ from those provided by their natural microenvironment.

5
Homing and Engraftment of Transplanted Mesenchymal Stem Cells

In vivo tracking of implanted MSCs is very important, because the success of cell and gene therapy protocols with these cells depends on their engraftment abilities. The analysis of MSC engraftment is also related to the exact nature of the grafted cells. Heterogeneous populations of adherent cells derived from mouse bone marrow engraft in multiple organs after systemic infusion (Pereira et al. 1995, 1998), and although there is strong evidence showing that the grafted cells are comprised of mainly MSCs, engraftment of other cell types can not be excluded.

More recently, studies using a well characterized and relatively homogeneous cell population comprised of murine bone marrow devoid of hematopoietic cells, were consistent with a successful in vivo engraftment of candidate MSCs in the central nervous system (Kopen et al. 1999; McBride et al. 2003). This cell population, in contrast to other murine MSCs, was not expandable in vitro (Baddoo et al. 2003; Meirelles and Nardi 2003; Gojo et al. 2003; Fang et al. 2004), and interspecies experiments were used to study MSC systemic engraftment in mice. For instance, when human MSCs were injected intraperitoneally into 13-day-old mouse embryos in uterus, multiorgan engraftment was detected 8 weeks after birth by real-time PCR (McBride et al. 2003). The sites analyzed included femur, heart, brain, liver, kidney, spleen, and lungs, where the highest level of human DNA was detected.

When cells obtained from bleomycin-resistant BALB/c mice, essentially as described by Kopen et al. (1999), were injected systemically into bleomycin-sensitive C57BL/6 mice, engraftment in the lungs was considerably higher in animals with lung injury than in animals without injury. Tissue damage, therefore, enhances MSC engraftment (Ortiz et al. 2003); however, murine MSC engraftment has also been demonstrated in noninjured animals. Gojo et al. (2003) reported the engraftment of in vitro-proliferative murine MSCs in the heart, lung, spleen, stomach, small intestine, and skeletal muscle of noninjured mice, where they differentiated locally into cardiomyocytes, vascular endothelial cells, and possibly vascular luminal cells. Selective sorting of an adherent fraction of passage two or three bone marrow cultures yielded nonhematopoietic cells that engrafted into several organs after systemic infusion (Anjos-Afonso et al. 2004). Engraftment in some organs was infrequent (brain, bone marrow), but in others (liver, lung, kidney), it exhibited higher levels of engrafted MSCs, and the presence of donor cells in circulating blood was also observed.

The deposition of MSCs in the lungs may represent a significant hurdle for engraftment therapies that employ systemic delivery of MSCs. This approach caused some animals to develop fibrosis and subsequent breathing difficulties. Gao et al. (2001) observed this phenomenon following systemic infusion of MSCs in rats, perhaps because the MSC diameter was larger than that of lung capillaries (20–24 μm vs 10–15 μm, respectively). The use of the vasodilator sodium nitroprusside at the time of injection, however, reduced entrapment of MSCs in the lungs. Murine MSCs, when detached from the dish, are also 20–25 μm wide (L. Meirelles, unpublished results), and if administered in large doses are likely to be trapped in lung capillaries before reaching important organs such as the brain and bone marrow.

In 2002, two groups (Ying et al. 2002; Terada et al. 2002) showed that stem cells can fuse with other cells in vitro and can acquire the characteristics of these cells, thus raising the possibility that the stem cell contribution to target tissues might be due to cell fusion rather than to (trans) differentiation. Fusion was also demonstrated between MSCs and epithelial cells in vitro (Spees et al. 2002); however, chromosomal analysis of xenografts indicate that fusion is not the principle mechanism responsible for the MSC contribution to multiple tissues in vivo (Pochampally et al. 2004; Sato et al. 2005). In a study describing the role of MSCs in the generation of gastric cancer in a mouse model, for example, it was observed that the percentage of tetraploid cells in affected and unaffected animals remained at the same levels (Houghton et al. 2004; see Sect. 8.1 for further information).

While the experimental study of MSC engraftment in humans is elusive, a recent paper describing microchimerism, possibly due to circulating fetal mesenchymal stem cells in pregnancy, in bone marrow and bone of women decades after giving birth to male fetuses has provided some insights into human MSC engraftment properties in vivo (O'Donoghue et al. 2004). A combined approach including immunocytochemistry, FISH, and PCR using rib sections and cultured MSCs derived from rib bone marrow was used. The results strongly suggest that circulating MSCs present in fetal blood (Campagnoli et al. 2001) crossed the placenta during pregnancy, entered the maternal circulation (O'Donoghue et al. 2003) and grafted with maternal bone and bone marrow. Khosrotehrani et al. (2004) also reported the detection of grafted male fetal cells in thyroid, cervix, intestine, liver, and lymph nodes when analyzing biopsy material of women who have had male pregnancies. The male cells were shown to express liver, hematopoietic, or epithelial markers, indicating tissue-specific incorporation.

Although fetal stem cells entering the maternal circulation include other cell populations, the results of experiments in animals suggest that MSCs are the main cell type that can engraft in maternal tissues. Human adult MSCs, therefore, can be expected to have multisite engraftment capabilities as well.

6
Characterization of Mesenchymal Stem Cells

Cultured MSCs have been extensively analyzed both morphologically and with respect to surface and molecular markers. None of these characteristics, however, is specific enough to adequately define this cell type, and mesenchymal stem cells are still operationally defined by the ultimate criteria used for identifying stem cells: prolonged proliferation and the potential to originate differentiated cell types. To abandon the term "operational MSC," it is necessary to show that these cells contribute to the formation of mesenchymal tissues after in vivo infusion (Verfaillie 2002).

A great number of surface markers have been described for committed mesenchymal progenitors (Otto and Rao 2004), and Deans and Moseley (2000) have compiled a long list of candidate markers, including CD44, CD29, and CD90, to define human MSCs. The expression of CD34 is not clearly defined in murine MSCs, but the marker is known to be absent from human and rat cells. More specific antigens such as Stro-1, SH2, SH3, and SH4 are also important markers for MSCs (reviewed in Barry and Murphy 2004), which are also positive for MHC-1 and Sca-1. None of these markers, however, seems to be a reliable parameter for the analysis of culture purity, since on the one hand even long-term cultures may exhibit some heterogeneity (maybe due to cell cycle-related marker expression) and, on the other, functionally different cultures may have similar immunophenotypic profiles.

Relatively little attention has been given to the morphology of the MSCs originating in culture. Two types of morphology can be observed—large, flat cells or elongated, fibroblastoid cells. The derivation of two types of adherent cell cultures from cord blood has already been pointed out by our group (Alfonso et al. 2000). The functional significance of these differences remains to be established.

In an earlier report (Meirelles and Nardi 2003), we described the isolation and long-term culture of murine MSCs without the need for any other medium supplementation than fetal calf serum. The cells exhibited a constant flat-type morphology (see Fig. 1), even when originating from other tissues such as spleen, lungs and brain (not published). In most publications, it is difficult to adequately assess cell morphology, but a review of the literature shows that in many cases the cells maintained a flattened shape, while others exhibited an elongated, fibroblastic phenotype (Table 2). The morphology of MAPCs also seems to be relatively flat (Reyes et al. 2001).

Still little is known about the profile of gene expression in mesenchymal stem cells. Tremain et al. (2001), in a study that also emphasized the heterogeneity of MSC cultures, reported over 2,000 expressed transcripts in a clone that originated from a stromal cell culture. In two recent studies, gene expression of bone marrow (Silva et al. 2003) and cord blood-derived MSCs (Panepucci et al. 2004; Jeong et al. 2005) was analyzed by serial analysis of gene expression (SAGE). A great number of genes were identified in the cultured cells, and an important contribution of extracellular protein products, adhesion molecules, cell motility, TGF-beta signaling, growth factor receptors, DNA repair, protein folding, and ubiquination as part of their transcriptome was observed.

Table 2 Reports of flat or elongated/fibroblastic morphology of cultured mesenchymal stem cells from different origins

Morphology	Species	Reference
Flat	Mouse	Meirelles and Nardi 2003 (Fig. 2)
	Human	Azizi et al. 1998 (Fig. 2a)
	Human	D'Ippolito et al. 2004 (Fig. 1)
	Human	Gronthos et al. 2003 (Fig. 2G)
	Human	Stute et al. 2004 (Fig. 6B)
	Human	Hung et al. 2004 (Fig. 1)
	Rat	Azizi et al. 1998 (Fig. 2c)
	Rat	Davani et al. 2003 (Fig. 1A)
	Rat	Kobayashi et al. 2004 (Fig. 1)
Fibroblastic	Human	Azizi et al. 1998 (Fig. 2b)
	Human	Koç et al. 2000 (Fig. 1)
	Human	Campagnoli et al. 2001 (Fig. 1)
	Human	Pittenger et al. 1999 (Fig. 1)
	Human	Pittenger and Martin 2004 (Fig. 1)
Other	Human	Seshi et al. 2000 (Fig. 1)

7
Differentiation of Mesenchymal Stem Cells

Although considered nondifferentiated cells, MSCs are nevertheless capable of performing at least one specialized function: they support hematopoiesis. This function is generally attributed to the bone marrow stroma, which is frequently confused with MSCs. Apparently homogeneous cultures of MSCs support hematopoietic stem cells with greater efficiency than conventionally established bone marrow stroma (Meirelles and Nardi 2003).

The in vitro differentiation of MSCs into several lineages is easily achieved. Representative examples of the protocols employed in a number of studies are shown in Table 3. Determination of the phenotype of differentiated cells depends on morphological, immunophenotypic, and functional criteria. The differentiation of osteoblasts, for instance, is determined by upregulation of alkaline phosphatase activity and deposition of a mineralized extracellular matrix in the culture plates that can be detected with Alizarin Red or other stains. Adipocytes are easily identified by their morphology and staining with Oil Red O. For identification of myocytes or neuronal cells, immunocytochemistry is performed with antibodies specific for antigens such as myosin and dystrophin, or Tau and GFAP, respectively.

Table 3 Examples of the culture protocols used for inducing in vitro differentiation of MSCs

Tissue	Species	Culture medium complement	Reference
Bone	Mouse	10^{-8} M dexamethasone, 5 µg/ml ascorbic acid 2-phosphate and 10 mM β-glycero-phosphate	Meirelles and Nardi 2003
Cartilage	Human	Transforming growth factor-β3 in serum-free medium, added to three-dimensional cultures	Pittenger et al. 1999
Fat	Human	1-methyl-3-isobutylxanthine, dexam-ethasone, insulin, and indomethacin	Pittenger et al. 1999
	Mouse	10^8 M dexamethasone and 5 µg/ml insulin	Meirelles and Nardi 2003
Neuron-like	Human	Isobutylmethylxanthine and dibutyryl cyclic AMP	Deng et al. 2001
	Mouse	50 ng/ml of basic fibroblast growth factor (bFGF) and 20 ng/ml of epidermal growth factor (EGF)	Anjos-Afonso et al. 2004
Muscle	Mouse	Amphotericin B	Phinney et al. 1999
	Rat	5-azacytidine	Wakitani et al. 1995
	Pig	5-azacytidine	Moscoso et al. 2005

In vitro cultured MSCs show great heterogeneity in their differentiation potential. Although the analysis of established MSC cultures show them to be pluripotent, with a tri-lineage (osteo/chondro/adipo, De Ugarte et al. 2003) or even higher (Anjos-Afonso et al. 2004) differentiation potential, clonal assays have shown that only one-third of the MSC clones derived from established cultures are pluripotent (Pittenger et al. 1999; Muraglia et al. 2000). Within established cultures, thus, a minority of cells seem to be pluripotent, with most of them having bi- or only uni-lineage differentiation capacity (Digirolamo et al. 1999). Models have been proposed to explain these results (Baksh et al. 2004), and it is possible that cultures are composed of a mixture of cells with different differentiation potentials. A small portion may correspond to authentic stem cells, whereas most may be committed to more differentiated phenotypes.

8
Applications of Mesenchymal Stem Cells in Cell and Gene Therapy

Although human MSCs can be immortalized through genetic modification using expression vectors carrying the catalytic subunit of human telomerase (Mihara et al. 2003), the study of murine MSCs in vitro is more attractive since they represent an unmodified natural population. They can also be promptly obtained by researchers who do not have access to a source of human cells or do not have adequate facilities for their manipulation. More importantly, murine MSCs can be directly applied to a wide range of murine models of diseases, where they can act as therapeutic agents per se or as vehicles for the delivery of therapeutic genes. Finally, MSCs obtained from rats, rabbits, pigs, and sheep will also be useful for the development of engineered tissues using autologous cells.

8.1
Study of Cancer Biology

The sustained proliferation of murine MSCs provides an interesting model for the evaluation of genetic and epigenetic factors involved in the maintenance of stemness, as well as the components responsible for the generation of tumors. Murine MSC self-renewal is not linked to neoplasia: experiments in which mice received intravenous or intraperitoneal MSC infusion do not develop donor-derived tumors (L. Meirelles and N. Nardi, unpublished results). Unraveling the genetic determinants of self-renewal may lead to the identification of candidate genes involved in tumorigenesis and to the development of drugs that can act specifically on their products. The fusion of murine MSCs and nonproliferative cells, for instance, would help with the mapping of genes involved in proliferation to specific chromosomes and chromosomal regions.

While studying the behavior of marrow-derived cells in a mouse model of gastric cancer induced by *Helicobacter pylori*, cells bearing the marker TFF2 could be associated with the predominant cell type present in this cancer (Houghton et al. 2004). In vitro studies using purified marrow-derived hematopoietic stem cells or MSCs exposed to cancerous tissue extracts showed that MSCs, but not HSCs, acquired expression of TFF2. The contribution of MSCs to tumor formation by cell fusion was ruled out by comparing the ploidy of stomach cells from infected and noninfected mice: the number of tetraploid cells in both groups did not differ significantly. Another recent study described the involvement of stem cells in human brain tumors (Singh et al. 2004). These results are consistent with an emerging view of cancer as a stem cell disorder, rather than a disease confined to fully or partially differentiated cells.

Besides their potential use for the study of basic cancer biology, modified MSCs may prove to be efficient antitumoral agents. Human MSCs have been shown to incorporate into tumor stroma (Studeny et al. 2002), a potentially useful tool for the delivery of gene products directly to tumors (see below).

8.2
Cell Therapy

Mesenchymal stem cells may participate in cell therapy protocols through two mechanisms. First, MSCs may contribute physically to injured sites when administered locally or systemically. Second, MSCs may have a supportive role through means of secreted factors. Examples of these applications are given below.

8.2.1
Fibrosis

As mentioned earlier, murine MSCs administered systemically to mice subjected to lung injury show superior lung engraftment rates relative to uninjured animals. Furthermore, MSC treatments performed immediately after antibiotic challenge reduces the fibrotic and inflammatory effects of the lesion significantly more than that in animals receiving the cells 7 days after the challenge (Ortiz et al. 2003). An earlier work, using a poorly characterized murine MSC population, showed that infusion of the cells in mice subjected to lung injury by bleomycin showed enhanced reproducibility of engraftment (Kotton et al. 2001). The injected cells were found to engraft as type I pneumocytes, but not type II pneumocytes. Similar results were reported by Ortiz et al. (2003). In the case of bleomycin-induced lung injury, this indicated that the main cellular contribution from the plastic-adherent fraction of bone marrow can be attributed to MSCs. This information may be valuable for future therapies aiming to reduce lung fibrosis in humans by autologous bone marrow transplantation.

MSCs have also been used to treat liver fibrosis. Fang et al. (2004) depleted murine bone marrow from $CD45^+$, $GlyA^+$, and $CD34^+$ cells to obtain adherent Flk^+ cells that are expandable in vitro for more than 30 passages. Using a murine model of tetrachloride-induced liver injury, they showed in the animals receiving MSCs systemically immediately after the challenge, but not 1 week later, that the fibrotic effects caused by the lesion were reduced. The presence of albumin-producing cells that exhibit donor-derived markers was also detected, although at a low frequency.

8.2.2
Cardiovasculogenesis

In a study originally designed to assess the contribution of murine MSCs to the cardiac tissue, Gojo et al. (2003) showed that a 5-azacytidine-responsive, $CD34^{low/-}$c-kit$^+$CD140a$^+$Sca-1^{high} clone transduced with an EGFP construct contributed to several sites when implanted in vivo. After injection into the ventricular myocardium, EGFP$^+$ cardiomyocytes were detected, along with EGFP$^+$CD31$^+$ cells lining the vessels surrounding the site of injection. The number of endothelial cells and cardiomyocytes grafted in the ventricle was estimated to be, respectively, 1,625 and 75 1 week after injection, and 275 and 25 3 months later. When MSCs were infused systemically through the inferior vena cava, the cells engrafted predominantly in the lungs 1 week after administration. Four weeks after the injection, the number of EGFP$^+$ cells in the lungs declined considerably. The grafted cells lacked CD31 expression, indicating that they had formed pericytes or smooth muscle cells. In addition to these results, EGFP$^+$ cells were found in the brain, thymus, uterus, and kidney. Engraftment in the stomach and small intestine was observed, and the number of donor-derived cells seemed to increase over time. When high cell numbers were implanted in the muscle, liver, or spleen, ectopic bone formation was observed, in contrast to the muscular and vascular fates adopted by cells delivered in low quantities. This finding cautions against experimental protocols involving the injection of large doses of MSCs directly in heart muscle, since they might differentiate into tissues other than those expected.

The use of purified MSCs to treat human heart diseases has not yet come into practice, despite the reported successes of blood or bone marrow-derived mononuclear cells (Assmus et al. 2002; Perin et al. 2003). Although studies demonstrating that bone marrow-derived c-kit$^+$lin$^-$ cells, a cellular fraction putatively enriched in HSCs, regenerate mouse infarcted myocardium (Orlic et al. 2001) these findings been challenged by others (Murry et al. 2004; Baslam et al. 2004). The plastic-adherent fraction of bone marrow has also improved cardiac performance in a rat model of heart infarction (Olivares et al. 2004). The CD34$^-$CD45$^-$cells collected for these latter experiments most likely comprised MSCs. Histological analyses indicated that the main contribution of the cells to the infarcted zone occurred through the formation of new myocardium and blood vessels.

Taken together, these studies indicate that the cell type most likely involved in cardiac regeneration is the MSC, possibly due more to its arteriogenic effects (see the next section) than to its cardiomyogenic properties.

8.2.3
Arteriogenic Effects

Kinnaird et al. (2004) induced unilateral hind limb ischemia in mice to demonstrate that murine bone marrow, devoid of CD34$^+$CD45$^+$ cells and delivered in situ 24 h after lesion, improved limb function despite little long-term cell engraftment. They found that medium conditioned by these cells contained several potent arteriogenic cytokines, such as basic fibroblast growth factor (bFGF), vascular endothelial growth factor (VEGF), placental growth factor (PlGF), and monocyte chemoattractant protein-1 (MCP-1). Animals that received the cells after injury contained donor-marked cells surrounded by bFGF and VEGF positive cells, indicating that the transplanted MSCs expressed these cytokines in situ. These findings support the hypothesis that factors secreted by MSCs have a significant role in limb recovery. Interestingly, MCP-1, which is secreted by cells present in the vascular wall, has been shown to recruit circulating monocytes that can differentiate into endothelial cells (Fujiyama et al. 2003). The arteriogenic effects of MSCs may thus involve the recruitment of circulating cells through the secretion of chemoattractant factors.

8.2.4
Immunosuppressive Effects

The subcutaneous co-injection of primary murine MSCs or of an embryonic mouse mesenchymal stem cell line (CH310T1/2) with a melanoma cell line (B16) was shown to favor tumor growth (Djouad et al. 2003). In vitro experiments in which activated murine splenocytes were co-cultured with CH310T1/2 cells in a transwell culture system indicated that soluble factors secreted by MSCs inhibit $CD8^+$ T cell proliferation. Even though the primary murine MSCs were not well characterized, the use of CH310T1/2 validated the hypothesis that MCSs favored tumor growth, since the results observed in vivo were similar for both cell types. These results indicated that the immunosuppressive effects should be considered whenever MSC transplantation takes place. Krampera et al. (2003) demonstrated even more clearly the immunosuppressive effects of MSCs by showing that culture-expanded murine MSCs are capable of inhibiting both naïve and memory antigen-specific T cell activation. The authors used a mixed lymphocyte reaction system in dose-dependent experiments, and determined that T cell inhibition was transient and independent of MHC antigen-presenting cells or $CD4^+CD25^+$ regulatory T cells. In contrast, the study by Djouad et al. (2003) showed that the MSC immunosuppressive effect required cell contact. Whether or not cell contact is required, it is clear that MSCs have immunomodulatory capabilities. Treatment of acute graft-versus-host disease in a human subject using third-party haploidentical MSCs can be taken as proof of this concept (Le Blanc et al. 2004).

The mechanisms involved in MSC-mediated immunosuppression are currently being investigated. Glennie et al. (2004) reported that MSCs suppress T cell effector function transiently, but the cells do not block activation. On the other hand, they induce an irreversible proliferation arrest not only in $CD4^+$ and $CD8^+$ T cells, but also in B cells, by downregulating cyclin-D2 expression. The interactions of MSCs and immune cells may have future implications not only for the knowledge of MSC biology, but also for the understanding of immune system homeostasis.

8.3
Mesenchymal Stem Cells and Tissue Engineering

In addition to systemic engraftment capabilities, MSCs show great potential for the replacement of damaged tissues such as bone, cartilage, tendon, and ligament. Although bone is capable of regeneration, the three other tissues often develop fibrous scar tissues when injured, which usually renders them unable to function properly. Large bone defects, however, do not heal spontaneously,

Table 4 Examples of tissues engineered with the use of MSCs

Engineered tissue	Methods	Reference
Respiratory mucosa	Human MSCs co-cultured with normal human bronchial epithelial cells, in vitro	Le Visage et al. 2004
Cartilage	Human MSCs cultured under chondrogenic conditions on 3D scaffold, in vitro	Chen et al. 2004a; Li et al. 2005
Bone	Critical-size cranial defect created in rabbit, repaired with BMP-2-expressing rabbit MSCs embedded in alginate	Chang et al. 2004
	Full-thickness mandibular defects created in pigs, and repaired with autologous MSCs previously seeded in poly-DL-lactic-coglycolic acid scaffolds and kept in osteo-inductive medium	Abukawa et al. 2004
Cardiac pacemakers	Human MSCs transfected with a cardiac pacemaker gene (*mHCN2*). Functional results observed in vitro by co-culture with neonatal rat ventricular myocytes, and in vivo by subepicardial injection into the canine left ventricular wall	Potapova et al. 2004

suggesting that MSC-based reconstitution may be feasible. The application of MSCs in the engineering of new tissue is dependent on the use of an appropriate scaffold to maintain an adequate three-dimensional distribution and on the use of specific molecules to drive their differentiation into cells that can restore the tissue-specific matrix (Huang et al. 2004).

The use of murine MSCs for tissue engineering is limited, due to the small size of the mouse. However, murine MSCs along with MSCs from other species are interesting candidates for the study of cell interactions with novel biomaterials, and the study of new molecules on differentiation. Examples of the use of MSCs for tissue engineering in larger animal models can be found in the literature, some of which are listed in Table 4.

8.4
Genetic Therapy

Genetic diseases can be generally classified into two categories: those caused by genetic alterations leading to loss of protein/gene function and those caused by a gain of function mutation. Other factors are involved such as the restriction of a disease phenotype to a specific organ as opposed to the whole body. When loss of function is the cause, introduction of genetic constructs expressing the missing product may be sufficient to revert or suppress the disease phenotype. When the disease involves gain of function, however, the insertion of vectors expressing healthy transcripts is not enough to correct the disorder, and some sort of genome or transcriptome editing is necessary.

The molecular tools currently used to address these issues include vectors derived from plasmids, virus, and even transposons (reviewed by Selkirk 2004 and Nathwani et al. 2004). Anti-sense RNA and interference RNA can also be used. Plasmid-derived vectors do not integrate into the host genome, and so do not last for the lifetime of the individual. On the other hand, virus-derived vectors can integrate into the genome of proliferating or nonproliferating cells, depending on the type of viral-based expression system. Sustained expression following integration makes them the vector system of choice. The systemic in vivo administration of viral vectors represents the main hurdle to their direct utilization, since they may elicit a strong host immune response that could lead to death (Kaiser 2004) or cause insertional mutagenesis resulting in cancer as reported recently in the X-SCID clinical trial (Hacein-Bey-Abina et al. 2003). The use of stem cells to deliver genetic material represents the best way to circumvent the first obstacle. Stem cells can be manipulated ex vivo and receive the genetic modifications necessary for correction of the disease, avoiding the need to expose the patient directly to vectors. When proliferative stem cells such as MSCs are used, there is also the possibility of selecting successfully altered clones for reinfusion, which might suffice to minimize insertional mutagenesis risks. This is in contrast to the use of HSCs, the stem cell type altered in the X-SCID trial, which are largely nonproliferative in vitro.

Systemic delivery of genetic constructs mediated by stem cells is feasible: stem cells engraft in vivo, and particularly in the case of MSCs, they engraft to multiple sites. When autologous cells are genetically corrected, they are likely to acquire a proliferative advantage over the patient's cells, increasing the like-lihood of engraftment and providing continued expression of the therapeutic construct. Moreover, if HLA-matched allogeneic stem cells are used there may be no need to use genetic manipulation tools, as the cells themselves may exert therapeutic effects through the expression of donor genes.

8.4.1
Correction of Genetic Disorders

The availability of homogeneous populations of murine MSCs has profound implications for the treatment of genetic diseases in mouse models, and by analogy to humans. The use of murine models is appropriate when trying to develop new therapeutic strategies. The cost of maintaining mice is not excessively high, and mouse genetics are well described. Moreover, knock-out mice can be generated by site-directed mutagenesis in embryonic stem cells, which means that many loss-of-function diseases, excluding those that lead to embryonic lethality, can be simulated in mice. The results obtained using a small animal model should, nevertheless, be validated using larger animals to avoid any unexpected effects when the therapy is applied to humans.

Table 5 Selected candidate mouse models of genetic disease for MSC-mediated therapy

Model	Expected role of transplanted MSCs	See also
Mucopolysaccharidosis type I	Production of α-L-iduronidase, particularly in the brain	Koç et al. 2002
Hemophilia A	Production and release into the blood of coagulation factor VIII	Van Damme et al. 2003
Niemann-Pick disease	Sphingomyelinase production, particularly in the brain	Jin et al. 2002
Osteogenesis imperfecta	Production of healthy collagen type I fibers	Pereira et al. 1995; Chamberlain et al. 2004

Reference: http://jaxmice.jax.org/jaxmice-cgi/jaxmicedb.cgi as of 03/28/2005 (mouse models database). See also complementary references for further information

In a search at The Jackson Laboratory mouse database (http://jaxmice.jax.org/jaxmice-cgi/jaxmicedb.cgi) using the term "genetic disease," 140 results were retrieved. Some of them were selected (Table 5) as examples of experimental models that could be used to test a MSC-based therapeutic approach, including the mouse model of mucopolysaccharidosis type I (Ohmi et al. 2003) that we currently study.

The application of MSC-mediated gene therapy in humans is still in its infancy, with no clinical trials reported so far. In vitro studies, however, show promise. Baxter et al. (2002) have successfully restored α-L-iduronidase expression by retroviral transduction of the human IDUA cDNA into MSCs obtained from patients affected by mucopolysaccharidosis type I. While this work demonstrates the possibility of reversing loss-of-function genetic disorders in humans, another study (Chamberlain et al. 2004) went even further. In this latter study, the correction of a gain-of-function genetic disease, osteogenesis imperfecta, was addressed. MSCs obtained from affected patients were genetically modified to disrupt the dominant-negative mutant allele of the COL1A1 gene. Because the site-directed mutagenesis method could affect both normal and mutant alleles and lead to inappropriate integration events in the genome, screening for correctly altered clones was performed. The investigators specifically screened several clones to identify those cells that had been appropriately modified. Once selected, these clones could generate cells that accumulated limited amounts of intracellular procollagen and could produce relatively normal collagen extracellular matrix.

8.4.2
Cancer Suppression

As mentioned earlier, the ability of MSCs to incorporate into tumor stroma could be used to design strategies to fight cancer. Studeny et al. (2002) transduced human MSCs with a construct expressing human IFN-β, which has immunomodulatory properties and antiproliferative effects over melanoma cell lines. The transduced MSCs were administered subcutaneously to nude mice together with the A375SM human melanoma cell line. The results showed that the tumor area was strikingly reduced even when only 10% IFN-β-expressing MSCs were co-injected with the melanoma cells, as compared to control animals that received the melanoma cells alone. The same effect was not achieved when nontransduced MSCs were used, indicating that IFN-β was the mediator of tumor suppression. Moreover, the tumor area was not reduced by IFN-β injection alone, indicating that MSCs were required. The survival period of treated animals, compared to controls, also significantly increased (i.e., 41–110 days for animals receiving different proportions of IFN-β-expressing MSCs vs 21–27 days for animals that received melanoma cells alone). A study examining tumor metastasis in lungs yielded similar results (Studeny et al. 2004). The results obtained using xenograft tumor models in immunoincompetent mice also show promise.

Equivalent studies with syngeneic or allogeneic murine MSCs in immunocompetent mice are required to evaluate the efficacy of this treatment in individuals with normal immune activity, since the development of anti-cancer protocols without the need for immunosuppression are highly desirable for application in humans.

9
Pharmacologic Aspects of Mesenchymal Stem Cell Biology

The pharmacological relevance of MSCs can be divided into four categories. First, the molecules secreted by MSCs may be employed as therapeutic agents or adjuvants in animal models. A long list of biologically important molecules secreted by MSCs (Majumdar et al. 1998; Kinnaird et al. 2004) include interleukins 6, 7, 8, 11, 12, 14, and 15, M-CSF, Flt-3 ligand, SCF, LIF, bFGF, VEGF, PlGF, and MCP-1. Second, specific receptors expressed by MSCs (Table 6) may be used as targets for drugs aimed at MSCs in vivo. These studies may provide information on homing mechanisms when systemically infused. Third, genetic constructs can be made that are preferentially expressed in MSCs by the incorporation of cell-specific regulatory regions, similar to that described earlier. Fourth, natural or artificial molecules may be used modify the natural behavior of MSCs and alter the MSC compartment in vivo.

While a set of natural and synthetic compounds have been shown to exert many biological effects, such as differentiation induction (Table 7), many other compounds remain to be discovered and/or fully characterized. For instance, a small molecule termed reversine (a 2-(4-morpholinoanilino)-6-cyclohexylaminopurine analog) has the ability to reprogram myogenesis-committed precursor cells (the murine cell line C2C12) into a less differentiated

Table 6 Receptors expressed by MSCs render them responsive to specific molecules

Category	Expressed	Nonexpressed
Cytokine receptors	IL-1R (CD121a)	IL-2R (CD25)
	IL-3Ra (CD123)	
	IL-4R (CDw124)	
	IL-6R (CD126)	
	IL-7R (CD127)	
Chemokine receptors	CXCR4	
Factor receptors	EGFR	EGFR-3
	IGF1 R (CD221)	Fas ligand (CD178)
	NGFR	
	IFNγR (CDw119)	
	TNFIR (CD120a)	
	TNFIIR (CD120b)	
	TGFβIR	
	TGFβIIR	
	bFGFR	
	PDGFR (CD140a)	
	Transferrin (CD71)	
Matrix receptors	ICAM-1 (CD54)	ICAM-3 (CD50)
	ICAM-2 (CD102)	E-selectin (CD62E)
	VCAM-1 (CD106)	P-selectin (CD62P)
	L-Selectin (CD62L)	PECAM-1 (CD31)
	LFA-3 (CD58)	vW factor
	ALCAM (CD166)	Cadherin 5 (CD144)
	Hyaluronate (CD44)	Lewis^x (CD15)
	Endoglin (CD105)	

References: Pittenger et al. 1999; Gronthos et al. 1998; Wynn et al. 2004

state equivalent to that of MSCs (Chen et al. 2004b). The resulting MSCs were shown to differentiate into osteoblastic and adipocytic cells upon appropriate stimulation.

10
Conclusions

Mesenchymal stem cells are finally attracting the attention of the scientific community, some 30 years after the first insights on the existence of non-hematopoietic stem cells in bone marrow. Their ease of derivation and manip-

Table 7 Specific molecules can direct MSC differentiation or modulate their expansion capacity

Molecule	Main effect	Reference
5-azacytidine	Myogenesis	Wakitani et al. 1995
All-trans-retinoic acid	Neurogenesis	Sanchez-Ramos et al. 2000
Amphotericin B	Myogenesis	Phinney et al. 1999
Ascorbic acid	Osteogenesis; chondrogenesis	Pittenger et al. 1999
Beta-glycerophosphate	Osteogenesis; chondrogenesis	Pittenger et al. 1999
Beta-mercaptoethanol	Neurogenesis	Woodbury et al. 2000
bFGF	Proliferation	Kuznetsov et al. 1997; Bianchi et al. 2003
BHA	Neurogenesis	Woodbury et al. 2000
Dexamethasone	Adipogenesis; osteogenesis; chondrogenesis	Pittenger et al. 1999
EGF	proliferation	Kuznetsov et al. 1997
ETYA	Adipogenesis	Kopen et al. 1999
Hydrocortisone	Myogenesis	Zuk et al. 2001
IBMX	Adipogenesis	Pittenger et al. 1999
Indomethacin	Adipogenesis	Pittenger et al. 1999
Insulin	Adipogenesis	Pittenger et al. 1999; Zuk et al. 2001
PDGF	Proliferation	Kuznetsov et al. 1997
TGF-beta family members (incl. BMPs)	Proliferation; differentiation Roelen and Dijke 2003	Kuznetsov et al. 1997;

ulation ex vivo, together with the growing body of information provided by studies on their characterization and differentiation potential, have generated excitement in the field of stem cell based therapies. Clinical applications with MSCs are also relatively close to realization, when compared with most other stem cells.

Most of the knowledge generated so far, however, concerns their behavior in vitro, because little is known about their properties in vivo. Although this does not necessarily hinder their application for the treatment of severe diseases or for the replacement of damaged tissues, it is clear that a comprehensive understanding of their biology is required to achieve maximal benefits. The task will not be easy, because at present, tracking the fates of ex vivo manipulated MSCs after their systemic delivery in animal models may lead to skewed results. In vitro manipulation seems to alter the original properties of the cells. The lack of definitive markers also does not allow the direct observation of MSCs in situ, so that putative MSCs should be functionally characterized in vitro prior to their use in the experiments. Ultimately, concrete data indicating that MSCs are present in multiple adult tissues together with findings suggesting the existence of a perivascular niche for mesenchymal precursors will help us to better understand the role of the mesenchymal stem cell in vivo and consequently will help in the development of more efficient strategies to treat a wide range of diseases.

Acknowledgements   The authors are indebted to Conselho Nacional de Desenvolvimento Cientifico e Tecnologico (CNPq) and Fundação de Amparo a Pesquisa do Estado do Rio Grande do Sul (FAPERGS) for funding.

References

Abukawa H, Shin M, Williams WB, Vacanti JP, Kaban LB, Troulis MJ (2004) Reconstruction of mandibular defects with autologous tissue-engineered bone. J Oral Maxillofac Surg 62:601–606

Alfonso ZZ, Forneck ED, Allebrandt WF, Nardi NB (2000) Establishment of an adherent cell layer from human umbilical cord blood. Genet Mol Biol 23:519–522

Anjos-Afonso F, Siapati EK, Bonnet D (2004) In vivo contribution of murine mesenchymal stem cells into multiple cell-types under minimal damage conditions. J Cell Sci 117:5655–5664

Assmus B, Schachinger V, Teupe C, Britten M, Lehmann R, Dobert N, Grunwald F, Aicher A, Urbich C, Martin H, Hoelzer D, Dimmeler S, Zeiher AM (2002) Transplantation of progenitor cells and regeneration enhancement in acute myocardial infarction (TOPCARE-AMI). Circulation 106:3009–3017

Azizi SA, Stokes D, Augelli BJ, DiGirolamo C, Prockop DJ (1998) Engraftment and migration of human bone marrow stromal cells implanted in the brains of albino rats—similarities to astrocyte grafts. Proc Natl Acad Sci U S A 95:3908–3913

Baddoo M, Hill K, Wilkinson R, Gaupp D, Hughes C, Kopen GC, Phinney DG (2003) Characterization of mesenchymal stem cells isolated from murine bone marrow by negative selection. J Cell Biochem 89:1235–1249

Baksh D, Song L, Tuan RS (2004) Adult mesenchymal stem cells: characterization, differentiation, and application in cell and gene therapy. J Cell Mol Med 8:301–316

Balsam LB, Wagers AJ, Christensen JL, Kofidis T, Weissman IL, Robbins RC (2004) Haematopoietic stem cells adopt mature haematopoietic fates in ischaemic myocardium. Nature 428:668–673

Barry FP, Murphy JM (2004) Mesenchymal stem cells: clinical applications and biological characterization. Int J Biochem Cell Biol 36:568–584

Baxter MA, Wynn RF, Deakin JA, Bellantuono I, Edington KG, Cooper A, Besley GT, Church HJ, Wraith JE, Carr TF, Fairbairn LJ (2002) Retrovirally mediated correction of bone marrow-derived mesenchymal stem cells from patients with mucopolysaccharidosis type I. Blood 99:1857–1859

Bianchi G, Banfi A, Mastrogiacomo M, Notaro R, Luzzatto L, Cancedda R, Quarto R (2003) Ex vivo enrichment of mesenchymal cell progenitors by fibroblast growth factor 2. Exp Cell Res 287:98–105

Bianco P, Cossu G (1999) Uno, nessuno e centomila: searching for the identity of mesodermal progenitors. Exp Cell Res 251:257–263

Bianco P, Riminucci M, Gronthos S, Robey PG (2001) Bone marrow stromal stem cells: nature, biology, and potential applications. Stem Cells 19:180–192

Breems DA, Blokland EAW, Siebel KE, Mayen AEM, Engels LJA, Ploemacher RE (1998) Stroma-contact prevents loss of hematopoietic stem cell quality during ex vivo expansion of CD34+ mobilized peripheral blood stem cells. Blood 91:111–117

Bruder SP, Jaiswal N, Haynesworth SE (1997) Growth kinetics, self-renewal, and the osteogenic potential of purified human mesenchymal stem cells during extensive subcultivation and following cryopreservation. J Cell Biochem 64:278–294

Campagnoli C, Roberts IA, Kumar S, Bennett PR, Bellantuono I, Fisk NM (2001) Identification of mesenchymal stem/progenitor cells in human first-trimester fetal blood, liver, and bone marrow. Blood 98:2396–2402

Caplan AI (1994) The mesengenic process. Clin Plast Surg 21:429–435

Chamberlain JR, Schwarze U, Wang PR, Hirata RK, Hankenson KD, Pace JM, Underwood RA, Song KM, Sussman M, Byers PH, Russell DW (2004) Gene targeting in stem cells from individuals with osteogenesis imperfecta. Science 303:1198–1201

Chang SC, Chuang H, Chen YR, Yang LC, Chen JK, Mardini S, Chung HY, Lu YL, Ma WC, Lou J (2004) Cranial repair using BMP-2 gene engineered bone marrow stromal cells. J Surg Res 119:85–91

Chen G, Liu D, Tadokoro M, Hirochika R, Ohgushi H, Tanaka J, Tateishi T (2004a) Chondrogenic differentiation of human mesenchymal stem cells cultured in a cobweb-like biodegradable scaffold. Biochem Biophys Res Commun 322:50–55

Chen S, Zhang Q, Wu X, Schultz PG, Ding S (2004b) Dedifferentiation of lineage-committed cells by a small molecule. J Am Chem Soc 126:410–411

Colter DC, Class R, DiGirolamo CM, Prockop DJ (2000) Rapid expansion of recycling stem cells in cultures of plastic-adherent cells from human bone marrow. Proc Natl Acad Sci U S A 97:3213–3218

Cordero EAA, Silla LMR, Cañedo AD, Allebrandt WF, Fogliatto L, Nardi NB (2004) Interaction between normal and CML hematopoietic progenitors and stroma influences abnormal hematopoietic development. Stem Cells Devel 13:225–228

Davani S, Marandin A, Mersin N, Royer B, Kantelip B, Herve P, Etievent JP, Kantelip JP (2003) Mesenchymal progenitor cells differentiate into an endothelial phenotype, enhance vascular density, and improve heart function in a rat cellular cardiomyoplasty model. Circulation 108 Suppl 1:II253–II258

De Bari C, Dell'Accio F, Vandenabeele F, Vermeesch JR, Raymackers J-M, Luyten FP (2003) Skeletal muscle repair by adult human mesenchymal stem cells from synovial membrane. J Cell Biol 160:909–918

De Ugarte DA, Morizono K, Elbarbary A, Alfonso Z, Zuk PA, Zhu M, Dragoo JL, Ashjian P, Thomas B, Benhaim P, Chen I, Fraser J, Hedrick MH (2003) Comparison of multi-lineage cells from human adipose tissue and bone marrow. Cells Tissues Organs 174:101–109

Deans RJ, Moseley AB (2000) Mesenchymal stem cells: biology and potential clinical uses. Exp Hematol 28:875–884

Deng W, Obrocka M, Fischer I, Prockop DJ (2001) In vitro differentiation of human marrow stromal cells into early progenitors of neural cells by conditions that increase intracellular cyclic AMP. Biochem Biophys Res Commun 282:148–152

Dexter TM, Allen TD, Lajtha LG (1976) Conditions controlling the proliferation of haemopoietic stem cells in vitro. J Cell Physiol 91:335–344

Digirolamo CM, Stokes D, Colter D, Phinney DG, Class R, Prockop DJ (1999) Propagation and senescence of human marrow stromal cells in culture: a simple colony-forming assay identifies samples with the greatest potential to propagate and differentiate. Br J Haematol 107:275–281

D'Ippolito G, Diabira S, Howard GA, Menei P, Roos BA, Schiller PC (2004) Marrow-isolated adult multilineage inducible (MIAMI) cells, a unique population of postnatal young and old human cells with extensive expansion and differentiation potential. J Cell Sci 117:2971–2981

Djouad F, Plence P, Bony C, Tropel P, Apparailly F, Sany J, Noel D, Jorgensen C (2003) Immunosuppressive effect of mesenchymal stem cells favors tumor growth in allogeneic animals. Blood 102:3837–3844

Fang B, Shi M, Liao L, Yang S, Liu Y, Zhao RC (2004) Systemic infusion of FLK1(+) mesenchymal stem cells ameliorate carbon tetrachloride-induced liver fibrosis in mice. Transplantation 78:83–88

Friedenstein AJ, Gorskaja UF, Julagina NN (1976) Fibroblast precursors in normal and irradiated mouse hematopoietic organs. Exp Hematol 4:267–274

Fuchs E, Tumbar T, Guasch G (2004) Socializing with the neighbors: stem cells and their niche. Cell 116:769–778

Fujiyama S, Amano K, Uehira K, Yoshida M, Nishiwaki Y, Nozawa Y, Jin D, Takai S, Miyazaki M, Egashira K, Imada T, Iwasaka T, Matsubara H (2003) Bone marrow monocyte lineage cells adhere on injured endothelium in a monocyte chemoattractant protein-1-dependent manner and accelerate reendothelialization as endothelial progenitor cells. Circ Res 93:980–989

Gao J, Dennis JE, Muzic RF, Lundberg M, Caplan AI (2001) The dynamic in vivo distribution of bone marrow-derived mesenchymal stem cells after infusion. Cells Tissues Organs 169:12–20

Glennie S, Soeiro I, Dyson PJ, Lam EW, Dazzi F (2004) Bone marrow mesenchymal stem cells induce division arrest anergy of activated T cells. Blood 105:2821–2827

Gojo S, Gojo N, Takeda Y, Mori T, Abe H, Kyo S, Hata J, Umezawa A (2003) In vivo cardiovasculogenesis by direct injection of isolated adult mesenchymal stem cells. Exp Cell Res 288:51–59

Goodell MA, Brose K, Paradis G, Conner AS, Mulligan RC (1996) Isolation and functional properties of murine hematopoietic stem cells that are replicating in vivo. J Exp Med 183:1797–1806

Gronthos S, Simmons PJ (1995) The growth factor requirements of STRO-1-positive human bone marrow stromal precursors under serum-deprived conditions in vitro. Blood 85:929–940

Gronthos S, Graves SE, Simmons PJ (1998) Isolation, purification and in vitro manipulation of human bone marrow stromal precursor cells. In: Beresford JN, Owen ME (eds) Marrow stromal cell culture. Cambridge University Press, New York, pp 26–42

Gronthos S, Zannettino AC, Hay SJ, Shi S, Graves SE, Kortesidis A, Simmons PJ (2003) Molecular and cellular characterisation of highly purified stromal stem cells derived from human bone marrow. J Cell Sci 116:1827–1835

Hacein-Bey-Abina S, von Kalle C, Schmidt M, Le Deist F, Wulffraat N, McIntyre E, Radford I, Villeval JL, Fraser CC, Cavazzana-Calvo M, Fischer A (2003) A serious adverse event after successful gene therapy for X-linked severe combined immunodeficiency. N Engl J Med 348:255–256

Houghton J, Stoicov C, Nomura S, Rogers AB, Carlson J, Li H, Cai X, Fox JG, Goldenring JR, Wang TC (2004) Gastric cancer originating from bone marrow-derived cells. Science 306:1568–1571

Hu Y, Liao L, Wang Q, Ma L, Ma G, Jiang X, Zhao RC (2003) Isolation and identification of mesenchymal stem cells from human fetal pancreas. J Lab Clin Med 141:342–349

Huang JI, Yoo JU, Goldberg VM (2004) Orthopaedic applications of stem cells. In: Blau H, Melton D, Moore M, Thomas ED, Verfaillie C, Weissman I, West M (eds) Handbook of stem cells. Vol. 2. Elsevier, New York, pp 773–784

Hung SC, Chen NJ, Hsieh SL, Li H, Ma HL, Lo WH (2002) Isolation and characterization of size-sieved stem cells from human bone marrow. Stem Cells 20:249–258

Hung SC, Chang CF, Ma HL, Chen TH, Low-Tone Ho L (2004) Gene expression profiles of early adipogenesis in human mesenchymal stem cells. Gene 340:141–150

In 't Anker PS, Scherjon SA, Kleijburg-van der Keur C, de Groot-Swings GM, Claas FH, Fibbe WE, Kanhai HH (2004) Isolation of mesenchymal stem cells of fetal or maternal origin from human placenta. Stem Cells 22:1338–1345

Javazon EH, Beggs KJ, Flake AW (2004) Mesenchymal stem cells: paradoxes of passaging. Exp Hematol 32:414–425

Jeong JA, Hong SH, Gang EJ, Ahn C, Hwang SH, Yang IH, Han H, Kim H (2005) Differential gene expression profiling of human umbilical cord blood-derived mesenchymal stem cells by DNA microarray. Stem Cells 23:584–593

Jiang Y, Vaessen B, Lenvik T, Blackstad M, Reyes M, Verfaillie CM (2002) Multipotent progenitor cells can be isolated from postnatal murine bone marrow, muscle and brain. Exp Hematol 30:896–904

Kaiser J (2004) Gene therapy. Side effects sideline hemophilia trial. Science 304:1423–1425

Kassem M, Kristiansen M, Abdallah BM (2004) Mesenchymal stem cells: cell biology and potential use in therapy. Basic Clin Pharmacol Toxicol 95:209–214

Khosrotehrani K, Johnson KL, Cha DH, Salomon RN, Bianchi DW (2004) Transfer of fetal cells with multilineage potential to maternal tissue. JAMA 292:75–80

Kinnaird T, Stabile E, Burnett MS, Shou M, Lee CW, Barr S, Fuchs S, Epstein SE (2004) Local delivery of marrow-derived stromal cells augments collateral perfusion through paracrine mechanisms. Circulation 109:1543–1549

Kobayashi N, Yasu T, Ueba H, Sata M, Hashimoto S, Kuroki M, Saito M, Kawakami M (2004) Mechanical stress promotes the expression of smooth muscle-like properties in marrow stromal cells. Exp Hematol 32:1238–1245

Koç ON, Gerson SL, Cooper BW, Dyhouse SM, Haynesworth SE, Caplan AI, Lazarus HM (2000) Rapid hematopoietic recovery after coinfusion of autologous-blood stem cells and culture-expanded marrow mesenchymal stem cells in advanced breast cancer patients receiving high-dose chemotherapy. J Clin Oncol 18:307–316

Koç ON, Day J, Nieder M, Gerson SL, Lazarus HM, Krivit W (2002) Allogeneic mesenchymal stem cell infusion for treatment of metachromatic leukodystrophy (MLD) and Hurler syndrome (MPS-IH). Bone Marrow Transplant 30:215–222

Kojima S (1998) Hematopoietic growth factors and marrow stroma in aplastic anemia. Int J Hematol 68:19–28

Kopen GC, Prockop DJ, Phinney DG (1999) Marrow stromal cells migrate throughout forebrain and cerebellum, and they differentiate into astrocytes after injection into neonatal mouse brains. Proc Natl Acad Sci U S A 96:10711–10716

Kotton DN, Ma BY, Cardoso WV, Sanderson EA, Summer RS, Williams MC, Fine A (2001) Bone marrow-derived cells as progenitors of lung alveolar epithelium. Development 128:5181–5188

Krampera M, Glennie S, Dyson J, Scott D, Laylor R, Simpson E, Dazzi F (2003) Bone marrow mesenchymal stem cells inhibit the response of naive and memory antigen-specific T cells to their cognate peptide. Blood 101:3722–3729

Kuznetsov SA, Friedenstein AJ, Robey PG (1997) Factors required for bone marrow stromal fibroblast colony formation in vitro. Br J Haematol 97:561–570

Kuwana M, Okazaki Y, Kodama H, Izumi K, Yasuoka H, Ogawa Y, Kawakami Y, Ikeda Y (2003) Human circulating CD14+ monocytes as a source of progenitors that exhibit mesenchymal cell differentiation. J Leukoc Biol 74:833–845

Le Blanc K, Rasmusson I, Sundberg B, Gotherstrom C, Hassan M, Uzunel M, Ringden O (2004) Treatment of severe acute graft-versus-host disease with third party haploidentical mesenchymal stem cells. Lancet 363:1439–1441

Le Visage C, Dunham B, Flint P, Leong KW (2004) Coculture of mesenchymal stem cells and respiratory epithelial cells to engineer a human composite respiratory mucosa. Tissue Eng 10:1426–1435

Li WJ, Tuli R, Okafor C, Derfoul A, Danielson KG, Hall DJ, Tuan RS (2005) A three-dimensional nanofibrous scaffold for cartilage tissue engineering using human mesenchymal stem cells. Biomaterials 26:599–609

Lodie TA, Blickarz CE, Devarakonda TJ, He C, Dash AB, Clarke J, Gleneck K, Shihabuddin L, Tubo R (2002) Systematic analysis of reportedly distinct populations of multipotent bone marrow-derived stem cells reveals a lack of distinction. Tissue Eng 8:739–751

Mackay AM, Beck SC, Murphy JM, Barry FP, Chichester CO, Pittenger MF (1998) Chondrogenic differentiation of cultured human mesenchymal stem cells from marrow. Tissue Eng 4:415–428

Majumdar MK, Thiede MA, Mosca JD, Moorman M, Gerson SL (1998) Phenotypic and functional comparison of cultures of marrow-derived mesenchymal stem cells (MSCs) and stromal cells. J Cell Physiol 176:57–66

Makino S, Fukuda K, Miyoshi S, Konishi F, Kodama H, Pan J, Sano M, Takahashi T, Hori S, Abe H, Hata J, Umezawa A, Ogawa S (1999) Cardiomyocytes can be generated from marrow stromal cells in vitro. J Clin Invest 103:697–705

McBride C, Gaupp D, Phinney DG (2003) Quantifying levels of transplanted murine and human mesenchymal stem cells in vivo by real-time PCR. Cytotherapy 5:7–18

Meirelles Lda S, Nardi NB (2003) Murine marrow-derived mesenchymal stem cell: isolation, in vitro expansion, and characterization. Br J Haematol 123:702–711

Mihara K, Imai C, Coustan-Smith E, Dome JS, Dominici M, Vanin E, Campana D (2003) Development and functional characterization of human bone marrow mesenchymal cells immortalized by enforced expression of telomerase. Br J Haematol 120:846–849

Moscoso I, Centeno A, Lopez E, Rodriguez-Barbosa JI, Santamarina I, Filgueira P, Sanchez MJ, Dominguez-Perles R, Penuelas-Rivas G, Domenech N (2005) Differentiation "in vitro" of primary and immortalized porcine mesenchymal stem cells into cardiomyocytes for cell transplantation. Transplant Proc 37:481–482

Muraglia A, Cancedda R, Quarto R (2000) Clonal mesenchymal progenitors from human bone marrow differentiate in vitro according to a hierarchical model. J Cell Sci 113:1161–1166

Murry CE, Soonpaa MH, Reinecke H, Nakajima H, Nakajima HO, Rubart M, Pasumarthi KB, Virag JI, Bartelmez SH, Poppa V, Bradford G, Dowell JD, Williams DA, Field LJ (2004) Haematopoietic stem cells do not transdifferentiate into cardiac myocytes in myocardial infarcts. Nature 428:664–668

Nardi NB (2005) All the adult stem cells, where do they all come from? An external source for organ-specific stem cell pools. Med Hypoth 64:811–817

Nardi NB, Alfonso ZZC (1999) The hematopoietic stroma. Braz J Med Biol Res 32:601–609

Nathwani AC, Davidoff AM, Tuddenham EG (2004) Prospects for gene therapy of haemophilia. Haemophilia 10:309–318

O'Donoghue K, Choolani M, Chan J, de la Fuente J, Kumar S, Campagnoli C, Bennett PR, Roberts IA, Fisk NM (2003) Identification of fetal mesenchymal stem cells in maternal blood: implications for non-invasive prenatal diagnosis. Mol Hum Reprod 9:497–502

O'Donoghue K, Chan J, de la Fuente J, Kennea N, Sandison A, Anderson JR, Roberts IA, Fisk NM (2004) Microchimerism in female bone marrow and bone decades after fetal mesenchymal stem-cell trafficking in pregnancy. Lancet 364:179–182

Ogawa M (1993) Differentiation and proliferation of hematopoietic stem cells. Blood 81:2844–2853

Ohmi K, Greenberg DS, Rajavel KS, Ryazantsev S, Li HH, Neufeld EF (2003) Activated microglia in cortex of mouse models of mucopolysaccharidoses I and IIIB. Proc Natl Acad Sci U S A 100:1902–1907

Olivares EL, Ribeiro VP, Werneck de Castro JP, Ribeiro KC, Mattos EC, Goldenberg RC, Mill JG, Dohmann HF, dos Santos RR, de Carvalho AC, Masuda MO (2004) Bone marrow stromal cells improve cardiac performance in healed infarcted rat hearts. Am J Physiol Heart Circ Physiol 287:H464–H470

Orlic D, Kajstura J, Chimenti S, Jakoniuk I, Anderson SM, Li B, Pickel J, McKay R, Nadal-Ginard B, Bodine DM, Leri A, Anversa P (2001) Bone marrow cells regenerate infarcted myocardium. Nature 410:701–705

Ortiz LA, Gambelli F, McBride C, Gaupp D, Baddoo M, Kaminski N, Phinney DG (2003) Mesenchymal stem cell engraftment in lung is enhanced in response to bleomycin exposure and ameliorates its fibrotic effects. Proc Natl Acad Sci U S A 100:8407–8411

Otto WR, Rao J (2004) Tomorrow's skeleton staff: mesenchymal stem cells and the repair of bone and cartilage. Cell Prolif 37:97–110

Owen M (1985) Lineage of osteogenic cells and their relationship to the stromal system. In: Peck WA (ed) Bone and mineral research. Vol. 3. Elsevier, New York, pp 1–25

Panepucci RA, Siufi JL, Silva WA Jr, Proto-Siquiera R, Neder L, Orellana M, Rocha V, Covas DT, Zago MA (2004) Comparison of gene expression of umbilical cord vein and bone marrow-derived mesenchymal stem cells. Stem Cells 22:1263–1278

Pereira RF, Halford KW, O'Hara MD, Leeper DB, Sokolov BP, Pollard MD, Bagasra O, Prockop DJ (1995) Cultured adherent cells from marrow can serve as long-lasting precursor cells for bone, cartilage, and lung in irradiated mice. Proc Natl Acad Sci U S A 92:4857–4861

Pereira RF, O'Hara MD, Laptev AV, Halford KW, Pollard MD, Class R, Simon D, Livezey K, Prockop DJ (1998) Marrow stromal cells as a source of progenitor cells for nonhematopoietic tissues in transgenic mice with a phenotype of osteogenesis imperfecta. Proc Natl Acad Sci U S A 95:1142–1147

Perin EC, Dohmann HF, Borojevic R, Silva SA, Sousa AL, Mesquita CT, Rossi MI, Carvalho AC, Dutra HS, Dohmann HJ, Silva GV, Belem L, Vivacqua R, Rangel FO, Esporcatte R, Geng YJ, Vaughn WK, Assad JA, Mesquita ET, Willerson JT (2003) Transendocardial, autologous bone marrow cell transplantation for severe, chronic ischemic heart failure. Circulation 107:2294–2302

Phinney DG (2002) Building a consensus regarding the nature and origin of mesenchymal stem cells. J Cell Biochem Suppl 38:7–12

Phinney DG, Kopen G, Isaacson RL, Prockop DJ (1999) Plastic adherent stromal cells from the bone marrow of commonly used strains of inbred mice: variations in yield, growth, and differentiation. J Cell Biochem 72:570–585

Pittenger MF, Martin BJ (2004) Mesenchymal stem cells and their potential as cardiac therapeutics. Circ Res 95:9–20

Pittenger MF, Mackay AM, Beck SC, Jaiswal RK, Douglas R, Mosca JD, Moorman MA, Simon-etti DW, Craig S, Marshak DR (1999) Multilineage potential of adult human mesenchymal stem cells. Science 284:143–147

Pochampally RR, Neville BT, Schwarz EJ, Li MM, Prockop DJ (2004) Rat adult stem cells (marrow stromal cells) engraft and differentiate in chick embryos without evidence of cell fusion. Proc Natl Acad Sci U S A 101:9282–9285

Potapova I, Plotnikov A, Lu Z, Danilo P Jr, Valiunas V, Qu J, Doronin S, Zuckerman J, Shlapakova IN, Gao J, Pan Z, Herron AJ, Robinson RB, Brink PR, Rosen MR, Cohen IS (2004) Human mesenchymal stem cells as a gene delivery system to create cardiac pacemakers. Circ Res 94:952–959

Pranke P, Failace RR, Allebrandt WF, Steibel G, Schmidt F, Nardi N (2001) Hematologic and immunophenotypic characterization of human umbilical cord blood. Acta Haematol 105:71–76

Prockop DJ (1997) Marrow stromal cells as stem cells for nonhematopoietic tissues. Science 276:71–74

Reyes M, Verfaillie CM (2001) Characterization of multipotent adult progenitor cells, a sub-population of mesenchymal stem cells. Ann N Y Acad Sci 938:231–233

Reyes M, Lund T, Lenvik T, Aguiar D, Koodie L, Verfaillie CM (2001) Purification and ex vivo expansion of postnatal human marrow mesodermal progenitor cells. Blood 98:2615–2625

Roelen BA, Dijke P (2003) Controlling mesenchymal stem cell differentiation by TGFbeta family members. J Orthop Sci 8:740–748

Rombouts WJ, Ploemacher RE (2003) Primary murine MSC show highly efficient homing to the bone marrow but lose homing ability following culture. Leukemia 17:160–170

Safford KM, Hicok KC, Safford SD, Halvorsen YD, Wilkison WO, Gimble JM, Rice HE (2002) Neurogenic differentiation of murine and human adipose-derived stromal cells. Biochem Biophys Res Commun 294:371–379

Salingcarnboriboon R, Yoshitake H, Tsuji K, Obinata M, Amagasa T, Nifuji A, Noda M (2003) Establishment of tendon-derived cell lines exhibiting pluripotent mesenchymal stem cell-like property. Exp Cell Res 287:289–300

Sanchez-Ramos J, Song S, Cardozo-Pelaez F, Hazzi C, Stedeford T, Willing A, Freeman TB, Saporta S, Janssen W, Patel N, Cooper DR, Sanberg PR (2000) Adult bone marrow stromal cells differentiate into neural cells in vitro. Exp Neurol 164:247–256

Sato Y, Araki H, Kato J, Nakamura K, Kawano Y, Kobune M, Sato T, Miyanishi K, Takayama T, Takahashi M, Takimoto R, Iyama S, Matsunaga T, Ohtani S, Matsuura A, Hamada H, Niitsu Y (2005) Human mesenchymal stem cells xenografted directly to rat liver differ-entiated into human hepatocytes without fusion. Blood Apr 7; [Epub ahead of print]

Sekiya I, Larson BL, Smith JR, Pochampally R, Cui JG, Prockop DJ (2002) Expansion of human adult stem cells from bone marrow stroma: conditions that maximize the yields of early progenitors and evaluate their quality. Stem Cells 20:530–541

Selkirk SM (2004) Gene therapy in clinical medicine. Postgrad Med J 80:560–570

Seshi B, Kumar S, Sellers D (2000) Human bone marrow stromal cell: coexpression of markers specific for multiple mesenchymal cell lineages. Blood Cells Mol Dis 26:234–246

Short B, Brouard N, Occhiodoro-Scott T, Ramakrishnan A, Simmons PJ (2003) Mesenchymal stem cells. Arch Med Res 34:565–571

Silva WA Jr, Covas DT, Panepucci RA, Proto-Siqueira R, Siufi JL, Zanette DL, Santos AR, Zago MA (2003) The profile of gene expression of human marrow mesenchymal stem cells. Stem Cells 21:661–669

Singh SK, Hawkins C, Clarke ID, Squire JA, Bayani J, Hide T, Henkelman RM, Cusimano MD, Dirks PB (2004) Identification of human brain tumour initiating cells. Nature 432:396–401

Spees JL, Olson SD, Ylostalo J, Lynch PJ, Smith J, Perry A, Peister A, Wang MY, Prockop DJ (2003) Differentiation, cell fusion, and nuclear fusion during ex vivo repair of epithelium by human adult stem cells from bone marrow stroma. Proc Natl Acad Sci U S A 100:2397–2402

Studeny M, Marini FC, Champlin RE, Zompetta C, Fidler IJ, Andreeff M (2002) Bone marrow-derived mesenchymal stem cells as vehicles for interferon-beta delivery into tumors. Cancer Res 62:3603–3608

Studeny M, Marini FC, Dembinski JL, Zompetta C, Cabreira-Hansen M, Bekele BN, Champlin RE, Andreeff M (2004) Mesenchymal stem cells: potential precursors for tumor stroma and targeted-delivery vehicles for anticancer agents. J Natl Cancer Inst 96:1593–1603

Stute N, Holtz K, Bubenheim M, Lange C, Blake F, Zander AR (2004) Autologous serum for isolation and expansion of human mesenchymal stem cells for clinical use. Exp Hematol 32:1212–1225

Tang DG, Tokumoto YM, Apperly JA, Lloyd AC, Raff MC (2001) Lack of replicative senescence in cultured rat oligodendrocyte precursor cells. Science 291:868–871

Tavassoli M (1984). Marrow adipose cells and hemopoiesis: an interpretative review. Exp Hematol 12:139–146

Terada N, Hamazaki T, Oka M, Hoki M, Mastalerz DM, Nakano Y, Meyer EM, Morel L, Petersen BE, Scott EW (2002) Bone marrow cells adopt the phenotype of other cells by spontaneous cell fusion. Nature 416:542–545

Tremain N, Korkko J, Ibberson D, Kopen GC, DiGirolamo C, Phinney DG (2001) MicroSAGE analysis of 2,353 expressed genes in a single cell-derived colony of undifferentiated human mesenchymal stem cells reveals mRNAs of multiple cell lineages. Stem Cells 19:408–418

Tuli R, Seghatoleslami MR, Tuli S, Wang ML, Hozack WJ, Manner PA, Danielson KG, Tuan RS (2003) A simple, high-yield method for obtaining multipotential mesenchymal progenitor cells from trabecular bone. Mol Biotechnol 23:37–49

Verfaillie CM (1992) Direct contact between human primitive hematopoietic progenitors and bone marrow stroma is not required for long-term in vitro hematopoiesis. Blood 79:2821–2826

Verfaillie CM (2002) Adult stem cells: assessing the case for pluripotency. Trends Cell Biol 12:502–508

Wakitani S, Saito T, Caplan AI (1995) Myogenic cells derived from rat bone marrow mesenchymal stem cells exposed to 5-azacytidine. Muscle Nerve 18:1417–1426

Wang Q-R, Yan Z-J, Wolf NS (1990) Dissecting the hematopoietic microenvironment. VI. The effects of several growth factors on the growth of murine bone marrow CFU-F. Exp Hematol 18:341–347

Watt FM, Hogan BL (2000) Out of Eden: stem cells and their niches. Science 287:1427–1430

Wexler SA, Donaldson C, Denning-Kendall P, Rice C, Bradley B, Hows JM (2003) Adult bone marrow is a rich source of human mesenchymal 'stem' cells but umbilical cord and mobilized adult blood are not. Br J Haematol 121:368–374

Whetton AD, Grahan GJ (1999) Homing and mobilization in the stem cell niche. Trends Cell Biol 9:233–238

Woodbury D, Schwarz EJ, Prockop DJ, Black IB (2000) Adult rat and human bone marrow stromal cells differentiate into neurons. J Neurosci Res 61:364–370

Wynn RF, Hart CA, Corradi-Perini C, O'Neill L, Evans CA, Wraith JE, Fairbairn LJ, Bellantuono I (2004) A small proportion of mesenchymal stem cells strongly expresses functionally active CXCR4 receptor capable of promoting migration to bone marrow. Blood 104:2643–2645

Ying QL, Nichols J, Evans EP, Smith AG (2002) Changing potency by spontaneous fusion. Nature 416:545–548

Young HE, Steele TA, Bray RA, Hudson J, Floyd JA, Hawkins K, Thomas K, Austin T, Edwards C, Cuzzourt J, Duenzl M, Lucas PA, Black AC Jr (2001) Human reserve pluripotent mesenchymal stem cells are present in the connective tissues of skeletal muscle and dermis derived from fetal, adult, and geriatric donors. Anat Rec 264:51–62

Zipori D (2004) Mesenchymal stem cells: harnessing cell plasticity to tissue and organ repair. Blood Cells Mol Dis 33:211–215

Zuk PA, Zhu M, Mizuno H, Huang J, Futrell JW, Katz AJ, Benhaim P, Lorenz HP, Hedrick MH (2001) Multilineage cells from human adipose tissue: implications for cell-based therapies. Tissue Eng 7:211–228

Zuk PA, Zhu M, Ashjian P, De Ugarte DA, Huang JI, Mizuno H, Alfonso ZC, Fraser JK, Benhaim P, Hedrick MH (2002) Human adipose tissue is a source of multipotent stem cells. Mol Biol Cell 13:4279–4295

HEP (2006) 174:283–298
© Springer-Verlag Berlin Heidelberg 2006

Neovascularization and Cardiac Repair by Bone Marrow-Derived Stem Cells

C. Badorff · S. Dimmeler (✉)

Department of Molecular Cardiology, University of Frankfurt, Theodor Stern-Kai 7,
60590 Frankfurt, Germany
Dimmeler@em.uni-frankfurt.de

Abstract Postinfarction congestive heart failure with impaired systolic left ventricular function is a loss of cardiomyocyte disease. Adult stem or progenitor cells from the bone marrow and the peripheral blood have been experimentally shown to differentiate towards endothelial cells and cardiomyocytes under the appropriate conditions. The use of autologous adult stem cells for neovascularization and cardiac regeneration is a promising concept and has shown benefit in pilot clinical trails enrolling postinfarction patients with coronary artery disease. Cell therapy may act through differentiation into and thus replacement of cardiomyocytes and/or neovascularization, the formation of new vessels in the adult organism. Moreover, the release of factors acting in a paracrine manner may contribute to neovascularization and scar remodelling. In this review, the experimental data regarding neovascularization and cardiomyocyte formation from adult stem/progenitor cells are discussed.

Keywords Endothelial progenitor cells · Neovascularization · Adult stem cells · Cardiomyogenesis · Cardiac regeneration

1
Introduction

Coronary artery disease and its sequelae, myocardial infarction and congestive heart failure, are major causes of mortality in industrialized nations. Myocardial infarction leads to a loss of cardiomyocytes, the contracting cells in the heart. Cardiomyocytes as terminally differentiated cells have a very limited ability to divide and hence the mammalian heart has a poor regenerative capacity and heals infarcts through scar formation. Fibrotic scars, however, are dysfunctional tissue since they are noncontracting and potentially prone to arrhythmia formation (Tomaselli and Zipes 2004). Thus, congestive heart failure with impaired systolic left ventricular function is now viewed as a loss of cardiomyocyte disease (Schneider 2004).

Although a number of pharmacological therapies, namely beta-blockers and inhibitors of the renin-angiotensin-aldosterone system, have been conclusively shown in large randomized clinical trials to improve symptoms and prognosis in patients with congestive heart failure, these drugs ameliorate rather than cure the disease (McMurray et al. 2004). In particular, no pharmacological substance to date has been shown to result in neovascularization or regeneration of cardiomyocytes, which would represent a causative therapy of congestive heart failure. Therefore, over the last years biological therapies aiming to repair and regenerate the failing heart have gained considerable scientific and public interest.

In particular, the use of stem or progenitor cells from a number of different sources, including but not limited to the bone marrow and the peripheral blood, for the purpose of neovascularization and cardiac regeneration is a promising biological concept and has shown clinical benefit in pilot clinical trails (Assmus et al. 2002; Strauer et al. 2002; Wollert et al. 2004). Cell therapy may act through a number of possible mechanisms which remain to be identified in man, but two prominent concepts, based on a wealth of experimental data, are that these cells may regenerate the heart through a differentiation into and thus replacement of cardiomyocytes and/or neovascularization, the formation of new vessels in the adult organism. Moreover, the release of factors acting in a paracrine manner may contribute to neovascularization and scar remodelling.

2
Neovascularization

Adult blood vessel formation occurs through arteriogenesis, angiogenesis or vasculogenesis (Carmeliet 2000). Arteriogenesis describes the growth of collateral vessels, whereas angiogenesis refers to the growth of new capillaries by sprouting of pre-existing vessels through migration and proliferation of mature endothelial cells. Recent studies suggested that vasculogenesis can also contribute to postnatal neovascularization after ischaemia (Asahara et al. 1997). Vasculogenesis includes the mobilization of bone marrow-derived progenitor cells, which home to sites of ischaemia and contribute to new blood vessel formation (Carmeliet 2000). The finding that vasculogenesis also contributes to postnatal neovascularization offers novel therapeutic strategies for the use of bone marrow-derived or ex vivo cultivated circulating endothelial progenitor cells for cell therapy of tissue ischaemia.

Endothelial precursor cells (EPCs) can be grown from purified populations of $CD34^+$ or $CD133^+$ haematopoietic cells, purified $CD14^+$ monocytes or total peripheral blood mononuclear cells (MNCs) (Asahara et al. 1997). Cultivated EPCs grown from different starting populations have been shown to express endothelial marker proteins such as von Willebrand factor, VEGF-receptor 2 (KDR), VE-cadherin, CD146, CD31 and eNOS (Asahara et al. 1997; Gehling et al. 2000; Kalka et al. 2000). Moreover, these cells were characterized by their functional capacity to form endothelial cell colonies and improve neovascularization in animal models of hind limb ischaemia and myocardial infarction (Kalka et al. 2000; Kawamoto et al. 2001; Kocher et al. 2001; Urbich et al. 2003).

Moreover, a recent clinical study suggests that intracoronary infusion of blood-derived EPCs or BMC can be used to improve coronary flow reserve and cardiac function in patients after acute myocardial infarction (Assmus et al. 2002). However, it is not clear at present to what extent the cell-mediated improvement of cardiac function in patients after acute myocardial infarction is due to an effect on vascularization (Assmus et al. 2002; Strauer et al. 2002; Wollert et al. 2004).

The number of bone marrow-derived incorporated cells in newly formed capillaries varies in the literature. Whereas several studies showed that up to 50% of the newly generated capillaries derive from bone marrow-derived cells, other studies failed to show an incorporation of circulating cells in the endothelial lining (for review see Urbich and Dimmeler 2004). This variation may reflect differences in experimental models (e.g. mice strains, tumours vs ischaemia, extent of injury, etc.). Despite a minor physical incorporation of cells in some models, clearly all studies showed a significant improvement of neovascularization after infusion of different progenitor cell populations. These data suggest that progenitor cells may act via an additional mechanism, which may include the release of growth factors acting in a paracrine manner (Heil et al. 2004).

3
Cardiac Repair

Numerous studies have experimentally addressed the potential of bone marrow-derived stem cells to differentiate into the cardiomyogenic lineage, partly with conflicting results. Here, we will review the current knowledge on the differentiation of bone marrow-derived stem or progenitor cells into cardiomyocytes. As a comparison to these adult cells, we will briefly discuss the results obtained with embryonic stem cells.

3.1
Differentiation of Embryonic Stem Cells into Cardiomyocytes In Vitro

Embryonic stem (ES) cells are derived from the inner cell mass or epiblast of preimplantation embryos and can be infinitely propagated in cell culture in an undifferentiated state. Induced by a change in the cultivation conditions, the so-called hanging drop technique, embryonic stem cells aggregate and form embryoid bodies, an early embryonic tissue with portions of all three germ layers.

Within an embryoid body, embryonic stem cells spontaneously differentiate into cardiomyocytes, which constitute approximately 5%–10% of all cells within an embryoid body (Wobus et al. 1991). Functionally active cardiomyocytes have been generated from mouse as well as human ES cells (Kehat et al. 2001; Boheler et al. 2002). ES cell-derived cardiomyocytes show macromolecular sarcomeric organization, calcium sparks, ionic currents, functional and anatomical integration with surrounding cardiomyocytes, propagation of electrical activity as well as pacemaker activity (Sauer et al. 2001; Boheler et al. 2002; Kehat et al. 2002, 2004). Collectively, these data demonstrate that ES cells spontaneously differentiate into fully functionally active, foetal-like cardiomyocytes in vitro.

Although these in vitro data would suggest that ES cells are ideal candidates for in vivo cardiac repair, animal studies have shown a dose-dependent incidence of tumour formation, in particular teratocarcinoma formation, after transplantation of ES cells into mice (Erdo et al. 2003). Therefore, the safety of ES cell transplantation into rodents and man remains an unsolved question to date.

3.2
Differentiation of Adult Stem and Progenitor Cells into Cardiomyocytes In Vitro

Due to safety concerns and legal restrictions in many countries, researchers have focussed on the potential of adult bone marrow-derived stem or progenitor cells to differentiate into the cardiomyogenic lineage.

In contrast to ES cells, adult stem or progenitor cells do not spontaneously differentiate into cardiomyocytes but rather require an adequate stimulus to do so. Over the past few years, it has become apparent that the local microenvironment determines the cell fate of adult stem cells (Blau et al. 2001). Therefore, a co-culture technique was developed where stem or progenitor cells are cultured together with rat neonatal ventricular cardiomyocytes in order to simulate a cardiac-like surrounding in vitro (Condorelli et al. 2001). Many researchers have used such a co-culture system to induce differentiation of adult stem or progenitor cells from various species and organs (summarized in Table 1). Indeed, several studies demonstrated that the physical contact with and the beating of neighbouring cardiomyocytes is indeed required for the differentiation process to occur (Badorff et al. 2003; Iijima et al. 2003; Rangappa et al. 2003a). Alternatively, the nonspecific transcriptional activator 5′-azacytidine or the neurohormone oxytocin have been employed to induce differentiation (Table 1).

It is important to note that in most in vitro studies the adult stem/progenitor cell-derived cardiomyocyte-like cells showed varying morphological, genetic, biochemical, structural and functional aspects of cardiomyocytes but were not fully mature and functionally competent adult cardiomyocytes. This indicates that in vitro the co-culture technique, albeit effective to initiate cardiomyogenic

Table 1 In vitro cardiomyogenic differentiation of adult stem/progenitor cells

Species	Model	Cells	Comment	Reference
Mouse	Co-culture	Foetal aortal mesangioblasts		Condorelli et al. 2001
Mouse	5′-Azacytidine	Bone marrow mesenchymal stem cells	Cells express functional adrenergic and muscarinic receptors	Hakuno et al. 2002; Makino et al. 1999
Mouse	Oxytocin	Cardiac Sca-1$^+$ cells		Matsuura et al. 2004a
Mouse	Co-culture	Skeletal muscle cells	Cardiomyocyte beating necessary for differentiation	Iijima et al. 2003
Rat	Co-culture	Hepatic stem cell line (WB F344)		Muller-Borer et al. 2004
Rabbit	Co-culture	Fatty tissue mesenchymal cells		Rangappa et al. 2003b
Human	Co-culture	Circulating endothelial progenitor cells and CD34$^+$ cells	Healthy controls and coronary artery disease patients	Badorff et al. 2003; Rupp et al. 2004
			Contact with cardiomyocytes necessary for differentiation	
Human	Co-culture	Bone-marrow mesenchymal cells	Contact with cardiomyocytes necessary for differentiation	Rangappa et al. 2003a
Human	5′-Azacytidine	Bone-marrow mesenchymal cells		Xu et al. 2004

differentiation, is not sufficient for full cardiomyocyte maturation. In this regard, ES cell-derived cardiomyocytes are superior to adult stem/progenitor cell-derived cardiomyocyte-like cells.

3.3
Molecular Mechanisms of Cardiomyogenic Stem Cell Differentiation

In most in vitro systems, the percentage of adult stem/progenitor cells differentiating into cardiomyocytes is rather low (Badorff et al. 2003). Therefore, attempts have been made to understand the underlying molecular mechanisms and, in particular, to identify extracellular ligands which enhance or are in themselves sufficient to induce cardiomyogenic differentiation (summarized in Table 2).

Initial studies used chicken precardiac mesodermal cells, a classical system to study cardiovascular development, and the long-established P19 mouse embryonic carcinoma cell line. These studies have identified a variety of molecular signals and pathways, including bone morphogenic proteins, oxytocin, the noncanonical Wnt signalling pathway and fibroblast growth factors, amongst others, which modulate cardiomyogenic differentiation (Lough et al. 1996; Schultheiss et al. 1997; Pandur et al. 2002; Paquin et al. 2002; van der Heyden and Defize 2003; Terami et al. 2004). Likewise, in embryonic stem cells, a platelet-derived growth factor was identified as cardiomyocyte differentiation-enhancing factor (Sachinidis et al. 2003).

While this role of oxytocin and platelet-derived growth factor was confirmed in experimental systems using adult stem and progenitor cells (Matsuura et al. 2004a; Xaymardan et al. 2004), the role of many other factors remain elusive in the differentiation process of adult stem or progenitor cells into cardiomyocytes. Although it is now clear that cardiomyogenic differentiation is a multifactorial biological process, the precise molecular orchestration regulating this phenotypic change in the adult organism remains poorly understood. This puzzle will be of prominent scientific interest in the future.

3.4
Differentiation Versus Cellular Fusion

The biological concept of adult stem or progenitor cell plasticity with the cellular ability to change the phenotype at the single-cell level (single cell-transdifferentiation) was recently challenged by the experimental observation that adult stem cells can fuse with other cells and thereby adopt a novel phenotype just mimicking single-cell differentiation. In fact, several reports questioned the plasticity of adult bone marrow cells or described cardiomyogenic differentiation as an extremely rare event (Balsam et al. 2004; Murry et al. 2004).

Table 2 Extracellular signals inducing cardiomyogenic differentiation

Species	Cells	Treatment	Comment	Reference
Mouse	Bone marrow mesenchymal stem cells	5′-Azacytidine	Nonspecific transcriptional activation	Makino et al. 1999; Hakuno et al. 2002
Mouse	Adult cardiac Sca-1$^+$ cardiac progenitor cells	5′-Azacytidine	Nonspecific transcriptional activation	Oh et al. 2003, 2004
Mouse	P19 embryonic carcinoma cells	DMSO BMPs		reviewed in van der Heyden and Defize 2003
Mouse	Cardiac Sca-1$^+$ cells	Oxytocin		Matsuura et al. 2004a
Mouse	P19 embryonic carcinoma cells	Oxytocin		Paquin et al. 2002
Mouse	Mononuclear bone marrow cells	PDGF-AB		Xaymardan et al. 2004
Mouse	Embryonic stem cells	PDGF-BB		Sachinidis et al. 2003
Mouse	P19 embryonic carcinoma cells	Wnt11	Activation of noncanonical Wnt pathway	Pandur et al. 2002; Terami et al. 2004
Human	Bone marrow mesenchymal stem cells	Insulin, dexamethasone and ascorbic acid		Shim et al. 2004
Human	Adipose tissue stem cells	Nuclear and cytoplasmic extracts of rat cardiomyocytes	Adipose tissue stem cells reversibly permeabilized	Gaustad et al. 2004
Chicken	Precardiac mesoderm	FGF-4 and BMP-2		Lough et al. 1996
Chicken	Precardiac mesoderm	BMP-2 and BMP-4		Schultheiss et al. 1997

The observation of cellular fusion between stem cells and other cell types was initially made for cell types other than cardiomyocytes, namely, hepatocytes and neurons (Ying et al. 2002; Wang et al. 2003), but several groups have now reported cellular fusion between bona-fide cardiomyocytes and bone marrow-derived cells in cell culture (summarized in Table 3). While all these studies were performed with murine bone marrow cells, it is less clear whether fusion also occurs with human cells. Initial results from our group (S. Dimmeler, unpublished results) indicate that human circulating progenitor cells can indeed fuse with rat neonatal cardiomyocytes upon co-culture in vitro.

Table 3 Fusion between cardiomyocytes and other cell types

Species	Model	Cells	Comment	Reference
Mouse	Co-culture with rat neonatal cardiomyoyctes	Bone marrow cells		Matsuura et al. 2004b
Mouse	Adult mouse heart, myocardial infarct	Bone marrow cells		Nygren et al. 2004
Mouse	Co-culture with rat neonatal cardiomyocytes	Bone marrow cells		Alvarez-Dolado et al. 2003
Mouse	Adult mouse heart, myocardial infarct	Adult cardiac Sca-1$^+$ cardiac progenitor cells		Oh et al. 2003
Human	Adult SCID mouse heart, myocardial infarct	Peripheral blood CD34$^+$ cells		Zhang et al. 2004

Interestingly, single cell differentiation and cellular fusion are not mutually exclusive, but can rather both occur and contribute roughly equally to the phenotype observed in one experimental system (Oh et al. 2003, 2004). Additionally, the rate of fusion events between stem cells and other cells types in well below 1% (Ying et al. 2002; Wang et al. 2003), a value too low to explain the reported differentiation rate in co-culture experiments (Badorff et al. 2003). Furthermore, by co-culturing human circulating progenitor cells with paraformaldehyde-fixed cardiomyocytes, we were able to demonstrate that cardiomyogenic differentiation can occur independent of a fusion event (Badorff et al. 2003). However, for many experimental reports, it remains to be determined to which degree single cell differentiation and fusion contribute to the cardiomyogenic phenotypic change.

3.5
Differentiation of Stem and Progenitor Cells into Cardiomyocytes in Animal Models

Following the observation that bone marrow cells can differentiate into cardiomyocytes in vitro, this question was addressed in animal models of myocardial ischaemia or myocardial infarction (summarized in Table 4). Myocardial infarction was either induced by cryoinjury to the left ventricular free wall or ligation of the left anterior descending coronary artery. Introduction of the syngenic bone marrow cells into the animal undergoing myocardial infarction was accomplished either by prior bone marrow transplantation or direct intracardiac injection into the peri-infarct border zone following myocardial infarction. The population of bone marrow cells used varied among the different studies, as depicted in Table 4.

Despite these differences in the experimental design and the type of cell used for transplantation, various groups have reported the occurrence of cardiomy-

Table 4 In vivo differentiation towards cardiomyocytes observed

Species	Model	Cells	Comment	Reference
Mouse	Myocardial infarct	Whole bone marrow	Bone marrow transplantation Mobilization with G-CSF	Kawada et al. 2004
Mouse	Myocardial ischaemia	Lin$^-$ c-kit$^+$ cardiac stem cells		Beltrami et al. 2003
Mouse	Myocardial infarct	Adult peripheral blood CD34+ cells		Yeh et al. 2003
Mouse	Myocardial infarct	Bone-marrow Lin$^-$ c-kit$^+$ cells	Improved LV haemodynamics	Orlic et al. 2001
Mouse	Myocardial infarct	Bone marrow cells (not specified)	Bone marrow transplantation	Kuramochi et al. 2003
Mouse	Myocardial infarct	Bone-marrow Lin$^-$ cells and mesenchymal cells		Kudo et al. 2003
Mouse	Myocardial infarct	Side population cells (CD34$^{-/low}$, c-Kit$^+$, Sca-1$^+$)	Bone marrow transplantation	Jackson et al. 2001
Mouse	Ischaemia/ Reperfusion	Adult cardiac Sca-1$^+$ cardiac progenitor cells	Genetic cell-fate tracking	Oh et al. 2003
SCID mouse	No infarct	Human bone-marrow mesenchymal cells		Toma et al. 2002
SCID mouse	Myocardial infarct	Human peripheral blood CD34$^+$ cells		Zhang et al. 2004
Rat	Myocardial infarct	Bone marrow cells ex vivo pretreated with 5′-Azacytidine	Intracardiac injection Improved systolic blood pressure	Tomita et al. 1999
Pig	Myocardial infarct	Bone marrow cells ex vivo pretreated with 5′-Azacytidine	Intracardiac injection Improved LV haemodynamics	Tomita et al. 2002

ocyte formation in the heart from the transplanted bone marrow cells. These studies were predominantly performed in mice, but confirmed in rats and pigs, suggesting that cardiomyogenic differentiation can occur across different species (Table 4). Cardiomyocyte differentiation was demonstrate predominantly by the expression and organization of sarcomeric proteins using immunohistological techniques (all references in Table 4) and, in some instances, ultrastructural analyses (Kawada et al. 2004). One study confirmed these results using a genetic cell fate tracking system based on a Cre/Lox donor/recipient pair (alphaMHC-Cre/R26R) (Oh et al. 2003).

Importantly, in some studies an improvement of left ventricular function was observed, indicating a "biological repair" of infarcted hearts (Tomita et al. 1999, 2002; Orlic et al. 2001; Kawamoto et al. 2003).

Taken together, these studies suggest that cardiomyocyte differentiation can occur in vivo from various bone marrow cell populations, albeit at varying frequency depending on the exact cell type and experimental condition used.

3.6
No Differentiation of Stem and Progenitor Cells into Cardiomyocytes in Animal Models

The plasticity of haematopoietic stem cells remains controversial because such plasticity could not be demonstrated in all experiments (Wagers et al. 2002; Wagers and Weissman 2004). In detail, the transdifferentiation of circulating haematopoietic stem cells and/or their progeny was described as an extremely rare event, if it occurs at all (Wagers et al. 2002).

With regard to cardiomyogenic differentiation of bone marrow-derived stem cells in intact animals, the referenced positive results depicted in Table 4 could not be reproduced by other groups. A number of recent publications in which no in vivo differentiation of bone marrow-derived cells into cardiomyocytes could be demonstrated are shown in Table 5.

Table 5 No in vivo differentiation towards cardiomyocytes observed

Species	Model	Cells	Comment	Reference
Mouse	Myocardial infarct	Lin^- c-kit^+ Lin^- c-kit^+ Sca-1^+ bone marrow cells Unfractionated bone marrow cells	Transplantation into peri-infarct zone and bone marrow transplantation Genetic cell fate tracking	Murry et al. 2004
Mouse	Myocardial infarct	Unfractionated bone marrow cells Lin^- c-kit^+ bone marrow cells	Bone marrow transplant and direct intracardiac injection Genetic cell fate tracking	Nygren et al. 2004
Mouse	Myocardial infarct	Lin^- c-kit^+ bone marrow cells c-kit^+ $Thy1.1^{low}$ Lin^- Sca-1^+ long-term reconstituting haematopoietic stem cells	Transplantation into peri-infarct zone and parabiotic mice Genetic cell fate tracking	Balsam et al. 2004
Human	Athymic nude rat	Human mobilized $CD34^+$ cells	Neovascularization observed	Kocher et al. 2001

3.7
Possible Explanations for the Divergent Experimental Results

At present and as discussed in the above-referenced manuscripts, it is not clear what the exact causes of the different experimental results are. One possibility is that the genetic cell fate tracking techniques are more stringent and thus less prone to false positive results when compared to immunohistological detection systems. In particular, the genetic techniques are able to distinguish cellular fusion (which was detected in at least two studies: Nygren et al. 2004; Zhang et al. 2004) from differentiation at the single cell level. However, even genetic tagging of differentiation and/or fusion events requires subsequent immunohistological staining and detection in the adult heart. Alternatively, it is conceivable that methodological differences in the isolation, purification, characterization and injection of the cells used are responsible for the discrepant experimental results obtained. The level of expertise with regard to these sophisticated techniques may indeed vary between individual laboratories. This issue remains unsolved at present but definitely warrants further investigation. It appears conceivable that differences in cell handling may influence epigenetic reprogramming such as histone modifications or DNA methylation, both of which are important parameters of early lineage decisions in mammalian cells (Morgan et al. 2005).

Importantly, bone marrow-derived stem cells do not necessarily need to differentiate themselves into cardiomyocytes to result in cardiac repair following myocardial infarction. An alternative concept is that these cells, through the local production of cytokines and growth factors, augment the endogenous cardiac repair program, either through the recruitment of and cardiomyogenic differentiation of cardiac stem cells or the proliferation of bona-fide cardiomyocytes at the sites of injury. Indeed, induction of proliferation and regeneration of endogenous cardiomyocytes was observed in an athymic rat model of myocardial infarction following transplantation of human CD34$^+$ stem cells mobilized from the bone marrow (Schuster et al. 2004). In line with this concept, circulating human endothelial progenitor cells produce a variety of cytokines known to be important for the biology of vascular and cardiac cells (S. Dimmeler, unpublished observation). It is noteworthy that such a mode of action may explain the observed improvement of left ventricular function in patients with acute myocardial infarction following autologous transplantation of at most a few million CD34$^+$ cells in clinical trials (Assmus et al. 2002; Strauer et al. 2002; Wollert et al. 2004).

4
Summary

In summary, a growing body of experimental evidence suggests that bone marrow-derived stem cells can, under the appropriate conditions, differentiate into cardiomyogenic cells in cell culture and also fuse with cardiomyocytes. In intact animal model systems, this issue still remains controversial but differentiation probably also can occur at a low frequency. Alternative modes of action, such as an augmentation of the endogenous cardiac repair program, are just beginning to be explored. Ultimately, the mechanisms of cellular therapies will have to be identified in humans to understand the benefits observed in early clinical trials. Such an understanding would greatly advance the field of cardiac repair therapy, one of the most dynamic fields in modern cardiology.

References

Alvarez-Dolado M, Pardal R, Garcia-Verdugo JM, Fike JR, Lee HO, Pfeffer K, Lois C, Morrison SJ, Alvarez-Buylla A (2003) Fusion of bone-marrow-derived cells with Purkinje neurons, cardiomyocytes and hepatocytes. Nature 425:968–973

Asahara T, Murohara T, Sullivan A, Silver M, van der Zee R, Li T, Witzenbichler B, Schatteman G, Isner JM (1997) Isolation of putative progenitor endothelial cells for angiogenesis. Science 275:964–967

Assmus B, Schachinger V, Teupe C, Britten M, Lehmann R, Dobert N, Grunwald F, Aicher A, Urbich C, Martin H, Hoelzer D, Dimmeler S, Zeiher AM (2002) Transplantation of progenitor cells and regeneration enhancement in acute myocardial infarction (TOPCARE-AMI). Circulation 106:3009–3017

Badorff C, Brandes RP, Popp R, Rupp S, Urbich C, Aicher A, Fleming I, Busse R, Zeiher AM, Dimmeler S (2003) Transdifferentiation of blood-derived human adult endothelial progenitor cells into functionally active cardiomyocytes. Circulation 107:1024–1032

Balsam LB, Wagers AJ, Christensen JL, Kofidis T, Weissman IL, Robbins RC (2004) Haematopoietic stem cells adopt mature haematopoietic fates in ischaemic myocardium. Nature 428:668–673

Beltrami AP, Barlucchi L, Torella D, Baker M, Limana F, Chimenti S, Kasahara H, Rota M, Musso E, Urbanek K, Leri A, Kajstura J, Nadal-Ginard B, Anversa P (2003) Adult cardiac stem cells are multipotent and support myocardial regeneration. Cell 114:763–776

Blau HM, Brazelton TR, Weimann JM (2001) The evolving concept of a stem cell: entity or function? Cell 105:829–841

Boheler KR, Czyz J, Tweedie D, Yang HT, Anisimov SV, Wobus AM (2002) Differentiation of pluripotent embryonic stem cells into cardiomyocytes. Circ Res 91:189–201

Carmeliet P (2000) Mechanisms of angiogenesis and arteriogenesis. Nat Med 6:389–395

Condorelli G, Borello U, De Angelis L, Latronico M, Sirabella D, Coletta M, Galli R, Balconi G, Follenzi A, Frati G, Cusella De Angelis MG, Gioglio L, Amuchastegui S, Adorini L, Naldini L, Vescovi A, Dejana E, Cossu G (2001) Cardiomyocytes induce endothelial cells to trans-differentiate into cardiac muscle: implications for myocardium regeneration. Proc Natl Acad Sci U S A 98:10733–10738

Erdo F, Buhrle C, Blunk J, Hoehn M, Xia Y, Fleischmann B, Focking M, Kustermann E, Kolossov E, Hescheler J, Hossmann KA, Trapp T (2003) Host-dependent tumorigenesis of embryonic stem cell transplantation in experimental stroke. J Cereb Blood Flow Metab 23:780–785

Gaustad KG, Boquest AC, Anderson BE, Gerdes AM, Collas P (2004) Differentiation of human adipose tissue stem cells using extracts of rat cardiomyocytes. Biochem Biophys Res Commun 314:420–427

Gehling UM, Ergun S, Schumacher U, Wagener C, Pantel K, Otte M, Schuch G, Schafhausen P, Mende T, Kilic N, Kluge K, Schafer B, Hossfeld DK, Fiedler W (2000) In vitro differentiation of endothelial cells from AC133-positive progenitor cells. Blood 95:3106–3112

Hakuno D, Fukuda K, Makino S, Konishi F, Tomita Y, Manabe T, Suzuki Y, Umezawa A, Ogawa S (2002) Bone marrow-derived regenerated cardiomyocytes (CMG Cells) express functional adrenergic and muscarinic receptors. Circulation 105:380–386

Heil M, Ziegelhoeffer T, Mees B, Schaper W (2004) A different outlook on the role of bone marrow stem cells in vascular growth: bone marrow delivers software not hardware. Circ Res 94:573–574

Iijima Y, Nagai T, Mizukami M, Matsuura K, Ogura T, Wada H, Toko H, Akazawa H, Takano H, Nakaya H, Komuro I (2003) Beating is necessary for transdifferentiation of skeletal muscle-derived cells into cardiomyocytes. FASEB J 17:1361–1363

Jackson KA, Majka SM, Wang H, Pocius J, Hartley CJ, Majesky MW, Entman ML, Michael LH, Hirschi KK, Goodell MA (2001) Regeneration of ischemic cardiac muscle and vascular endothelium by adult stem cells. J Clin Invest 107:1395–1402

Kalka C, Masuda H, Takahashi T, Kalka-Moll WM, Silver M, Kearney M, Li T, Isner JM, Asahara T (2000) Transplantation of ex vivo expanded endothelial progenitor cells for therapeutic neovascularization. Proc Natl Acad Sci U S A 97:3422–3427

Kawada H, Fujita J, Kinjo K, Matsuzaki Y, Tsuma M, Miyatake H, Muguruma Y, Tsuboi K, Itabashi Y, Ikeda Y, Ogawa S, Okano H, Hotta T, Ando K, Fukuda K (2004) Nonhematopoietic mesenchymal stem cells can be mobilized and differentiate into cardiomyocytes after myocardial infarction. Blood 104:3581–3587

Kawamoto A, Gwon HC, Iwaguro H, Yamaguchi JI, Uchida S, Masuda H, Silver M, Ma H, Kearney M, Isner JM, Asahara T (2001) Therapeutic potential of ex vivo expanded endothelial progenitor cells for myocardial ischemia. Circulation 103:634–637

Kawamoto A, Tkebuchava T, Yamaguchi J, Nishimura H, Yoon YS, Milliken C, Uchida S, Masuo O, Iwaguro H, Ma H, Hanley A, Silver M, Kearney M, Losordo DW, Isner JM, Asahara T (2003) Intramyocardial transplantation of autologous endothelial progenitor cells for therapeutic neovascularization of myocardial ischemia. Circulation 107:461–468

Kehat I, Gepstein A, Spira A, Itskovitz-Eldor J, Gepstein L (2002) High-resolution electrophysiological assessment of human embryonic stem cell-derived cardiomyocytes: a novel in vitro model for the study of conduction. Circ Res 91:659–661

Kehat I, Kenyagin-Karsenti D, Snir M, Segev H, Amit M, Gepstein A, Livne E, Binah O, Itskovitz-Eldor J, Gepstein L (2001) Human embryonic stem cells can differentiate into myocytes with structural and functional properties of cardiomyocytes. J Clin Invest 108:407–414

Kehat I, Khimovich L, Caspi O, Gepstein A, Shofti R, Arbel G, Huber I, Satin J, Itskovitz-Eldor J, Gepstein L (2004) Electromechanical integration of cardiomyocytes derived from human embryonic stem cells. Nat Biotechnol 22:1282–1289

Kocher AA, Schuster MD, Szabolcs MJ, Takuma S, Burkhoff D, Wang J, Homma S, Edwards NM, Itescu S (2001) Neovascularization of ischemic myocardium by human bone-marrow-derived angioblasts prevents cardiomyocyte apoptosis, reduces remodeling and improves cardiac function. Nat Med 7:430–436

Kudo M, Wang Y, Wani MA, Xu M, Ayub A, Ashraf M (2003) Implantation of bone marrow stem cells reduces the infarction and fibrosis in ischemic mouse heart. J Mol Cell Cardiol 35:1113–1119

Kuramochi Y, Fukazawa R, Migita M, Hayakawa J, Hayashida M, Uchikoba Y, Fukumi D, Shimada T, Ogawa S (2003) Cardiomyocyte regeneration from circulating bone marrow cells in mice. Pediatr Res 54:319–325

Lough J, Barron M, Brogley M, Sugi Y, Bolender DL, Zhu X (1996) Combined BMP-2 and FGF-4, but neither factor alone, induces cardiogenesis in non-precardiac embryonic mesoderm. Dev Biol 178:198–202

Makino S, Fukuda K, Miyoshi S, Konishi F, Kodama H, Pan J, Sano M, Takahashi T, Hori S, Abe H, Hata J, Umezawa A, Ogawa S (1999) Cardiomyocytes can be generated from marrow stromal cells in vitro. J Clin Invest 103:697–705

Matsuura K, Nagai T, Nishigaki N, Oyama T, Nishi J, Wada H, Sano M, Toko H, Akazawa H, Sato T, Nakaya H, Kasanuki H, Komuro I (2004a) Adult cardiac Sca-1-positive cells differentiate into beating cardiomyocytes. J Biol Chem 279:11384–11391

Matsuura K, Wada H, Nagai T, Iijima Y, Minamino T, Sano M, Akazawa H, Molkentin JD, Kasanuki H, Komuro I (2004b) Cardiomyocytes fuse with surrounding noncardiomy- ocytes and reenter the cell cycle. J Cell Biol 167:351–363

McMurray JJ, Pfeffer MA, Swedberg K, Dzau VJ (2004) Which inhibitor of the renin-angiotensin system should be used in chronic heart failure and acute myocardial in- farction? Circulation 110:3281–3288

Morgan HD, Santos F, Green K, Dean W, Reik W (2005) Epigenetic reprogramming in mammals. Hum Mol Genet 14:R47–R58

Muller-Borer BJ, Cascio WE, Anderson PA, Snowwaert JN, Frye JR, Desai N, Esch GL, Brackham JA, Bagnell CR, Coleman WB, Grisham JW, Malouf NN (2004) Adult-derived liver stem cells acquire a cardiomyocyte structural and functional phenotype ex vivo. Am J Pathol 165:135–145

Murry CE, Soonpaa MH, Reinecke H, Nakajima H, Nakajima HO, Rubart M, Pasumarthi KB, Virag JI, Bartelmez SH, Poppa V, Bradford G, Dowell JD, Williams DA, Field LJ (2004) Haematopoietic stem cells do not transdifferentiate into cardiac myocytes in myocardial infarcts. Nature 428:664–668

Nygren JM, Jovinge S, Breitbach M, Sawen P, Roll W, Hescheler J, Taneera J, Fleischmann BK, Jacobsen SE (2004) Bone marrow-derived hematopoietic cells generate cardiomyocytes at a low frequency through cell fusion, but not transdifferentiation. Nat Med 10:494–501

Oh H, Bradfute SB, Gallardo TD, Nakamura T, Gaussin V, Mishina Y, Pocius J, Michael LH, Behringer RR, Garry DJ, Entman ML, Schneider MD (2003) Cardiac progenitor cells from adult myocardium: homing, differentiation, and fusion after infarction. Proc Natl Acad Sci U S A 100:12313–12318

Oh H, Chi X, Bradfute SB, Mishina Y, Pocius J, Michael LH, Behringer RR, Schwartz RJ, Entman ML, Schneider MD (2004) Cardiac muscle plasticity in adult and embryo by heart-derived progenitor cells. Ann N Y Acad Sci 1015:182–189

Orlic D, Kajstura J, Chimenti S, Jakoniuk I, Anderson SM, Li B, Pickel J, McKay R, Nadal-Ginard B, Bodine DM, Leri A, Anversa P (2001) Bone marrow cells regenerate infarcted myocardium. Nature 410:701–705

Pandur P, Lasche M, Eisenberg LM, Kuhl M (2002) Wnt-11 activation of a non-canonical Wnt signalling pathway is required for cardiogenesis. Nature 418:636–641

Paquin J, Danalache BA, Jankowski M, McCann SM, Gutkowska J (2002) Oxytocin induces differentiation of P19 embryonic stem cells to cardiomyocytes. Proc Natl Acad Sci U S A 99:9550–9555

Rangappa S, Entwistle JW, Wechsler AS, Kresh JY (2003a) Cardiomyocyte-mediated contact programs human mesenchymal stem cells to express cardiogenic phenotype. J Thorac Cardiovasc Surg 126:124–132

Rangappa S, Fen C, Lee EH, Bongso A, Sim EK, Wei EK (2003b) Transformation of adult mesenchymal stem cells isolated from the fatty tissue into cardiomyocytes. Ann Thorac Surg 75:775–779

Rupp S, Badorff C, Koyanagi M, Urbich C, Fichtlscherer S, Aicher A, Zeiher AM, Dimmeler S (2004) Statin therapy in patients with coronary artery disease improves the impaired endothelial progenitor cell differentiation into cardiomyogenic cells. Basic Res Cardiol 99:61–68

Sachinidis A, Gissel C, Nierhoff D, Hippler-Altenburg R, Sauer H, Wartenberg M, Hescheler J (2003) Identification of plateled-derived growth factor-BB as cardiogenesis-inducing factor in mouse embryonic stem cells under serum-free conditions. Cell Physiol Biochem 13:423–429

Sauer H, Theben T, Hescheler J, Lindner M, Brandt MC, Wartenberg M (2001) Characteristics of calcium sparks in cardiomyocytes derived from embryonic stem cells. Am J Physiol Heart Circ Physiol 281:H411–H421

Schneider MD (2004) Regenerative medicine: prometheus unbound. Nature 432:451–453

Schultheiss TM, Burch JB, Lassar AB (1997) A role for bone morphogenetic proteins in the induction of cardiac myogenesis. Genes Dev 11:451–462

Schuster MD, Kocher AA, Seki T, Martens TP, Xiang G, Homma S, Itescu S (2004) Myocardial neovascularization by bone marrow angioblasts results in cardiomyocyte regeneration. Am J Physiol Heart Circ Physiol 287:H525–H532

Shim WS, Jiang S, Wong P, Tan J, Chua YL, Tan YS, Sin YK, Lim CH, Chua T, Teh M, Liu TC, Sim E (2004) Ex vivo differentiation of human adult bone marrow stem cells into cardiomyocyte-like cells. Biochem Biophys Res Commun 324:481–488

Strauer BE, Brehm M, Zeus T, Kostering M, Hernandez A, Sorg RV, Kogler G, Wernet P (2002) Repair of infarcted myocardium by autologous intracoronary mononuclear bone marrow cell transplantation in humans. Circulation 106:1913–1918

Terami H, Hidaka K, Katsumata T, Iio A, Morisaki T (2004) Wnt11 facilitates embryonic stem cell differentiation to Nkx2.5-positive cardiomyocytes. Biochem Biophys Res Commun 325:968–975

Toma C, Pittenger MF, Cahill KS, Byrne BJ, Kessler PD (2002) Human mesenchymal stem cells differentiate to a cardiomyocyte phenotype in the adult murine heart. Circulation 105:93–98

Tomaselli GF, Zipes DP (2004) What causes sudden death in heart failure? Circ Res 95:754–763

Tomita S, Li RK, Weisel RD, Mickle DA, Kim EJ, Sakai T, Jia ZQ (1999) Autologous transplantation of bone marrow cells improves damaged heart function. Circulation 100:II247–II256

Tomita S, Mickle DA, Weisel RD, Jia ZQ, Tumiati LC, Allidina Y, Liu P, Li RK (2002) Improved heart function with myogenesis and angiogenesis after autologous porcine bone marrow stromal cell transplantation. J Thorac Cardiovasc Surg 123:1132–1140

Urbich C, Dimmeler S (2004) Endothelial progenitor cells: characterization and role in vascular biology. Circ Res 95:343–353

Urbich C, Heeschen C, Aicher A, Sasaki KI, Bruhl T, Farhadi MR, Vajkoczy P, Hofmann WK, Peters C, Pennacchio LA, Abolmaali ND, Chavakis E, Reinheckel T, Zeiher AM, Dimmeler S (2005) Cathepsin L is required for endothelial progenitor cell-induced neovascularization. Nat Med 11:206–213

Urbich C, Heeschen C, Aicher A, Hofmann WK, Peters C, Reinheckel T, Zeiher AM, Dimmeler S (2003) Cathepsins are essential for endothelial progenitor cell-induced neovascularization. submitted

Van der Heyden MA, Defize LH (2003) Twenty-one years of P19 cells: what an embryonal carcinoma cell line taught us about cardiomyocyte differentiation. Cardiovasc Res 58:292–302

Wagers AJ, Sherwood RI, Christensen JL, Weissman IL (2002) Little evidence for developmental plasticity of adult hematopoietic stem cells. Science 297:2256–2259

Wagers AJ, Weissman IL (2004) Plasticity of adult stem cells. Cell 116:639–648

Wang X, Willenbring H, Akkari Y, Torimaru Y, Foster M, Al-Dhalimy M, Lagasse E, Finegold M, Olson S, Grompe M (2003) Cell fusion is the principal source of bone-marrow-derived hepatocytes. Nature 422:897–901

Wobus AM, Wallukat G, Hescheler J (1991) Pluripotent mouse embryonic stem cells are able to differentiate into cardiomyocytes expressing chronotropic responses to adrenergic and cholinergic agents and Ca^{2+} channel blockers. Differentiation 48:173–182

Wollert KC, Meyer GP, Lotz J, Ringes-Lichtenberg S, Lippolt P, Breidenbach C, Fichtner S, Korte T, Hornig B, Messinger D, Arseniev L, Hertenstein B, Ganser A, Drexler H (2004) Intracoronary autologous bone-marrow cell transfer after myocardial infarction: the BOOST randomised controlled clinical trial. Lancet 364:141–148

Xaymardan M, Tang L, Zagreda L, Pallante B, Zheng J, Chazen JL, Chin A, Duignan I, Nahirney P, Rafii S, Mikawa T, Edelberg JM (2004) Platelet-derived growth factor-AB promotes the generation of adult bone marrow-derived cardiac myocytes. Circ Res 94:E39–E45

Xu W, Zhang X, Qian H, Zhu W, Sun X, Hu J, Zhou H, Chen Y (2004) Mesenchymal stem cells from adult human bone marrow differentiate into a cardiomyocyte phenotype in vitro. Exp Biol Med (Maywood) 229:623–631

Yeh ET, Zhang S, Wu HD, Korbling M, Willerson JT, Estrov Z (2003) Transdifferentiation of human peripheral blood CD34+-enriched cell population into cardiomyocytes, endothelial cells, and smooth muscle cells in vivo. Circulation 108:2070–2073

Ying QL, Nichols J, Evans EP, Smith AG (2002) Changing potency by spontaneous fusion. Nature 416:545–548

Zhang S, Wang D, Estrov Z, Raj S, Willerson JT, Yeh ET (2004) Both cell fusion and transdifferentiation account for the transformation of human peripheral blood CD34-positive cells into cardiomyocytes in vivo. Circulation 110:3803–3807

HEP (2006) 174:299–317
© Springer-Verlag Berlin Heidelberg 2006

The Potential Use of Myogenic Stem Cells in Regenerative Medicine

G. Grenier · M. A. Rudnicki (✉)

Molecular Medicine Program and Centre for Stem Cell and Gene Therapy, Ottawa Health Research Institute, 501 Smyth Road , Ottawa Ontario, K1H 8L6, Canada
mrudnicki@ohri.ca

Abstract More than a century after the initial description of muscular dystrophy, no curative treatment is currently available. To date, clinical trials with myogenic stem cell transplantation have met with only modest success. There are multiple factors behind these failures, yet they provide powerful insights for improvement. In this chapter, we review the different myogenic stem cell populations that have been reported to be potential vectors for the treatment of myopathies in a context of regenerative medicine.

Keywords Skeletal muscle · Myogenic stem cells · Regeneration

Abbreviations

DMD	Duchenne muscular dystrophy
MPC	Muscle progenitor cell
MTT	Myoblast transplantation therapy
BM	Bone marrow
MDSC	Muscle-derived stem cell
SP	Side population

1
Introduction

Muscular dystrophies form a heterogeneous group of neuromuscular disorders, characterized by a progressive muscle weakness resulting in ambulatory deficiency that leads to death by respiratory insufficiency in some cases (Blake et al. 2002; Emery 2002; Nishino and Ozawa 2002). Furthermore, muscle fiber necrosis, chronic inflammation, and muscle wasting due to the exhaustion of the pool of muscle progenitor cells, the satellite cells, are commonly observed (for a review see Dalkilic and Kunkel 2003). Although muscular dystrophies were described more than 150 years ago, therapies remain only supportive rather than curative.

Recently, the field of regenerative medicine has exploded following the discovery of stem cells possessing an exceptional capacity for growth and differentiation. Stem cells present in a variety of tissues are capable of generating blood, liver, heart, skin and muscle. The use of stem cells for the treatment of myopathies provides significant advantages: it offers the possibility to deliver cells containing a normal genome and to potentially replenish the number of myogenic cells, thereby reducing muscle wasting. However, the successful use of stem cells as a treatment for myopathies has yet to be demonstrated.

In this chapter, we review the literature pertaining to the different myogenic stem cell populations that have been reported and could potentially be used for the treatment of myopathies in the context of regenerative medicine.

2
Muscle Regeneration

To fulfill its role of contraction, adult skeletal muscle tissue is comprised of multinucleated basic contractile units, the myofibers, that are in contact with motor neurons. The myofiber is surrounded by a basal lamina and grouped into bundles within the perimysium to form a skeletal muscle that is itself contained by the epimysium (for a review see Charge and Rudnicki 2004). A vast network of capillaries is also found tightly associated and oriented between the myofibers as muscle requires a high level of energy consumption. Localized beneath the basal lamina of myofibers is a population of quiescent muscle progenitor cells, the satellite cells, that are required for muscle maintenance.

Recently, our laboratory has described an important role for Pax7, a paired box transcription factor, in the specification of satellite cells (Seale et al. 2000). Our studies revealed that Pax7$^{-/-}$ mice display a markedly reduced number of satellite cells. Consequently, Pax7$^{-/-}$ adult mice display tremendous muscle wasting, with a striking impairment for regeneration following injury. Other reports suggest that Pax7 might also be involved in the self-renewal of satellite cells. Indeed, neonatal-derived satellite cells from Pax7$^{-/-}$ mice display poor proliferative capacity in vitro (Olguin and Olwin 2004). Myofibers within adult skeletal muscle tissue are generally mitotically quiescent, as demonstrated by the low turnover of myonuclei. According to Schmalbruch and Lewis, only 1–2% of the myonuclei are replaced every week under physiological conditions (Schmalbruch and Lewis 2000).

However, muscles that are injured following intensive exercise or trauma, display a rapid and high capacity to regenerate. Muscle regeneration is made up of two main phases.

The magnitude of the first phase is determined by the severity of the damage. Following muscle injury, degeneration of the tissue is characterized by the presence of necrosed myofibers that release chemotaxic agents inducing inflammatory cell recruitment to the wounded site. Hence, leukocytes present in the circulation adhere to the endothelium, penetrate the tissue and migrate to the site of injury (Gute et al. 1998; Figarella-Branger et al. 2003). The primary inflammatory response occurs within a few hours and reaches a plateau 4 days after injury. This plateau is maintained for the next 3 days and decreases slowly, disappearing after 14 days (Grenier, unpublished observations). The function of inflammatory cells is to phagocytose cell debris and because of their presence, a wide variety of cytokines are secreted, initiating the second phase of the regeneration process.

The second phase of muscle regeneration concerns de novo formation of myofibers. It is characterized by the activation of satellite cells and the differentiation of their daughter cells. During the inflammatory response, mitotically quiescent satellite cells become activated, cross the basal lamina and migrate to the site of injury (Bischoff 1997). At the site of injury, the satellite cells proliferate and their descendants, the myogenic precursor cells (MPCs), undergo multiple rounds of division prior to fusing with existing or new myofibers (Fig. 1).

Activation of satellite cells is characterized by the initial upregulation of two members of the myogenic regulatory factor family (MRFs), *Myf5* and *MyoD*. Normally, these MRFs are expressed at low levels in satellite cells, but highly expressed during the activation and subsequent proliferation stage of MPCs following muscle injury. Developmental analysis revealed that Myf5 and MyoD knockout mice are viable and display no muscle abnormalities in normal adult mice (Kablar and Rudnicki 2000), but MyoD$^{-/-}$ mice display lower regenerative abilities (Megeney et al. 1996). Moreover, cultured primary myoblasts derived from MyoD$^{-/-}$ mice display a higher proliferative capability and lower index of fusion compared to wild type cells, suggesting a differentiation role for MyoD (Sabourin et al. 1999). The role of Myf5 is more complex, with several lines of evidence implicating it in the self-renewal of satellite cells. For example, when human satellite cells or C2C12 cells (a murine cell line) are induced to differentiate, a small population of undifferentiated Myf5^{+}/MyoD^{-} cells persist and retain the capacity to self-renew and to give rise to differentiation-competent progeny (Baroffio et al. 1996; Yoshida et al. 1998).

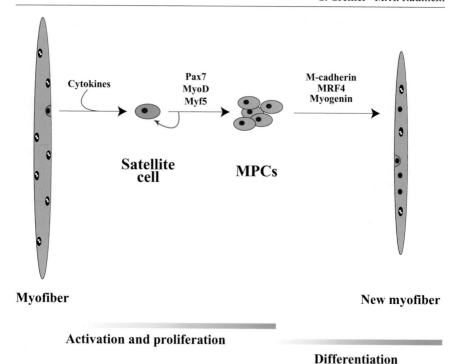

Myofiber   **New myofiber**

Activation and proliferation

Differentiation

Fig. 1 Schematic diagram of muscle regeneration with satellite cells. Muscle regeneration
is characterized by the activation of the quiescent satellite cells beneath the basal lamina
of the myofibers after muscle injury. This activation is due in part by the presence of
cytokines secreted by inflammatory cells. Most of the activated satellite cells or myogenic
progenitor cells (*MPCs*) proliferate and fuse to newly formed multinucleated myofibers.
Others replenish the pool of satellite cells within skeletal muscle tissue

At the end of their proliferation phase, MPCs initiate a program of differentiation leading to the formation of myotubes/myofibers. At this point, two
other important MRFs, myogenin and MRF4, are upregulated and the cell
cycle is arrested via the hypophosphorylation of pRb (Corbeil and Branton
1997; Huh et al. 2004). This is followed by the expression of a myriad of proteins promoting the specific differentiation and fusion of MPCs. The resulting
fusion between MPCs leads to the formation of multinucleated cells, called
myotubes or myofibers. At the end of its maturation, differentiated myotubes
will express a large quantity of myosin heavy chain (MHC) that interacts with
actin, allowing the contraction of multinucleated myotubes.

To accomplish fusion, semi-stable intercellular junction structures that mediate cell–cell adhesion and regulate intracellular cytoskeleton architecture
are required. Cell–cell interactions are promoted by the cadherin family of
transmembrane proteins (see review by Geiger and Ayalon 1992; Kaufmann
et al. 1999). Muscle-specific M-cadherin is thought to be essential for MPC fu-

sion because it is almost exclusively expressed in developing and regenerating skeletal muscles, as well as in skeletal muscle cell lines and in satellite cells cultured in vitro (myoblasts) (Rose et al. 1994; Kaufmann et al. 1999). In vitro its expression is upregulated during the first phase of cell differentiation and downregulated after myofiber formation, suggestive of a key role during the fusion process (Donalies et al. 1991). However, the central role for M-cadherin in myoblast fusion has recently been revised by the generation of an M-cadherin targeted gene disruption in mice (Hollnagel et al. 2002). M-cadherin$^{-/-}$ mice developed normal skeletal musculature and exhibited normal kinetics of muscle regeneration (Hollnagel et al. 2002). The discrepancy between the in vitro results and those obtained in vivo may be due to a compensatory mechanism in the M-cadherin$^{-/-}$ mice. Indeed, it appears that other cadherins present in skeletal muscle, particularly N-cadherin and R-cadherin, might substitute for M-cadherin function (Charlton et al. 1997; Hollnagel et al. 2002).

3
Myogenic Stem Cells

Stem cells participate in organ development within embryos and contribute to tissue healing within adults. During tissue regeneration, adult stem cells that are normally quiescent became activated. From a low number of stem cells residing within tissues, a high number of daughter cells emerge and commit to a specific cell lineage, whilst some return to a quiescent state in order to maintain the pool of stem cells. This essential feature corresponds to the self-renewing character of stem cells, allowing their continuity during life expectancy (Fig. 2).

Although their plasticity remains controversial, their potential differentiation is defined by four categories:

1. Totipotent stem cells are able to give rise to the three germ layers, the placenta (trophoblast), and the primordial germ cells.

2. Pluripotent stem cells can give rise only to all three germ layers.

3. Multipotent stem cells can also give rise to various cell types of only one germ layer but not to the trophoblast.

4. Progenitor, or committed stem cells, can give rise only to a tissue-specific cell type.

No totipotent stem cells have been found within adult tissues. However, it is possible to establish totipotent stem cell lines from adult differentiated cells by using nuclear transfer technology (Kato et al. 2004).

For many years, it was thought that the only source of myogenic stem cells present in the muscle were the satellite cells. However, with the use of techniques

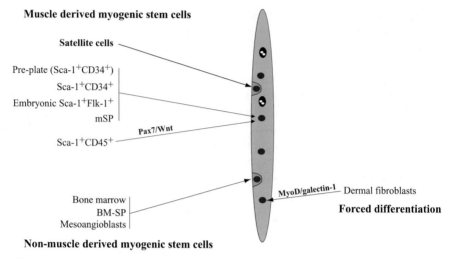

Fig. 2 Schematic diagram showing potential contribution of myogenic stem cells to muscle regeneration. Myogenic stem cells are muscle or nonmuscle-derived. The most important source of myogenic stem cells originates from the satellite cells. Cells infected with MyoD or treated with galectin-1 can be forced to differentiate

such as flow cytometry and cell culture methodology, it has become possible to fractionate the tissue and to identify other potential myogenic stem cells. These resident or muscle-derived stem cells (MDSCs) showcase a broad potential of differentiation, suggesting that some are multipotent rather than committed to the muscle lineage. The existence of nonmuscle-derived stem cells have also been described that participate in myogenesis or do so under forced conditions.

3.1
Muscle-Derived Myogenic Stem Cells

3.1.1
Satellite Cells

As mentioned, satellite cells are the most important source of adult myogenic stem cells within skeletal muscle. When satellite cells are isolated from skeletal muscle and cultured in vitro, we defined them as primary myoblasts. Interestingly, primary myoblasts display some plasticity and are capable of differentiating into other cell types when induced to do so. Indeed, we and others have demonstrated that primary myoblasts in culture can express pparγ2 and C/EBPα, CBFa1, and MyoD and Myf5, representing the master genes that regulate adipogenic, osteogenic and myogenic differentiation, respectively (Asakura et al. 2001). This implies that satellite cells are not committed progenitors, but rather multipotent stem cells (Asakura et al. 2001; Wada et al. 2002; Komaki et al. 2004).

Primary myoblasts can provide a ready source of cells for cell therapy and tissue engineering applications because they are numerous and easily obtained from a small biopsy. The injection of myoblasts into muscles is known as myoblast transplantation therapy (MTT). In the late 1970s, Partridge et al. set the basis for myoblast transplantation, making the first successful myoblast transplantation in mouse (Partridge et al. 1978). Wild type myoblasts were able to generate dystrophin positive myofibers in mice lacking the dystrophin gene, the mdx mouse, used as a model for studying muscular dystrophy (Morgan et al. 1988; Partridge et al. 1989). More recently, other groups have used MTT in other mouse models for muscular dystrophy, showing merosin and dysferlin positive myofibers in deficient mice (Vilquin et al. 1996; Leriche-Guerin et al. 2002).

MTT with other animal models has not been as successful, thus highlighting serious limitations of this procedure for human applications. One of the limitations is due to the low migration ability of myoblasts in muscle recipients. For example, in a careful experiment conducted with monkeys, results showed that injection of myoblasts every millimeter in muscle tissue allows about 25%–65% of donor cell-myofiber integration (Skuk et al. 2002). If injections were made every 2 mm, this percentage fell to 5%–15%. Positive myofibers were present in muscle biopsy for up to 12 months following their transplantation as long as an effective immunotherapy was maintained (Skuk et al. 2002). One approach to circumvent this problem was to pretreat host muscle with metalloproteinases (MMPs) (Torrente et al. 2000). In this way, the modification of the extracellular matrix significantly improved the migration and the fusion of donor myoblasts within host muscle (Torrente et al. 2000).

Another drawback to MTT is that microinjection causes an acute immunological response by the host such that over 90% of donor myoblasts are eliminated within 1 h (Beauchamp et al. 1997), the majority being killed within minutes following transplantation (Hodgetts et al. 2000). Possible factors and pathways causing the rapid and massive death have been recently reviewed by Smythe et al. (2000, 2001). The host immune response is thought to act through three main pathways. The first might be due to the presence of pre-existing "natural" host antibodies, inducing a proteolytic cascade of the complement system, which ultimately leads to the rapid lysis of the donor cells. The second is represented by direct interaction with host T cells through expression by donor myoblasts of cell-surface molecules. As an example, recognition of the major histocompatibility complex (MHC) results in a direct interaction with the host $CD4^+$ helper T cells. The third is the indirect activation of host T cells by the binding of cell-surface molecules to the host antigen-presenting cells, which present donor antigen to host T cells.

An important point to address for MTT is whether a genetically deficient myofiber be functionally restored by a donor nucleus from an MTT procedure. For example, gene complementation produced by the fusion of normal myoblasts to a dystrophin-deficient myofiber does not ensure expression of dystrophin throughout the myofiber. In fact, most intracellular proteins coded by a single nucleus in a myofiber remain localized to a region known as the nuclear domain (Pavlath et al. 1989). This restriction depends on three main factors. One is a physicochemical constraint that is linked to the diffusion ability of a protein throughout its environment. The second restriction is that some diffused proteins will remain anchored with other components of the myofiber. Finally, mRNA will diffuse only 100 µm from the nucleus that expresses it within a myofiber (Hall and Ralston 1989; Ralston and Hall 1992). For example, cultured myoblasts from normal mice and transgenic mice overexpressing 50-fold dystrophin (Tg-MDA), were transplanted into dystrophin-deficient mdx mouse muscles. Four weeks after their transplantation, four times more dystrophin-positive fibers were observed in cross-sections of muscles injected with Tg-MDA as compared to those injected with normal myoblasts. Moreover, the fiber length displaying dystrophin was about 500 µm using normal myoblasts as compared to 1,500 µm with Tg-MDA myoblasts. These experiments demonstrate that the membrane area over which dystrophin was expressed increased only threefold despite the transplant of myoblasts overexpressing dystrophin 50-fold (Kinoshita et al. 1998).

Human clinical trials employing MTT have been initiated with dystrophin-deficient patients. In one study, only a few host myofibers expressed dystrophin despite the injection of millions of myoblasts. In another, Gussoni et al. reported some encouraging results, revealing that muscle biopsies made from three patients that received MTT 6 months previously displayed more than 10% of the original number of donor cells. Half of the surviving donor cells fused to the host myofibers, and nearly 50% produced dystrophin (Gussoni et al. 1997). These results suggest that more work should be done to ensure an optimized MTT treatment strategy for potential patients.

3.1.2
Muscle-Derived Side Population Cells

MDSCs displaying hematopoietic characteristics can be enriched by FACS relying on the unique property of these cells to actively exclude dyes such as Hoechst 33342, due to the activity at the cell surface of multidrug resistance-like proteins such as BCRP1/ABCG2 (Goodell et al. 1996; Gussoni et al. 1999; Jackson et al. 1999; Zhou et al. 2001, 2002; Asakura et al. 2002). Somewhat less effective than their bone marrow (BM) counterparts, muscle side population (mSP) cells are capable of reconstituting all hematopoietic blood cell lineages after intravenous injection into lethally irradiated mice (Gussoni et al. 1999). More importantly, mSP can commit to myogenic conversion in vivo. Indeed, when injected intravenously into mdx mice, mSP can convert to myogenic cells. Seventeen days after their injection, 9% of total myofibers were dystrophin-positive, and among them, 3% of their myonuclei were Y-chromosome-positive (Gussoni et al. 1999). Our laboratory has also shown that Pax7$^{-/-}$ mice lacking satellite cells possess mSP in their musculature (Seale et al. 2000; Asakura et al.

2002). These results suggest that mSP cells and satellite cells are distinct cell populations (Seale et al. 2000). However, mSP cells might actually represent satellite cell progenitors. Indeed, mSP isolated from Pax7$^{-/-}$ mice preferentially form hematopoietic colonies, whereas mSP cells isolated from wild type muscle form satellite cells in the host muscle (Gussoni et al. 1999; Seale et al. 2000; Asakura et al. 2002). Myogenic conversion for mSP fraction might be regulated via cell–cell interactions because it requires co-culture with primary myoblasts in vitro (Asakura et al. 2002). Thus, these results clearly illustrate the presence of progenitor cells with myogenic potential other than satellite cells within skeletal muscles.

The SP fraction represents a mixed cellular population. Hence it is important to further characterize them on the basis of cell surface markers. The analysis of mSP cell surface markers were based on those previously used to define murine bone marrow SP, primarily Sca-1, CD34 and CD45. In this study, 92% of mSP express Sca-1, whereas only 16% express CD45 consisting of both Sca-1$^+$ (57.5%) and Sca-1$^-$ (42.5%) (Asakura et al. 2002). Moreover, it was shown that the hematopoietic activity of mSP cells are mainly due to CD45$^+$ cells, but not CD45$^-$ (Asakura et al. 2002; McKinney-Freeman et al. 2002). In vivo, the myogenic potential of mSP was shown to be greater in CD45$^-$ than CD45$^+$ muscle-derived cells following intramuscular injection (McKinney-Freeman et al. 2002). However, in vitro analysis indicates as many as 9% of CD45$^+$ mSP cells undergo myogenic conversion when co-cultured with myoblasts (Asakura et al. 2002).

3.1.3
Muscle Resident Sca-1$^+$CD45$^+$ Stem Cells

CD45$^+$ was first defined as a hematopoietic cell-specific marker (Trowbridge and Thomas 1994). CD45$^+$ cells isolated from uninjured muscle or other tissues do not display any intrinsic myogenic potential (Asakura et al. 2002; McKinney-Freeman et al. 2002; Polesskaya and Rudnicki 2002). However, myogenic differentiation of CD45$^+$ cells isolated from muscle does occur following their intramuscular injection as well as in co-culture with primary myoblasts (Asakura et al. 2002; Polesskaya and Rudnicki 2002). Following muscle cardiotoxin-induced injury, muscle-resident Sca1$^+$CD45$^+$ cells enter the cell cycle and increase 30-fold in number. Interestingly, a high proportion of these cells, isolated from regenerating muscle, acquire myogenic potential and are capable of differentiating into myotubes (Polesskaya et al. 2003). Taken together, these results provide the first experimental evidence that muscle-resident CD45$^+$ adult stem cells have a normal physiological role in tissue regeneration (Polesskaya and Rudnicki 2002).

One intriguing question is which signals trigger the myogenic specification of muscle-resident Sca1$^+$CD45$^+$ cell population during muscle regeneration.

Some of the answers can be found during embryonic development, when muscle cell precursors are specified in the somite in response to proteins secreted from the neural tube and notochord (Christ and Ordahl 1995). Sonic hedgehog (Shh), secreted by the notochord, and several proteins of the Wingless family of proteins (Wnt), secreted by the dorsal neural tube and surface ectoderm, are required for the induction of myogenesis (Munsterberg et al. 1995; Tajbakhsh et al. 1998). These signals induce the expression of developmental control transcription factors such as Pax3 and the myogenic regulatory factors Myf5 and MyoD, which enforce commitment to the myogenic cell lineage. Our experiments confirm an autologous role for Wnts in adult myogenesis. Injection of the Wnt antagonists, soluble Frizzled receptor protein (sFRP2/3), into regenerating muscle markedly reduced CD45$^+$ stem cell proliferation and their myogenic differentiation (Polesskaya et al. 2003).

Primary myoblasts also express high levels of Wnts, suggesting that Wnts mediate their ability to induce the myogenic specification of muscle-resident CD45$^+$ stem cells. Stimulation of the Wnt signaling canonical pathway with lithium chloride in freshly isolated muscle-resident Sca1$^+$CD45$^+$ cells is sufficient to induce myogenic specification. Moreover, co-culture with cells ectopically expressing Wnt proteins induced expression of Pax7 and their myogenic commitment. Therefore, these findings unequivocally establish that Wnt-signaling is the mechanism triggering myogenic specification of muscle-derived CD45$^+$ adult stem cells both in vivo and following co-culture with primary myoblasts. These observations underscore the parallels that exist in the regulation of embryonic vs regenerative myogenesis by demonstrating that developmentally appropriate pathways regulate the participation of CD45$^+$ stem cells in muscle regeneration.

The molecular mechanism that induces myogenic conversion of muscle-resident Sca-1$^+$CD45$^+$ cell population was further assessed in vitro (Seale et al. 2004). Results show that the myogenic potential of Sca-1$^+$CD45$^+$ stem cells isolated from uninjured muscle is due to the expression of Pax7. Sca-1$^+$CD45$^+$ isolated from injured Pax7$^{-/-}$ muscle showcase no myogenic conversion, yet when retrovirally infected with Pax7 they efficiently activated their myogenic program. The resulting myoblasts expressed Myf5 and MyoD and differentiated into myotubes that expressed myogenin and myosin heavy chain. Notably, infection of Pax7$^{-/-}$ muscle in vivo with adenoviral Pax7 resulted in an increased formation of regenerated myofibers. Taken together, these results indicate that Pax7 is necessary and sufficient to induce the myogenic specification of adult-derived Sca-1$^+$CD45$^+$ muscle cells.

3.1.4
Adult Muscle-Derived CD34$^+$

Another MDSC population is the Sca-1$^+$CD34$^+$ fraction (Torrente et al. 2001; Jankowski et al. 2002; Qu-Petersen et al. 2002). CD34 is a sialylated transmembrane glycoprotein that is expressed in myeloid progenitors and endothelial cells (Krause et al. 1994; Fennie et al. 1995; Morel et al. 1996). A muscle culture system of successive preplating combined with FACS sorting facilitated the enrichment and purification of Sca-1$^+$CD34$^+$ cells having both myogenic and hematopoietic differentiation potential (Torrente et al. 2001). Torrente et al. show that when these cells were isolated from newborn mice expressing muscle-specific LacZ and injected intra-arterially into mdx mice, they were able to attach firmly to the endothelium. Eight weeks after transplantation, β-gal$^+$ staining co-localized with dystrophin in all recipient muscles. Interestingly, the migration of the MSDC Sca-1$^+$CD34$^+$ donor cells from the vasculature and their incorporation to the recipient musculature was increased following muscle injury. In this case, up to 12% of the myofibers were β-gal$^+$ (Torrente et al. 2001). These data suggest that bi-potential stem cells present within the vasculature may be activated to enter the myogenic lineage when the muscle receives extensive damage. However, the potential of the Sca-1$^+$CD34$^+$ cells to replenish the pool of the satellite cells is not known.

Sca-1$^+$CD34$^+$ cells derived from adult mouse muscle were also grown as continuous cell culture using a preplating technique (Qu-Petersen et al. 2002). These plated cells have characteristics usually associated with noncommitted progenitor cells such as the capacity to self-renew and proliferate as well as multiple differentiation abilities (Qu-Petersen et al. 2002). Interestingly, these MDSC are c-Kit$^-$CD45$^-$, eliminating their potential hematopoietic origin. Moreover, they also have a high potential for myogenic conversion in vitro and in vivo, and can also spontaneously express myogenic markers, MyoD and desmin. They also have similar phenotypic characteristics to Sca-1$^+$M-cadherin$^-$ cells that have been identified as satellite cells in situ (Qu-Petersen et al. 2002).

3.1.5
Embryonic Muscle-Derived CD34$^+$

Myogenic stem cells have also been found in embryonic muscle vasculature. Published data by Le grand et al. show that FACS-sorted CD34$^+$FLK1$^+$ cell populations isolated from the muscle of E17 embryos have the propensity to differentiate in vitro into endothelial cells as well as skeletal muscle cells (Le Grand et al. 2004). Interestingly, these cells cultured in muscle medium activate myogenic-related genes that were not expressed at the time of their isolation. In myogenic differentiation medium, activated cells express muscle-specific genes such as desmin, MyoD, Pax3 and MHC, and also fuse to form multinucleated myotubes. The efficiency of these cells for transplantation was shown by isolating CD34$^+$Flk1$^+$ cells from muscle of E17 transgenic mice expressing β-gal under the control of the desmin promoter. Isolated cells were then transplanted into the tibialis anterior (TA) muscle of mdx mice after local irradiation. Eight days after transplantation, muscle recipients displayed β-gal positive myofibers representing 60% of the total muscle length, suggesting an enhanced ability of the cells to disperse within the recipient muscle. Moreover, 18% of the total myofibers within the mdx muscle recipient were dystrophin-positive (Le Grand et al. 2004).

The above data, for the marker CD34, suggests its importance for providing a method for isolating myogenic progenitors. However, a sub-population of satellite cells express CD34, suggesting the possible contamination of CD34$^+$ satellite cells. This highlights the need for multiple markers for identification of MDSC(Beauchamp et al. 1999; Lee et al. 2000).

3.2
Non-Muscle-Derived Myogenic Stem Cells

3.2.1
Bone Marrow-Derived Myogenic Stem Cells

The contribution of nonresident myogenic stem cells during muscle regeneration was first reported by Ferrari (1998). In this seminal study, BM donor cells derived from a transgenic mouse expressing β-gal driven by a muscle-specific promoter, were transplanted into an immunodeficient mouse. After 3 weeks, β-gal$^+$ staining originating from donor cells was observed within the musculature of the recipient. However, the frequency of donor cells that contribute to muscle regeneration was about 100–500 β-gal$^+$ cells per muscle, much lower than the endogenous contribution of satellite cells. Moreover, in order to improve the integration of BM-derived cells to the host musculature, extensive muscle regeneration induced by cardiotoxin was required, thereby creating a nonphysiological environment. LaBarge et al. demonstrated the integration of BM-derived cells following exercise, being more relevant physiologically (LaBarge and Blau 2002). In this study, GFP$^+$ BM-derived cells behaved as satellite cells expressing muscle-specific proteins in vivo and in vitro and exhibited self-renewal potential in tissue culture. Following exercise, they contributed as much as 3.5% of the muscle fibers (LaBarge and Blau 2002). In addition, clonal progenies of GFP$^+$ satellite cell isolated from recipient muscles contributed to new fiber formation when re-injected in TA muscles of a secondary recipient mouse.

To assess the integration of BM-derived myogenic stem cells in a model that reflects the physiopathology of muscular dystrophy, several groups used the mdx mouse as a host (Bittner et al. 1999; Gussoni et al. 1999). BM-derived cells that possess myogenic activity were found in the small subpopulation of the BM SP (Gussoni et al. 1999). These BM SP cells are stem cell antigen-1 (Sca-1)$^+$, cKit$^+$, CD43$^+$, CD45$^+$, lineage marker (B220, Mac-1, Gr-1, CD4, CD5, CD8) negative and CD34$^-$, and accounted for about 100–500 cells per mouse (Gussoni et al. 1997). Following tail vein injection, BM SP cells were capable of integrating into the host musculature, as shown by the presence of donor cells that express dystrophin and by FISH analysis of the Y-chromosome in serial sections of the recipient muscle. Five weeks following BM SP cell transplantation, less than 1% of the myofibers expressed dystrophin, as was the case with recipients engrafted with an unfractionated BM-derived cells. After 12 weeks, up to 4% of the myofibers were dystrophin-positive, with 10±30% of these containing fused BM SP-derived donor nuclei.

The observations made with the mdx mouse model recapitulate the results obtained in a human DMD patient who received a BM transplantation at 1 year of age (Gussoni et al. 2002). In this study, the presence of donor nuclei represented 0.5%–0.9% within a small number of muscle myofibers 13 years after transplantation. Interestingly, the majority of these myofibers stained positively for dystrophin (Gussoni et al. 2002). These findings highlight the inefficient and slow incorporation of such BM-derived cells into the musculature, as compared to myoblasts, making them at present an ineffective therapeutic intervention (Ferrari et al. 1998; Wernig et al. 2000; Heslop et al. 2001). Further studies are necessary to establish the optimal cellular and environmental conditions to promote recruitment and myogenic conversion of nonmuscle stem cells for therapeutic use.

3.2.2
Mesoangioblasts

Embryonically derived cells that possess myogenic activity have been also reported by the Cossu laboratory (De Angelis et al. 1999). These cells, mesoangioblasts, were isolated by the explant method from the dorsal aorta of E9.5 mouse embryos. In culture, mesoangioblasts can be grown clonally, expanding to over 50 passages, and do not demonstrate any tumoral activity when injected into nude mice. Moreover, when exposed to certain cytokines, mesoangioblasts can differentiate into several mesodermal cell types, but not other germ layers, indicating a multipotent ability (Minasi et al. 2002). In vivo experiments with a mouse model for skeletal muscle wasting, α-sarcoglycan (α-SG)-null mice, show the important contribution of these cells for muscle restoration. Indeed, intra-arterial delivery of wild type mesoangioblasts into 1-month-old immunocompetent α-SG-null mice revealed that the quadriceps, tibialis anterior, soleus, gastrocnemius, and EDL muscle expressed α-SG after 2 months, indicating donor cell engraftment (Sampaolesi et al. 2003). In order to verify that α-SG-null mice could be rescued by mesoangioblasts, three functional analyses were made: cross-sectional area (CSA), specific force (Po/CSA), and maximum shortening velocity (Vo) measurements. Results show that CSAs of type 2B fibers were increased in size for α-SG null mice treated with mesoangioblasts. In addition, the Po/CSA from single muscle fibers demonstrated a significant recovery with no differences in Vo. The lack of difference for Vo suggests that neither muscular dystrophy nor mesoangioblast treatment affected the kinetics of acto-myosin interaction.

This study also revealed that the method of delivering cells is important for the success of the cell engraftment. Indeed, 24 h after their delivery, 30±7% of the injected mesoangioblasts were detected in the muscles downstream of the injected artery, whereas less than 3% of donor cells were detected in the same muscles when injection had occurred through the tail vein or intramuscularly. Therefore, the success of the protocol relies on the widespread distribution of donor cells through the capillary network.

3.2.3
Adult Fibroblasts

Other cell types possess myogenic activity. It has been reported that fibroblasts are particularly inclined to form myoblasts under forced conditions. This was first demonstrated by retroviral infection of fibroblasts and other cell lines with MyoD (Weintraub et al. 1989). The myogenic potential of fibroblasts depends on its tissue derivation. By using an adenoviral delivery system for MyoD, dermal compared to muscle-derived fibroblasts had higher myogenic conversion efficiencies as defined by the activation of muscle-specific genes and their fusion into contractile myotubes. Moreover, MHC staining demonstrated that between 42% and 70% of dermal-derived fibroblasts display myogenic conversion as compared to muscle-derived fibroblasts, which account for only 32%–44% (Lattanzi et al. 1998). Converted fibroblasts also have an in vivo ability to regenerate muscle. Twenty-four hours after adenoviral exposure with MyoD, converted cultures of human dermal fibroblasts that were retrovirally infected with a vector expressing β-gal were injected into regenerating muscle of immunodeficient mice. Donor cells were subsequently capable of giving rise to β-gal[+] myofibers expressing human myosin heavy chains (Lattanzi et al. 1998).

Murine dermal fibroblasts can also become myogenic in vitro by culturing with galectin-1 (Goldring et al. 2000). Myogenic conversion in this case could reach 100%, as defined by desmin expression (Goldring et al. 2002). Forced myogenic conversion of such easily isolated cells could be useful for ex vivo gene correction and therefore could be a particularly attractive source of cells for clinical applications (Partridge 1991).

4
Conclusion

Since their description a century ago, muscular dystrophies have challenged the scientific community for the development of an efficient treatment. To date, no treatment has been found. Whilst the use of myogenic stem cells as therapy is promising, the first attempts using MTT indicate that we are far from an adequate treatment. Despite this shortcoming, MTT has permitted us to make significant advances in understanding the factors that limit its use. Three hurdles have to be overcome: the appropriate way to deliver stem cells, their subsequent survival in the host, and a better comprehension of basic molecular mechanisms underlying the induction of myogenic commitment and differentiation of stem cells. Indeed, findings related to these aspects of biology will permit the improvement of isolation and ex vivo amplification of myogenic stem cells prior to their transplantation.

Acknowledgements We thank Dr. Anthony Scime and Dr. Iain McKinnell for critical review of the manuscript. This work was supported by grants from the Canadian Institute of Health Research (CIHR) to M.A.R. was a recipient of the CIHR and a Canadian Research Chair on Stem Cells. G.G. is the recipient of a postdoctoral fellowship from the Fonds de la Recherche en Santé du Québec.

References

Asakura A, Komaki M, Rudnicki M (2001) Muscle satellite cells are multipotential stem cells that exhibit myogenic, osteogenic, and adipogenic differentiation. Differentiation 68:245–253

Asakura A, Seale P, Girgis-Gabardo A, Rudnicki MA (2002) Myogenic specification of side population cells in skeletal muscle. J Cell Biol 159:123–134

Baroffio A, Hamann M, Bernheim L, Bochaton-Piallat ML, Gabbiani G, Bader CR (1996) Identification of self-renewing myoblasts in the progeny of single human muscle satellite cells. Differentiation 60:47–57

Beauchamp JR, Pagel CN, Partridge TA (1997) A dual-marker system for quantitative studies of myoblast transplantation in the mouse. Transplantation 63:1794–1797

Beauchamp JR, Morgan JE, Pagel CN, Partridge TA (1999) Dynamics of myoblast transplantation reveal a discrete minority of precursors with stem cell-like properties as the myogenic source. J Cell Biol 144:1113–1122

Bischoff R (1997) Chemotaxis of skeletal muscle satellite cells. Dev Dyn 208:505–515

Bittner RE, Schofer C, Weipoltshammer K, Ivanova S, Streubel B, Hauser E, Freilinger M, Hoger H, Elbe-Burger A, Wachtler F (1999) Recruitment of bone-marrow-derived cells by skeletal and cardiac muscle in adult dystrophic mdx mice. Anat Embryol (Berl) 199:391–396

Blake DJ, Weir A, Newey SE, Davies KE (2002) Function and genetics of dystrophin and dystrophin-related proteins in muscle. Physiol Rev 82:291–329

Charge SB, Rudnicki MA (2004) Cellular and molecular regulation of muscle regeneration. Physiol Rev 84:209–238

Charlton CA, Mohler WA, Radice GL, Hynes RO, Blau HM (1997) Fusion competence of myoblasts rendered genetically null for N-cadherin in culture. J Cell Biol 138:331–336

Christ B, Ordahl CP (1995) Early stages of chick somite development. Anat Embryol (Berl) 191:381–396

Corbeil HB, Branton PE (1997) Characterization of an E2F-p130 complex formed during growth arrest. Oncogene 15:657–668

Dalkilic I, Kunkel LM (2003) Muscular dystrophies: genes to pathogenesis. Curr Opin Genet Dev 13:231–238

De Angelis L, Berghella L, Coletta M, Lattanzi L, Zanchi M, Cusella-De Angelis MG, Ponzetto C, Cossu G (1999) Skeletal myogenic progenitors originating from embryonic dorsal aorta coexpress endothelial and myogenic markers and contribute to postnatal muscle growth and regeneration. J Cell Biol 147:869–878

Donalies M, Cramer M, Ringwald M, Starzinski-Powitz A (1991) Expression of M-cadherin, a member of the cadherin multigene family, correlates with differentiation of skeletal muscle cells. Proc Natl Acad Sci U S A 88:8024–8028

Emery AE (2002) The muscular dystrophies. Lancet 359:687–695

Fennie C, Cheng J, Dowbenko D, Young P, Lasky LA (1995) CD34+ endothelial cell lines derived from murine yolk sac induce the proliferation and differentiation of yolk sac CD34+ hematopoietic progenitors. Blood 86:4454–4467

Ferrari G, Cusella-De Angelis G, Coletta M, Paolucci E, Stornaiuolo A, Cossu G, Mavilio F (1998) Muscle regeneration by bone marrow-derived myogenic progenitors. Science 279:1528–1530

Figarella-Branger D, Civatte M, Bartoli C, Pellissier JF (2003) Cytokines, chemokines, and cell adhesion molecules in inflammatory myopathies. Muscle Nerve 28:659–682

Geiger B, Ayalon O (1992) Cadherins. Annu Rev Cell Biol 8:307–332

Goldring K, Jones GE, Watt DJ (2000) A factor implicated in the myogenic conversion of nonmuscle cells derived from the mouse dermis. Cell Transplant 9:519–529

Goldring K, Jones GE, Sewry CA, Watt DJ (2002) The muscle-specific marker desmin is expressed in a proportion of human dermal fibroblasts after their exposure to galectin-1. Neuromuscul Disord 12:183–186

Goodell MA, Brose K, Paradis G, Conner AS, Mulligan RC (1996) Isolation and functional properties of murine hematopoietic stem cells that are replicating in vivo. J Exp Med 183:1797–1806

Gussoni E, Blau HM, Kunkel LM (1997) The fate of individual myoblasts after transplantation into muscles of DMD patients. Nat Med 3:970–977

Gussoni E, Soneoka Y, Strickland CD, Buzney EA, Khan MK, Flint AF, Kunkel LM, Mulligan RC (1999) Dystrophin expression in the mdx mouse restored by stem cell transplantation. Nature 401:390–394

Gussoni E, Bennett RR, Muskiewicz KR, Meyerrose T, Nolta JA, Gilgoff I, Stein J, Chan YM, Lidov HG, Bonnemann CG, Von Moers A, Morris GE, Den Dunnen JT, Chamberlain JS, Kunkel LM, Weinberg K (2002) Long-term persistence of donor nuclei in a Duchenne muscular dystrophy patient receiving bone marrow transplantation. J Clin Invest 110:807–814

Gute DC, Ishida T, Yarimizu K, Korthuis RJ (1998) Inflammatory responses to ischemia and reperfusion in skeletal muscle. Mol Cell Biochem 179:169–187

Hall ZW, Ralston E (1989) Nuclear domains in muscle cells. Cell 59:771–772

Heslop L, Beauchamp JR, Tajbakhsh S, Buckingham ME, Partridge TA, Zammit PS (2001) Transplanted primary neonatal myoblasts can give rise to functional satellite cells as identified using the Myf5nlacZl+ mouse. Gene Ther 8:778–783

Hodgetts SI, Beilharz MW, Scalzo AA, Grounds MD (2000) Why do cultured transplanted myoblasts die in vivo? DNA quantification shows enhanced survival of donor male myoblasts in host mice depleted of CD4+ and CD8+ cells or Nk1.1+ cells. Cell Transplant 9:489–502

Hollnagel A, Grund C, Franke WW, Arnold HH (2002) The cell adhesion molecule M-cadherin is not essential for muscle development and regeneration. Mol Cell Biol 22:4760–4770

Huh MS, Parker MH, Scime A, Parks R, Rudnicki MA (2004) Rb is required for progression through myogenic differentiation but not maintenance of terminal differentiation. J Cell Biol 166:865–876

Jackson KA, Mi T, Goodell MA (1999) Hematopoietic potential of stem cells isolated from murine skeletal muscle. Proc Natl Acad Sci U S A 96:14482–14486

Jankowski RJ, Deasy BM, Cao B, Gates C, Huard J (2002) The role of CD34 expression and cellular fusion in the regeneration capacity of myogenic progenitor cells. J Cell Sci 115:4361–4374

Kablar B, Rudnicki MA (2000) Skeletal muscle development in the mouse embryo. Histol Histopathol 15:649–656

Kato Y, Imabayashi H, Mori T, Tani T, Taniguchi M, Higashi M, Matsumoto M, Umezawa A, Tsunoda Y (2004) Nuclear transfer of adult bone marrow mesenchymal stem cells: developmental totipotency of tissue-specific stem cells from an adult mammal. Biol Reprod 70:415–418

Kaufmann U, Martin B, Link D, Witt K, Zeitler R, Reinhard S, Starzinski-Powitz A (1999) M-cadherin and its sisters in development of striated muscle. Cell Tissue Res 296:191–198

Kawada H, Ogawa M (2001a) Bone marrow origin of hematopoietic progenitors and stem cells in murine muscle. Blood 98:2008–2013

Kawada H, Ogawa M (2001b) Hematopoietic progenitors and stem cells in murine muscle. Blood Cells Mol Dis 27:605–609

Kinoshita I, Vilquin JT, Asselin I, Chamberlain J, Tremblay JP (1998) Transplantation of myoblasts from a transgenic mouse overexpressing dystrophin produced only a relatively small increase of dystrophin-positive membrane. Muscle Nerve 21:91–103

Komaki M, Asakura A, Rudnicki MA, Sodek J, Cheifetz S (2004) MyoD enhances BMP7-induced osteogenic differentiation of myogenic cell cultures. J Cell Sci 117:1457–1468

Krause DS, Ito T, Fackler MJ, Smith OM, Collector MI, Sharkis SJ, May WS (1994) Characterization of murine CD34, a marker for hematopoietic progenitor and stem cells. Blood 84:691–701

LaBarge MA, Blau HM (2002) Biological progression from adult bone marrow to mononucleate muscle stem cell to multinucleate muscle fiber in response to injury. Cell 111:589–601

Lattanzi L, Salvatori G, Coletta M, Sonnino C, Cusella De Angelis MG, Gioglio L, Murry CE, Kelly R, Ferrari G, Molinaro M, Crescenzi M, Mavilio F, Cossu G (1998) High efficiency myogenic conversion of human fibroblasts by adenoviral vector-mediated MyoD gene transfer. An alternative strategy for ex vivo gene therapy of primary myopathies. J Clin Invest 101:2119–2128

Le Grand F, Auda-Boucher G, Levitsky D, Rouaud T, Fontaine-Perus J, Gardahaut MF (2004) Endothelial cells within embryonic skeletal muscles: a potential source of myogenic progenitors. Exp Cell Res 301:232–241

Lee JY, Qu-Petersen Z, Cao B, Kimura S, Jankowski R, Cummins J, Usas A, Gates C, Robbins P, Wernig A, Huard J (2000) Clonal isolation of muscle-derived cells capable of enhancing muscle regeneration and bone healing. J Cell Biol 150:1085–1100

Leriche-Guerin K, Anderson LV, Wrogemann K, Roy B, Goulet M, Tremblay JP (2002) Dysferlin expression after normal myoblast transplantation in SCID and in SJL mice. Neuromuscul Disord 12:167–173

McKinney-Freeman SL, Jackson KA, Camargo FD, Ferrari G, Mavilio F, Goodell MA (2002) Muscle-derived hematopoietic stem cells are hematopoietic in origin. Proc Natl Acad Sci U S A 99:1341–1346

Megeney LA, Kablar B, Garrett K, Anderson JE, Rudnicki MA (1996) MyoD is required for myogenic stem cell function in adult skeletal muscle. Genes Dev 10:1173–1183

Minasi MG, Riminucci M, De Angelis L, Borello U, Berarducci B, Innocenzi A, Caprioli A, Sirabella D, Baiocchi M, De Maria R, Boratto R, Jaffredo T, Broccoli V, Bianco P, Cossu G (2002) The meso-angioblast: a multipotent, self-renewing cell that originates from the dorsal aorta and differentiates into most mesodermal tissues. Development 129:2773–2783

Morel F, Szilvassy SJ, Travis M, Chen B, Galy A (1996) Primitive hematopoietic cells in murine bone marrow express the CD34 antigen. Blood 88:3774–3784

Morgan JE, Watt DJ, Sloper JC, Partridge TA (1988) Partial correction of an inherited biochemical defect of skeletal muscle by grafts of normal muscle precursor cells. J Neurol Sci 86:137–147

Munsterberg AE, Kitajewski J, Bumcrot DA, McMahon AP, Lassar AB (1995) Combinatorial signaling by Sonic hedgehog and Wnt family members induces myogenic bHLH gene expression in the somite. Genes Dev 9:2911–2922

Nishino I, Ozawa E (2002) Muscular dystrophies. Curr Opin Neurol 15:539–544

Olguin HC, Olwin BB (2004) Pax-7 up-regulation inhibits myogenesis and cell cycle progression in satellite cells: a potential mechanism for self-renewal. Dev Biol 275:375–388

Partridge TA (1991) Invited review: myoblast transfer: a possible therapy for inherited myopathies? Muscle Nerve 14:197–212

Partridge TA, Grounds M, Sloper JC (1978) Evidence of fusion between host and donor myoblasts in skeletal muscle grafts. Nature 273:306–308

Partridge TA, Morgan JE, Coulton GR, Hoffman EP, Kunkel LM (1989) Conversion of mdx myofibers from dystrophin-negative to -positive by injection of normal myoblasts. Nature 337:176–179

Pavlath GK, Rich K, Webster SG, Blau HM (1989) Localization of muscle gene products in nuclear domains. Nature 337:570–573

Polesskaya A, Rudnicki MA (2002) A MyoD-dependent differentiation checkpoint: ensuring genome integrity. Dev Cell 3:757–758

Polesskaya A, Seale P, Rudnicki MA (2003) Wnt signaling induces the myogenic specification of resident CD45+ adult stem cells during muscle regeneration. Cell 113:841–852

Qu-Petersen Z, Deasy B, Jankowski R, Ikezawa M, Cummins J, Pruchnic R, Mytinger J, Cao B, Gates C, Wernig A, Huard J (2002) Identification of a novel population of muscle stem cells in mice: potential for muscle regeneration. J Cell Biol 157:851–864

Ralston E, Hall ZW (1992) Restricted distribution of mRNA produced from a single nucleus in hybrid myotubes. J Cell Biol 119:1063–1068

Rose O, Rohwedel J, Reinhardt S, Bachmann M, Cramer M, Rotter M, Wobus A, Starzinski-Powitz A (1994) Expression of M-cadherin protein in myogenic cells during prenatal mouse development and differentiation of embryonic stem cells in culture. Dev Dyn 201:245–259

Sabourin LA, Girgis-Gabardo A, Seale P, Asakura A, Rudnicki MA (1999) Reduced differentiation potential of primary MyoD–/– myogenic cells derived from adult skeletal muscle. J Cell Biol 144:631–643

Sampaolesi M, Torrente Y, Innocenzi A, Tonlorenzi R, D'Antona G, Pellegrino MA, Barresi R, Bresolin N, De Angelis MG, Campbell KP, Bottinelli R, Cossu G (2003) Cell therapy of alpha-sarcoglycan null dystrophic mice through intra-arterial delivery of mesoangioblasts. Science 301:487–492

Schmalbruch H, Lewis DM (2000) Dynamics of nuclei of muscle fibers and connective tissue cells in normal and denervated rat muscles. Muscle Nerve 23:617–626

Seale P, Sabourin LA, Girgis-Gabardo A, Mansouri A, Gruss P, Rudnicki MA (2000) Pax7 is required for the specification of myogenic satellite cells. Cell 102:777–786

Seale P, Ishibashi J, Scime A, Rudnicki MA (2004) Pax7 is necessary and sufficient for the myogenic specification of CD45+:Sca1+ stem cells from injured muscle. PLoS Biol 2:E130

Skuk D, Goulet M, Roy B, Tremblay JP (2002) Efficacy of myoblast transplantation in nonhuman primates following simple intramuscular cell injections: toward defining strategies applicable to humans. Exp Neurol 175:112–126

Smythe GM, Hodgetts SI, Grounds MD (2000) Immunobiology and the future of myoblast transfer therapy. Mol Ther 1:304–313

Smythe GM, Hodgetts SI, Grounds MD (2001) Problems and solutions in myoblast transfer therapy. J Cell Mol Med 5:33–47

Tajbakhsh S, Borello U, Vivarelli E, Kelly R, Papkoff J, Duprez D, Buckingham M, Cossu G (1998) Differential activation of Myf5 and MyoD by different Wnts in explants of mouse paraxial mesoderm and the later activation of myogenesis in the absence of Myf5. Development 125:4155–4162

Torrente Y, El Fahime E, Caron NJ, Bresolin N, Tremblay JP (2000) Intramuscular migration of myoblasts transplanted after muscle pretreatment with metalloproteinases. Cell Transplant 9:539–549

Torrente Y, Tremblay JP, Pisati F, Belicchi M, Rossi B, Sironi M, Fortunato F, El Fahime M, D'Angelo MG, Caron NJ, Constantin G, Paulin D, Scarlato G, Bresolin N (2001) Intraarterial injection of muscle-derived CD34(+)Sca-1(+) stem cells restores dystrophin in mdx mice. J Cell Biol 152:335–348

Trowbridge IS, Thomas ML (1994) CD45: an emerging role as a protein tyrosine phosphatase required for lymphocyte activation and development. Annu Rev Immunol 12:85–116

Vilquin JT, Kinoshita I, Roy B, Goulet M, Engvall E, Tome F, Fardeau M, Tremblay JP (1996) Partial laminin alpha2 chain restoration in alpha2 chain-deficient dy/dy mouse by primary muscle cell culture transplantation. J Cell Biol 133:185–197

Wada MR, Inagawa-Ogashiwa M, Shimizu S, Yasumoto S, Hashimoto N (2002) Generation of different fates from multipotent muscle stem cells. Development 129:2987–2995

Weintraub H, Tapscott SJ, Davis RL, Thayer MJ, Adam MA, Lassar AB, Miller AD (1989) Activation of muscle-specific genes in pigment, nerve, fat, liver, and fibroblast cell lines by forced expression of MyoD. Proc Natl Acad Sci U S A 86:5434–5438

Wernig A, Zweyer M, Irintchev A (2000) Function of skeletal muscle tissue formed after myoblast transplantation into irradiated mouse muscles. J Physiol 522:333–345

Yoshida N, Yoshida S, Koishi K, Masuda K, Nabeshima Y (1998) Cell heterogeneity upon myogenic differentiation: down-regulation of MyoD and Myf-5 generates 'reserve cells'. J Cell Sci 111:769–779

Zhou S, Schuetz JD, Bunting KD, Colapietro AM, Sampath J, Morris JJ, Lagutina I, Grosveld GC, Osawa M, Nakauchi H, Sorrentino BP (2001) The ABC transporter Bcrp1/ABCG2 is expressed in a wide variety of stem cells and is a molecular determinant of the side-population phenotype. Nat Med 7:1028–1034

Zhou S, Morris JJ, Barnes Y, Lan L, Schuetz JD, Sorrentino BP (2002) Bcrp1 gene expression is required for normal numbers of side population stem cells in mice, and confers relative protection to mitoxantrone in hematopoietic cells in vivo. Proc Natl Acad Sci U S A 99:12339–12344

HEP (2006) 174:319–360
© Springer-Verlag Berlin Heidelberg 2006

Neural Stem Cells: On Where They Hide, in Which Disguise, and How We May Lure Them Out

B. Berninger (✉) · M. A. Hack · M. Götz (✉)

Institute of Stem Cell Research, GSF-National Research Center for Environment and
Health, Ingolstädter Landstrasse 1, 85764 Neuherberg, Germany
benedikt.berninger@gsf.de
magdalena.goetz@gsf.de

Ταρασσει τους ανθρωπους ου τα πραγματα αλλα τα περι των πραγματων δογματα
Not the facts but the opinions about the facts trouble men (from the *Handbook of Epictetus*)

Abstract In contrast to the haematopoietic system in which each cell type is subject to constant turnover, thus endowing this system with the permanent ability to reconstitute itself, the nervous system has long been known as an organ devoid of spontaneous cellular reconstitution. Yet the discovery that certain regions of the mammalian central nervous system do sustain neurogenesis throughout life, together with the fact that cells can be isolated from the adult brain that generate neurons in vitro, has led to the idea that the nervous tissue harbours neural stem cells. The term "neural stem cell" has now become associated with enormous expectations for curing diseases of the nervous system. Yet many of the biological fundamentals of neural stem cells need to be revealed before these expectations can be properly judged or even fulfilled. This begins with the question of whether the neural stem cell corresponds to a real entity or rather represents an in vitro dedifferentiation phenomenon. In this chapter we attempt to give an overview of our current knowledge of the biology of the presumable adult neural stem cell. This is followed by a comparative assessment of the possibilities of using adult neural stem cells and embryonic stem cells for therapeutic approaches in the context of neurodegenerative diseases. Finally, we will look at the "evil side" of stemness by discussing the evidence that brain cancers may originate from cells with stem cell-like properties.

Keywords Adult neurogenesis · Stem cell niche · Neuronal differentiation · Cell replacement therapy · Brain cancer

1
Introductory Remarks

Even though continuous generation of neurons in specific regions of the adult central nervous system was already observed several decades ago (Altman and Das 1965; Altman 1969; Kaplan and Bell 1984), it was first met with strong scepticism. But recent years have vindicated these early observations and a new field has emerged devoted to the study of the biology and function of adult neural "stem cells". These developments also have nurtured the idea that adult neural stem cells may ultimately allow for the regeneration of neurons that die as a consequence of disease or trauma. Obviously, in order to build a safe fundament for such hopes, we need to have a thorough knowledge of these still quite mysterious cells. Mysterious above all because there is still no way to identify them prospectively either in vivo or in vitro. Therefore, we must start with a discussion of what we actually know about the biology of the adult neural stem cell and to which extent the term "stem cell" is appropriate or not.

2
The Biology of the Adult Neural Stem Cell

2.1
What, If Anything, Is a Neural Stem Cell?

The hallmarks that characterize a stem cell are as follows: (a) the ability to self renew, i.e. to give rise to progeny with identical properties and (b) multipotency, i.e. to give rise to progeny of distinct cellular lineages (Weissman 2000). Accordingly, the stem cell is placed at the base of a lineage tree (Fig. 1), presupposing a hierarchy of cells of ever more restricted fate and largely assuming that progressive specifications are not reversible. Part of a tentative definition may also include (c) the idea that a stem cell must be able to replicate itself ad infinitum

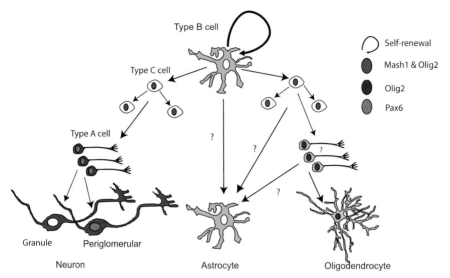

Fig. 1 A scheme illustrating the hierarchical specification of distinct neural progeny of adult olfactory neurogenesis. Stem cells (type B cells) with self-renewal capacity give rise to fast proliferating transit-amplifying (type C) cells and these in turn into fate-restricted progenitors, i.e. neuroblasts (type A cells) and may be also glioblasts that ultimately generate neurons, oligodendrocytes and possibly astrocytes. Shown is the expression of key fate determinants, where known. Pax6 is required for specifying neuronal fate at the neuroblast stage, while at later postmitotic stages Pax6 instructs a dopaminergic fate. The proneural gene Mash1 is expressed in transit-amplifying precursors and some neuroblasts and plays a role for specification of both neuronal and oligodendroglial lineages. Olig2 is expressed in all transit-amplifying precursors and plays a crucial role in their specification and maintenance. Downregulation of Olig2 is necessary for progression along the neuronal lineages, while its maintenance imparts an oligodendroglial fate at subsequent stages

(or at least during the entire life time of the animal) without loss of its developmental potential, yet there is evidence of an age-dependent decline of stem cells in many organs, such as the skeletal muscle (Conboy and Rando 2005) and liver (Iakova et al. 2003), ultimately leading to exhaustion of regenerative capacity.

Do cells that meet these criteria really exist in the adult mammalian nervous system? Indeed there are regions in the adult brain where neurogenesis persists throughout adulthood (Gage 2000; Alvarez-Buylla et al. 2002), suggestive of the presence of multipotent stem cells. Moreover, these regions harbour precursors that in principle have the potential to generate cells of all three neural, i.e. neuronal, astroglial and oligodendroglial, lineages (Reynolds and Weiss 1992; Rietze et al. 2001). Yet in vivo these cells give rise foremost to progenitors that already express many neuronal traits and appear to be firmly restricted to this lineage (Luskin 1993, 1998), following a similar cascade of hierarchical fate restrictions that takes place during development (Price and Thurlow 1988; Grove et al. 1993; Walsh and Cepko 1993). Thus, the starting point of our discussion will be the question of which cells in the adult brain meet the stringent criteria listed above. As we will see, these criteria are more easily defined than verified.

2.2
The "Who's Who" of Adult Neurogenesis

In the adult brain of most mammalian species, two regions have been identified where neurogenesis takes place at a surprisingly significant rate throughout life, including in humans (Eriksson et al. 1998; Bedard and Parent 2004; Sanai et al. 2004). One of these is the adult dentate gyrus of the hippocampal formation, where new neurons are born in the subgranular zone (SGZ) (Altman and Das 1965; Kaplan and Bell 1984) and then migrate a few cell diameters upward into the granular layer, where they differentiate into bona fide granule neurons (Cameron et al. 1993). The other example of adult neurogenesis appears to be more elaborate: here neurons are derived from progenitors residing in the lateral wall of the lateral ventricle, commonly called subependymal (SEZ) or subventricular zone (Altman 1969; Lois and Alvarez-Buylla 1993; Lois and Alvarez-Buylla 1994). Within this SEZ, morphological and molecular characterization has resulted in the classification of four cell types (Doetsch et al. 1997):

1. The ependymal or type E cell that lines the ventricle surface

2. A cell commonly called type B cell that displays ultra-structural and molecular features of an astrocyte

3. The so-called type C or transit amplifying cells

4. The neuroblasts or type A cells that already exhibit neuronal features such as β III-tubulin expression (Luskin 1998)

These type A cells migrate in chains through tunnels created by type B cells along the rostral migratory stream (RMS) towards the olfactory bulb (Doetsch and Alvarez-Buylla 1996; Lois et al. 1996), where they differentiate into different classes of neurons (Doetsch and Alvarez-Buylla 1996; Carleton et al. 2003). It has been a matter of controversy as to which cell type is the genuine stem cell that gives rise to these distinct cells. Originally, arguments for both a subpopulation of ependymal cells (Johansson et al. 1999) as well as type B cells (Doetsch et al. 1999a) were raised, but the evidence for the former could not be reproduced (Chiasson et al. 1999; Laywell et al. 2000; Capela and Temple 2002). Studies in which the SEZ was temporarily depleted of fast-proliferating cells using the anti-mitotic agent cytosine-β-D-arabinofuranoside (Ara-C), thereby deleting neurogenesis completely, revealed that cells positive for glial fibrillary acidic protein (GFAP) and displaying ultra-structural astrocyte characteristics were able to reconstitute all other adult precursors and re-establish neurogenesis (Doetsch et al. 1999a). This data clearly demonstrates that astrocytes are able to reconstitute the other types of precursors and, hence, reside at the base of the lineage tree. While in the presence of Ara-C the SEZ was devoid of both type C and type A cells, removal of the drug resulted first in the reappearance of type C cells and subsequently type A cells (Doetsch et al. 1999b), consistent with the premise that type B cells generate the transit-amplifying type C cells, which in turn give rise to type A cells (Fig. 1). Moreover, lineage tracing using the replication competent avian leukosis (RCAS) virus in transgenic mice expressing the viral receptor TVA under control of the human GFAP promoter revealed that GFAP-positive cells give rise to neurons in the olfactory bulb (Doetsch et al. 1999a). This conclusion was recently corroborated by the fact that elimination of the GFAP-positive cell population in the adult SEZ by genetically targeted thymidine kinase expression (which sensitizes these cells to the pro-drug ganciclovir) also eliminates adult neurogenesis in the olfactory bulb (Garcia et al. 2004).

When do type B cells first appear in the brain and from where do they originate? Interestingly, it has been shown that the subependymal astrocyte and its progeny are derived from radial gliaof the early postnatal ventral pallium/dorsal subpallium (Alvarez-Buylla et al. 2001; Stenman et al. 2003; Tramontin et al. 2003; Merkle et al. 2004). Radial glia were genetically marked at birth by means of local transduction with adenoviral vectors encoding the Cre-recombinase in reporter mice that allow for the visualization of Cre-recombinase activity (Merkle et al. 2004). These experiments showed that the Cre-induced genetic modification was inherited to type B and to type C cells as well as to adult neuroblasts in the RMS and adult-born neurons within the olfactory bulb. Notably, labelled radial glial cells gave rise not only to the precursors of adult neurons and their progeny, but also to ependymal cells lining the ventricle wall and oligodendrocytes residing in the corpus callosum and the striatum, consistent with previous data of radial glial cells genetically labelled at yet earlier stages (Malatesta et al. 2003). It will be interesting to know in more detail how this metamorphosis from radial glia to specific types of astrocytes that remain in the subependyma takes place. Notably, many radial glial cells transform into astrocytes at the end of neurogenesis, but only a few remain in the subependyma and only subependymal astrocytes lining the lateral wall of the lateral ventricle seemingly retain the potential to generate neurons throughout life. For the earlier role of radial glial cells in neurogenesis, see the review by Götz et al. (2002).

2.3
The Stem Cell Character of the Astrocyte

2.3.1
The Subependymal Zone Stem Cell

Given that the most widely accepted model of adult subependymal neurogenesis currently proposes that it is a subpopulation of GFAP-positive astrocytes that functions as stem cells (Fig. 1), we may briefly examine whether these cells fulfil the general criteria of a stem cell. The fact that GFAP-positive astrocytes can reconstitute the entire compartment of dividing cells in the SEZ (Doetsch et al. 1999a) suggests that these cells do indeed possess the ability of self-renewal. Whether these cells have an "infinite" self-renewal capacity, however, is not known. Like other tissue-specific stem cells, there is evidence for an age-related decrease in progenitor proliferation (Enwere et al. 2004). Finally, there is no direct in vivo proof that these cells are truly multipotent, i.e. that a single GFAP-positive astrocyte can give rise to a clone consisting of neurons, astrocytes and oligodendrocytes (tripotent precursor). All evidence for the multipotency of SEZ stem cells has been derived in vitro using the so-called neurosphere assay system (Reynolds and Weiss 1992). In this assay, cells are cultured in nonadherent conditions at clonal density in the presence of mitogens such as epidermal growth factor (EGF) and fibroblast growth factor-2 (FGF2). Under these conditions, presumable stem cells generate clonal aggregates called neurospheres. The multipotency of the original stem cell is then assessed by allowing cells derived from a single sphere to differentiate. If progeny of all three neural cell types, i.e. astrocytes, oligodendrocytes and neurons, is produced, this is taken as evidence for multipotency of the cell of origin. Likewise, when a neurosphere can give rise to secondary neurospheres upon dissociation, this is taken as proof for self-renewal capacity of the founder cell of the primary neurosphere. From the adult SEZ neurospheres can indeed be obtained that possess a long-term self-renewal capacity (forming secondary, tertiary, etc. neurospheres) and multipotency (giving rise to neurons, astrocytes and oligodendrocytes when allowed to differentiate) (Reynolds and Weiss 1992; Rietze et al. 2001; Seaberg and van der Kooy 2002). Yet cells are severely altered in the neurosphere assay and hence may acquire multipotency only in vitro (Gabay et al. 2003; Hack et al. 2004). Finally, there is a controversy whether the actual neurosphere-forming cell is the GFAP-positive type B cell (Morshead et al. 2003) or rather the fast-proliferating type C cell (Doetsch et al. 2002). Type C cells can be distinguished from type B cells by their expression of the transcription factor Dlx2, which allowed Doetsch and colleagues to selectively kill type C cells by genetic targeting of thymidine kinase to these cells (Doetsch et al. 2002). The result was a drastic reduction in the number of neurospheres. These data were further supported by the fact that in vivo EGF seemingly acts on the rapidly dividing type C cells, which express high levels of EGF receptor (Doetsch et al. 2002). EGF not only promoted proliferation of these cells, but also steered progeny towards an astroglial fate at the expense of neurogenesis. Yet using a similar genetic approach, Morshead and colleagues were able to eliminate neurosphere formation by ablation of GFAP-positive type B cells (Morshead et al. 2003). The crucial problem hampering the precise interpretation of these contradictory results may stem from the experimental read out: neurospheres can be discerned as such only upon having reached a certain size. Thus, even though a sphere may be originally initiated by a slow-dividing GFAP-positive cell, the bulk of the cells within a sphere are likely to be fast-proliferating type C-like cells and hence elimination of these cells interferes with neurosphere formation. Consistent with abundance of type C cells in neurospheres is the observation that they contain many cells positive for the basic helix-loop-helix transcription factor Olig2, which is expressed within the SEZ in fast-proliferating type C cells (Hack et al. 2004), while only low levels of GFAP can be detected in neurospheres (Morshead et al. 2003). Thus, the bulk of neurosphere cells may reflect the fast-proliferating transit-amplifying precursors in vivo. Moreover, many regions of the central nervous system (CNS) without any apparent levels of adult neurogenesis can also give rise to neurosphere-forming cells (Weiss et al. 1996; Johansson et al. 1999; Palmer et al. 1999; Nunes et al. 2003). This indicates that the potential to form neurospheres does not necessarily reflect the presence of stem cells or their behaviour in vivo. Indeed, Olig2 expression in neurosphere cells in vitro and in type C cells in the adult SEZ is crucial for the specification of these cells as transit-amplifying precursors. Interference with Olig2 expression via short interfering RNA in vitro drastically reduces the number of neurosphere-forming cells (Hack et al. 2004) and retrovirally mediated expression of a dominant-negative construct of Olig2 in the adult SEZ in vivo virtually deletes all transit-amplifying precursor cells (Hack et al. 2005). Conversely, Olig2 overexpression in the adult SEZ expands the number of transit-amplifying precursors (Hack et al. 2005). Taken together, neurosphere cells are fast proliferating undifferentiated precursors that resemble the transit-amplifying precursors more than the slow-dividing stem cells seen in vivo.

2.3.2
The Subgranular Zone Stem Cell

Like in the SEZ, when actively dividing cells were killed in the hippocampal SGZ with Ara-C, GFAP-positive cells were capable of restoring neurogenesis upon removal of the drug (Seri et al. 2001), suggesting that these cells also have self-renewal capacity in vivo, even though their neurosphere-forming capacity has limitations (Seaberg and van der Kooy 2002). As in the SEZ, deletion of GFAP-positive cells by transgenic expression of thymidine kinase also abrogated the generation of new neurons (Garcia et al. 2004), indicating that also in the SGZ newly generated neurons are derived from astrocytes. Yet, the stem cell character of these GFAP-positive cells has been contested and it has been suggested that the SGZ harbours restricted progenitors instead of multipotent cells with long-term self-renewal capacity (Seaberg and van der Kooy 2002). This suggestion was based on the finding that primary adult SGZ neurospheres cannot give rise to secondary spheres and their progeny appear to be fate-restricted, generating clones comprised of only neuronal or glial cells. Yet, as we have seen above, the neurosphere assay is not really adequate to assess the presence of stem cells within a tissue. Curiously enough, type C cells that may be the actual neurosphere-forming cells from SEZ tissue (Doetsch et al. 2002) seem to be absent from the SGZ, in which exclusively GFAP-positive astrocytes and precursors with neuronal traits have been identified (Seri et al. 2001, 2004). Moreover, the growth factors EGF or FGF2 used to expand neurosphere cells may simply fail to induce multipotency in these cells. Ultimately it is not clear which mitogens are the ones that would make the real stem cell proliferate. The devil's advocate will have an easy pleading when claiming that the neurosphere assay will not provide the definitive answer to the question of whether or not a given cell may be a stem cell. A more appropriate assay would have to mimic more closely the local environment in which stem cells find themselves in vivo.

In conclusion, if neural stem cells are defined as potentially uni- or bipotent precursors with self-renewal capacity in the adult mammalian brain, we may call GFAP-positive cells in the SEZ and SGZ neural stem cells. While no definite dogma on the stem cell nature of GFAP-positive astrocytes or their direct descendants can yet be promulgated at this point, we are dealing here certainly with remarkable cells, as they are able to generate and regenerate neurons throughout life. In this regard, we will refer to them henceforth as neural stem cells. Importantly, generation of new neurons has been observed both in the adult human SGZ (Eriksson et al. 1998) and the olfactory bulb (Bedard and Parent 2004). However, the cellular organization of the human SEZ departs radically from the architecture observed in other mammalian species, including nonhuman primates (Kornack and Rakic 2001b; Pencea et al. 2001): within the human SEZ, there are no chains of migrating neuroblasts, but instead a dense ribbon of GFAP-positive astrocytes that are spatially separated from the ependyma by a gap (Sanai et al. 2004). Yet these ribbon astrocytes proliferate in vivo and neurosphere-forming cells can be isolated from the human SEZ that exhibit multipotency (Sanai et al. 2004). Since a RMS as found in other mammalian species cannot be discerned in the human brain, the lineage relationship between the GFAP-positive cells in the human SEZ and the adult-born neurons in the olfactory bulb remains elusive.

2.3.3
Searching for a Stem Cell Marker

As will have become obvious from the preceding discussion, the entire field would greatly benefit from the discovery of specific and unambiguous stem cell markers allowing for the prospective isolation of neural stem cells. GFAP expression cannot be used to identify stem cells, as many GFAP-positive astrocytes exist throughout the adult brain that do not possess stem cell properties. Likewise, the intermediate filament protein nestin is expressed by all kinds of neural progenitors including type B, C and A cells, hence precluding specific isolation of putative stem cells (Gritti et al. 2002). A method adopted from the haematopoiesis field to make out stem cells is called side population analysis. It is based on the happenstance that haematopoietic stem cells possess a transport mechanism that results in the high efflux of Hoechst dye (a DNA-binding dye), which allows isolation of these cells due to their low fluorescence intensity from the bulk population (Goodell et al. 1996; Goodell et al. 1997). Side population analysis performed on adult derived neurospheres likewise results in a marked enrichment of cells forming secondary neurospheres (Kim and Morshead 2003). More recently, the carbohydrate LewisX(LeX)/ssea-1 was shown to be expressed on the surface of a rare population of SEZ cells in vivo and in vitro and isolating LeX-positive cells again resulted in an enrichment of neurosphere-forming cells (Capela and Temple 2002). Notably, however, LeX immunoreactivity is localized mostly to transit-amplifying precursors. Other criteria such as low levels of proteins binding peanut agglutinin and of heat stable antigen (mCD24a) were also reported to enrich for cells with neurosphere-forming activity (Rietze et al. 2001). However, the problem with all these methods is that they are based on the assumption that stem and neurosphere-forming cells are the very same cells. As pointed out above, such an assumption is highly questionable.

The identification of the GFAP-positive astrocytes in the adult SEZ and SGZ as the source of adult neurogenesis and the fact that radial glia also act as neuronal precursors during development (Malatesta et al. 2000, 2003; Noctor et al. 2001) has led to the concept that astrocytes may not represent terminally differentiated cells, but rather highly plastic cells that can be driven towards various cell fates depending on extrinsic and intrinsic contexts (Heins et al. 2002). Yet most astrocytes do not act as adult neural stem cells, since in most regions of the adult brain neurogenesis does not take place even though astrocytes are the most prominent cellular component. Furthermore, even in neurogenic regions such as the SEZ and SGZ, it is not clear whether all the dividing GFAP-positive cells have neural stem cell characteristics. Thus, we must now turn to the question of why significant neurogenesis is restricted to some regions by asking what makes the environment, in which adult neurogenesis continues, so special.

2.4
The Stem Cell Niche

From a plethora of different tissue-specific stem cell systems and organisms, the concept of a so-called stem cell niche has emerged (Spradling et al. 2001; Fuchs et al. 2004). The stem cell niche represents a local environment which provides the extrinsic signals to maintain a certain part of the total stem cell pool in a quiescent state while permitting the other to enter the cell cycle and undergo either symmetric or asymmetric cell divisions, thereby contributing to stem cell self-renewal and generation of a differentiated progeny. What factors determine whether a stem cell stays quiescent or undergoes self-renewal or cellular differentiation? These questions embody some of the most fascinating and unresolved issues of stem cell biology. What are the mechanisms that ensure the maintenance of a stem cell pool and prevent it from premature exhaustion? The key question then is how extrinsic factors provided by the niche act on the intrinsic machinery within the stem cell to determine subsequent fate decisions. But let's first ask the question, what are the cellular components that make up the niche for neurogenesis in the adult brain.

2.4.1
Creating a Niche for Neurogenesis: Ependyma, Astrocytes and Endothelial Cells

Besides the above-mentioned protagonists, i.e. the putative stem cells, transit-amplifying precursors and more fate-restricted progeny, distinct cell types appear to play an important role in creating the local milieu necessary for the maintaining the SEZ and SGZ as germinal zones for adult neurogenesis (Doetsch 2003; Alvarez-Buylla and Lim 2004). Within these germinal zones, neural precursors maintain close contact with astrocytes, blood vessels, and in case of the SEZ, with the ependyma (Doetsch 2003). Moreover, some of the type B cells, i.e. the presumable stem cells, maintain physical contact to the ventricular fluid and often extend a single cilium lacking a central pair of microtubules, a structural motif shared with early neuroepithelial cells (Doetsch et al. 1999b). This may suggest that some substances present in the cerebrospinal fluid, e.g. molecules secreted by the choroid plexus, participate in the regulation of adult neurogenesis.

A cell type with good credentials to play an important role in setting the stage for adult neurogenesis is the astrocyte itself. Dividing precursors maintain very close physical contact with astrocytes in the SEZ and the SGZ (Lim and Alvarez-Buylla 1999; Song et al. 2002a). Consistent with a functional meaning of these contacts, astrocytes have been shown to exert an, albeit modest, neurogenic influence in vitro on adult progenitor cells (Lim and Alvarez-Buylla 1999; Song et al. 2002a). The fact that the stem cell itself can also be considered an astrocyte begs the interesting question about the lineage relationship between the "stem cell"-astrocyte and the fate instructing "tutor"-astrocyte. Does the "tutor"-astrocyte also possess stem cell potential or is it itself an adult-born progeny of a stem cell? It is worth mentioning here that a similar dual nature, as precursor and as "tutor", is typical of radial glia during embryonic cortical development (Campbell and Götz 2002).

Images of striking beauty show the most intimate relationship of neural precursors with microcapillaries (Palmer et al. 2000). Surprisingly, in the SGZ of the dentate gyrus, endothelial cells were found not only to serve as a passive scaffold for the dividing neural precursors, but to be actively engaged in cell division, suggesting local angiogenesis and vascular remodeling concomitant with neurogenesis (Palmer et al. 2000). Based on such observations, the term of a "vascular niche" for neurogenesis was coined (Palmer et al. 2000). Direct evidence for a role of angiogenesis in the regulation of neurogenesis stems from studies on adult canaries. It was found that testosterone, which stimulates neurogenesis in the higher vocal centre of the bird neostriatum, also promoted angiogenesis, and this effect was mediated through upregulation of vascular endothelial growth factor (VEGF) and its receptor on endothelial cells, which led to the production of the neurotrophin brain-derived neurotrophic factor (BDNF) (Louissaint et al. 2002). However, VEGF appears also to exert direct effects on neural precursors. VEGF administration increased bromod-eoxyuridine (BrdU) incorporation both in the SEZ and the SGZ (Jin et al. 2002; Schanzer et al. 2004). Interestingly, it has been shown that endothelial cells can suppress the differentiation of embryonic cortical and adult SEZ progenitors, promoting symmetric cell divisions (Shen et al. 2004). When inserts of endothelial cells were cultured above neural progenitors, proliferation of the latter was enhanced and they remained in an undifferentiated state. Upon removal of the endothelial insert, progenitors started to differentiate. Importantly, they produced more neurons than progenitors grown in the absence of endothelial cells, thus suggesting that the latter might also be involved in providing neurogenic signals.

2.4.2
Extrinsic Factors Regulating Neurogenesis

The molecular mechanisms by which the distinct cells comprising the stem cell niche regulate the behaviour of stem and progenitor cells are poorly understood, yet a number of molecules have been implicated. We will briefly introduce only some of those thought to be among the protagonists.

2.4.2.1
EGF and FGF2 Receptor Signalling

Neurosphere formation in vitro depends on the presence of mitogens such as EGF and FGF2 in the media. Yet the extent to which EGF and FGF2 signal in the adult SEZ or SGZ in vivo is not clear. In vivo EGF receptor signalling may be elicited not by EGF itself but by its alternative ligand transforming growth factor-α (TGF-α) (Wilcox and Derynck 1988; Weickert and Blum 1995). Both TGF-$\alpha^{-/-}$ and Waved-1 mutant mice, TGF-α hypomorphs, show reduced levels of proliferation within the SEZ and olfactory neurogenesis (Tropepe et al. 1997; Enwere et al. 2004). Intraventricular injection of EGF receptor ligands induces massive proliferation in the SEZ (Craig et al. 1996; Kuhn et al. 1997; Doetsch et al. 2002), but does not enhance olfactory neurogenesis (Kuhn et al. 1997; Doetsch et al. 2002). Exogenous EGF appears to act primarily on type C cells, which express high amounts of EGF receptor (Doetsch et al. 2002). Surprisingly, however, type C cells drastically stray from their normal behaviour under the influence of exogenous EGF in that neuronal commitment is inhibited and instead astrocyte-like cells are generated that invade the parenchyma (Kuhn et al. 1997; Doetsch et al. 2002). As discussed below, EGF receptor gene amplification is a common feature of many brain cancers. These data thus suggest that under normal conditions EGF receptor activation is likely to be tightly controlled. In contrast to EGF, exogenous administration of FGF2 enhances neurogenesis of olfactory bulb interneurons (Kuhn et al. 1997). In FGF2-deficient mice, proliferation in the SEZ and olfactory neurogenesis is reduced, suggesting a role for endogenous FGF2 in the adult SEZ (Zheng et al. 2004).

2.4.2.2
Notch

Signalling through Notch receptors inhibits neurogenesis (Nye et al. 1994; Morrison et al. 2000; Tanigaki et al. 2001). Upon ligand-dependent activation and proteolytic cleavage of the Notch receptor, an intracellular portion translocates to the nucleus where it stimulates Notch-dependent gene transcription (Artavanis-Tsakonas et al. 1999). Notch signalling blocks neuronal differentiation via the induction of the mammalian hairy/enhancer-of-split homologues Hes1 and Hes5, which encode for basic helix-loop-helix transcription factors (Kageyama and Ohtsuka 1999; Ohtsuka et al. 1999). Controversy has arisen as to whether Notch signalling maintains stem cell multipotency or actively instructs a glial cell fate (Morrison et al. 2000; Tanigaki et al. 2001; Hitoshi et al. 2002). Transient Notch activation induced by exogenous Notch ligand has been reported to cause a rapid and irreversible loss of neurogenic capacity accompanied by accelerated glial differentiation in neural crest cells (Morrison et al. 2000). Likewise, activated Notch1 or Notch3 were found to induce GFAP-expression in FGF2-expanded adult hippocampal progenitors, a finding that was interpreted as evidence for a commitment towards an astroglial fate, even though the cells continued to express high levels of nestin (Tanigaki et al. 2001). Yet, neurosphere-forming cells are depleted in mice deficient in Notch1 or key regulators of Notch signalling activity such as RBK-Jκ or presenilin (Hitoshi et al. 2002). Likewise simultaneous deficiency in both Hes1 and Hes5 results in a drastic reduction of neurosphere-forming cells (Ohtsuka et al. 2001). Moreover, transient misexpression of Hes1 and Hes5 maintains embryonic cortical progenitors in an undifferentiated state, but it does not prevent subsequent neuronal differentiation when forced Hes expression ceases, arguing that Notch signalling does not instruct gliogenesis but serves to maintain neural precursors in a self-renewing state (Ohtsuka et al. 2001). Such an interpretation is consistent with findings showing that Hes1 can preserve long-term reconstituting activity of haematopoietic stem cells in vitro (Kunisato et al. 2003). Forced expression of activated Notch1 in mouse embryonic forebrain by retroviral transduction revealed that Notch-infected cells acquire morphological and molecular characteristics of radial glia (Gaiano et al. 2000). While originally thought to be part of the glial lineage, it has been firmly established that proliferative radial glial function as neuronal precursors in the developing brain (Malatesta et al. 2000, 2003; Noctor et al. 2001). Hence the finding that activated Notch induces a radial glial phenotype in early neural progenitors is again consistent with the possibility that Notch signalling maintains cells in a precursor state rather than promoting terminal differentiation into astrocytes. During postnatal development, many of the Notch-infected cells eventually were found to become periventricular astrocytes (i.e. type B cells) (Gaiano et al. 2000), which may not come as a surprise given the fact that type B cells of the SEZ are generated from radial glia (Merkle et al. 2004). In skeletal muscle, an age-related decline in Notch signalling has been shown to underlie the progressive decrease in proliferation and myogenic lineage progression of satellite cells and reduced muscle repair (Conboy et al. 2003). Remarkably, the decline in Notch signalling appears to be due to systemic serum factors and exposure to a young systemic environment can "rejuvenate" aged satellite cells (Conboy et al. 2005). It remains to be established whether the age-dependent decline in neural progenitor proliferation (Kuhn et al. 1996; Enwere et al. 2004) is similarly due to systemic changes affecting Notch signalling, rather than due to a cell-autonomous loss of progenitor function.

2.4.2.3
Bone Morphogenetic Proteins

The most striking property of the neurogenic niches of the SEZ and SGZ is that they are permissive for neurogenesis in contrast to all other regions of the adult mammalian CNS. If we understood the underlying molecular mechanisms we would also have a clue how to allow for neurogenesis in most of the other, non-neurogenic regions in the adult mammalian brain. One molecular mechanism proposed to be involved in creating a neurogenic niche in the SEZ is the local antagonistic interplay between noggin or related molecules and the various members of the bone morphogenetic proteins (BMPs) (Lim et al. 2000). Noggin counteracts the effects of BMPs by binding and thereby scavenging BMPs, hence preventing the signal cascade elicited by binding of BMPs to their cognate receptors (Balemans and Van Hul 2002). Within the SEZ BMP-2, -4 and 7 are strongly expressed (Lim et al. 2000; Liu et al. 2004; Peretto et al. 2004), particularly in astroglial, hence type B cells (Peretto et al. 2004). The primary effect of these BMPs is to inhibit neurogenesis and promote an astroglial fate, both in vivo and in vitro (Lim et al. 2000; Gomes et al. 2003). Yet, these anti-neurogenic effects of BMPs are counteracted by the local secretion of the BMP antagonist noggin from ependymal cells (Lim et al. 2000) and may be also type B cells (Peretto et al. 2004). These findings suggest a model in which neurogenesis occurs within the narrow range of a local noggin source (Lim et al. 2000). Interestingly, BMPs and noggin are also expressed along the RMS (Peretto et al. 2004), suggesting that the RMS may not only serve as a migratory highway towards the olfactory bulb, but it may also harbour stem cells and permit neurogenesis (Gritti et al. 2002). Whether the same scenario also plays a role in creating a neurogenic niche within the hippocampus has not been experimentally tested, but there is strong noggin expression in the dentate gyrus (Peretto et al. 2004). An exciting therapeutic implication of the antagonism between BMPs and noggin or related molecules is the possibility that it may enable us to create a permissive environment for neurogenesis in a priori non-neurogenic regions of the adult brain by local delivery of BMP antagonists (Lim et al. 2000; Chmielnicki et al. 2004).

2.4.2.4
Sonic Hedgehog

Often signals that play an important role during development are reemployed in adulthood. A classical example is sonic hedgehog (Shh), a molecule that performs important patterning functions during development and is known to promote cell proliferation in external granule cells of the cerebellum (see also Sect. 4 for discussion on Shh signalling in brain cancers) (Ho and Scott 2002). Shh was also shown to influence cell proliferation in the SGZ and SEZ (Lai et al. 2003; Machold et al. 2003; Palma et al. 2005) by acting not only on transit-amplifying precursors, but more importantly also on GFAP-positive cells, i.e. the presumable SVZ stem cell (Palma et al. 2005). Low levels of Shh mRNA and Gli1 mRNA expression, the latter being an indicator of active Shh signalling, were detected in the lateral wall of the lateral ventricles. Notably, only about 20% of the GFAP-positive cells expressed Gli1. Provided that the other 80% GFAP-positive cells indeed comprised part of the stem cell population, this might hint at the possibility that stem cell proliferation could be tightly controlled by assigning Shh responsiveness only to a subpopulation of the total stem cell pool whilst maintaining the other in a quiescent state. The physiological relevance of these findings were further underscored by the fact that cyclopamine treatment, an inhibitor of Shh signalling, reduced BrdU incorporation in the adult SEZ and caused a marked reduction in the number of newly generated granule neurons in the olfactory bulb. Shh may play a similar role in the adult hippocampus where it is expressed in the hilus, thus close to the site where hippocampal stem cells reside (Dahmane et al. 2001; Lai et al. 2003; Machold et al. 2003). Alternatively, Shh might be provided to the hippocampus via axonal projections from the septum (Traiffort et al. 1999). Finally, given the fact that components of the self-renewal machinery of stem cells are commonly implicated in carcinogenesis, it is not surprising that in many brain cancers elements of the Shh signalling pathway are affected (see Sect. 4).

2.4.3
Intrinsic Molecular Machinery Underlying Stem Cell Self-Renewal

Our knowledge of the intrinsic molecular machinery responsible for preserving the pool of neural stem cells is at best fragmentary. While essentially nothing is known about the mechanisms that maintain part of the neural stem cells in a quiescent state, some preliminary progress has been made regarding our understanding of the molecular components responsible for stem cell self-renewal. For instance, it has been suggested that the orphan nuclear receptor tailless/TLX is part of the self-renewal process of adult neural progenitors and deficiency in the TLX gene is associated with a reduction in nestin-positive precursor cells in the adult SGZ and SEZ (Shi et al. 2004). Interestingly, during cortical development the Tlx gene appears to regulate the timing of neurogenesis by influencing the decision of precursor cells to proliferate or differentiate through a mechanism that may involve the regulation of cell cycle transit time (Roy et al. 2004). For instance, precocious neurogenesis observed in the cortex of Tlx-deficient mice may lead to shortened cell cycle of precursors in order to replenish the depleting precursor pool (Roy et al. 2004) (see also later in this section, the discussion on cell cycle length and asymmetric cell division).

The polycomb group transcriptional repressor Bmi-1 has also been suggested to regulate stem cell renewal. First, it had been shown that Bmi-1 is required for the maintenance of adult haematopoietic stems cells (HSCs) (Lessard and Sauvageau 2003; Park et al. 2003). Deficiency in Bmi-1 leads to an upregulation (due to de-repression) of the cell cycle inhibitors p16Ink4a and p19Arf and thereby causes proliferative arrest in HSCs, ultimately resulting in depletion of the HSC pool. Importantly, transplantation of Bmi-1-deficient HSCs into secondary recipients permitted only transient reconstitution of haematopoiesis, presumably because the Bmi-1-deficient cells failed to sustain the precursor pool, i.e. stem cells capable of self-renewal were missing. Recently, Molofsky and colleagues have suggested a similar role of Bmi-1 in the self-renewal of adult neural stem cells (Molofsky et al. 2003). The authors used the neurosphere assay to assess multipotency, proliferation and self-renewal. The lack of Bmi-1 resulted in a reduced number of neurosphere-forming cells and this phenotype further worsened during development into adulthood (Molofsky et al. 2003). Moreover, neurospheres were also smaller and generated less secondary neurospheres in the absence of Bmi-1. These data indicate that both the number and proliferation of neurosphere-forming cells is affected by Bmi-1. Since, however, the identity of the neurosphere-forming cells is not known (either stem cells or transit-amplifying precursors), these data may be explained by depletion and reduced proliferation of either or both cell types. Indeed, fast-proliferating precursors in the adult (P30) SEZ labelled by a short pulse of BrdU were reduced in Bmi-1 mutant mice, consistent with an increase in the expression of the cyclin-dependent kinase inhibitors p16Inka and p19Arf. Most interestingly, these inhibitors are only upregulated in Bmi-1 mutant mice at postnatal stages and thus represent one of the few molecular correlates of differences between embryonic and adult precursors. Consistent with a role of Bmi-1 in fast-proliferating precursors, Bmi-1 is also contained in fast-proliferating and even fate-committed precursors in the external granule layer of the developing cerebellum (Leung et al. 2004). Accordingly, the cerebellum of Bmi-1 mutant mice is reduced in size and the animals are ataxic

(Jacobs et al. 1999; Leung et al. 2004). Notably, Shh rapidly upregulates Bmi-1 expression (Leung et al. 2004) and lack of Bmi-1 also dampens the proliferative action of Shh on progenitors of cerebellar granule neurons. Thus it is conceivable that some of the above-discussed effect of Shh on neural stem cells in the adult SEZ and SGZ may be mediated by Bmi-1.

Thus, the molecules regulating specifically self-renewal remain elusive, but many factors affect proliferation of adult neural precursors, indicating that there is a tight control of this parameter. One possible mechanism to achieve self-renewal is via asymmetric cell division. In this scenario, a stem cell divides and generates two distinct daughter cells: a stem cell identical to itself (self-renewal) and a more differentiated precursor cell, e.g. a transit-amplifying precursor. However, stem cell self-renewal may as well be achieved by symmetric cell division of a pool of stem cells, some of which then generate again two stem cells, while others produce two already fate-restricted descendants. Both models can explain the plasticity of stem cell self-renewal upon a lesion when more precursors generate offspring undergoing differentiation, if required. In the first setting, stem cells may simply divide more often symmetrically than asymmetrically, while in the second case, in which most stem cells divide symmetrically, more of them would generate two transit-amplifying precursors. Interestingly, a recent study examined the orientation of cell division along the adult SEZ in rats subjected to stroke (Zhang et al. 2004). The authors of this study observed an apparent change in the orientation of cell division from predominantly horizontal to vertical cleavage planes. These data would be consistent with an asymmetric cell division of adult neural precursors occurring horizontally by separating fate determinants distributed unequally along the apico-basal axis. While the unequal distribution of apico-basal fate determinants by cell division orthogonal to the apico-basal axis (i.e. horizontally) is a well-described mechanism of asymmetric cell division in the developing nervous system from *Drosophila* to vertebrates (Huttner and Brand 1997; Wodarz and Huttner 2003; Götz and Huttner 2005), there is no direct evidence for this mechanism in adult neural stem cells yet. Notably, however, adult neural stem cells seem to be the only cells in the adult SEZ with access to the ventricle, except the nondividing ependymal cells (Doetsch et al. 1999b, 2002; Capela and Temple 2002), where apical membrane specializations may occur (Kosodo et al. 2004). This may allow these astrocytes with access to the ventricle to divide asymmetrically by unequally distributing their apical membrane. Typically, astrocytes in the parenchyma have contact to the basement membrane surrounding the blood vessels. Future experiments will have to address which of these potential sources of apico-basal polarity is indeed functionally relevant and whether or not access to the ventricle may hold the key to understanding the difference between astrocytes acting as adult neural stem cells and the ordinary astrocytes in the parenchyma (for discussion see Götz and Steindler 2003).

Interestingly, a common cell biological hallmark of self-renewing stem cells in various organs seems to be their slow cell cycle. Indeed, label-retaining cells dividing so slowly that they retain a label incorporated during cell division that is diluted by all other much faster dividing precursors are considered as stem cells in several organ systems (Cotsarelis et al. 1990; Clarke et al. 2003; Bickenbach 2005). This raises the cell biology issue of whether cell cycle length and the mode of cell division are linked. Indeed, there is experimental evidence from the developing nervous system that a slower cell cycle may be associated with an asymmetric cell division while fast-dividing precursors tend to divide symmetrically (Qian et al. 1998, 2000; Lukaszewicz et al. 2002; Calegari and Huttner 2003). Thus, cell cycle length may be *the* defining and crucial difference between a self-renewing stem cell and a transit-amplifying, non-self renewing cell. If this is the case, then understanding the mechanisms of cell cycle regulation and self-renewal may answer many, if not most of the issues about stem cell vs transit-amplifying precursor identity, an issue also of crucial importance for our understanding of brain cancers.

2.4.4
Intrinsic Fate Determinants of Adult Neurogenesis

When a stem cell divides in such a way as to give rise to more differentiated progeny, a program is elicited within the latter that restricts its future cell fate. We are just starting to understand the molecular determinants controlling fate decisions in adult neurogenesis. Again we may learn important lessons from similar processes during development (Bertrand et al. 2002), as many of the transcriptional regulators involved in neural cell fate specification in the developing CNS are also encountered in zones of adult neurogenesis, such as the paired box transcription factor Pax6 or the basic helix-loop helix transcription factors Olig2 and Mash1 (Hack et al. 2004; Parras et al. 2004) (Fig. 1). Mash1 is a proneural transcription factor required for the production of neuronal precursors in the ventral telencephalon (Casarosa et al. 1999). In the adult SEZ, Mash1 is predominantly expressed in transit-amplifying precursors and to a lesser degree also in neuroblasts, where it may be only transiently retained (Parras et al. 2004). Treatment with the anti-mitotic drug Ara-C resulted in the ablation of Mash1-positive cells and control levels of Mash1-positive cells were found 48 h after cessation of drug treatment consistent with the presence of Mash1 in fast proliferating precursors. Since Mash1 mutant mice die at birth, no direct evidence for a proneural function in the adult SEZ could be obtained, but analysis at birth revealed that the mutant RMS contained fewer proliferating cells. Most remarkably, a dramatic reduction of neurons in the granular layer of the olfactory bulb was observed in neonatal Mash1 mutant mice, while formation of periglomerular cells was only slightly affected (Parras et al. 2004), suggesting that Mash1 might also be involved in specifying the generation of granule neurons in the adult SEZ. Another transcription factor crucially

involved in the neuronal commitment of adult precursors is Pax6 (Fig. 1).
It is expressed in type A cells (Hack et al. 2004) and retrovirally mediated
interference with normal Pax6 function drastically reduces neurogenesis of
the transduced precursors in the adult SEZ (Hack et al. 2005). Notably, Pax6
expression is turned off in the postmitotic neurons in the olfactory bulb,
except in a subpopulation of postmitotic periglomerular neurons, namely
those expressing the neurotransmitter dopamine. Indeed, forced expression of
Pax6 drives newly generated neurons to assume dopaminergic identity. These
data suggest a model in which Pax6 acts in two succeeding phases of fate
decision, namely when precursors are specified towards a (possibly generic)
neuronal fate and subsequently in the specification of a subpopulation of these
cells towards a dopaminergic phenotype (Fig. 1).

2.5
Fine Tuning of Adult Neurogenesis upon Demand

Adult neurogenesis appears to be a highly regulated process. In the adult
dentate gyrus, there is compelling evidence that the degree of neurogenesis is
dependent on activation of hippocampal circuitry (Kempermann et al. 1997;
Deisseroth et al. 2004). For instance, neurogenesis can be stimulated by physical
exercise such as running (van Praag et al. 1999) and by exposure to an enriched
environment (Kempermann et al. 1997). Both effects may be mediated by
VEGF signalling (Fabel et al. 2003; Cao et al. 2004). Furthermore, seizure
activity strongly upregulates dentate neurogenesis (Parent et al. 1997), an effect
that might be due to what has been called neurogenesis-excitation coupling
(Deisseroth et al. 2004), or it may be due to consequences of the post-seizure
lesion. In case of the adult SEZ, it has been shown that the rapidly dividing
type C cells express dopamine receptors (D2L type) and receive dopaminergic
innervation (Höglinger et al. 2004). Experimentally induced dopaminergic
denervation reduces proliferation in the adult SEZ and SGZ and neurogenesis
in the adult olfactory bulb. Importantly, a similar reduction is observed in
post-mortem brains of Parkinson disease patients (Höglinger et al. 2004).

By virtue of such regulation, adult neurogenesis may be amenable to pharmacological manipulations. In particular, antidepressant drugs such as the
serotonin reuptake inhibitor fluoxetine have been shown to increase the degree of dentate neurogenesis (Malberg et al. 2000). A recent important study
has indeed associated the antidepressant effects of fluoxetine with its ability to
enhance neurogenesis (Santarelli et al. 2003). X-irradiation induced ablation of
dentate neurogenesis prevented the behavioural responses to fluoxetine. The
idea that antidepressants may act by enhancing dentate neurogenesis is particularly attractive considering the fact that their action typically requires several
weeks of treatment until their beneficial effects become manifest, possibly the
time also required for the maturation and functional integration of newborn
neurons into the network. Thus, if confirmed, these findings would imply that

constant reconstruction of hippocampal circuitry by insertion of new dentate granule cells may be of importance for controlling an animal's and possibly a human's motivational state. Interestingly, antidepressants may not so much cause an increase in net numbers of neurons, but rather enhance their turnover since they not only stimulate proliferation, but also apoptosis (Sairanen et al. 2005). For the right appreciation of this finding, however, it would be important to know whether the cells that commit apoptosis include mature or only newly generated granule neurons, the survival of which appears to be dependent on BDNF signalling (Sairanen et al. 2005).

2.6
Incorporation of Adult-Born Neurons into the Preexisting Circuitry

This leads us to the more general question of whether newborn neurons fulfil a specific role with respect to neuronal information processing or simply take over the function of older neurons that have died. The fact that neural activity may affect the production of new neurons, has led to the hypothesis that adult neurogenesis could play a role in learning and memory (Carleton et al. 2002; Schinder and Gage 2004). Notably, it has been reported that adult neurogenesis may be required for the formation of trace memories, i.e. the association of stimuli that are separated in time, a process that is known to depend on the hippocampus (Shors et al. 2002). It was also suggested that adult dentate neurogenesis may be involved in the clearance of memories (Feng et al. 2001) and increased olfactory bulb neurogenesis appears to improve odor memory (Rochefort et al. 2002). Thus, it will be critical to understand what newly generated neurons can contribute to signal processing in the hippocampus or olfactory bulb that cannot be achieved by the preexisting neurons.

To serve as a secure fundament for more elaborate hypotheses on the function of adult-born neurons, it was necessary to show that newborn neurons do in fact functionally integrate into the preexisting neuronal circuitry. Labelling of progenitors undergoing cell division in the adult subgranular zone of the dentate gyrus with GFP encoding retroviruses allowed Van Praag and colleagues to record from newborn neurons (van Praag et al. 2002). This study revealed that newborn neurons do in fact receive functional synaptic input from the perforant path (PP), similar to their more mature sister neurons. A subsequent study, however, showed that the PP input into newborn neurons may exhibit a higher degree of synaptic plasticity (Schmidt-Hieber et al. 2004). In contrast to the previous study, newborn neurons were identified by their immunoreactivity for the early neuronal marker polysialylated neural cell adhesion molecule (PSA-NCAM) and their significantly higher input resistance compared to mature neurons. When the PP was repetitively stimulated with a theta burst temporally coupled with a single postsynaptic spike in the granule neuron (due to current injection), synaptic potentiation was selectively induced in newborn neurons, while more mature neurons did not show a change in synaptic efficacy. The authors suggested that the enhanced synaptic plasticity might be attributable to greater membrane excitability based on the fact that in these cells sodium-driven spikes were often boosted by calcium spikes mediated by low-voltage activated T-type calcium channels. Yet many other mechanisms might have contributed to this effect, for instance differences in synaptic inhibition. It is not known at what stage input mediated by γ-aminobutyric acid (GABA) becomes functionally inhibitory, considering the fact that developing neurons commonly display a reverse chloride gradient that renders GABAergic input excitatory (Kaila 1994). Thus, newly integrated neurons may be excited rather than inhibited by GABAergic input at early stages, which would facilitate synaptic potentiation. With respect to the possible role of the enhanced synaptic plasticity of the PP input into newborn granule neurons, one can only speculate, given that the recorded neurons were only a few weeks of age. It seems unlikely that this enhanced plasticity is indicative of greater involvement of the newborn neuron in learning and memory, but relative to mature granule neurons, it may reflect a greater need to stabilize new synaptic connections or face cell death in the absence of functional integration. In the case of the olfactory bulb, many newborn granule neurons die, but surprisingly only after appropriate insertion into the granule cell layer and acquirement of mature morphological characteristics (Petreanu and Alvarez-Buylla 2002), suggesting that at this advanced stage a selection process may take place that ensures that only functionally incorporated neurons may survive. This is corroborated by observations that survival of newly generated neurons in the olfactory bulb is regulated by olfaction, i.e. functional input (Petreanu and Alvarez-Buylla 2002; Rochefort et al. 2002; Mechawar et al. 2004). Prior to functional integration in the olfactory bulb, adult born neurons gradually acquire neuronal properties (Carleton et al. 2003). While still migrating in the rostral extension of the RMS, newborn neurons acquire responsiveness first to the transmitter GABA and subsequently to glutamate activating α-amino-3-hydroxy-5-methyl-4-isoxazolepropionic acid (AMPA)/kainate type receptors. Finally, at the point when neurons start to migrate radially into the bulb, N-methyl-d-aspartate (NMDA) -type glutamate responses can be recorded. Along with the morphological maturation such as dendritic development and formation of spines, inhibitory and excitatory synaptic responses can be recorded from these cells. Surprisingly, active sodium conductances and the ability of spiking are acquired only after synaptic innervation has been established. Cell death at this final stage of maturation may then serve as a mechanism to eliminate inappropriately integrated neurons.

While these studies have shown that newborn neurons in the hippocampus and the olfactory bulb do receive functional input (Carlen et al. 2002; van Praag et al. 2002; Belluzzi et al. 2003; Carleton et al. 2003), they have not revealed so far whether these neurons also produce a functional output. This is technically challenging as it requires simultaneous recording of a presynaptic neurons identified as newborn and a postsynaptic target cell. However, with regard to the problem of whether newborn neurons contribute a unique function to the neuronal circuitry, this is of foremost interest. It is conceivable that the development of a functional output is a highly controlled process, since it must take place without interfering with the stability of the network activity of the preexisting circuitry. The fact that the circuitry of the hippocampus plays a crucial role in the development of temporal lobe epilepsies underlines the potential dangers of uncontrolled functional integration. The surprising observation that newborn granule neurons in the olfactory bulb receive functional synaptic input prior to acquiring the ability to fire sodium-driven action potentials suggests that the onset of functional output of these newborn neurons may be a highly controlled step within the integration process (Carleton et al. 2003). This sequence of first receiving functional input and subsequently maturing membrane excitability sharply contrasts the reverse order of events during early postnatal development (Carleton et al. 2003). This hints to the possibility that functional integration in the adult vs the developing neural circuitry is fundamentally different. More specifically, it may indicate that the mature olfactory bulb provides inhibitory signals that halt maturation of membrane excitability of newborn neurons, for instance by suppressing expression of voltage-sensitive sodium channels, thus enforcing a functional "embargo" that is only lifted when appropriate synaptic integration has taken place.

3
The Perspectives of Cell Replacement Therapy

The existence of adult neural stem or progenitor cells has raised great hopes that it might be in principle possible to replace neurons that have died due to an injury or a neurodegenerative disease by new neurons. Here essentially two approaches can be taken: (a) replacement of dead cells by in vitro expanded and differentiated cells and (b) replacement by recruitment of endogenous progenitors. While it is too early to weigh these different approaches against each other, we would like to briefly illustrate the achievements and problems with each.

3.1
In Vitro Expanded Neural Stem Cells as a Source for Cell Replacement Therapy

With regard to the first strategy, i.e. to expand a suitable cell source in vitro and transplant the desired progeny into a lesioned area, two main sources of cells are currently being investigated: (a) neural stem cells isolated from the embryonic or adult brain and expanded in vitro or (b) embryonic stem (ES) cells. While neural stem cells could in principle be isolated even from the patient himself, their differentiation into neurons has proven more difficult than expected. Expansion as neurosphere cells in high concentrations of EGF and

FGF2, a prerequisite for large numbers of transplantable cells, also abolishes many region-specific characteristics of neural precursors (Gabay et al. 2003; Hack et al. 2004), but see Parmar et al. (2003) for evidence that expanded precursors may retain some regional specification. This growth factor-induced dedifferentiation may also result in reduction of neurogenic competence, as most expanded adult neural precursor cells differentiate into astrocytes, both in culture (Song et al. 2002a; Hack et al. 2004) and after transplantation (Cao et al. 2002; Hofstetter et al. 2005). However, the problem of low-level neurogenesis from expanded precursors can be in principle overcome by transduction with key neurogenic fate determinants, such as Pax6 or neurogenin-2, resulting in the generation of 90% or 40% neurons, respectively (Hack et al. 2004; Hofstetter et al. 2005). Yet it remains to be seen whether it is also possible to direct these still poorly regionalized neurons towards highly specified neuronal subtypes, such as midbrain dopaminergic neurons. So far the differentiation of neurons derived from in vitro expanded precursors is mostly directed towards a GABAergic phenotype, and it has not yet been possible to unravel mechanisms to direct them in considerable numbers towards other neuronal subtypes. Moreover, it is not fully understood to what extent they form functional synapses. Adult SEZ precursors expanded in neurosphere culture and subsequently allowed to differentiate develop into neurons that acquire the ability to fire action potentials and receive functional synaptic input, when co-cultured with neurons from the embryonic olfactory bulb, but fail to establish a functional presynaptic compartment (Berninger et al., unpublished observation). Directly plated SEZ neuroblasts, in contrast, are capable of forming both pre- and postsynaptic specializations, indicating that like the loss of regional specification the competence to assemble a functional presynaptic terminal is severely affected upon exposure to mitogens. Importantly, however, it is possible to overcome this loss of competence, at least in vitro, by treatment with the neurotrophin BDNF (Berninger et al., unpublished observation). Similar findings were obtained studying neurons derived from a hippocampal stem cell line expanded in FGF2 (Song et al. 2002b). It was shown that these neurons can receive functional synapses when co-cultured with embryonic hippocampal neurons, but again their competence to provide functional synaptic output was rather low. Interestingly, though, evidence for secretion of both neurotransmitters glutamate and GABA was obtained. However, the relative abundance of glutamatergic vs GABAergic neurons in these cultures was not assessed, and it is not at all clear whether these neurons truly resemble dentate granule neurons or rather represent a type of generic neuron. Given the fact that the cell line had been extensively passaged before and expanded in the presence of FGF2, it would be critical to know how much of the regional specification of the original mother cell is retained by these cells or has been lost.

For therapy of neurodegenerative diseases or traumatic lesions by cell replacement, ultimately neural stem cells or their in vitro predifferentiated descendants must be delivered to the afflicted region. There is evidence that neurosphere-derived cells may spontaneously migrate to sites of brain lesion (Pluchino et al. 2003), yet widespread distribution of neural precursors throughout the nervous system may have undesired side effects. Furthermore, the migration potential of more committed precursors is largely unknown. The reason why one would prefer to transplant already committed precursors is that most regions of the brain are in fact not permissive to neurogenesis. For instance, when adult hippocampal progenitors or adult spinal cord stem cells were transplanted into a young adult brain, neuronal differentiation was only observed upon grafting into the RMS or the dentate gyrus, the two main neurogenic regions of the adult mammalian brain (Suhonen et al. 1996; Shihabuddin et al. 2000). In contrast, the same progenitors failed to generate neurons in other regions (Suhonen et al. 1996). One way to overcome the restraints of a non-neurogenic environment may be to locally block BMP signalling by delivery of BMP antagonists such as noggin. When precursors from the adult SEZ were grafted into the adult striatum, no cells expressing neuronal markers such as TuJ1 were present and only astrocytic cells were found (Lim et al. 2000). However, when the striatum was "primed" by local delivery of an adenovirus encoding for noggin, TuJ1-positive cell clusters were encountered, suggesting that the environment had been made permissive at least for the most early steps of neurogenesis (Lim et al. 2000). The problem associated with a non-neurogenic environment has also been underscored by a recent study showing that adult neurosphere cells locally grafted into sites of spinal cord trauma largely differentiate into astrocytes (Hofstetter et al. 2005). Although such treatment results in some functional recovery from the spinal cord injury, it is accompanied by massive allodynia, a phenomenon of pain hypersensitivity often found in patients suffering from spinal cord injury and possibly due to aberrant fibre sprouting. Interestingly, however, Hofstetter and colleagues also showed that prior retroviral transduction of neurosphere cells with neurogenin-2 repressed astroglial differentiation, thereby also reducing the allodynia. Surprisingly, the positive effect of the forced neurogenin-2 expression may have resulted from the fact that many neurosphere cells now differentiated into oligodendrocytes, which may have promoted remyelination of nerve fibres within the afflicted tissue.

Whether local grafting of neural precursors is successful or not will furthermore depend on whether the local environment can provide the cues necessary for the appropriate integration into the preexisting circuitry. We have learned already that functional integration of endogenously produced neurons in the adult olfactory bulb is a complex sequence of events that substantially deviates from those underlying circuit assembly during development (Carleton et al. 2003), warranting caution with regard to the notion that appropriate integration may take place spontaneously.

3.2
The Alternative to the Adult Neural Stem Cell: Guided Neuronal Differentiation of Embryonic Stem Cells

Embryonic stem (ES) cells comprise another potential source for neuronal cell replacement (Kim et al. 2003a). Surprisingly, when transplanted in vivo, ES cells become readily committed towards a neural fate and such neural precursors differentiate and become functionally incorporated (Björklund et al. 2002; Wernig et al. 2004). The fact that grafted neurons derived from ES cells readily received functional synaptic input from host tissue has been rightly considered a great benevolence of nature towards the investigator, but whether this will mean the same to the patient remains to be determined. Once again, the devil may reveal itself in the details of such functional integration. To give an example, neurons derived from ES cells that were grafted onto hippocampal slice cultures have been shown to display functional glutamatergic and GABAergic input (Benninger et al. 2003). Yet glutamatergic synapses established on the grafted neurons exhibited a conspicuous absence of an NMDA-receptor-mediated component as well as differences in short-term plasticity. While such discrepancies between synapses onto grafted and endogenous neurons may be caused by the different maturational state of the respective postsynaptic neurons, it may also indicate that the grafted neurons may not fully phenocopy endogenous neurons on all functional aspects. Given the fact that NMDA receptor activation plays a crucial role in long-term synaptic modifications, the absence of a notable NMDA receptor component may render these grafted neurons unable to fulfil their function appropriately. The key problem is that ES-derived neurons are not fully specified, even though they may become functionally integrated (Wernig et al. 2004).

To circumvent inappropriate differentiation of ES cells within a host tissue, it might be necessary to induce these cells to become specified towards the desired neuronal phenotype. Indeed, protocols have been developed that allow for the selective generation of various types of neurons, such as midbrain dopaminergic and serotonergic neurons (Kawasaki et al. 2000; Kim et al. 2003b; Perrier et al. 2004), cholinergic motor neurons (Wichterle et al. 2002) and glutamatergic neurons (Bibel et al. 2004; Watanabe et al. 2005). Underlying all these protocols has been the idea that ES cells might adopt the desired neuronal type when exposed to the same signals that are relevant for specifying these cell types during embryogenesis. Following this hypothesis, Wichterle et al. established an experimental protocol to drive the specification of mouse ES cells into spinal progenitor cells and subsequently into motor neurons (Wichterle et al. 2002). ES cells were grown as aggregates, so-called embryoid bodies (EBs), in the presence of a fibroblast monolayer. Treatment of these EBs with retinoic acid (RA), an agent that besides its neuralizing effect also acts as a caudalizing signal, induced expression of markers of postmitotic neurons as well as markers indicating a spinal cord identity such as Hoxc5 and Hoxc6 in these aggregates.

When EBs were simultaneously treated with RA and sonic hedgehog (Shh), neurons adopted either a more dorsal or ventral spinal fate dependent on the concentration of Shh used, consistent with Shh's function as a morphogen during development (Roelink et al. 1995; Ericson et al. 1996, 1997). When grown at relatively high Shh concentrations, neurons expressed transcription factors typical of spinal motor neurons (Wichterle et al. 2002). Finally, when grafted into chick embryos, motor neurons derived from RA- and Shh-treated EBs extended axons via the ventral root towards the periphery, apparently innervating muscle tissue. Furthermore, on arrival at the target, such ES cell-derived motor neurons showed signs of cholinergic presynaptic differentiation, suggesting that they form functional endplates. Somewhat surprising was the observation that, whereas these ES-derived motor neurons expressed a LIM transcription factor profile, indicating a rostral cervical positional identity, their peripheral axonal projection was still dependent on which segment of the spinal cord they had been grafted. Thus molecular specification did not obstruct the positional influence, indicating a remarkable degree of plasticity. Notably, also ES cells, differentiating into neurons using a rather different protocol, developed into motor neurons upon transplantation in the developing chick spinal cord (Plachta et al. 2004).

A similar approach has been chosen by investigators to generate midbrain dopaminergic neurons from ES cells (Kim et al. 2003b; Perrier et al. 2004). Death of midbrain dopaminergic neurons is one of the major hallmarks of Parkinson's disease and there is evidence based on transplantation of foetal midbrain cells that cell replacement might in principle work to alleviate the disease symptoms (Björklund et al. 2003). During embryonic development the isthmic organizer, a signalling centre located at the midbrain/hindbrain boundary provides signals such as fibroblast growth factor-8 (FGF8) and Shh that instruct rostrally located precursors to adopt a dopaminergic phenotype (Ye et al. 1998). Indeed, the same factors are capable of driving mouse ES cells towards a midbrain dopaminergic phenotype which can be further enhanced by ectopic expression of Nurr1, an orphan member of the hormone receptor family of transcriptions factors known to be required for the generation of dopaminergic neurons (Kim et al. 2003b). When transplanted into the striatum of 6-hydoxy dopamine (6-OH-DA) lesioned rats, an animal model for Parkinson's disease, tyrosine hydroxylase-positive cells not only survived, but also received functional input from adjacent host tissue and extended their axonal projection over considerable distances. Finally, grafting also ameliorated the motor deficits caused by the 6-OH-DA lesion. More recently, a protocol was developed for the selective and high-yield differentiation of human ES cells into midbrain dopaminergic neurons (Perrier et al. 2004). When cultured on a stromal feeder cell line, human ES cells adopted a neural fate, generating neuroepithelial structures (so-called rosettes) consisting of neural precursors expressing Sox1 and Pax6. For efficient commitment of these precursors towards a midbrain dopaminergic fate, precursors had to be passaged twice and be exposed to FGF8 and Shh prior to differentiation in medium containing glial cell-derived neurotrophic factor (GDNF), dibutyryl cAMP, and TGF-β3. After a total of 50 days in vitro, up to 50% of the cells were TuJ1-positive, and of these, 80% expressed tyrosine hydroxylase. Consistent with a specification towards a midbrain dopaminergic phenotype, first expression of the transcription factors Pax2 and Pax5 was detected, followed by that of engrailed-1. Efficient dopamine release was detected only upon additional weeks of differentiation.

For generation of glutamatergic neurons, ES cells were cultured transiently as EBs, again treated with retinoic acid, but in the absence of feeder cells (Bibel et al. 2004). These cells started then to express markers of neurogenic radial glia cells, such as nestin, RC2, GLAST and most intriguingly virtually all cells were Pax6-immunoreactive. During development Pax6-positive radial glial cells serve as precursors in a variety of regions including the neocortex where they generate glutamatergic neurons (Heins et al. 2002; Malatesta et al. 2003; Haubst et al. 2004). Consistent with the hypothesis that the ES cells were driven to a similar cell fate, the majority of the progeny appeared to be indeed of a glutamatergic nature and formed typical glutamatergic synapses. Yet a small percentage of these cells were GABAergic. In a subsequent study, the authors aimed to characterize the developmental potential of these in vitro specified ES cell-derived progenitors by transplanting them to different tissues in the developing chick (Plachta et al. 2004). When grafted into a segment of the neural tube of chick embryos, these cells generated neurons that expressed markers of interneurons and motor neurons of the spinal cord and extended axons into the ventral root. Moreover, some of the cells grafted into the embryonic neural tube behaved like neural crest cells and populated dorsal root ganglia (DRGs). These cells were capable of generating neurons, but failed to express the appropriate markers of DRG neurons and did not extend axons towards the periphery. By contrast, cells grafted into the DRG without prior specification with RA were capable of responding to the local cues and differentiated in neurons expressing the appropriate markers. These data show that prior specification of ES cells restricts the fate of neuronal progenitors generated from ES cells in the respective in vivo environment.

In an attempt to specifically generate forebrain neurons from ES cells, Watanabe et al. (2005) developed a protocol that omitted RA, a molecule that not only exerts neuralizing, but also exhibits caudalizing activities. Interestingly, they found that blocking Wnt signalling (by applying the endogenous Wnt antagonist Dkk1) and Nodal signalling promoted neural specification in ES cells. Notably, a substantial portion of Dkk1-treated precursors expressed Foxg1, a marker for telencephalic neurons. Once this stage was reached, activation of Wnt signalling (by addition of Wnt3a) now induced Pax6 expression, suggesting specification towards a dorsal telencephalic fate. Conversely, treatment with the ventralizing factor Shh induced expression of ventral telencephalic markers such as Islet1.

In summary, knowledge of the molecular events that underly specification of neural precursors towards a given neuronal/glial fate appears to provide us with the tools to generate in principle any desired neural cell type from ES cells. In vitro differentiation of ES cells prior to grafting may also reduce the risk for teratoma formation (Björklund et al. 2002; Kim et al. 2003b). However, appropriate functional incorporation of ES cell-derived neurons establishing the proper type of synaptic connections with neighbouring cells remains to be demonstrated.

3.3
Recruitment of Endogenous Neural Stem Cells

The fact that neurosphere-forming cells can be isolated from many other regions than the two major neurogenic regions, the SEZ and the SGZ (Weiss et al. 1996; Johansson et al. 1999; Palmer et al. 1999; Nunes et al. 2003), suggests the possibility that the CNS may contain resident stem or precursor cells that in principle could be stimulated to generate neurons in case of disease or trauma-induced neurodegeneration. Alternatively, nonresident stem or precursor cells may become recruited towards a site of neuronal degeneration. The first evidence for degeneration-induced activation of a neurogenic program was provided by a study from Magavi and colleagues (2000). Layer VI corticothalamic projection neurons were selectively ablated by chromophore-targeted neuronal apoptosis. While no neurogenesis occurs in the intact neocortex (Magavi et al. 2000; Kornack and Rakic 2001a), cells both positive for BrdU and the neuronal marker NeuN extending long-range axons towards the thalamus were encountered within the damaged cortical layer, indicating that degenerated neurons had been replaced by newborn neurons, albeit to a limited degree (Magavi et al. 2000). Similar findings were made in cases of focal ablation of corticospinal projection neurons (Chen et al. 2004). While in both cases local generation of neurons cannot be excluded, there was evidence of migration of BrdU- and doublecortin-positive young neurons from the SEZ across the corpus callosum towards the lesioned cortical layer. In an experimental model of stroke, a similar recruitment of neuronal precursors from the SEZ towards the lesioned adult striatum was observed (Arvidsson et al. 2002). Newly generated cells within the ischaemic area expressed markers of mature striatal medium-sized spiny neurons, although the mechanism for this appropriate fate commitment remains unclear given that the local microenvironment upon the ischaemic insult is severely damaged. Unfortunately, the majority of the newly generated neurons appeared to be very short-lived, which may not be surprising, given that they must dwell in a highly unfavourable environment. As we have discussed above, functional integration may be key to preventing apoptotic cell death of adult-born neurons in the olfactory bulb (Petreanu and Alvarez-Buylla 2002). Notably, adult genesis of medium-sized spiny neurons from SEZ precursors can be also elicited in the adult striatum in the absence of injury by adenoviral expression of the BMP antagonist noggin and the neurotrophin BDNF (Chmielnicki et al. 2004). These neurons survived for more than 2 months and were capable of projecting to the globus pallidus, their natural target structure.

The most striking example of replacement of degenerated neurons by newly generated cells is a study conducted by Nakatomi and colleagues (Nakatomi et al. 2002). In a stroke model which results in the total loss of CA1 pyramidal neurons, a spontaneous, albeit very modest repopulation of the damaged area was observed. However, neuronal recovery could be massively boosted upon intraventricular delivery of the growth factors EGF and FGF2. There was again evidence that neuronal precursors had been recruited from outside of the afflicted region, namely the periventricular zone just above the hippocampal CA fields. Anatomical recovery in growth factor-treated animals was accompanied by functional amelioration, as demonstrated by the presence of a measurable CA1 field potential upon Schaffer collateral stimulation (which was totally gone in controls) and even behavioural tasks that require an intact hippocampus.

Thus, recruitment of endogenous precursors depends on appropriate signals. Indeed, migrating neuroblasts can also be rerouted from the RMS by the extracellular matrix protein tenascin-R (Saghatelyan et al. 2004). Tenascin-R plays a critical role within the olfactory bulb by initiating detachment of neuroblasts from chains and inducing radial migration. Ectopic expression of tenascin-R within the striatum reroutes migrating neuroblasts towards this tissue. This may provide means to recruit these cells to damaged areas that cannot provide the necessary signals on their own (Saghatelyan et al. 2004). Finally, SEZ precursors can also be mobilized to periventricular white matter by experimental autoimmune encephalomyelitis, where they generate astrocytes and oligodendrocytes (Picard-Riera et al. 2002). Clearly, the more we know about the properties of adult stem cells and their progeny, the more tools we will acquire to employ them to their fullest potential.

4
When Stem Cells Turn Awry

While the presence of stem cells in the brain has raised many hopes that these may become therapeutically useful, there is also justified suspicion that in some cases they might themselves be the origin of a highly deadly disease, namely brain cancer. Actually over the last couple of years, the hypothesis has taken momentum that many forms of tumours arise from rare cancer stem cells that give rise to a hierarchy of more differentiated progeny whose behaviour resembles normal tissue stem cells (Reya et al. 2001; Beachy et al. 2004). While the more differentiated progeny constitutes the majority of the tumour cells, it is the cancer stem cell that is responsible for tumour propagation. This hypothesis has been experimentally verified in case of acute myelogenous leukaemia: a subpopulation of cells, isolated from leukaemic patients bearing characteristics of haematopoietic stem cells, e.g. with self-renewal capacity, unlimited replication and similar antigenic properties, were the only cells that could reconstitute tumours upon transfer into the NOD/SCID (nonobese diabetic/severe combined immunodeficient) mice (Lapidot et al. 1994; Bonnet and Dick 1997; Hope et al. 2004). Recent findings point to a quite similar scenario in case of breast cancer (Al-Hajj et al. 2003). Even more recently, the same concept has been successfully applied to brain cancers. A large variety of brain tumours such as medulloblastoma and glioblastoma contain a subpopulation of cells which can give rise to clonal aggregates resembling neurospheres that can further generate secondary clonal aggregates, suggesting the ability for self-renewal (Hemmati et al. 2003; Singh et al. 2003; Yuan et al. 2004). Furthermore, when allowed to differentiate, tumour-derived progenitors developed into the different neural lineages based on marker expression. Notably, however, tumour-derived progenitors can differentiate into abnormal progeny that co-express markers of distinct neural lineages such as TuJ1 and GFAP (Hemmati et al. 2003; Singh et al. 2003) (Fig. 2).

Recently it has been found that self-renewal ability may be specifically found in a subpopulation of the tumour cells that express the surface protein CD133/prominin (Singh et al. 2004), a molecule localized asymmetrically also on neural precursors in the developing brain (Kosodo et al. 2004). Most importantly, when CD133-positive cells were isolated from patients and transplanted into the brain of NOD/SCID mice, only a hundred of these cells were required to induce tumour formation, while 1,000-fold higher numbers of CD133-negative brain tumour cells were ineffective in causing a secondary brain cancer.

Two more aspects of these studies are of interest. First, while CD133-positive cells are crucial for the propagation of the tumour, they also give rise to CD133-negative offspring, indicating a second key feature of stem cells, namely the ability not only of self-renewal but also to give rise to more differentiated progeny. Secondly, analysis of the tumours reconstituted in the mouse brain showed that these tumours histologically resembled the original tumour obtained from the human patient bearing typical features of medulloblastoma or glioblastoma.

These findings can be essentially interpreted in two ways: the cancer originally arises from a proper stem cell or, alternatively, from a more differentiated cell that reacquired properties of a stem cell by de-differentiation (Fig. 2). There is evidence that in case of high-grade malignant gliomas both scenarios may occur (Dai et al. 2001; Bachoo et al. 2002). In glioblastoma, the loss of the cell cycle inhibitors Ink4a/Arf is frequently associated with activation of EGF receptor signalling, pointing to the possibility that these mutations may interact to cause cellular transformation. A proof of principle study showed that combined loss of p16Ink4a and p19Arf and concomitant activation of the EGF receptor drives astrocytes to de-differentiate into nestin-positive progenitors in vitro (Bachoo et al. 2002). Moreover, when a constitutively active EGF recep-

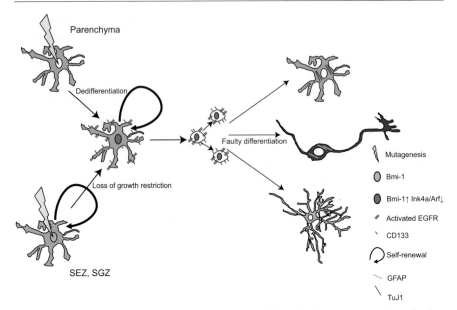

Fig. 2 A model illustrating the role of tumour stem cells in brain cancerogenesis. Whether the tumour stem cell indeed resembles more the type B cell as shown here or rather the transit-amplifying precursors is not clear. In any case, tumour stem cells (identified by the expression of CD133) may arise from at least two distinct sources: (a) stem cells such as those residing in the SEZ or SGZ or from (b) parenchymal glial cells or precursors that have undergone dedifferentiation as a consequence of a mutagenizing event that results in the gain of self-renewal capacity (as exemplified by the upregulation of Bmi-1) and unrestricted proliferation (for instance by EGF receptor gene amplification). Self-renewal capacity is crucial for the propagation of the tumour. Progeny of cancer stem cells are typically found to exhibit a faulty differentiation, as exemplified by co-expression of the astroglial marker GFAP in neuron-like cells (as illustrated by the *green lines* in the *red neuron*) and the neuronal marker TuJ1 in astroglial-like cells (*red lines* in the *green astrocyte*)

tor was expressed in p16Ink4a- and p19Arf-deficient astrocytes and these were orthotopically transplanted into brains of SCID mice, high-grade gliomas were induced. Interestingly, primary neural progenitors bearing the same genetic modifications were equally tumorigenic, thus indicating that both differentiated cells as well as undifferentiated progenitors may serve as the cell of tumour origin. Finally, upon EGF injection into the adult SEZ, proliferation was massively enhanced in Ink/Arf mutant adult mice compared to wild types, causing lesions that were cytologically similar to the tumours provoked by transplantation of mutant astrocytes or neural progenitors. It is worth remembering here again the data by Doetsch et al. (2002) that showed that EGF treatment in the intact adult SEZ does not only dramatically enhance proliferation of type C cells, but also interferes with the appropriate differentiation program in that it diverts progeny away from a neuronal towards an "activated" astroglial fate (Doetsch et al. 2002). Notably, these dedifferentiated astrocytes leave their usual position in the SEZ and RMS and invade the parenchyma of the striatum, cortex and corpus callosum, therein resembling cancerous cells. The fact that malignant glioblastoma are very often associated with a gene amplification of the EGF receptor (Ekstrand et al. 1991; von Deimling et al. 1992; Hayashi et al. 1997) suggests that tumour cells in glioblastomas may be molecularly very similar to the transit-amplifying type C cells, which are the cells expressing the highest amount of EGF receptor within the SEZ compartment (Doetsch et al. 2002) (Figs. 1 and 2).

We have previously encountered the cell cycle inhibitors Ink/Arf in the context of discussing the molecular mechanisms underlying stem cell self-renewal (Sect. 2.4.3). We have seen that they are targets of the transcriptional repressor Bmi-1 thought to be a critical component of the machinery regulating cell division of adult neural precursors. Interestingly, Bmi-1 overexpression occurs frequently in human medulloblastomas (Leung et al. 2004). Medulloblastomas are highly malignant brain tumours which arise from uncontrolled proliferation of granule cell precursors in the extragranule cell layer (EGL) (Wechsler-Reya and Scott 2001; Pomeroy et al. 2002). Many of these medulloblastomas exhibit aberrant Shh signalling due to mutations in the Shh receptors Ptch (Dong et al. 2000; Zurawel et al. 2000) or smoothened and suppressor of Fused (SUFU), a regulator of Shh signalling (Taylor et al. 2002). Also Bmi-1 upregulation is accompanied by higher levels of Ptch and SUFU (Leung et al. 2004), suggesting that Bmi-1 activation may occur downstream of Shh signalling in these tumours.

In conclusion, a detailed knowledge of the molecular mechanisms regulating stem cell renewal and fate specification will not only allow us to understand the intricate processes that underlie adult neurogenesis, hopefully providing us with means to develop novel therapies for neurodegenerative diseases, but also pave the way for new strategies to cure brain cancer.

References

Al-Hajj M, Wicha MS, Benito-Hernandez A, Morrison SJ, Clarke MF (2003) Prospective identification of tumorigenic breast cancer cells. Proc Natl Acad Sci U S A 100:3983–3988

Altman J (1969) Autoradiographic and histological studies of postnatal neurogenesis. IV. Cell proliferation and migration in the anterior forebrain, with special reference to persisting neurogenesis in the olfactory bulb. J Comp Neurol 137:433–457

Altman J, Das GD (1965) Autoradiographic and histological evidence of postnatal hippocampal neurogenesis in rats. J Comp Neurol 124:319–335

Alvarez-Buylla A, Garcia-Verdugo JM, Tramontin AD (2001) A unified hypothesis on the lineage of neural stem cells. Nat Rev Neurosci 2:287–293

Alvarez-Buylla A, Lim DA (2004) For the long run: maintaining germinal niches in the adult brain. Neuron 41:683–686

Alvarez-Buylla A, Seri B, Doetsch F (2002) Identification of neural stem cells in the adult vertebrate brain. Brain Res Bull 57:751–758

Artavanis-Tsakonas S, Rand MD, Lake RJ (1999) Notch signaling: cell fate control and signal integration in development. Science 284:770–776

Arvidsson A, Collin T, Kirik D, Kokaia Z, Lindvall O (2002) Neuronal replacement from endogenous precursors in the adult brain after stroke. Nat Med 8:963–970

Bachoo RM, Maher EA, Ligon KL, Sharpless NE, Chan SS, You MJ, Tang Y, DeFrances J, Stover E, Weissleder R, Rowitch DH, Louis DN, DePinho RA (2002) Epidermal growth factor receptor and Ink4a/Arf: convergent mechanisms governing terminal differentiation and transformation along the neural stem cell to astrocyte axis. Cancer Cell 1:269–277

Balemans W, Van Hul W (2002) Extracellular regulation of BMP signaling in vertebrates: a cocktail of modulators. Dev Biol 250:231–250

Beachy PA, Karhadkar SS, Berman DM (2004) Tissue repair and stem cell renewal in carcinogenesis. Nature 432:324–331

Bedard A, Parent A (2004) Evidence of newly generated neurons in the human olfactory bulb. Brain Res Dev Brain Res 151:159–168

Belluzzi O, Benedusi M, Ackman J, LoTurco JJ (2003) Electrophysiological differentiation of new neurons in the olfactory bulb. J Neurosci 23:10411–10418

Benninger F, Beck H, Wernig M, Tucker KL, Brustle O, Scheffler B (2003) Functional integration of embryonic stem cell-derived neurons in hippocampal slice cultures. J Neurosci 23:7075–7083

Bertrand N, Castro DS, Guillemot F (2002) Proneural genes and the specification of neural cell types. Nat Rev Neurosci 3:517–530

Bibel M, Richter J, Schrenk K, Tucker KL, Staiger V, Korte M, Goetz M, Barde YA (2004) Differentiation of mouse embryonic stem cells into a defined neuronal lineage. Nat Neurosci 7:1003–1009

Bickenbach JR (2005) Isolation, characterization, and culture of epithelial stem cells. Methods Mol Biol 289:97–102

Björklund A, Dunnett SB, Brundin P, Stoessl AJ, Freed CR, Breeze RE, Levivier M, Peschanski M, Studer L, Barker R (2003) Neural transplantation for the treatment of Parkinson's disease. Lancet Neurol 2:437–445

Björklund LM, Sanchez-Pernaute R, Chung S, Andersson T, Chen IY, McNaught KS, Brownell AL, Jenkins BG, Wahlestedt C, Kim KS, Isacson O (2002) Embryonic stem cells develop into functional dopaminergic neurons after transplantation in a Parkinson rat model. Proc Natl Acad Sci U S A 99:2344–2349

Bonnet D, Dick JE (1997) Human acute myeloid leukemia is organized as a hierarchy that originates from a primitive hematopoietic cell. Nat Med 3:730–737

Calegari F, Huttner WB (2003) An inhibition of cyclin-dependent kinases that lengthens, but does not arrest, neuroepithelial cell cycle induces premature neurogenesis. J Cell Sci 116:4947–4955

Cameron HA, Woolley CS, McEwen BS, Gould E (1993) Differentiation of newly born neurons and glia in the dentate gyrus of the adult rat. Neuroscience 56:337–344

Campbell K, Götz M (2002) Radial glia: multi-purpose cells for vertebrate brain development. Trends Neurosci 25:235–238

Cao L, Jiao X, Zuzga DS, Liu Y, Fong DM, Young D, During MJ (2004) VEGF links hippocampal activity with neurogenesis, learning and memory. Nat Genet 36:827–835

Cao Q, Benton RL, Whittemore SR (2002) Stem cell repair of central nervous system injury. J Neurosci Res 68:501–510

Capela A, Temple S (2002) LeX/ssea-1 is expressed by adult mouse CNS stem cells, identifying them as nonependymal. Neuron 35:865–875

Carlen M, Cassidy RM, Brismar H, Smith GA, Enquist LW, Frisen J (2002) Functional integration of adult-born neurons. Curr Biol 12:606–608

Carleton A, Petreanu LT, Lansford R, Alvarez-Buylla A, Lledo PM (2003) Becoming a new neuron in the adult olfactory bulb. Nat Neurosci 6:507–518

Carleton A, Rochefort C, Morante-Oria J, Desmaisons D, Vincent JD, Gheusi G, Lledo PM (2002) Making scents of olfactory neurogenesis. J Physiol Paris 96:115–122

Casarosa S, Fode C, Guillemot F (1999) Mash1 regulates neurogenesis in the ventral telencephalon. Development 126:525–534

Chen J, Magavi SS, Macklis JD (2004) Neurogenesis of corticospinal motor neurons extending spinal projections in adult mice. Proc Natl Acad Sci U S A 101:16357–16362

Chiasson BJ, Tropepe V, Morshead CM, van der Kooy D (1999) Adult mammalian forebrain ependymal and subependymal cells demonstrate proliferative potential, but only subependymal cells have neural stem cell characteristics. J Neurosci 19:4462–4471

Chmielnicki E, Benraiss A, Economides AN, Goldman SA (2004) Adenovirally expressed noggin and brain-derived neurotrophic factor cooperate to induce new medium spiny neurons from resident progenitor cells in the adult striatal ventricular zone. J Neurosci 24:2133–2142

Clarke RB, Anderson E, Howell A, Potten CS (2003) Regulation of human breast epithelial stem cells. Cell Prolif 36 [Suppl 1]:45–58

Conboy I, Rando T (2005) Aging, stem cells and tissue regeneration: lessons from muscle. Cell Cycle 4:407–410

Conboy IM, Conboy MJ, Smythe GM, Rando TA (2003) Notch-mediated restoration of regenerative potential to aged muscle. Science 302:1575–1577

Conboy IM, Conboy MJ, Wagers AJ, Girma ER, Weissman IL, Rando TA (2005) Rejuvenation of aged progenitor cells by exposure to a young systemic environment. Nature 433:760–764

Cotsarelis G, Sun TT, Lavker RM (1990) Label-retaining cells reside in the bulge area of pilosebaceous unit: implications for follicular stem cells, hair cycle, and skin carcinogenesis. Cell 61:1329–1337

Craig CG, Tropepe V, Morshead CM, Reynolds BA, Weiss S, van der Kooy D (1996) In vivo growth factor expansion of endogenous subependymal neural precursor cell populations in the adult mouse brain. J Neurosci 16:2649–2658

Dahmane N, Sanchez P, Gitton Y, Palma V, Sun T, Beyna M, Weiner H, Ruiz i Altaba A (2001) The Sonic Hedgehog-Gli pathway regulates dorsal brain growth and tumorigenesis. Development 128:5201–5212

Dai C, Celestino JC, Okada Y, Louis DN, Fuller GN, Holland EC (2001) PDGF autocrine stimulation dedifferentiates cultured astrocytes and induces oligodendrogliomas and oligoastrocytomas from neural progenitors and astrocytes in vivo. Genes Dev 15:1913–1925

Deisseroth K, Singla S, Toda H, Monje M, Palmer TD, Malenka RC (2004) Excitation-neurogenesis coupling in adult neural stem/progenitor cells. Neuron 42:535–552

Doetsch F (2003) A niche for adult neural stem cells. Curr Opin Genet Dev 13:543–550

Doetsch F, Alvarez-Buylla A (1996) Network of tangential pathways for neuronal migration in adult mammalian brain. Proc Natl Acad Sci U S A 93:14895–14900

Doetsch F, Caille I, Lim DA, Garcia-Verdugo JM, Alvarez-Buylla A (1999a) Subventricular zone astrocytes are neural stem cells in the adult mammalian brain. Cell 97:703–716

Doetsch F, Garcia-Verdugo JM, Alvarez-Buylla A (1997) Cellular composition and three-dimensional organization of the subventricular germinal zone in the adult mammalian brain. J Neurosci 17:5046–5061

Doetsch F, Garcia-Verdugo JM, Alvarez-Buylla A (1999b) Regeneration of a germinal layer in the adult mammalian brain. Proc Natl Acad Sci U S A 96:11619–11624

Doetsch F, Petreanu L, Caille I, Garcia-Verdugo JM, Alvarez-Buylla A (2002) EGF converts transit-amplifying neurogenic precursors in the adult brain into multipotent stem cells. Neuron 36:1021–1034

Dong J, Gailani MR, Pomeroy SL, Reardon D, Bale AE (2000) Identification of PATCHED mutations in medulloblastomas by direct sequencing. Hum Mutat 16:89–90

Ekstrand AJ, James CD, Cavenee WK, Seliger B, Pettersson RF, Collins VP (1991) Genes for epidermal growth factor receptor, transforming growth factor alpha, and epidermal growth factor and their expression in human gliomas in vivo. Cancer Res 51:2164–2172

Enwere E, Shingo T, Gregg C, Fujikawa H, Ohta S, Weiss S (2004) Aging results in reduced epidermal growth factor receptor signaling, diminished olfactory neurogenesis, and deficits in fine olfactory discrimination. J Neurosci 24:8354–8365

Ericson J, Briscoe J, Rashbass P, van Heyningen V, Jessell TM (1997) Graded sonic hedgehog signaling and the specification of cell fate in the ventral neural tube. Cold Spring Harb Symp Quant Biol 62:451–466

Ericson J, Morton S, Kawakami A, Roelink H, Jessell TM (1996) Two critical periods of Sonic Hedgehog signaling required for the specification of motor neuron identity. Cell 87:661–673

Eriksson PS, Perfilieva E, Bjork-Eriksson T, Alborn AM, Nordborg C, Peterson DA, Gage FH (1998) Neurogenesis in the adult human hippocampus. Nat Med 4:1313–1317

Fabel K, Tam B, Kaufer D, Baiker A, Simmons N, Kuo CJ, Palmer TD (2003) VEGF is necessary for exercise-induced adult hippocampal neurogenesis. Eur J Neurosci 18:2803–2812

Feng R, Rampon C, Tang YP, Shrom D, Jin J, Kyin M, Sopher B, Miller MW, Ware CB, Martin GM, Kim SH, Langdon RB, Sisodia SS, Tsien JZ (2001) Deficient neurogenesis in forebrain-specific presenilin-1 knockout mice is associated with reduced clearance of hippocampal memory traces. Neuron 32:911–926

Fuchs E, Tumbar T, Guasch G (2004) Socializing with the neighbors: stem cells and their niche. Cell 116:769–778

Gabay L, Lowell S, Rubin LL, Anderson DJ (2003) Deregulation of dorsoventral patterning by FGF confers trilineage differentiation capacity on CNS stem cells in vitro. Neuron 40:485–499

Gage FH (2000) Mammalian neural stem cells. Science 287:1433–1438

Gaiano N, Nye JS, Fishell G (2000) Radial glial identity is promoted by Notch1 signaling in the murine forebrain. Neuron 26:395–404

Garcia AD, Doan NB, Imura T, Bush TG, Sofroniew MV (2004) GFAP-expressing progenitors are the principal source of constitutive neurogenesis in adult mouse forebrain. Nat Neurosci 7:1233–1241

Gomes WA, Mehler MF, Kessler JA (2003) Transgenic overexpression of BMP4 increases astroglial and decreases oligodendroglial lineage commitment. Dev Biol 255:164–177

Goodell MA, Brose K, Paradis G, Conner AS, Mulligan RC (1996) Isolation and functional properties of murine hematopoietic stem cells that are replicating in vivo. J Exp Med 183:1797–1806

Goodell MA, Rosenzweig M, Kim H, Marks DF, DeMaria M, Paradis G, Grupp SA, Sieff CA, Mulligan RC, Johnson RP (1997) Dye efflux studies suggest that hematopoietic stem cells expressing low or undetectable levels of CD34 antigen exist in multiple species. Nat Med 3:1337–1345

Götz M, Hartfuss E, Malatesta P (2002) Radial glial cells as neuronal precursors: a new perspective on the correlation of morphology and lineage restriction in the developing cerebral cortex of mice. Brain Res Bull 57:777–788

Götz M, Huttner WB (2005) The cell biology of neurogenesis. Nat Rev Neurosci, in press

Götz M, Steindler D (2003) To be glial or not: how glial are the precursors of neurons in development and adulthood? Glia 43:1–3

Gritti A, Bonfanti L, Doetsch F, Caille I, Alvarez-Buylla A, Lim DA, Galli R, Verdugo JM, Herrera DG, Vescovi AL (2002) Multipotent neural stem cells reside into the rostral extension and olfactory bulb of adult rodents. J Neurosci 22:437–445

Grove EA, Williams BP, Li DQ, Hajihosseini M, Friedrich A, Price J (1993) Multiple restricted lineages in the embryonic rat cerebral cortex. Development 117:553–561

Hack MA, Saghatelyan A, de Chevigny A, Ashery-Padan R, Lledo PM, Götz M (2005) Neuronal fate determinants of adult olfactory bulb neurogenesis. Nat Neurosci, 8:865–872

Hack MA, Sugimori M, Lundberg C, Nakafuku M, Götz M (2004) Regionalization and fate specification in neurospheres: the role of Olig2 and Pax6. Mol Cell Neurosci 25:664–678

Haubst N, Berger J, Radjendirane V, Graw J, Favor J, Saunders GF, Stoykova A, Götz M (2004) Molecular dissection of Pax6 function: the specific roles of the paired domain and homeodomain in brain development. Development 131:6131–6140

Hayashi Y, Ueki K, Waha A, Wiestler OD, Louis DN, von Deimling A (1997) Association of EGFR gene amplification and CDKN2 (p16/MTS1) gene deletion in glioblastoma multiforme. Brain Pathol 7:871–875

Heins N, Malatesta P, Cecconi F, Nakafuku M, Tucker KL, Hack MA, Chapouton P, Barde YA, Götz M (2002) Glial cells generate neurons: the role of the transcription factor Pax6. Nat Neurosci 5:308–315

Hemmati HD, Nakano I, Lazareff JA, Masterman-Smith M, Geschwind DH, Bronner-Fraser M, Kornblum HI (2003) Cancerous stem cells can arise from pediatric brain tumors. Proc Natl Acad Sci U S A 100:15178–15183

Hitoshi S, Alexson T, Tropepe V, Donoviel D, Elia AJ, Nye JS, Conlon RA, Mak TW, Bernstein A, van der Kooy D (2002) Notch pathway molecules are essential for the maintenance, but not the generation, of mammalian neural stem cells. Genes Dev 16:846–858

Ho KS, Scott MP (2002) Sonic hedgehog in the nervous system: functions, modifications and mechanisms. Curr Opin Neurobiol 12:57–63

Hofstetter CP, Holmstrom NA, Lilja JA, Schweinhardt P, Hao J, Spenger C, Wiesenfeld-Hallin Z, Kurpad SN, Frisen J, Olson L (2005) Allodynia limits the usefulness of intraspinal neural stem cell grafts; directed differentiation improves outcome. Nat Neurosci 8:346–353

Höglinger GU, Rizk P, Muriel MP, Duyckaerts C, Oertel WH, Caille I, Hirsch EC (2004) Dopamine depletion impairs precursor cell proliferation in Parkinson disease. Nat Neurosci 7:726–735

Hope KJ, Jin L, Dick JE (2004) Acute myeloid leukemia originates from a hierarchy of leukemic stem cell classes that differ in self-renewal capacity. Nat Immunol 5:738–743

Huttner WB, Brand M (1997) Asymmetric division and polarity of neuroepithelial cells. Curr Opin Neurobiol 7:29–39

Iakova P, Awad SS, Timchenko NA (2003) Aging reduces proliferative capacities of liver by switching pathways of C/EBPalpha growth arrest. Cell 113:495–506

Jacobs JJ, Kieboom K, Marino S, DePinho RA, van Lohuizen M (1999) The oncogene and Polycomb-group gene bmi-1 regulates cell proliferation and senescence through the ink4a locus. Nature 397:164–168

Jin K, Zhu Y, Sun Y, Mao XO, Xie L, Greenberg DA (2002) Vascular endothelial growth factor (VEGF) stimulates neurogenesis in vitro and in vivo. Proc Natl Acad Sci U S A 99:11946–11950

Johansson CB, Momma S, Clarke DL, Risling M, Lendahl U, Frisen J (1999) Identification of a neural stem cell in the adult mammalian central nervous system. Cell 96:25–34

Kageyama R, Ohtsuka T (1999) The Notch-Hes pathway in mammalian neural development. Cell Res 9:179–188

Kaila K (1994) Ionic basis of GABAA receptor channel function in the nervous system. Prog Neurobiol 42:489–537

Kaplan MS, Bell DH (1984) Mitotic neuroblasts in the 9-day-old and 11-month-old rodent hippocampus. J Neurosci 4:1429–1441

Kawasaki H, Mizuseki K, Nishikawa S, Kaneko S, Kuwana Y, Nakanishi S, Nishikawa SI, Sasai Y (2000) Induction of midbrain dopaminergic neurons from ES cells by stromal cell-derived inducing activity. Neuron 28:31–40

Kempermann G, Kuhn HG, Gage FH (1997) More hippocampal neurons in adult mice living in an enriched environment. Nature 386:493–495

Kim JH, Panchision D, Kittappa R, McKay R (2003a) Generating CNS neurons from embryonic, fetal, and adult stem cells. Methods Enzymol 365:303–327

Kim JY, Koh HC, Lee JY, Chang MY, Kim YC, Chung HY, Son H, Lee YS, Studer L, McKay R, Lee SH (2003b) Dopaminergic neuronal differentiation from rat embryonic neural precursors by Nurr1 overexpression. J Neurochem 85:1443–1454

Kim M, Morshead CM (2003) Distinct populations of forebrain neural stem and progenitor cells can be isolated using side-population analysis. J Neurosci 23:10703–10709

Kornack DR, Rakic P (2001a) Cell proliferation without neurogenesis in adult primate neocortex. Science 294:2127–2130

Kornack DR, Rakic P (2001b) The generation, migration, and differentiation of olfactory neurons in the adult primate brain. Proc Natl Acad Sci U S A 98:4752–4757

Kosodo Y, Roper K, Haubensak W, Marzesco AM, Corbeil D, Huttner WB (2004) Asymmetric distribution of the apical plasma membrane during neurogenic divisions of mammalian neuroepithelial cells. EMBO J 23:2314–2324

Kuhn HG, Dickinson-Anson H, Gage FH (1996) Neurogenesis in the dentate gyrus of the adult rat: age-related decrease of neuronal progenitor proliferation. J Neurosci 16:2027–2033

Kuhn HG, Winkler J, Kempermann G, Thal LJ, Gage FH (1997) Epidermal growth factor and fibroblast growth factor-2 have different effects on neural progenitors in the adult rat brain. J Neurosci 17:5820–5829

Kunisato A, Chiba S, Nakagami-Yamaguchi E, Kumano K, Saito T, Masuda S, Yamaguchi T, Osawa M, Kageyama R, Nakauchi H, Nishikawa M, Hirai H (2003) HES-1 preserves purified hematopoietic stem cells ex vivo and accumulates side population cells in vivo. Blood 101:1777–1783

Lai K, Kaspar BK, Gage FH, Schaffer DV (2003) Sonic hedgehog regulates adult neural progenitor proliferation in vitro and in vivo. Nat Neurosci 6:21–27

Lapidot T, Sirard C, Vormoor J, Murdoch B, Hoang T, Caceres-Cortes J, Minden M, Paterson B, Caligiuri MA, Dick JE (1994) A cell initiating human acute myeloid leukaemia after transplantation into SCID mice. Nature 367:645–648

Laywell ED, Rakic P, Kukekov VG, Holland EC, Steindler DA (2000) Identification of a multipotent astrocytic stem cell in the immature and adult mouse brain. Proc Natl Acad Sci U S A 97:13883–13888

Lessard J, Sauvageau G (2003) Bmi-1 determines the proliferative capacity of normal and leukaemic stem cells. Nature 423:255–260

Leung C, Lingbeek M, Shakhova O, Liu J, Tanger E, Saremaslani P, Van Lohuizen M, Marino S (2004) Bmi1 is essential for cerebellar development and is overexpressed in human medulloblastomas. Nature 428:337–341

Lim DA, Alvarez-Buylla A (1999) Interaction between astrocytes and adult subventricular zone precursors stimulates neurogenesis. Proc Natl Acad Sci U S A 96:7526–7531

Lim DA, Tramontin AD, Trevejo JM, Herrera DG, Garcia-Verdugo JM, Alvarez-Buylla A (2000) Noggin antagonizes BMP signaling to create a niche for adult neurogenesis. Neuron 28:713–726

Liu SY, Zhang ZY, Song YC, Qiu KJ, Zhang KC, An N, Zhou Z, Cai WQ, Yang H (2004) SVZa neural stem cells differentiate into distinct lineages in response to BMP4. Exp Neurol 190:109–121

Lois C, Alvarez-Buylla A (1993) Proliferating subventricular zone cells in the adult mammalian forebrain can differentiate into neurons and glia. Proc Natl Acad Sci U S A 90:2074–2077

Lois C, Alvarez-Buylla A (1994) Long-distance neuronal migration in the adult mammalian brain. Science 264:1145–1148

Lois C, Garcia-Verdugo JM, Alvarez-Buylla A (1996) Chain migration of neuronal precursors. Science 271:978–981

Louissaint A Jr, Rao S, Leventhal C, Goldman SA (2002) Coordinated interaction of neurogenesis and angiogenesis in the adult songbird brain. Neuron 34:945–960

Lukaszewicz A, Savatier P, Cortay V, Kennedy H, Dehay C (2002) Contrasting effects of basic fibroblast growth factor and neurotrophin 3 on cell cycle kinetics of mouse cortical stem cells. J Neurosci 22:6610–6622

Luskin MB (1993) Restricted proliferation and migration of postnatally generated neurons derived from the forebrain subventricular zone. Neuron 11:173–189

Luskin MB (1998) Neuroblasts of the postnatal mammalian forebrain: their phenotype and fate. J Neurobiol 36:221–233

Machold R, Hayashi S, Rutlin M, Muzumdar MD, Nery S, Corbin JG, Gritli-Linde A, Dellovade T, Porter JA, Rubin LL, Dudek H, McMahon AP, Fishell G (2003) Sonic hedgehog is required for progenitor cell maintenance in telencephalic stem cell niches. Neuron 39:937–950

Magavi SS, Leavitt BR, Macklis JD (2000) Induction of neurogenesis in the neocortex of adult mice. Nature 405:951–955

Malatesta P, Hack MA, Hartfuss E, Kettenmann H, Klinkert W, Kirchhoff F, Götz M (2003) Neuronal or glial progeny: regional differences in radial glia fate. Neuron 37:751–764

Malatesta P, Hartfuss E, Götz M (2000) Isolation of radial glial cells by fluorescent-activated cell sorting reveals a neuronal lineage. Development 127:5253–5263

Malberg JE, Eisch AJ, Nestler EJ, Duman RS (2000) Chronic antidepressant treatment increases neurogenesis in adult rat hippocampus. J Neurosci 20:9104–9110

Mechawar N, Saghatelyan A, Grailhe R, Scoriels L, Gheusi G, Gabellec MM, Lledo PM, Changeux JP (2004) Nicotinic receptors regulate the survival of newborn neurons in the adult olfactory bulb. Proc Natl Acad Sci U S A 101:9822–9826

Merkle FT, Tramontin AD, Garcia-Verdugo JM, Alvarez-Buylla A (2004) Radial glia give rise to adult neural stem cells in the subventricular zone. Proc Natl Acad Sci U S A 101:17528–17532

Molofsky AV, Pardal R, Iwashita T, Park IK, Clarke MF, Morrison SJ (2003) Bmi-1 dependence distinguishes neural stem cell self-renewal from progenitor proliferation. Nature 425:962–967

Morrison SJ, Perez SE, Qiao Z, Verdi JM, Hicks C, Weinmaster G, Anderson DJ (2000) Transient Notch activation initiates an irreversible switch from neurogenesis to gliogenesis by neural crest stem cells. Cell 101:499–510

Morshead CM, Garcia AD, Sofroniew MV, van Der Kooy D (2003) The ablation of glial fibrillary acidic protein-positive cells from the adult central nervous system results in the loss of forebrain neural stem cells but not retinal stem cells. Eur J Neurosci 18:76–84

Nakatomi H, Kuriu T, Okabe S, Yamamoto S, Hatano O, Kawahara N, Tamura A, Kirino T, Nakafuku M (2002) Regeneration of hippocampal pyramidal neurons after ischemic brain injury by recruitment of endogenous neural progenitors. Cell 110:429–441

Noctor SC, Flint AC, Weissman TA, Dammerman RS, Kriegstein AR (2001) Neurons derived from radial glial cells establish radial units in neocortex. Nature 409:714–720

Nunes MC, Roy NS, Keyoung HM, Goodman RR, McKhann G 2nd, Jiang L, Kang J, Nedergaard M, Goldman SA (2003) Identification and isolation of multipotential neural progenitor cells from the subcortical white matter of the adult human brain. Nat Med 9:439–447

Nye JS, Kopan R, Axel R (1994) An activated Notch suppresses neurogenesis and myogenesis but not gliogenesis in mammalian cells. Development 120:2421–2430

Ohtsuka T, Ishibashi M, Gradwohl G, Nakanishi S, Guillemot F, Kageyama R (1999) Hes1 and Hes5 as notch effectors in mammalian neuronal differentiation. EMBO J 18:2196–2207

Ohtsuka T, Sakamoto M, Guillemot F, Kageyama R (2001) Roles of the basic helix-loop-helix genes Hes1 and Hes5 in expansion of neural stem cells of the developing brain. J Biol Chem 276:30467–30474

Palma V, Lim DA, Dahmane N, Sanchez P, Brionne TC, Herzberg CD, Gitton Y, Carleton A, Alvarez-Buylla A, Ruiz i Altaba A (2005) Sonic hedgehog controls stem cell behavior in the postnatal and adult brain. Development 132:335–344

Palmer TD, Markakis EA, Willhoite AR, Safar F, Gage FH (1999) Fibroblast growth factor-2 activates a latent neurogenic program in neural stem cells from diverse regions of the adult CNS. J Neurosci 19:8487–8497

Palmer TD, Willhoite AR, Gage FH (2000) Vascular niche for adult hippocampal neurogenesis. J Comp Neurol 425:479–494

Parent JM, Yu TW, Leibowitz RT, Geschwind DH, Sloviter RS, Lowenstein DH (1997) Dentate granule cell neurogenesis is increased by seizures and contributes to aberrant network reorganization in the adult rat hippocampus. J Neurosci 17:3727–3738

Park IK, Qian D, Kiel M, Becker MW, Pihalja M, Weissman IL, Morrison SJ, Clarke MF (2003) Bmi-1 is required for maintenance of adult self-renewing haematopoietic stem cells. Nature 423:302–305

Parmar M, Sjoberg A, Björklund A, Kokaia Z (2003) Phenotypic and molecular identity of cells in the adult subventricular zone in vivo and after expansion in vitro. Mol Cell Neurosci 24:741–752

Parras CM, Galli R, Britz O, Soares S, Galichet C, Battiste J, Johnson JE, Nakafuku M, Vescovi A, Guillemot F (2004) Mash1 specifies neurons and oligodendrocytes in the postnatal brain. Embo J 23:4495–4505

Pencea V, Bingaman KD, Freedman LJ, Luskin MB (2001) Neurogenesis in the subventricular zone and rostral migratory stream of the neonatal and adult primate forebrain. Exp Neurol 172:1–16

Peretto P, Dati C, De Marchis S, Kim HH, Ukhanova M, Fasolo A, Margolis FL (2004) Expression of the secreted factors noggin and bone morphogenetic proteins in the subependymal layer and olfactory bulb of the adult mouse brain. Neuroscience 128:685–696

Perrier AL, Tabar V, Barberi T, Rubio ME, Bruses J, Topf N, Harrison NL, Studer L (2004) Derivation of midbrain dopamine neurons from human embryonic stem cells. Proc Natl Acad Sci U S A 101:12543–12548

Petreanu L, Alvarez-Buylla A (2002) Maturation and death of adult-born olfactory bulb granule neurons: role of olfaction. J Neurosci 22:6106–6113

Picard-Riera N, Decker L, Delarasse C, Goude K, Nait-Oumesmar B, Liblau R, Pham-Dinh D, Evercooren AB (2002) Experimental autoimmune encephalomyelitis mobilizes neural progenitors from the subventricular zone to undergo oligodendrogenesis in adult mice. Proc Natl Acad Sci U S A 99:13211–13216

Plachta N, Bibel M, Tucker KL, Barde YA (2004) Developmental potential of defined neural progenitors derived from mouse embryonic stem cells. Development 131:5449–5456

Pluchino S, Quattrini A, Brambilla E, Gritti A, Salani G, Dina G, Galli R, Del Carro U, Amadio S, Bergami A, Furlan R, Comi G, Vescovi AL, Martino G (2003) Injection of adult neurospheres induces recovery in a chronic model of multiple sclerosis. Nature 422:688–694

Pomeroy SL, Tamayo P, Gaasenbeek M, Sturla LM, Angelo M, McLaughlin ME, Kim JY, Goumnerova LC, Black PM, Lau C, Allen JC, Zagzag D, Olson JM, Curran T, Wetmore C, Biegel JA, Poggio T, Mukherjee S, Rifkin R, Califano A, Stolovitzky G, Louis DN, Mesirov JP, Lander ES, Golub TR (2002) Prediction of central nervous system embryonal tumour outcome based on gene expression. Nature 415:436–442

Price J, Thurlow L (1988) Cell lineage in the rat cerebral cortex: a study using retroviral-mediated gene transfer. Development 104:473–482

Qian X, Goderie SK, Shen Q, Stern JH, Temple S (1998) Intrinsic programs of patterned cell lineages in isolated vertebrate CNS ventricular zone cells. Development 125:3143–3152

Qian X, Shen Q, Goderie SK, He W, Capela A, Davis AA, Temple S (2000) Timing of CNS cell generation: a programmed sequence of neuron and glial cell production from isolated murine cortical stem cells. Neuron 28:69–80

Reya T, Morrison SJ, Clarke MF, Weissman IL (2001) Stem cells, cancer, and cancer stem cells. Nature 414:105–111

Reynolds BA, Weiss S (1992) Generation of neurons and astrocytes from isolated cells of the adult mammalian central nervous system. Science 255:1707–1710

Rietze RL, Valcanis H, Brooker GF, Thomas T, Voss AK, Bartlett PF (2001) Purification of a pluripotent neural stem cell from the adult mouse brain. Nature 412:736–739

Rochefort C, Gheusi G, Vincent JD, Lledo PM (2002) Enriched odor exposure increases the number of newborn neurons in the adult olfactory bulb and improves odor memory. J Neurosci 22:2679–2689

Roelink H, Porter JA, Chiang C, Tanabe Y, Chang DT, Beachy PA, Jessell TM (1995) Floor plate and motor neuron induction by different concentrations of the amino-terminal cleavage product of sonic hedgehog autoproteolysis. Cell 81:445–455

Roy K, Kuznicki K, Wu Q, Sun Z, Bock D, Schutz G, Vranich N, Monaghan AP (2004) The Tlx gene regulates the timing of neurogenesis in the cortex. J Neurosci 24:8333–8345

Saghatelyan A, de Chevigny A, Schachner M, Lledo PM (2004) Tenascin-R mediates activity-dependent recruitment of neuroblasts in the adult mouse forebrain. Nat Neurosci 7:347–356

Sairanen M, Lucas G, Ernfors P, Castren M, Castren E (2005) Brain-derived neurotrophic factor and antidepressant drugs have different but coordinated effects on neuronal turnover, proliferation, and survival in the adult dentate gyrus. J Neurosci 25:1089–1094

Sanai N, Tramontin AD, Quinones-Hinojosa A, Barbaro NM, Gupta N, Kunwar S, Lawton MT, McDermott MW, Parsa AT, Manuel-Garcia Verdugo J, Berger MS, Alvarez-Buylla A (2004) Unique astrocyte ribbon in adult human brain contains neural stem cells but lacks chain migration. Nature 427:740–744

Santarelli L, Saxe M, Gross C, Surget A, Battaglia F, Dulawa S, Weisstaub N, Lee J, Duman R, Arancio O, Belzung C, Hen R (2003) Requirement of hippocampal neurogenesis for the behavioral effects of antidepressants. Science 301:805–809

Schanzer A, Wachs FP, Wilhelm D, Acker T, Cooper-Kuhn C, Beck H, Winkler J, Aigner L, Plate KH, Kuhn HG (2004) Direct stimulation of adult neural stem cells in vitro and neurogenesis in vivo by vascular endothelial growth factor. Brain Pathol 14:237–248

Schinder AF, Gage FH (2004) A hypothesis about the role of adult neurogenesis in hippocampal function. Physiology (Bethesda) 19:253–261

Schmidt-Hieber C, Jonas P, Bischofberger J (2004) Enhanced synaptic plasticity in newly generated granule cells of the adult hippocampus. Nature 429:184–187

Seaberg RM, van der Kooy D (2002) Adult rodent neurogenic regions: the ventricular subependyma contains neural stem cells, but the dentate gyrus contains restricted progenitors. J Neurosci 22:1784–1793

Seri B, Garcia-Verdugo JM, Collado-Morente L, McEwen BS, Alvarez-Buylla A (2004) Cell types, lineage, and architecture of the germinal zone in the adult dentate gyrus. J Comp Neurol 478:359–378

Seri B, Garcia-Verdugo JM, McEwen BS, Alvarez-Buylla A (2001) Astrocytes give rise to new neurons in the adult mammalian hippocampus. J Neurosci 21:7153–7160

Shen Q, Goderie SK, Jin L, Karanth N, Sun Y, Abramova N, Vincent P, Pumiglia K, Temple S (2004) Endothelial cells stimulate self-renewal and expand neurogenesis of neural stem cells. Science 304:1338–1340

Shi Y, Chichung Lie D, Taupin P, Nakashima K, Ray J, Yu RT, Gage FH, Evans RM (2004) Expression and function of orphan nuclear receptor TLX in adult neural stem cells. Nature 427:78–83

Shihabuddin LS, Horner PJ, Ray J, Gage FH (2000) Adult spinal cord stem cells generate neurons after transplantation in the adult dentate gyrus. J Neurosci 20:8727–8735

Shors TJ, Townsend DA, Zhao M, Kozorovitskiy Y, Gould E (2002) Neurogenesis may relate to some but not all types of hippocampal-dependent learning. Hippocampus 12:578–584

Singh SK, Clarke ID, Terasaki M, Bonn VE, Hawkins C, Squire J, Dirks PB (2003) Identification of a cancer stem cell in human brain tumors. Cancer Res 63:5821–5828

Singh SK, Hawkins C, Clarke ID, Squire JA, Bayani J, Hide T, Henkelman RM, Cusimano MD, Dirks PB (2004) Identification of human brain tumour initiating cells. Nature 432:396–401

Song H, Stevens CF, Gage FH (2002a) Astroglia induce neurogenesis from adult neural stem cells. Nature 417:39–44

Song HJ, Stevens CF, Gage FH (2002b) Neural stem cells from adult hippocampus develop essential properties of functional CNS neurons. Nat Neurosci 5:438–445

Spradling A, Drummond-Barbosa D, Kai T (2001) Stem cells find their niche. Nature 414:98–104

Stenman J, Toresson H, Campbell K (2003) Identification of two distinct progenitor populations in the lateral ganglionic eminence: implications for striatal and olfactory bulb neurogenesis. J Neurosci 23:167–174

Suhonen JO, Peterson DA, Ray J, Gage FH (1996) Differentiation of adult hippocampus-derived progenitors into olfactory neurons in vivo. Nature 383:624–627

Tanigaki K, Nogaki F, Takahashi J, Tashiro K, Kurooka H, Honjo T (2001) Notch1 and Notch3 instructively restrict bFGF-responsive multipotent neural progenitor cells to an astroglial fate. Neuron 29:45–55

Taylor MD, Liu L, Raffel C, Hui CC, Mainprize TG, Zhang X, Agatep R, Chiappa S, Gao L, Lowrance A, Hao A, Goldstein AM, Stavrou T, Scherer SW, Dura WT, Wainwright B, Squire JA, Rutka JT, Hogg D (2002) Mutations in SUFU predispose to medulloblastoma. Nat Genet 31:306–310

Traiffort E, Charytoniuk D, Watroba L, Faure H, Sales N, Ruat M (1999) Discrete localizations of hedgehog signalling components in the developing and adult rat nervous system. Eur J Neurosci 11:3199–3214

Tramontin AD, Garcia-Verdugo JM, Lim DA, Alvarez-Buylla A (2003) Postnatal development of radial glia and the ventricular zone (VZ): a continuum of the neural stem cell compartment. Cereb Cortex 13:580–587

Tropepe V, Craig CG, Morshead CM, van der Kooy D (1997) Transforming growth factor-alpha null and senescent mice show decreased neural progenitor cell proliferation in the forebrain subependyma. J Neurosci 17:7850–7859

Van Praag H, Kempermann G, Gage FH (1999) Running increases cell proliferation and neurogenesis in the adult mouse dentate gyrus. Nat Neurosci 2:266–270

Van Praag H, Schinder AF, Christie BR, Toni N, Palmer TD, Gage FH (2002) Functional neurogenesis in the adult hippocampus. Nature 415:1030–1034

Von Deimling A, Louis DN, von Ammon K, Petersen I, Hoell T, Chung RY, Martuza RL, Schoenfeld DA, Yasargil MG, Wiestler OD et al (1992) Association of epidermal growth factor receptor gene amplification with loss of chromosome 10 in human glioblastoma multiforme. J Neurosurg 77:295–301

Walsh C, Cepko CL (1993) Clonal dispersion in proliferative layers of developing cerebral cortex. Nature 362:632–635

Watanabe K, Kamiya D, Nishiyama A, Katayama T, Nozaki S, Kawasaki H, Watanabe Y, Mizuseki K, Sasai Y (2005) Directed differentiation of telencephalic precursors from embryonic stem cells. Nat Neurosci 8:288–296

Wechsler-Reya R, Scott MP (2001) The developmental biology of brain tumors. Annu Rev Neurosci 24:385–428

Weickert CS, Blum M (1995) Striatal TGF-alpha: postnatal developmental expression and evidence for a role in the proliferation of subependymal cells. Brain Res Dev Brain Res 86:203–216

Weiss S, Dunne C, Hewson J, Wohl C, Wheatley M, Peterson AC, Reynolds BA (1996) Multipotent CNS stem cells are present in the adult mammalian spinal cord and ventricular neuroaxis. J Neurosci 16:7599–7609

Weissman IL (2000) Stem cells: units of development, units of regeneration, and units in evolution. Cell 100:157–168

Wernig M, Benninger F, Schmandt T, Rade M, Tucker KL, Bussow H, Beck H, Brustle O (2004) Functional integration of embryonic stem cell-derived neurons in vivo. J Neurosci 24:5258–5268

Wichterle H, Lieberam I, Porter JA, Jessell TM (2002) Directed differentiation of embryonic stem cells into motor neurons. Cell 110:385–397

Wilcox JN, Derynck R (1988) Localization of cells synthesizing transforming growth factor-alpha mRNA in the mouse brain. J Neurosci 8:1901–1904

Wodarz A, Huttner WB (2003) Asymmetric cell division during neurogenesis in Drosophila and vertebrates. Mech Dev 120:1297–1309

Ye W, Shimamura K, Rubenstein JL, Hynes MA, Rosenthal A (1998) FGF and Shh signals control dopaminergic and serotonergic cell fate in the anterior neural plate. Cell 93:755–766

Yuan X, Curtin J, Xiong Y, Liu G, Waschsmann-Hogiu S, Farkas DL, Black KL, Yu JS (2004) Isolation of cancer stem cells from adult glioblastoma multiforme. Oncogene 23:9392–9400

Zhang R, Zhang Z, Zhang C, Zhang L, Robin A, Wang Y, Lu M, Chopp M (2004) Stroke transiently increases subventricular zone cell division from asymmetric to symmetric and increases neuronal differentiation in the adult rat. J Neurosci 24:5810–5815

Zheng W, Nowakowski RS, Vaccarino FM (2004) Fibroblast growth factor 2 is required for maintaining the neural stem cell pool in the mouse brain subventricular zone. Dev Neurosci 26:181–196

Zurawel RH, Allen C, Chiappa S, Cato W, Biegel J, Cogen P, de Sauvage F, Raffel C (2000) Analysis of PTCH/SMO/SHH pathway genes in medulloblastoma. Genes Chromosomes Cancer 27:44–51

HEP (2006) 174:361–388
© Springer-Verlag Berlin Heidelberg 2006

Cell Transplantation for Patients with Parkinson's Disease

G. Paul

Neuronal Survival Unit, Experimental Medical Sciences, Wallenberg Neurocentrum,
University of Lund, BMC A10, 22184 Lund, Sweden
gesine.paul@mphy.lu.se

Abstract This chapter focuses on cell replacement therapies in Parkinson's disease (PD) and describes experimental data leading to clinical trials, as well as the methodology and efficacy of grafts of human embryonic nigral tissue in patients with PD. It also highlights some of the clinical problems the procedure presents and considers future alternative sources of donor tissue, including various forms of stem cells.

Keywords Parkinson's disease · Neurotransplantation · Dyskinesia · Stem cells

Abbreviations

AADC	L-aromatic amino acid decarboxylase
ASC	Adult stem cell
CAPIT	Core Assessment Protocol for Intracerebral Transplantations
CAPSIT	Core Assessment Program for Surgical interventions and Transplantation
CMV	Cytomegalovirus
CNS	Central nervous system
DA	Dopaminergic
DAT	Dopamine transporter
DOPA	Dihydroxyphenylalanine
F-DOPA	Fluoro-DOPA
Gpi	Globus pallidus internus
En	Engrailed
ES	Embryonic stem
bFGF	Basic fibroblast growth factor
c-Ret	Protein kinase receptor, ligand is glial cell line-derived neurotrophic factor (GDNF)
MRI	Magnetic resonance imaging
NIH	National Institute of Health
Nurr	Nur(nuclear receptor)-related factor
6-OHDA	6-Hydroxydopamine
PET	Positron-emission tomography
PERV	Porcine endogenous retrovirus
PD	Parkinson's disease
Ptx	Paired-like homeodomain transcription factor
SN	Substantia nigra
SNc	Substantia nigra pars compacta
STN	Subthalamic nucleus
SVZ	Subventricular zone
TGF α	Transforming growth factor alpha
TH	Tyrosine hydroxylase
UPDRS	Unified Parkinson's Disease Rating Scale
VM	Ventral mesencephalon
VMAT	Vesicle membrane-associated transporter
VTA	Ventral tegmental area

1
Introduction: Parkinson's Disease

Parkinson's disease is the second most common neurodegenerative disorder and affects almost 1% of the population above the age of 60 (Inzelberg et al. 2002). Patients primarily suffer from motor symptoms such as bradykinesia (slowness of movement), rigidity (muscle stiffness) and tremor at rest (for review see Lang and Lozano 1998a, 1998b; Samii et al. 2004). These symptoms progress over time and, in addition, most patients eventually exhibit vegetative disturbances, depression (Oertel et al. 2001), and dementia in the course of the disease (Mayeux et al. 1990; Aarsland et al. 1996).

The main neuropathologic finding in PD is the progressive loss of dopaminergic (DA) neurons in the substantia nigra pars compacta (SNc). These neurons project to the striatum and their loss results in a reduction of striatal dopamine (DA) levels (Kish et al. 1988; Agid 1991; Fearnley and Lees 1991). The precise etiology of the cell loss is still not known. There are several hypotheses regarding the pathogenetic mechanisms in PD such as mitochondrial dysfunction, oxidative stress, exogenous toxins, intracellular accumulation of toxic metabolites, viral infections, excitotoxicity, deficient trophic support and immune mechanisms; additionally a genetic predisposition may play a role (for review see Schapira 1997; Samii et al. 2004).

Due to the lack of understanding of PD etiology and pathogenesis, there is still no treatment that can prevent or retard the progression of the disease. The following chapter will briefly summarize currently available symptomatic treatments for Parkinson's disease and then focus on cell replacement strategies as a still experimental approach to treat PD. The experimental background, the grafting technique, clinical trials, and current problems will be described. Future directions using stem cells as a cell source for transplantation or endogenous cell repair are illustrated.

2
Treatment of Parkinson's Disease

2.1
Pharmacological Treatment

Since the late 1960s, the main approach to treating PD has been the pharmacological alleviation of the striatal DA deficit by administration of the DA precursor L-Dopa in combination with drugs inhibiting L-Dopa breakdown and/or drugs enhancing dopaminergic transmission by blocking the breakdown of DA. There are also several DA agonists that act by direct binding on postsynaptic receptor sites. Nondopaminergic medications include anticholinergic agents and amantadine, which blocks a class of glutamatergic receptors (for review see Rascol et al. 2002; Samii et al. 2004).

Pharmacological treatment of PD has been remarkably successful in reducing motor symptoms in PD early in the course of the disease, but at later stages patients often develop one or several treatment complications. The loss of drug efficacy is apparent in "wearing-off" symptoms; as a result, increasing and more frequent doses of medication are required. Later, psychiatric disturbances such as hallucinations may develop, probably as a consequence of stimulation of DA receptors outside the striatum. Another major problem is the partly unpredictable fluctuation between immobility and an increased ability to move (the so called on-off phenomenon). During the "on" phases, when the drug allows the patients to move, they typically exhibit disturbing involuntary movements, termed dyskinesias.

2.2
Surgical Treatment

Due to the problems associated with long-term pharmacological DA replacement therapy, new treatments have been developed. Three different neurosurgical approaches have been tested in PD patients: first, ablative procedures, thalamotomy, pallidotomy and subthalamotomy; second, functional lesions using electrical currents (deep brain stimulation, DBS), aiming at the ventral intermediate nucleus (VIM) of the thalamus, the subthalamic nucleus (STN), or the internal segment of the globus pallidus (Gpi) (for review see Walter and Vitek 2004). These interventions attempt to restore functional imbalance in the basal ganglia and are based on observations that imply a hyperactivity of structures such as the STN and the GPi as a result of the dopaminergic deficit (Alexander and Crutcher 1990; DeLong 1990). The third surgical approach aims at the replacement of the lost cell type by transplantation of different cell types to the brain (Bjorklund and Lindvall 2000) and is discussed further in this chapter.

Transplantation attempts to restore function of the diseased cells or organ by replacing lost cells. This is clinical practice for several organs; however, cell replacement in the brain remains experimental. Repairing the diseased brain has been the dream of physicians and scientists for decades, even though at first glance it seems unrealistic to attempt functional recovery by replacing lost neurons in such a complex structure as the brain. Parkinson's disease is a good candidate for cell replacement therapy primarily because the symptoms result from a progressive loss of dopaminergic cells in a circumscribed region, the SNc, albeit not exclusively (Braak et al. 2004). Replenishment of lost dopaminergic neurons by grafting immature neurons seems obvious and studies in animal models of PD have demonstrated that neuronal replacement and partial reconstruction of the diseased neuronal circuitry is indeed possible.

3
Animal Experiments: The Proof of Principle

Cell-based therapies for experimental and clinical PD have undergone considerable development over the past three decades (Dunnett et al. 2001). Experiments in animal models of PD have shown the proof of concept and helped to understand the neurobiological principles that underlie the integration and function of grafted cells in the damaged nervous system.

Olson and co-workers were the first to graft catecholamine-secreting cells in the nervous system. They transplanted adrenal chromaffin cells and embryonic dopaminergic neurons into the anterior eye chamber of the rat (Olson and Malmfors 1970; Olson and Seiger 1972). These studies revealed that developing embryonic neurons are needed to achieve survival and neurite outgrowth from grafted neurons. Therefore cells have to be dissected during a critical stage of development when neurons are already determined to become dopaminergic but are not yet fully differentiated. A few years later, it was demonstrated that embryonic DA neurons could also be grafted to the brain (Bjorklund et al. 1976; Stenevi et al. 1976) and that grafts can lead to functional recovery in hemiparkinsonian rats (Bjorklund and Stenevi 1979; Perlow et al. 1979). In these experiments, rats were injected unilaterally into the nigrostriatal pathway with 6-hydroxydopamine (6-OHDA) that causes an ipsilateral depletion of striatal DA due to cell loss in the SN. The imbalance in striatal DA leads to motor asymmetry that can be amplified as rotational behavior by administration of drugs that affect the DA system such as amphetamine or apomorphine (Ungerstedt and Arbuthnott 1970) Fig. 1 a,b). In these pioneering studies, graft tissue was dissected from the ventral mesencephalon (VM) of rat embryos, a region that contains a large number of immature dopaminergic neurons in the developing SN, and ventral tegmental area (VTA). The tissue was transplanted in two ways: as solid grafts of nigral tissue into the ventricle adjacent to the denervated striatum (Perlow et al. 1979) or into pre-made cortical cavities overlying the striatum (Bjorklund and Stenevi 1979). Nigral tissue grafts reversed motor asymmetry in the rats and extended axons into the denervated host striatum.

Shortly thereafter, cell suspension grafting technology, a dissociated neuronal culture technique, was introduced. Donor tissue is enzymatically digested and mechanically dissociated to a single cell suspension that can be drawn into a microsyringe and stereotactically injected into any desired brain region

Table 1 Conclusions from experimental studies grafting cells into the brain in animals model of Parkinson's disease

Immature (embryonic) neurons are needed to achieve survival and neurite outgrowth.
Grafted immature dopaminergic neurons:

Survive transplantation

Reinnervate the lesioned striatum (the target structure of dopaminergic neurons)

Make synaptic contacts with the host striatum

Release dopamine in a regulated fashion

Restore baseline dopamine synthesis

Are tonically active

Receive inputs from host neurons and partially reverse several different motor deficits in animal models of Parkinson's disease

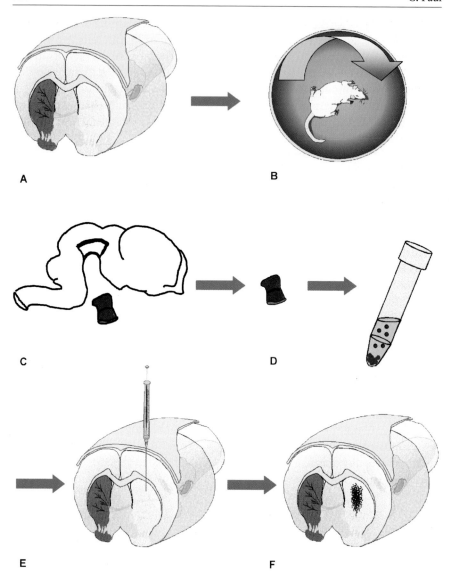

Fig. 1a–f Illustration of intracerebral grafting in a rat model of PD. **a** Unilateral lesion of the nigrostriatal pathway leads to DA depletion in the striatum. **b** Animals exhibit rotational behavior as a result of striatal DA imbalance. **c** The ventral mesencephalon (VM) is dissected out from the midbrain of a rat embryo and is (**d**) enzymatically and mechanically dissociated. **e** The cell suspension is stereotactically injected into the DA depleted striatum. **f** The grafted cells survive, integrate into the host brain and express TH

(Schmidt et al. 1981; Bjorklund et al. 1983a, 1983b; Dunnett et al. 1983a, 1983b; Schmidt et al. 1983) (see Fig. 1, illustrating experimental methodology).

Grafted dopaminergic neurons make synaptic contacts with the host striatum (Freund et al. 1985; Mahalik et al. 1985) and release DA in a regulated fashion (Zetterstrom et al. 1986; Strecker et al. 1987). Moreover, transplanted neurons receive inputs from host neurons (Arbuthnott et al. 1985; Doucet et al. 1989) and partially reverse several different motor deficits in animal models of PD (for conclusions from experimental studies, see Table 1). Graft effects were examined using several different motor tests. Grafts have been shown to reverse many of the simple sensorimotor deficits in PD models, however, more complex motor behaviors have not been as readily ameliorated (for review, see Brundin et al. 1994).

4
Clinical Trials in Parkinson's Disease: What Cells to Graft?

4.1
Initial Transplantations Using Different Cell Sources

The first clinical trials in PD used catecholaminergic cells from the adrenal medulla (Backlund et al. 1985). In this procedure, the relevant cells were dissected from one adrenal medulla of the patient and transplanted back into the brain. Several hundred patients received such grafts in the late 1980s in a series of rather poorly controlled clinical trials (Backlund et al. 1985; Lindvall et al. 1987; Madrazo et al. 1987, 1988, 1990a, 1990b). However, these surgical procedures not only failed to produce beneficial effects, but some were also accompanied by an unacceptable level of mortality and morbidity (Goetz et al. 1991). Other sources of catecholaminergic donor cells such as carotid body cells (Espejo et al. 1998; Luquin et al. 1999) and superior cervical ganglion cells (Itakura et al. 1994, 1997) have been grafted to patients without major clinical benefit. A small number of patients have received human retinal pigment epithelium cells (Subramanian 2001; Bakay et al. 2004) and 6 months after implantation some improvement has been reported (Bakay et al. 2004). However, we await the results of long-term studies.

4.2
Transplanting Human Embryonic/Fetal Mesencephalic Tissue

In the late 1980s, the first systematic clinical transplantation trials using embryonic dopaminergic neurons in patients with PD were conducted (Lindvall et al. 1988, 1989; Madrazo et al. 1988, 1990a, 1990b). Those cells are derived from embryonic VM, the region in the developing CNS that is rich in immature dopaminergic neurons. The neural transplantation surgery protocol varies between different centers regarding donor age, tissue storage and preparation, numbers and location of injections, and the use of immunosuppression.

5
The Grafting Technique

At Lund University, Sweden, 18 patients have been transplanted to date. Cells were taken from the VM during embryonic development between the 5th and 8th week after fertilization, at a time when the neurons are undergoing terminal differentiation (Freeman et al. 1991; Brundin 1992). The embryos are collected from routine elective abortions with informed consent of the women undergoing abortion, in accordance with strict ethical guidelines (Boer 1994). The embryo is rinsed in sterile balanced salt solution and the VM dissected. Some centers have employed a tissue storage step, which has either taken place in explant culture for 1–4 weeks (Freed et al. 1990) or at 4 °C in a hibernation medium for 1–8 days (Petersen et al. 2000). Typically the VM from multiple embryonic donors are collected, enzymatically digested, and mechanically dissociated into a near single cell suspension. Some centers chose to implant strand-like cell clusters after a storage time in vitro (Clarkson et al. 1998; Freed et al. 2001) or implant VM tissue pieces (Olanow et al. 2003). Using magnet resonance tomography (MRI)-guided stereotactic neurosurgery, grafts are placed along three to seven trajectories in the putamen and in some cases along two trajectories into the head of the caudate nucleus. Different centers have opted for different policies on the use of immunosuppression, varying from no immunosuppression (Freed et al. 1990, 2001), immunosuppression with cyclosporine A for 6 months (Olanow et al. 2003) to using three different drugs (cyclosporin A, steroids, and azathioprine) (Wenning et al. 1997; Piccini et al. 2000) (see Fig. 2 for illustration of methodology of grafting).

6
Grafting Embryonic Tissue: Does It Improve the Patient's Symptoms?

6.1
Open-Labeled Trials

The first reports on fetal nigral grafts in PD patients (Lindvall et al. 1988, 1989; Madrazo et al. 1988) were soon followed by evidence for graft survival and function in these PD patients (Lindvall et al. 1990). Since then, it is estimated that over 400 PD patients worldwide have been grafted with nigral tissue (Brundin 2001). There are multiple reports of long-lasting symptomatic improvement (Defer et al. 1996; Hagell et al. 1999; Hauser et al. 1999; Brundin et al. 2000b; Mendez et al. 2002), (for review, see Lindvall and Hagell 2000; Hagell and

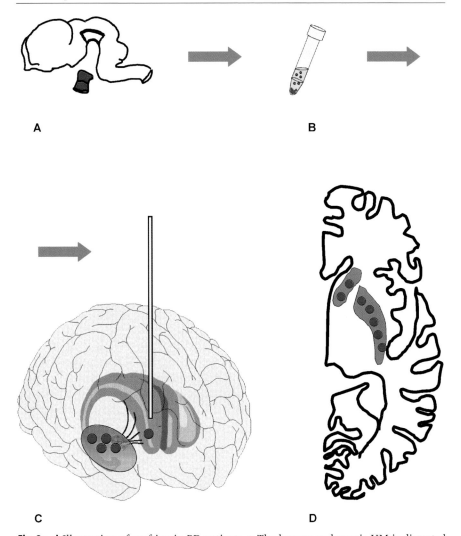

Fig. 2a–d Illustration of grafting in PD patients. **a** The human embryonic VM is dissected from embryos from routine abortions after informed consent of the woman undergoing abortion and according to ethical guidelines. **b** The tissue is enzymatically and mechanically dissociated in some centers, in others the tissue is stored for several weeks and implanted as tissue strands, or the tissue is grafted in pieces. **c** The cells are stereotactically injected into the putamen and caudate. Patients have been grafted uni- and bilaterally. Immunosuppression of the patient varies between centers. **d** The cells are injected along several trajectories. Tissue from two to four embryos/side of the brain is needed to achieve a sufficient number of surviving DA neurons

Brundin 2001). All these transplantations were performed in an open-labeled fashion: only a small group of patients is treated with a transplant, with no control placebo group or blinding procedure. Transplanted cells may require many months to mature and integrate into the host brain circuitry and graft effects are therefore not straightforward to evaluate. Unfortunately, functional improvement is assessed in different ways at different centers, making a comparison of the results between centers difficult. Therefore, a consortium of European and US centers has developed a standardized Core Assessment Protocol for Intracerebral Transplantations (CAPIT) and later the revised form, the Core Assessment Program for Surgical interventions and Transplantation (CAPSIT), that defines regular neurological examination and imaging assessments at designated time intervals before and after the transplantation. This provides a baseline over a minimum of 3 months before operation and 1–2 years after operation (Langston et al. 1992; Defer et al. 1999). Open-labeled trials provided convincing evidence that embryonic human nigral tissue can survive transplantation into the adult human brain, integrate, and function over a long time. Grafted cells reinnervate the surrounding host striatum, release DA and provide significant improvement of motor function. Symptomatic improvement of between 30%–50% has been reported on the motor part of the unified Parkinson's disease rating scale (UPDRS) (for review, see Lindvall et al. 1990, 1994; Widner et al. 1992; Hagell et al. 1999; Brundin et al. 2000b; Dunnett et al. 2001; Winkler et al. 2005). These improvements have been maintained in some patients for over 10 years. Some patients have been able to reduce or even stop medication and resume an independent life (Wenning et al. 1997). Interestingly, not all symptoms are clearly improved by transplantation. For example, impaired postural function, swallowing, and speech do not seem to improve as dramatically as limb hypokinesia and rigidity (Baker et al. 1997; Lindvall and Hagell 2000). Patients received regular ^{18}F-DOPA positron-emission tomography (PET). ^{18}F-DOPA is a substance taken up by presynaptic dopaminergic terminals in the striatum and is therefore an indicator for surviving grafts and fiber outgrowth. Uptake values reached between 48% and 68% of the values of normal controls in most of the open-labeled studies (for review, see Dunnett et al. 2001; Winkler et al. 2005). In one patient, restitution of F-DOPA uptake reached 100% (Piccini et al. 1999). Functional improvement seems to correlate with neuroradiological evidence of surviving graft tissue (Remy et al. 1995; Piccini et al. 1999, 2000; Hagell and Brundin 2001; Cochen et al. 2003).

6.2
Double-Blind Placebo Controlled Trials

The functional improvements seen in patients from open-labeled trials have been questioned because of possible placebo effects. Therefore, two double-blind, placebo-controlled studies were initiated and funded by the NIH to investigate whether transplantation of embryonic nigral tissue has an effect in patients suffering from PD. Both trials had a sham group: the patients received anesthesia, a burr hole was made into the skull but the dura was not penetrated, and no tissue implanted. The patient and examiner were blinded to the condition of the patient.

In the Denver/New York Surgical Trial (Freed et al. 2001) 40 patients were included, 19 of whom received a transplant, the remaining underwent sham surgery as described above. Cells were stored for several days in vitro and implanted as "tissue strands" using a frontal surgical approach; no immunosuppression was given. Patients were assessed for using a subjective global rating scale (self-assessment) rather than a motor examination by a neurologist, up to 1 year after grafting. At 1 year, there was no improvement in the sham group, but modest improvement in two neurological rating scales, especially in younger (< 60 years) patients. The ^{18}F-DOPA-PET showed around 40% improvement. Fifteen percent of the patients developed severe off-dyskinesias (involuntary movements that also persist after cessation of medication) between 1–3 years after grafting.

The Tampa /Mount Sinai Surgical Trial was the second randomized, double-blind, placebo-controlled study to be conducted. Solid pieces of embryonic VM from one donor (11 patients) or from four donors (12 patients) were implanted into the putamen on each side of the patient's brain. Eleven patients received sham surgery. Patients were immunosuppressed with cyclosporine A for 6 months. In this study, patients were followed up for 2 years, however, there was no significant difference between the groups at 2 years measured by the UPDRS. Patients who had received cells from four donors showed progressive improvement up to 6 months. The loss in improvement of symptoms occurred at the same time as the discontinuation of immunosuppression, suggesting an immune response to the graft and maybe a late rejection. Striatal ^{18}F-DOPA uptake was significantly increased after transplantation, indicating survival of grafted neurons. Robust survival of DA neurons but also microglial cells could be observed at postmortem examination. Fifty-six percent of the transplanted patients developed off-dyskinesias that persisted upon drug withdrawal (Olanow et al. 2003).

6.3
Problems

Overall, these two studies failed to show an effect of cell transplantation in PD. This is in contrast to the case reports from open-labeled trials and may be attributed to several factors: clinical assessment was not conducted according to the CAPSIT protocol and therefore it makes it difficult to compare the results of this study with those from other centers. Endpoint measures were undertaken up to 1 or 2 years after transplantation, respectively, which seems a short follow-up considering the slowness of graft maturation. Furthermore, the first study (Freed et al. 2001) differed from most others in the technique of tissue preparation, long-term storage in vitro, absence of immunosuppression, and an unusual surgical approach. The appearance of dyskinesias is a worrying side effect of this treatment, and has been attributed to a possible overproduction of DA in the striatum by the grafts (Freed et al. 2001). However, the patients who died showed a low number of surviving dopaminergic neurons (7,000–40,000) as compared to grafts from open-labeled trials (80,000–135,000, per side) (Kordower et al. 1995), which argues against an overproduction of DA (Brundin et al. 2001).

The second study (Olanow et al. 2003) reports an even higher number of patients suffering from off-dyskinesias. Solid pieces of VM have been transplanted in this study and immunosuppression was only given for 6 months. Four cases have come to autopsy and show activated microglia in and around the graft deposits. The postmortem cases from the Denver/NewYork trial also showed infiltration of the graft with immune cells similar to an earlier study, where low-dose cyclosporine was terminated at 6 months after grafting (Kordower et al. 1997). The observed dyskinesias may reflect partial, but inadequate graft survival, that is producing, storing, and releasing low levels of DA insufficient to induce an antiparkinsonian response (Olanow et al. 2003). This is hypothetical but could have implications for further transplant protocols. Retrospective analysis of some of the patients analyzed in Lund, who were usually immunosuppressed for at least 18 months with the triple regimen (see above), showed some involuntary movements (7% of the patients), however, none of the dyskinesias reached the severity described in the Denver/New York or Tampa/Mount Sinai study (Hagell et al. 2002) (for a summary of hypotheses regarding the cause of dyskinesias in transplanted patients, see Table 2).

However, taken together, these studies suggest that patients have to be carefully selected and undergo detailed clinical evaluation before and after neurotransplantation. The choice of rating scale is crucial, as certain evaluations are more susceptible to placebo effects than others (McRae et al. 2004). The sham controlled double-blind studies illustrate that the present cell replacement procedures are far from optimal and that further research is necessary

Table 2 Hypothetical causes of dyskinesias

Correlated to L-dopa dyskinesias prior to grafting
Excessive dopamine release from the grafts
Patchy striatal reinnervation
Altered synapse formation
Partial graft rejection
Presence of non-dopaminergic neurons in grafts
Insufficient graft size
Extent of pre-operative loss of striatal dopaminergic terminals

Table 3 Conclusions from clinical trials grafting embryonic ventral mesencephalon in Parkinsonian patients

---

1. Cells from human embryonic ventral mesencephalon survive grafting
    a. Patients show increase in striatal F-Dopa uptake
    b. Postmortem examination shows surviving grafts
2. There is no evidence that grafted cells are affected by ongoing disease process
3. The clinical improvement can be long lasting
4. There is high variability in clinical improvement between patients
5. There is no agreement regarding immunosuppression between centers
6. Patient selection is crucial for the benefit
    a. Younger, less affected patients may benefit more
    b. L-dopa responsiveness prior to grafting is predictive for outcome of graft
7. Dyskinesias are still an unresolved side effect
8. Graft tissue may be an important factor for benefit and dyskinesias (preparation, storage, number of donors, precise donor age)
9. Graft location within the striatum may be crucial for dyskinesias and/or behavioral recovery

---

to optimize selection of patients and transplantation procedures (see Table 3 for conclusions from clinical trials).

7
Alternative Cell Sources

Human nigral grafts are only made up of 5%–10% of neurons that are destined to become dopaminergic neurons; the rest of the cells are other neuronal and glial cell types. Furthermore, only around 5%–10% of the cells destined to become DA neurons survive the grafting procedure (Brundin et al. 2000a). It has been proposed that at least 100,000 grafted DA neurons need to survive in the putamen to obtain behavioral effects in PD patients (Hagell and Brundin 2001). The number of embryos required to achieve this number of surviving cells depends on the donor age of the tissue, preparation of the cells and the surgical technique; and ranges between two to four embryos per side of the brain (each embryonic VM contains approximately 500,000–1,000,000 dopaminergic neurons, of which 5% survive). There are obvious logistic problems connected with the number of donors needed for each patient, and ethical concerns have been raised regarding the use of cells obtained from aborted embryos. These factors are restricting the wider application of embryonic tissue for neural transplantation and make it necessary to develop alternative sources of donor tissue (see Table 4). Attempts are made to generate neurons with a dopaminerigc phenotype from a variety of tissues, as discussed in the final sections of this chapter.

Table 4 Demands on a cell used for transplantation in Parkinson's disease

Large scale production
Standardized
Survival in vivo
No tumour formation
Genomic stability
Stable phenotype in vivo
Dopamine release in a regulated fashion
Should show molecular, morphological and electrophysiological
properties of dopaminergic neurons in the substantia nigra pars compacta
Synaptic functional integration into host circuitry
Functional effects in vivo in terms of behavioral recovery

7.1
Porcine Embryonic Dopaminergic Cells

Grafting of embryonic neuroblasts from the nervous system of a different mammalian species has long been considered (Freeman et al. 1988). The use of porcine tissue has several advantages: pigs are easy to breed and they are not an endangered species (Barker et al. 2000). Porcine tissue has already been considered for other organ transplants, and donor tissue can be genetically modified to, for example, increase cell survival (Cozzi and White 1995) or to knock out some of the dominating antigens responsible for the acute immunorejection (saccharide epitopes of the α-Gal on pig tissue) by naturally occurring xenoreactive antibodies. From animal experiments, it is known that embryonic porcine neural tissue transplanted into hemiparkinsonian immunosuppressed rats not only grows anatomically correct connections (Isacson et al. 1995) but also restores behavioral deficits (Galpern et al. 1996; Larsson and Widner 2000).

What are the problems using porcine tissue? There is a potential risk of infection by zoonotic organisms, especially by porcine endogenous retrovirus (PERV) and particularly in the context of immunosuppression (Michaels et al. 1994). The second major problem is the immune host response. An immunosuppressive regimen (probably life-long) needs to be established that ensures long-term graft survival while minimizing the risk of side effects associated with such therapy. Clinical trials have already commenced using porcine embryonic DA neurons. Twelve patients were grafted in a phase I study (Diacrin) with no clinical benefit and evidence of poor graft survival (Deacon et al. 1997; Schumacher et al. 2000). In a second study, 18 patients (Genzyme/Diacrin, phase II) were either assigned to graft or sham treatment. There was no significant improvement in the UPDRS at 18 months after grafting, however, and no disabling dyskinesias have been reported (Freeman et al. 2002).

In summary, porcine neural xenografts might offer some hope, but there are major problems with this approach, which have led to a moratorium on all clinical studies in the UK and some other countries.

7.2
Dopaminergic Neurons Derived from Embryonic Stem Cells

Mouse (Kawasaki et al. 2000), primate (Kawasaki et al. 2002; Takagi et al. 2005), and now also human ES cells (Perrier et al. 2004; Zeng et al. 2004) have been shown to differentiate into dopaminergic neurons using a co-culture system with mouse stromal cell lines (PA6 and MS5). Other epigenetic factors such as transforming growth factor α (TGFα) (Park et al. 2004) or a complex sequence of different factors (Perrier et al. 2004) also result in dopaminergic differentiation of human ES cells, probably by simulating the patterning and differentiation factors of midbrain development. A problem is the fact that both studies (Park et al. 2004; Perrier et al. 2004) employed mouse feeder layers for maintenance of human ES cells, a concern for clinical therapy where a xeno-free system is required. Furthermore, there is no published study to date showing that human ES cell-derived dopaminergic neurons can survive grafting, keep a stable phenotype in vivo (continue to express TH), integrate into the host brain without forming tumors, release DA in a regulated fashion, and lead to substantial behavioral recovery in animal models of PD.

Genetic modification using transcription factors to induce a DA phenotype has also been explored (Burbach et al. 2003; Simon et al. 2003; Wallen and Perlmann 2003). For example, Nurr1, a member of the steroid/thyroid hormone receptor family, is expressed in DA neurons and may be required for the survival and commitment of late dopaminergic precursors (Saucedo-Cardenas et al. 1998). Kim et al. (2002) used a cytomegalovirus plasmid (pCMV) driving expression of a rat Nurr1 cDNA to establish stable Nurr1 mouse ES cell lines. The yield of TH positive neurons was ten times that of wild type cells. Additionally, the cells possess several characteristics of midbrain dopaminergic neurons such as AADC, DAT, c-RET, Ptx3, and En-1 besides tyrosinhydroxylase (TH). Most importantly, when grafted to the striatum, they could reverse both drug-induced and spontaneous motor deficits in the unilateral 6-OHDA-lesion rat model of PD (Kim et al. 2002). No ongoing mitosis or tumor formation was found in the grafts. The safety issues surrounding ES cell transplants are of particular concern, especially after an earlier published report (Bjorklund et al. 2002). Undifferentiated mouse ES cells grafted into a rat PD model differentiated spontaneously into dopaminergic neurons and led to partial behavioral recovery. These data were intriguing because there was no special protocol to induce differentiation of dopaminergic neurons from the ES cells. However, the study reported a worryingly high frequency (25%) of teratomas in animals with a surviving graft, and a further 16% of the grafted animals contained non-neuronal cells that were positive for mesodermal markers (Bjorklund et al. 2002).

ES cells show promise regarding their therapeutic potential. However, long-term experiments need to be conducted to test the safety of ES cells in vivo. Until ES cells have been proven to be safe in terms of tumor formation and stable gene expression, clinical studies will remain a distant prospect.

7.3
Dopaminergic Cells Derived from Fetal Neural Progenitors

Neural progenitor cells are isolated from the developing embryo at later stages than ES cells. They have the ability to differentiate into neurons, oligodendro-cytes, and astrocytes. Several groups have explored the possibilities of using expanded progenitors from fetal tissue stem cells to generate DA cells.

Embryonic rodent mesencephalic precursors can be expanded and differ-entiate into cells with characteristics of DA neurons (Ling et al. 1998; Studer et al. 1998, 2000; Potter et al. 1999; Carvey et al. 2001; Yan et al. 2001; Storch et al. 2003). Upon transplantation, generated DA neurons survive and restore behavioral deficits in a rat Parkinson model (Studer et al. 1998). Although this suggested that expansion of DA precursors could reduce amounts of donor tissue needed for transplantation, there is a loss of about 95%–97% of differ-entiated DA neurons in the grafting step (Brundin and Bjorklund 1998).

Human fetal mesencephalic precursor cells can also be expanded for an extended time in vitro and generate DA neurons; however, the number is still low (Storch et al. 2001). Currently, cell survival of grafted progenitor cells is not sufficient to introduce the transplantation of progenitor cells into the clinical setting.

7.4
Dopaminergic Cells from Adult Stem Cells

Stem cells have also been identified in a variety of adult tissues such as bone marrow and blood as well as within the skin, liver, muscle, and even the adult brain.

Adult-derived stem cells (ASC) are pluripotent and have the ability of self-renewal. Furthermore, in comparison to ES cells, ASCs are easier to access and devoid of serious ethical issues because they can be, for example, harvested from the patient. This would also make immunosuppressive treatment after transplantation unnecessary.

7.4.1
Adult Neural Stem Cells

Neural stem cells can be isolated from various regions of the adult brain such as the subgranular zone of the dentate gyrus of the hippocampus, the subventricular zone (SVZ) and the spinal cord (for review, see Gage 2000). Adult neural stem cells can be grown as neurospheres in culture and differentiate into all three major CNS cell types (neurons, astrocytes, and oligodendrocytes). There is currently only one report on the derivation of a very low number of TH-positive cells from the adult rodent SVZ (Daadi and Weiss 1999). Attempts to transfect adult neural stem cells with Nurr-1 did not result in the induction of DA neurons (Sakurada et al. 1999).

Given their expected capacity to self-renew and differentiate efficiently into a desired cell type, clonal populations of neural stem cells promise to produce high numbers of DA neurons if they can be propagated, enriched, and manipulated to differentiate along the DA lineage. However, to date it is not clear whether and to what extent this is possible.

7.4.2
Bone Marrow-Derived Stem Cells

Cells expressing some markers of dopaminergic neurons have also been generated from tissues other than the brain (for review, see Paul et al. 2002). Adult rodent mesenchymal stem cells differentiate not only into mesenchymal cells, but also cells with visceral mesoderm, neuroectoderm, and endoderm characteristics in vitro and in vivo (Jiang et al. 2002a, 2002b, 2003). A subtype of these mesenchymal stem cells was isolated and termed multipotent adult progenitor cell (MAPC). Remarkably, as many as 30% of mouse MAPCs differentiated into TH-expressing neurons in vitro. The authors provide evidence that these cells are pluripotent, which suggests that mesenchymal stem cells could serve as an ideal cell source for neurotransplantation in PD. Another group found human bone marrow stromal cells could be converted into a neural stem cell-like population that can be differentiated into cells expressing neuronal markers. Interestingly, around 11% of the cells expressed TH using a neuronal differentiation protocol and cells released dopamine upon membrane depolarization (Hermann et al. 2004).These findings are interesting and clinically relevant. Future studies are warranted to see whether these cells can also show functional properties in animal models of PD.

7.5
Genetic Modification of Stem Cells

Stem cells could serve as carriers to deliver growth factors or DA, or for example could be genetically modified to generate DA neurons.

Different cell types can thereby be used as a vehicle, for example by transducing cells in vitro to release DA upon transplantation in vivo. This has been shown by introducing TH, the rate-limiting enzyme for DA synthesis, into several cell lines such as fibroblastic 3T3 cells, endocrine RIN cells, neuroblastoma NS20-Y, and neuroendocrine AtT-20 cells using a recombinant retrovirus encoding for human TH (Horellou et al. 1990 1991). Even though cells expressed TH and secreted high amounts of DOPA or even DA upon transplantation into the striatum of hemiparkinsonian rats, there was only partial or no behavioral recovery (Horellou et al. 1990, 1991). Similarly, human neural progenitors genetically modified with human TH under the control of a tetracycline responsive regulatory system were grafted, but no behavioral improvement by transplanted cells was reported (Corti et al. 1996, 1999).

Several studies have attempted DA neuron conversion of neural stem cells and precursor cells via overexpression of Nurr1. Wagner and colleagues induced a ventral mesencephalic DA phenotype in an immortalized multipotent neural stem cell line in vitro (Snyder et al. 1992; Wagner et al. 1999). Upon transfection with Nurr-1, 30% of the cells expressed a neuronal phenotype, and could be induced to express a DA phenotype in combination with a co-culture system using astrocytes from the E16 (embryonic stage 16) rat VM and bFGF. Neurons expressed TH and several markers of a DA phenotype. However, again, upon transplantation only a few surviving cells were found, and of those a small proportion expressed TH.

McKay and co-workers demonstrated that Nurr1 is sufficient to induce DA differentiation in rat CNS precursors from various developmental stages and regions of origin (cortex, VM, lateral ganglionic eminence) (Kim et al. 2003). Nurr1 transfection induced TH expression and TH-positive neurons showed characteristics of DA phenotypes (AADC, DAT, VMAT, Ptx3-expression) as well as spontaneous and evoked DA release. However, cells from other than mesencephalic regions were less mature and secreted lower levels of DA than those derived from mesencephalic precursors. Transplantation of Nurr1-induced DA neuron precursors resulted in limited survival and in vivo differentiation. No behavioral improvement was observed (Kim et al. 2003) in contrast to studies performed on mouse ES cells (Kim et al. 2002) (see Sect. 7.2).

The difference in the effect of Nurr1 overexpression may be due to the use of varied cell types and levels of overexpression. However, Nurr1-transfected cells show a lack of in vivo function when using fetal-derived stem cells (Wagner et al. 1999; Kim et al. 2003). This may be due to insufficient maturation and differentiation, preventing necessary synaptic interaction with the host brain to allow long-term graft function.

8
Harvesting Endogenous Stem Cells: Self-Repair of the Brain?

Another alternative option for cell therapy in PD would be to recruit endogenous neural stem cells in the patient's brain. There is consensus that new neurons are continuously generated in defined areas of the adult normal brain: in the SVZ and the dentate gyrus of the hippocampus (for review, see Gage

2000). Whether endogenous stem cells in the brain can give rise to new DA neurons in the brain is currently debated.

It has been claimed that the substantia nigra is a site of ongoing neurogenesis and continuous formation of newly differentiated DA-ergic neurons (Zhao et al. 2003). The authors describe an even further increase in newborn DA-ergic neurons in a lesion model of PD. However, this view has now been challenged by others in carefully conducted studies (Cooper and Isacson 2004; Frielingsdorf et al. 2004). In some studies, only a glial response in the SNc was observed after lesion of the nigrostriatal system (Lie et al. 2002).

The striatum is the second site where newborn cells might contribute to brain repair in PD. Fallon and colleagues (Fallon et al. 2000) reported the appearance of a small number of newborn cells expressing dopaminergic markers in the striatum following TGFα infusion into the striatum of hemiparkinsonian rats. Although this study was the first to suggest that adult neurogenesis in the striatum could contribute to behavioral recovery in an animal model of PD, caution is warranted. Other authors have recently failed to reproduce this finding (Cooper and Isacson 2004). However, this challenged the classical view that there are no TH-positive cells in the striatum but only fibers from projecting DA neurons in the SNc.

The occurrence of TH-positive neurons in the striatum has previously been reported (Dubach et al. 1987; Tashiro et al. 1989a, 1989b; Betarbet et al. 1997; Porritt et al. 2000; Palfi et al. 2002) and was claimed to be due to an apparent phenotypic switch in striatal neurons, whereby a small subpopulation of the striatal neurons changed their transmitter phenotype. However, loss of striatal DA innervation or administration of growth factors might further increase their numbers. Whether these cells are derived from stem cells in the SVZ stimulated by the lesion or whether they are of other origin remains unclear.

This self-repair mechanism after brain injury, if it exists, seems limited and is currently insufficient to restore normal function. Clinically these findings are very interesting, it may be possible to stimulate endogenous stem cells to proliferate, migrate to the site of lesion, and replace the lost neurons, possibly, for example, by infusion of defined factors. The challenge lies in differentiating those neurons into DA neurons that release DA and integrate into the host circuitry.

9
Conclusions

The proof of principle that cell transplantation can work in PD has been shown. However, there are several issues that need to be resolved. It is a challenge for scientists to develop a new DA cell type using genetic modification or to coax different stem cell types into a DA fate in order to obtain cells to be grafted in

PD. Research in this field is advancing fast and the recent findings raise hope for the development of stem cell therapy for PD in the near future.

However, before any of these cell types can enter clinical trials, issues such as cell survival, appropriate synaptic integration into the host brain, behavioral recovery, and tumor formation need to be resolved. Even though alternative cell sources might resolve ethical and logistic issues connected with the use of embryonic tissue, the strategies employed in the grafting of embryonic tissue will be the same for DA stem cell transplants. Therefore, the problem of dyskinesias in this context is a major issue that needs to be investigated in parallel, as research is ongoing for new cell sources.

References

Aarsland D, Tandberg E, Larsen JP, Cummings JL (1996) Frequency of dementia in Parkinson disease. Arch Neurol 53:538–542

Agid Y (1991) Parkinson's disease: pathophysiology. Lancet 337:1321–1324

Alexander GE, Crutcher MD (1990) Functional architecture of basal ganglia circuits: neural substrates of parallel processing. Trends Neurosci 13:266–271

Arbuthnott G, Dunnett S, MacLeod N (1985) Electrophysiological properties of single units in dopamine-rich mesencephalic transplants in rat brain. Neurosci Lett 57:205–210

Backlund EO, Granberg PO, Hamberger B, Knutsson E, Martensson A, Sedvall G, Seiger A, Olson L (1985) Transplantation of adrenal medullary tissue to striatum in parkinsonism. First clinical trials. J Neurosurg 62:169–173

Bakay RA, Raiser CD, Stover NP, Subramanian T, Cornfeldt ML, Schweikert AW, Allen RC, Watts R (2004) Implantation of Spheramine in advanced Parkinson's disease (PD). Front Biosci 9:592–602

Baker KK, Ramig LO, Johnson AB, Freed CR (1997) Preliminary voice and speech analysis following fetal dopamine transplants in 5 individuals with Parkinson disease. J Speech Lang Hear Res 40:615–626

Barker RA, Kendall AL, Widner H (2000) Neural tissue xenotransplantation: what is needed prior to clinical trials in Parkinson's disease? Neural Tissue Xenografting Project. Cell Transplant 9:235–246

Betarbet R, Turner R, Chockkan V, DeLong MR, Allers KA, Walters J, Levey AI, Greenamyre JT (1997) Dopaminergic neurons intrinsic to the primate striatum. J Neurosci 17:6761–6768

Bjorklund A, Stenevi U (1979) Reconstruction of the nigrostriatal dopamine pathway by intracerebral nigral transplants. Brain Res 177:555–560

Bjorklund A, Lindvall O (2000) Cell replacement therapies for central nervous system disorders. Nat Neurosci 3:537–544

Bjorklund A, Stenevi U, Svendgaard N (1976) Growth of transplanted monoaminergic neurones into the adult hippocampus along the perforant path. Nature 262:787–790

Bjorklund A, Stenevi U, Schmidt RH, Dunnett SB, Gage FH (1983a) Intracerebral grafting of neuronal cell suspensions. I. Introduction and general methods of preparation. Acta Physiol Scand Suppl 522:1–7

Bjorklund A, Stenevi U, Schmidt RH, Dunnett SB, Gage FH (1983b) Intracerebral grafting of neuronal cell suspensions. II. Survival and growth of nigral cell suspensions implanted in different brain sites. Acta Physiol Scand Suppl 522:9–18

Bjorklund LM, Sanchez-Pernaute R, Chung S, Andersson T, Chen IY, McNaught KS, Brownell AL, Jenkins BG, Wahlestedt C, Kim KS, Isacson O (2002) Embryonic stem cells develop into functional dopaminergic neurons after transplantation in a Parkinson rat model. Proc Natl Acad Sci U S A 99:2344–2349

Boer GJ (1994) Ethical guidelines for the use of human embryonic or fetal tissue for experimental and clinical neurotransplantation and research. Network of European CNS Transplantation and Restoration (NECTAR). J Neurol 242:1–13

Braak H, Ghebremedhin E, Rub U, Bratzke H, Del Tredici K (2004) Stages in the development of Parkinson's disease-related pathology. Cell Tissue Res 318:121–134

Brundin P (1992) Dissection, preparation and implantation of human embryonic brain tissue. In: Dunnett S (ed) Neural transplantation, a practical approach. Oxford University Press, Oxford, pp 139–160

Brundin P, Bjorklund A (1998) Survival of expanded dopaminergic precursors is critical for clinical trials. Nat Neurosci 1:537

Brundin P, Hagell P (2001) The neurobiology of cell transplantation in Parkinsons's disease. Clin Neurosci Res 1:507–520

Brundin P, Duan W, Sauer H (1994) Functional effects of mesencephalic dopamine neurons and adrenal chromaffin cells grafted to the rodent striatum. In: Dunnett S (ed) Functional neural transplantation. Raven Press, New York, pp 9–46

Brundin P, Karlsson J, Emgard M, Schierle GS, Hansson O, Petersen A, Castilho RF (2000a) Improving the survival of grafted dopaminergic neurons: a review over current approaches. Cell Transplant 9:179–195

Brundin P, Pogarell O, Hagell P, Piccini P, Widner H, Schrag A, Kupsch A, Crabb L, Odin P, Gustavii B, Bjorklund A, Brooks DJ, Marsden CD, Oertel WH, Quinn NP, Rehncrona S, Lindvall O (2000b) Bilateral caudate and putamen grafts of embryonic mesencephalic tissue treated with lazaroids in Parkinson's disease. Brain 123:1380–1390

Brundin P, Dunnett S, Bjorklund A, Nikkhah G (2001) Transplanted dopaminergic neurons: more or less? Nat Med 7:512–513

Burbach JP, Smits S, Smidt MP (2003) Transcription factors in the development of midbrain dopamine neurons. Ann N Y Acad Sci 991:61–68

Carvey PM, Ling ZD, Sortwell CE, Pitzer MR, McGuire SO, Storch A, Collier TJ (2001) A clonal line of mesencephalic progenitor cells converted to dopamine neurons by hematopoietic cytokines: a source of cells for transplantation in Parkinson's disease. Exp Neurol 171:98–108

Clarkson ED, Zawada WM, Adams FS, Bell KP, Freed CR (1998) Strands of embryonic mesencephalic tissue show greater dopamine neuron survival and better behavioral improvement than cell suspensions after transplantation in parkinsonian rats. Brain Res 806:60–68

Cochen V, Ribeiro MJ, Nguyen JP, Gurruchaga JM, Villafane G, Loc'h C, Defer G, Samson Y, Peschanski M, Hantraye P, Cesaro P, Remy P (2003) Transplantation in Parkinson's disease: PET changes correlate with the amount of grafted tissue. Mov Disord 18:928–932

Cooper O, Isacson O (2004) Intrastriatal transforming growth factor alpha delivery to a model of Parkinson's disease induces proliferation and migration of endogenous adult neural progenitor cells without differentiation into dopaminergic neurons. J Neurosci 24:8924–8931

Corti O, Horellou P, Colin P, Cattaneo E, Mallet J (1996) Intracerebral tetracycline-dependent regulation of gene expression in grafts of neural precursors. Neuroreport 7:1655–1659

Corti O, Sanchez-Capelo A, Colin P, Hanoun N, Hamon M, Mallet J (1999) Long-term doxycycline-controlled expression of human tyrosine hydroxylase after direct adeno-virus-mediated gene transfer to a rat model of Parkinson's disease. Proc Natl Acad Sci U S A 96:12120–12125

Cozzi E, White DJ (1995) The generation of transgenic pigs as potential organ donors for humans. Nat Med 1:964–966

Daadi MM, Weiss S (1999) Generation of tyrosine hydroxylase-producing neurons from precursors of the embryonic and adult forebrain. J Neurosci 19:4484–4497

Deacon T, Schumacher J, Dinsmore J, Thomas C, Palmer P, Kott S, Edge A, Penney D, Kassissieh S, Dempsey P, Isacson O (1997) Histological evidence of fetal pig neural cell survival after transplantation into a patient with Parkinson's disease. Nat Med 3:350–353

Defer GL, Geny C, Ricolfi F, Fenelon G, Monfort JC, Remy P, Villafane G, Jeny R, Samson Y, Keravel Y, Gaston A, Degos JD, Peschanski M, Cesaro P, Nguyen JP (1996) Long-term outcome of unilaterally transplanted parkinsonian patients. I. Clinical approach. Brain 119:41–50

Defer GL, Widner H, Marie RM, Remy P, Levivier M (1999) Core assessment program for surgical interventional therapies in Parkinson's disease (CAPSIT-PD). Mov Disord 14:572–584

DeLong MR (1990) Primate models of movement disorders of basal ganglia origin. Trends Neurosci 13:281–285

Doucet G, Murata Y, Brundin P, Bosler O, Mons N, Geffard M, Ouimet CC, Bjorklund A (1989) Host afferents into intrastriatal transplants of fetal ventral mesencephalon. Exp Neurol 106:1–19

Dubach M, Schmidt R, Kunkel D, Bowden DM, Martin R, German DC (1987) Primate neostriatal neurons containing tyrosine hydroxylase: immunohistochemical evidence. Neurosci Lett 75:205–210

Dunnett SB, Bjorklund A, Schmidt RH, Stenevi U, Iversen SD (1983a) Intracerebral grafting of neuronal cell suspensions. IV. Behavioural recovery in rats with unilateral 6-OHDA lesions following implantation of nigral cell suspensions in different forebrain sites. Acta Physiol Scand Suppl 522:29–37

Dunnett SB, Bjorklund A, Schmidt RH, Stenevi U, Iversen SD (1983b) Intracerebral grafting of neuronal cell suspensions. V. Behavioural recovery in rats with bilateral 6-OHDA lesions following implantation of nigral cell suspensions. Acta Physiol Scand Suppl 522:39–47

Dunnett SB, Bjorklund A, Lindvall O (2001) Cell therapy in Parkinson's disease—stop or go? Nat Rev Neurosci 2:365–369

Espejo EF, Montoro RJ, Armengol JA, Lopez-Barneo J (1998) Cellular and functional recovery of Parkinsonian rats after intrastriatal transplantation of carotid body cell aggregates. Neuron 20:197–206

Fallon J, Reid S, Kinyamu R, Opole I, Opole R, Baratta J, Korc M, Endo TL, Duong A, Nguyen G, Karkehabadhi M, Twardzik D, Patel S, Loughlin S (2000) In vivo induction of massive proliferation, directed migration, and differentiation of neural cells in the adult mammalian brain. Proc Natl Acad Sci U S A 97:14686–14691

Fearnley JM, Lees AJ (1991) Ageing and Parkinson's disease: substantia nigra regional selectivity. Brain 114:2283–2301

Freed CR, Breeze RE, Rosenberg NL, Schneck SA, Wells TH, Barrett JN, Grafton ST, Huang SC, Eidelberg D, Rottenberg DA (1990) Transplantation of human fetal dopamine cells for Parkinson's disease. Results at 1 year. Arch Neurol 47:505–512

Freed CR, Greene PE, Breeze RE, Tsai WY, DuMouchel W, Kao R, Dillon S, Winfield H, Culver S, Trojanowski JQ, Eidelberg D, Fahn S (2001) Transplantation of embryonic dopamine neurons for severe Parkinson's disease. N Engl J Med 344:710–719

Freeman T, Watts RL, Hauser RA, Bakay RA, Elias SA. Stoessl AJ, Eidelberg D, Dinsmore JH, Fink SJ (2002) A prospective, randomized, double-blind, surgical placebo-controlled trial of intrastriatal transplantation of fetal porcine ventral mesencephalic tissue (neurocell-PD) in subjects with Parkinson's disease (abstract 8.3). Exp Neurol 175:426

Freeman TB, Wojak JC, Brandeis L, Michel JP, Pearson J, Flamm ES (1988) Cross-species intracerebral grafting of embryonic swine dopaminergic neurons. Prog Brain Res 78:473–477

Freeman TB, Spence MS, Boss BD, Spector DH, Strecker RE, Olanow CW, Kordower JH (1991) Development of dopaminergic neurons in the human substantia nigra. Exp Neurol 113:344–353

Freund TF, Bolam JP, Bjorklund A, Stenevi U, Dunnett SB, Powell JF, Smith AD (1985) Efferent synaptic connections of grafted dopaminergic neurons reinnervating the host neostriatum: a tyrosine hydroxylase immunocytochemical study. J Neurosci 5:603–616

Frielingsdorf H, Schwarz K, Brundin P, Mohapel P (2004) No evidence for new dopaminergic neurons in the adult mammalian substantia nigra. Proc Natl Acad Sci U S A 101:10177–10182

Gage FH (2000) Mammalian neural stem cells. Science 287:1433–1438

Galpern WR, Burns LH, Deacon TW, Dinsmore J, Isacson O (1996) Xenotransplantation of porcine fetal ventral mesencephalon in a rat model of Parkinson's disease: functional recovery and graft morphology. Exp Neurol 140:1–13

Goetz CG, Stebbins GT 3rd, Klawans HL, Koller WC, Grossman RG, Bakay RA, Penn RD (1991) United Parkinson Foundation Neurotransplantation Registry on adrenal medullary transplants: presurgical, and 1- and 2-year follow-up. Neurology 41:1719–1722

Hagell P, Brundin P (2001) Cell survival and clinical outcome following intrastriatal transplantation in Parkinson disease. J Neuropathol Exp Neurol 60:741–752

Hagell P, Schrag A, Piccini P, Jahanshahi M, Brown R, Rehncrona S, Widner H, Brundin P, Rothwell JC, Odin P, Wenning GK, Morrish P, Gustavii B, Bjorklund A, Brooks DJ, Marsden CD, Quinn NP, Lindvall O (1999) Sequential bilateral transplantation in Parkinson's disease: effects of the second graft. Brain 122:1121–1132

Hagell P, Piccini P, Bjorklund A, Brundin P, Rehncrona S, Widner H, Crabb L, Pavese N, Oertel WH, Quinn N, Brooks DJ, Lindvall O (2002) Dyskinesias following neural transplantation in Parkinson's disease. Nat Neurosci 5:627–628

Hauser RA, Freeman TB, Snow BJ, Nauert M, Gauger L, Kordower JH, Olanow CW (1999) Long-term evaluation of bilateral fetal nigral transplantation in Parkinson disease. Arch Neurol 56:179–187

Hermann A, Gastl R, Liebau S, Popa MO, Fiedler J, Boehm BO, Maisel M, Lerche H, Schwarz J, Brenner R, Storch A (2004) Efficient generation of neural stem cell-like cells from adult human bone marrow stromal cells. J Cell Sci 117:4411–4422

Horellou P, Brundin P, Kalen P, Mallet J, Bjorklund A (1990) In vivo release of dopa and dopamine from genetically engineered cells grafted to the denervated rat striatum. Neuron 5:393–402

Horellou P, Lundberg C, Le Bourdelles B, Wictorin K, Brundin P, Kalen P, Bjorklund A, Mallet J (1991) Behavioural effects of genetically engineered cells releasing dopa and dopamine after intracerebral grafting in a rat model of Parkinson's disease. J Physiol (Paris) 85:158–170

Inzelberg R, Schechtman E, Paleacu D (2002) Onset age of Parkinson disease. Am J Med Genet 111:459–460; author reply 461

Isacson O, Deacon TW, Pakzaban P, Galpern WR, Dinsmore J, Burns LH (1995) Transplanted xenogeneic neural cells in neurodegenerative disease models exhibit remarkable axonal target specificity and distinct growth patterns of glial and axonal fibres. Nat Med 1:1189–1194

Itakura T, Komai N, Ryujin Y, Ooiwa Y, Nakai M, Yasui M (1994) Autologous transplantation of the cervical sympathetic ganglion into the parkinsonian brain: case report. Neurosurgery 35:155–157; discussion 157–158

Itakura T, Uematsu Y, Nakao N, Nakai E, Nakai K (1997) Transplantation of autologous sympathetic ganglion into the brain with Parkinson's disease. Long-term follow-up of 35 cases. Stereotact Funct Neurosurg 69:112–115

Jiang Y, Jahagirdar BN, Reinhardt RL, Schwartz RE, Keene CD, Ortiz-Gonzalez XR, Reyes M, Lenvik T, Lund T, Blackstad M, Du J, Aldrich S, Lisberg A, Low WC, Largaespada DA, Verfaillie CM (2002a) Pluripotency of mesenchymal stem cells derived from adult marrow. Nature 418:41–49

Jiang Y, Vaessen B, Lenvik T, Blackstad M, Reyes M, Verfaillie CM (2002b) Multipotent progenitor cells can be isolated from postnatal murine bone marrow, muscle, and brain. Exp Hematol 30:896–904

Jiang Y, Henderson D, Blackstad M, Chen A, Miller RF, Verfaillie CM (2003) Neuroectodermal differentiation from mouse multipotent adult progenitor cells. Proc Natl Acad Sci U S A 100 [Suppl 1]:11854–11860

Kawasaki H, Mizuseki K, Nishikawa S, Kaneko S, Kuwana Y, Nakanishi S, Nishikawa SI, Sasai Y (2000) Induction of midbrain dopaminergic neurons from ES cells by stromal cell-derived inducing activity. Neuron 28:31–40

Kawasaki H, Mizuseki K, Sasai Y (2002) Selective neural induction from ES cells by stromal cell-derived inducing activity and its potential therapeutic application in Parkinson's disease. Methods Mol Biol 185:217–227

Kim JH, Auerbach JM, Rodriguez-Gomez JA, Velasco I, Gavin D, Lumelsky N, Lee SH, Nguyen J, Sanchez-Pernaute R, Bankiewicz K, McKay R (2002) Dopamine neurons derived from embryonic stem cells function in an animal model of Parkinson's disease. Nature 418:50–56

Kim JY, Koh HC, Lee JY, Chang MY, Kim YC, Chung HY, Son H, Lee YS, Studer L, McKay R, Lee SH (2003) Dopaminergic neuronal differentiation from rat embryonic neural precursors by Nurr1 overexpression. J Neurochem 85:1443–1454

Kish SJ, Shannak K, Hornykiewicz O (1988) Uneven pattern of dopamine loss in the striatum of patients with idiopathic Parkinson's disease. Pathophysiologic and clinical implications. N Engl J Med 318:876–880

Kordower JH, Freeman TB, Snow BJ, Vingerhoets FJ, Mufson EJ, Sanberg PR, Hauser RA, Smith DA, Nauert GM, Perl DP et al (1995) Neuropathological evidence of graft survival and striatal reinnervation after the transplantation of fetal mesencephalic tissue in a patient with Parkinson's disease. N Engl J Med 332:1118–1124

Kordower JH, Styren S, Clarke M, DeKosky ST, Olanow CW, Freeman TB (1997) Fetal grafting for Parkinson's disease: expression of immune markers in two patients with functional fetal nigral implants. Cell Transplant 6:213–219

Lang AE, Lozano AM (1998a) Parkinson's disease. First of two parts. N Engl J Med 339:1044–1053

Lang AE, Lozano AM (1998b) Parkinson's disease. Second of two parts. N Engl J Med 339:1130–1143

Langston JW, Widner H, Goetz CG, Brooks D, Fahn S, Freeman T, Watts R (1992) Core assessment program for intracerebral transplantations (CAPIT). Mov Disord 7:2–13

Larsson LC, Widner H (2000) Neural tissue xenografting. Scand J Immunol 52:249–256

Lie DC, Dziewczapolski G, Willhoite AR, Kaspar BK, Shults CW, Gage FH (2002) The adult substantia nigra contains progenitor cells with neurogenic potential. J Neurosci 22:6639–6649

Lindvall O, Hagell P (2000) Clinical observations after neural transplantation in Parkinson's disease. Prog Brain Res 127:299–320

Lindvall O, Backlund EO, Farde L, Sedvall G, Freedman R, Hoffer B, Nobin A, Seiger A, Olson L (1987) Transplantation in Parkinson's disease: two cases of adrenal medullary grafts to the putamen. Ann Neurol 22:457–468

Lindvall O, Rehncrona S, Gustavii B, Brundin P, Astedt B, Widner H, Lindholm T, Bjorklund A, Leenders KL, Rothwell JC et al (1988) Fetal dopamine-rich mesencephalic grafts in Parkinson's disease. Lancet 2:1483–1484

Lindvall O, Rehncrona S, Brundin P, Gustavii B, Astedt B, Widner H, Lindholm T, Bjorklund A, Leenders KL, Rothwell JC et al (1989) Human fetal dopamine neurons grafted into the striatum in two patients with severe Parkinson's disease. A detailed account of methodology and a 6-month follow-up. Arch Neurol 46:615–631

Lindvall O, Brundin P, Widner H, Rehncrona S, Gustavii B, Frackowiak R, Leenders KL, Sawle G, Rothwell JC, Marsden CD et al (1990) Grafts of fetal dopamine neurons survive and improve motor function in Parkinson's disease. Science 247:574–577

Lindvall O, Sawle G, Widner H, Rothwell JC, Bjorklund A, Brooks D, Brundin P, Frackowiak R, Marsden CD, Odin P et al (1994) Evidence for long-term survival and function of dopaminergic grafts in progressive Parkinson's disease. Ann Neurol 35:172–180

Ling ZD, Potter ED, Lipton JW, Carvey PM (1998) Differentiation of mesencephalic progenitor cells into dopaminergic neurons by cytokines. Exp Neurol 149:411–423

Luquin MR, Montoro RJ, Guillen J, Saldise L, Insausti R, Del Rio J, Lopez-Barneo J (1999) Recovery of chronic parkinsonian monkeys by autotransplants of carotid body cell aggregates into putamen. Neuron 22:743–750

Madrazo I, Drucker-Colin R, Diaz V, Martinez-Mata J, Torres C, Becerril JJ (1987) Open microsurgical autograft of adrenal medulla to the right caudate nucleus in two patients with intractable Parkinson's disease. N Engl J Med 316:831–834

Madrazo I, Leon V, Torres C, Aguilera MC, Varela G, Alvarez F, Fraga A, Drucker-Colin R, Ostrosky F, Skurovich M et al (1988) Transplantation of fetal substantia nigra and adrenal medulla to the caudate nucleus in two patients with Parkinson's disease. N Engl J Med 318:51

Madrazo I, Franco-Bourland R, Ostrosky-Solis F, Aguilera M, Cuevas C, Alvarez F, Magallon E, Zamorano C, Morelos A (1990a) Neural transplantation (auto-adrenal, fetal nigral and fetal adrenal) in Parkinson's disease: the Mexican experience. Prog Brain Res 82:593–602

Madrazo I, Franco-Bourland R, Ostrosky-Solis F, Aguilera M, Cuevas C, Zamorano C, Morelos A, Magallon E, Guizar-Sahagun G (1990b) Fetal homotransplants (ventral mesencephalon and adrenal tissue) to the striatum of parkinsonian subjects. Arch Neurol 47:1281–1285

Mahalik TJ, Finger TE, Stromberg I, Olson L (1985) Substantia nigra transplants into denervated striatum of the rat: ultrastructure of graft and host interconnections. J Comp Neurol 240:60–70

Mayeux R, Chen J, Mirabello E, Marder K, Bell K, Dooneief G, Cote L, Stern Y (1990) An estimate of the incidence of dementia in idiopathic Parkinson's disease. Neurology 40:1513–1517

McRae C, Cherin E, Yamazaki TG, Diem G, Vo AH, Russell D, Ellgring JH, Fahn S, Greene P, Dillon S, Winfield H, Bjugstad KB, Freed CR (2004) Effects of perceived treatment on quality of life and medical outcomes in a double-blind placebo surgery trial. Arch Gen Psychiatry 61:412–420

Mendez I, Dagher A, Hong M, Gaudet P, Weerasinghe S, McAlister V, King D, Desrosiers J, Darvesh S, Acorn T, Robertson H (2002) Simultaneous intrastriatal and intranigral fetal dopaminergic grafts in patients with Parkinson disease: a pilot study. Report of three cases. J Neurosurg 96:589–596

Michaels MG, McMichael JP, Brasky K, Kalter S, Peters RL, Starzl TE, Simmons RL (1994) Screening donors for xenotransplantation. The potential for xenozoonoses. Transplantation 57:1462–1465

Oertel WH, Hoglinger GU, Caraceni T, Girotti F, Eichhorn T, Spottke AE, Krieg JC, Poewe W (2001) Depression in Parkinson's disease. An update. Adv Neurol 86:373–383

Olanow CW, Goetz CG, Kordower JH, Stoessl AJ, Sossi V, Brin MF, Shannon KM, Nauert GM, Perl DP, Godbold J, Freeman TB (2003) A double-blind controlled trial of bilateral fetal nigral transplantation in Parkinson's disease. Ann Neurol 54:403–414

Olson L, Malmfors T (1970) Growth characteristics of adrenergic nerves in the adult rat. Fluorescence histochemical and 3H-noradrenaline uptake studies using tissue transplantations to the anterior chamber of the eye. Acta Physiol Scand Suppl 348:1–112

Olson L, Seiger A (1972) Brain tissue transplanted to the anterior chamber of the eye. 1. Fluorescence histochemistry of immature catecholamine and 5-hydroxytryptamine neurons reinnervating the rat iris. Z Zellforsch Mikrosk Anat 135:175–194

Palfi S, Leventhal L, Chu Y, Ma SY, Emborg M, Bakay R, Deglon N, Hantraye P, Aebischer P, Kordower JH (2002) Lentivirally delivered glial cell line-derived neurotrophic factor increases the number of striatal dopaminergic neurons in primate models of nigrostriatal degeneration. J Neurosci 22:4942–4954

Park S, Lee KS, Lee YJ, Shin HA, Cho HY, Wang KC, Kim YS, Lee HT, Chung KS, Kim EY, Lim J (2004) Generation of dopaminergic neurons in vitro from human embryonic stem cells treated with neurotrophic factors. Neurosci Lett 359:99–103

Paul G, Li JY, Brundin P (2002) Stem cells: hype or hope? Drug Discov Today 7:295–302

Perlow MJ, Freed WJ, Hoffer BJ, Seiger A, Olson L, Wyatt RJ (1979) Brain grafts reduce motor abnormalities produced by destruction of nigrostriatal dopamine system. Science 204:643–647

Perrier AL, Tabar V, Barberi T, Rubio ME, Bruses J, Topf N, Harrison NL, Studer L (2004) Derivation of midbrain dopamine neurons from human embryonic stem cells. Proc Natl Acad Sci U S A 101:12543–12548

Petersen A, Hansson O, Emgard M, Brundin P (2000) Grafting of nigral tissue hibernated with tirilazad mesylate and glial cell line-derived neurotrophic factor. Cell Transplant 9:577–584

Piccini P, Brooks DJ, Bjorklund A, Gunn RN, Grasby PM, Rimoldi O, Brundin P, Hagell P, Rehncrona S, Widner H, Lindvall O (1999) Dopamine release from nigral transplants visualized in vivo in a Parkinson's patient. Nat Neurosci 2:1137–1140

Piccini P, Lindvall O, Bjorklund A, Brundin P, Hagell P, Ceravolo R, Oertel W, Quinn N, Samuel M, Rehncrona S, Widner H, Brooks DJ (2000) Delayed recovery of movement-related cortical function in Parkinson's disease after striatal dopaminergic grafts. Ann Neurol 48:689–695

Porritt MJ, Batchelor PE, Hughes AJ, Kalnins R, Donnan GA, Howells DW (2000) New dopaminergic neurons in Parkinson's disease striatum. Lancet 356:44–45

Potter ED, Ling ZD, Carvey PM (1999) Cytokine-induced conversion of mesencephalic-derived progenitor cells into dopamine neurons. Cell Tissue Res 296:235–246

Rascol O, Goetz C, Koller W, Poewe W, Sampaio C (2002) Treatment interventions for Parkinson's disease: an evidence based assessment. Lancet 359:1589–1598

Remy P, Samson Y, Hantraye P, Fontaine A, Defer G, Mangin JF, Fenelon G, Geny C, Ricolfi F, Frouin V et al (1995) Clinical correlates of [18F]fluorodopa uptake in five grafted parkinsonian patients. Ann Neurol 38:580–588

Sakurada K, Ohshima-Sakurada M, Palmer TD, Gage FH (1999) Nurr1, an orphan nuclear receptor, is a transcriptional activator of endogenous tyrosine hydroxylase in neural progenitor cells derived from the adult brain. Development 126:4017–4026

Samii A, Nutt JG, Ransom BR (2004) Parkinson's disease. Lancet 363:1783–1793

Saucedo-Cardenas O, Quintana-Hau JD, Le WD, Smidt MP, Cox JJ, De Mayo F, Burbach JP, Conneely OM (1998) Nurr1 is essential for the induction of the dopaminergic phenotype and the survival of ventral mesencephalic late dopaminergic precursor neurons. Proc Natl Acad Sci U S A 95:4013–4018

Schapira AH (1997) Pathogenesis of Parkinson's disease. Baillieres Clin Neurol 6:15–36

Schmidt RH, Bjorklund A, Stenevi U (1981) Intracerebral grafting of dissociated CNS tissue suspensions: a new approach for neuronal transplantation to deep brain sites. Brain Res 218:347–356

Schmidt RH, Bjorklund A, Stenevi U, Dunnett SB, Gage FH (1983) Intracerebral grafting of neuronal cell suspensions. III. Activity of intrastriatal nigral suspension implants as assessed by measurements of dopamine synthesis and metabolism. Acta Physiol Scand Suppl 522:19–28

Schumacher JM, Ellias SA, Palmer EP, Kott HS, Dinsmore J, Dempsey PK, Fischman AJ, Thomas C, Feldman RG, Kassissieh S, Raineri R, Manhart C, Penney D, Fink JS, Isacson O (2000) Transplantation of embryonic porcine mesencephalic tissue in patients with PD. Neurology 54:1042–1050

Simon HH, Bhatt L, Gherbassi D, Sgado P, Alberi L (2003) Midbrain dopaminergic neurons: determination of their developmental fate by transcription factors. Ann N Y Acad Sci 991:36–47

Snyder EY, Deitcher DL, Walsh C, Arnold-Aldea S, Hartwieg EA, Cepko CL (1992) Multipotent neural cell lines can engraft and participate in development of mouse cerebellum. Cell 68:33–51

Stenevi U, Bjorklund A, Svendgaard NA (1976) Transplantation of central and peripheral monoamine neurons to the adult rat brain: techniques and conditions for survival. Brain Res 114:1–20

Storch A, Paul G, Csete M, Boehm BO, Carvey PM, Kupsch A, Schwarz J (2001) Long-term proliferation and dopaminergic differentiation of human mesencephalic neural precursor cells. Exp Neurol 170:317–325

Storch A, Lester HA, Boehm BO, Schwarz J (2003) Functional characterization of dopaminergic neurons derived from rodent mesencephalic progenitor cells. J Chem Neuroanat 26:133–142

Strecker RE, Sharp T, Brundin P, Zetterstrom T, Ungerstedt U, Bjorklund A (1987) Autoregulation of dopamine release and metabolism by intrastriatal nigral grafts as revealed by intracerebral dialysis. Neuroscience 22:169–178

Studer L, Tabar V, McKay RD (1998) Transplantation of expanded mesencephalic precursors leads to recovery in parkinsonian rats. Nat Neurosci 1:290–295

Studer L, Csete M, Lee SH, Kabbani N, Walikonis J, Wold B, McKay R (2000) Enhanced proliferation, survival, and dopaminergic differentiation of CNS precursors in lowered oxygen. J Neurosci 20:7377–7383

Subramanian T (2001) Cell transplantation for the treatment of Parkinson's disease. Semin Neurol 21:103–115

Takagi Y, Takahashi J, Saiki H, Morizane A, Hayashi T, Kishi Y, Fukuda H, Okamoto Y, Koyanagi M, Ideguchi M, Hayashi H, Imazato T, Kawasaki H, Suemori H, Omachi S, Iida H, Itoh N, Nakatsuji N, Sasai Y, Hashimoto N (2005) Dopaminergic neurons generated from monkey embryonic stem cells function in a Parkinson primate model. J Clin Invest 115:102–109

Tashiro Y, Kaneko T, Sugimoto T, Nagatsu I, Kikuchi H, Mizuno N (1989a) Striatal neurons with aromatic L-amino acid decarboxylase-like immunoreactivity in the rat. Neurosci Lett 100:29–34

Tashiro Y, Sugimoto T, Hattori T, Uemura Y, Nagatsu I, Kikuchi H, Mizuno N (1989b) Tyrosine hydroxylase-like immunoreactive neurons in the striatum of the rat. Neurosci Lett 97:6–10

Ungerstedt U, Arbuthnott GW (1970) Quantitative recording of rotational behavior in rats after 6-hydroxy-dopamine lesions of the nigrostriatal dopamine system. Brain Res 24:485–493

Wagner J, Akerud P, Castro DS, Holm PC, Canals JM, Snyder EY, Perlmann T, Arenas E (1999) Induction of a midbrain dopaminergic phenotype in Nurr1-overexpressing neural stem cells by type 1 astrocytes. Nat Biotechnol 17:653–659

Wallen A, Perlmann T (2003) Transcriptional control of dopamine neuron development. Ann N Y Acad Sci 991:48–60

Walter BL, Vitek JL (2004) Surgical treatment for Parkinson's disease. Lancet Neurol 3:719–728

Wenning GK, Odin P, Morrish P, Rehncrona S, Widner H, Brundin P, Rothwell JC, Brown R, Gustavii B, Hagell P, Jahanshahi M, Sawle G, Bjorklund A, Brooks DJ, Marsden CD, Quinn NP, Lindvall O (1997) Short- and long-term survival and function of unilateral intrastriatal dopaminergic grafts in Parkinson's disease. Ann Neurol 42:95–107

Widner H, Tetrud J, Rehncrona S, Snow B, Brundin P, Gustavii B, Bjorklund A, Lindvall O, Langston JW (1992) Bilateral fetal mesencephalic grafting in two patients with parkinsonism induced by 1-methyl-4-phenyl-1,2,3,6-tetrahydropyridine (MPTP). N Engl J Med 327:1556–1563

Winkler C, Kirik D, Bjorklund A (2005) Cell transplantation in Parkinson's disease: how can we make it work? Trends Neurosci 28:86–92

Yan J, Studer L, McKay RD (2001) Ascorbic acid increases the yield of dopaminergic neurons derived from basic fibroblast growth factor expanded mesencephalic precursors. J Neurochem 76:307–311

Zeng X, Cai J, Chen J, Luo Y, You ZB, Fotter E, Wang Y, Harvey B, Miura T, Backman C, Chen GJ, Rao MS, Freed WJ (2004) Dopaminergic differentiation of human embryonic stem cells. Stem Cells 22:925–940

Zetterstrom T, Brundin P, Gage FH, Sharp T, Isacson O, Dunnett SB, Ungerstedt U, Bjorklund A (1986) In vivo measurement of spontaneous release and metabolism of dopamine from intrastriatal nigral grafts using intracerebral dialysis. Brain Res 362:344–349

Zhao M, Momma S, Delfani K, Carlen M, Cassidy RM, Johansson CB, Brismar H, Shupliakov O, Frisen J, Janson AM (2003) Evidence for neurogenesis in the adult mammalian substantia nigra. Proc Natl Acad Sci U S A 100:7925–7930

HEP (2006) 174:389–408
© Springer-Verlag Berlin Heidelberg 2006

Postmodern Biology: (Adult) (Stem) Cells Are Plastic, Stochastic, Complex, and Uncertain

N. D. Theise[1] (✉) · R. Harris[2]

[1]Department of Medicine, Division of Digestive Diseases, Beth Israel Medical Center, First Avenue at 16th Street, New York NY, 10003, USA
ntheise@chpnet.org

[2]Department of Laboratory Medicine, Yale University Medical School, New Haven CT, USA

Abstract This chapter will discuss recent findings regarding cell plasticity and stem cell behavior, focusing on ways in which experimental design, observer interference, and inherent stochasticity and complexity are serving to create a new, postmodern biology. The chapter will summarize: (a) the four recognized pathways whereby cell plasticity occurs physiologically; (b) recent findings regarding unexpected epigenetic reversibility of gene restrictions that provide the mechanistic core of plasticity; (c) current evidence for the stochastic nature of gene expression and, therefore, of cell fate decisions. It will be noted that stochastic, however, does not imply completely random; rather, constrained randomness, intermediate between rigid determinism and complete disorder is what is usually seen experimentally. Possible sources of such constrained disorder, from a biomolecular point of view, will be discussed. The chapter will conclude with discussions of how these findings contribute to a Complexity Theory formulation of the body as self-organizing emergence of interacting biomolecules and the implications of such concepts for design and interpretation of experimental results (i.e., a cellular version of Heisenbergian uncertainty).

Keywords Stem cells · Plasticity · Stochasticity · Complexity · Uncertainty principle

1
Introduction

Nearly every field of academic studies has been made slippery for tradition-
alists by introduction of "postmodern" analyses that highlight the observer
dependence and uncertainty of nearly any investigated phenomenon. Biology,
however, in its glory with the modern successes of molecular and cell biology
has remained relatively unchallenged in this regard.

However, studies of adult stem cell plasticity in combination with contem-
poraneous findings from other fields, demand reconsideration of long-held
dogmas. Up for revision are doctrines about reversibility of gene restrictions,
the role of stochasticity in cell fate decisions, and the ability of cell biologic
experiments, in vivo and ex vivo, to accurately reflect physiologic phenomena (Theise 2002; Theise and Krause 2001, 2002). Biology begins to get more
slippery in a postmodernist (parenthetical) sort of way.

We begin with the fact that the increasing intricacy of adult stem cell plasticity's phenomenology and of our gradually expanding appreciation of its
underlying mechanisms requires a clarification of language. This is where
postmodern approaches encroach upon orthodox certainties. A revisionist
approach to language is often the first postmodern shot across the bow.

A full discussion of the terminology issues is beyond the scope of this
chapter; however, for clarity of discourse, two labels, usually linked in a single,
politically potent phrase, require extrication from each other. These are the
terms "stem cells" and "plasticity." While they are related in some situations,
they are not to be treated like conjoined twins.

As Helen Blau has eloquently discussed, stem cells are not cellular "entities,"
but, rather, cells that perform certain stem cell "functions" (Blau et al. 2001).
The classical definition of a stem cell is still useful: a stem cell has capacities
for self-renewal and for asymmetric division leading to generation of other
differentiated cell types (either with each cell division or, in aggregate, when
populations are studied over time). Whether a stem cell is always a stem cell,
however, and whether non-stem cells can ever be recruited or induced to
behave like stem cells will be one of the topics addressed in this review. This is
the point of one set of parentheses in the title of this chapter: while the ideas
to be discussed arose in the context of stem cell research, we now understand
that they are not restricted to stem cells, per se.

Meanwhile, the word "plasticity" has been used to describe differentiative
events (or capacities), which are unexpected according to accepted standard
definitions of various cell lineages. Thus, hematopoietic stem cells give rise
to the full array of hematopoietic lineages, but this is not generally referred
to as plasticity; rather, plasticity is invoked when an unexpected differentiation event is revealed. Examples from 1999, when *Science* declared "Stem
cell plasticity" to be the Breakthrough of the Year, included marrow-derived
cells becoming skeletal muscle and liver and neural stem cells giving rise to

hematopoiesis (Bjornson et al. 1999; Ferrari et al. 1998; Petersen et al. 1999). The term "plasticity" is used in these contexts because cells are unexpectedly crossing organ boundaries or even embryonic lineage boundaries.

One must question, though, whether the experimental confirmation of plasticity events then eliminates the need for the word: if a differentiation pathway is considered normative, i.e., unsurprising, is it still plasticity? Or must the notion of plasticity be invoked when hypothetical embryonic trilaminar lineage boundaries are breached? Or must we consider something in between, such as when organ boundaries are breached? And is it only stem cells that can be plastic? Or is plasticity something that might be demonstrated by a wide variety (or perhaps all) cells, differentiated or otherwise?

These questions are up for discussion and will be among the topics of this review. To address them we will proceed through consideration of five experimental and/or conceptual sub-topics:

1. We will briefly summarize the four recognized pathways whereby cell plasticity occurs physiologically (for our purposes, in this review, "plasticity" will imply a more generalized sense of "differentiative potential"). The experimental data demonstrating these pathways, though somewhat scattershot and mechanistically undefined, point to the need for alternate models for the nature and behavior of cells.

2. Recent findings regarding unexpected epigenetic reversibility of gene restrictions, the underlying molecular events at the core of plasticity, will be updated for the reader. These more systematically acquired data provide the mechanistic core of plasticity.

3. Current evidence for the stochastic nature of gene expression and, therefore, of cell fate decisions will be considered. It will be noted that stochastic, however, does not imply completely random; rather, constrained randomness, intermediate between rigid determinism and complete disorder is what is usually seen experimentally. Possible sources of such constrained disorder, from a biomolecular point of view, will be discussed.

4. Taking these data together, we will then extend our prior discussion of how a complex systems analysis may be applied to cell behavior. We have argued previously that cells, in vivo, behave as interacting agents giving rise to emergent self-organization of cell lineages, tissues, organs, and bodies. Here we will consider that they are actually located within a hierarchy of complex systems and that they, themselves, are emergent phenomena self-organizing from the biomolecules which they comprise.

5. The implications of such concepts for design and interpretation of experimental results (i.e., a cellular version of Heisenbergian uncertainty) will complete the review.

All of these diverse strands of thought have been considered in prior papers, by us and by other investigators, but it is perhaps time to weave them together, to better imagine the emerging tapestry that may well turn out to be a new biology for this new millennium.

2
Pathways of Plasticity

Physiologic, in vivo expressions of differentiative potential can be seen in four flexibly employed processes or pathways (Theise and Wilmut 2003). First, of course, is the classic hierarchical, unidirectional concept of lineage commitment. In embryonic/fetal development, this begins with an embryonic stem cell or with a fetal stem cell. In adults, one is speaking of normative, tissue maintenance or repair after injury. In all these cases, one begins with a multi- or totipotent stem cell which, through asymmetric division, self renews and also gives rise to more differentiated cell types. These more differentiated daughter cells mature in an ordered, hierarchical, unidirectional fashion.

This model is certainly the dominant pathway for development and tissue maintenance, if not, perhaps the only pathway. As such, it was the most readily demonstrable experimentally. Detailed transplantation experiments established the hierarchical, unidirectional aspects. In moving cells from one part of the embryo to another, they would be influenced by the new microenvironment to change differentiative pathways until a certain temporal point in development, after which they would be "committed" and not respond to the new environmental cues. Even before the structure of DNA revealed how genetic encoding took place, these observations led to the idea of a restriction of gene expression that eventually confined a cell to a "terminally differentiated" state, from which it could not be coaxed.

The second pathway of plasticity is one of "dedifferentiation", i.e., reversion of a differentiated cell into a progenitor, often blast-like (i.e., primitive or undifferentiated) phenotype, which can then give rise to different lineages. In mammals, this has only been confidently recognized in neoplasia, in particular in malignancy, in the context of genetic mutations and other genomic derangements. While metaplastic phenomena may also include such a process, they are usually hypothesized to represent activation of an alternate pathway of a multipotent, intraorgan stem cell (Theise and Krause 2002). Examples of this would include osseous metaplasia within skeletal muscle, when mature bone forms after mechanical injury, or the squamous metaplasia of respiratory lining cells in the lungs of smokers. However, in limb-regenerating amphibians, there appear to be proteins which can induce a mature cell to reverse differentiative direction, giving rise to blasts which then give rise to the necessary mature cells in the regrowing limb (Endo et al. 2004).

The third and fourth pathways are those which currently capture the most controversial attention. The third is that of cells from one lineage directly differentiating into cells of another lineage (Krause et al. 2001) (This has often been referred to as "transdifferentiation," a term which engenders still more unnecessary debate and we now feel is best avoided.). Such direct differentiative events which jump between (dogmatically) hypothesized lineage or organ boundaries have now been convincingly demonstrated in vivo and ex vivo and are induced by local microenvironmental effects that lead to alterations in gene expression (Harris et al. 2004; Ianus et al. 2003; Ishikawa et al. 2003; Jang et al. 2004; Newsome et al. 2003).

The fourth pathway is that of cell–cell fusion, sometimes followed by nuclear–nuclear fusion. The idea of cell fusion was originally suggested as part of a critique of the findings regarding plasticity arising from direct differentiation, used to polemically dismiss those new findings as "artifact" (Newsome et al. 2003; Willenbring and Grompe 2003). However, it is now not merely a rhetorical or theoretical challenge for undermining one set of new, controversial findings, but is, itself, established as yet another alternate and surprising physiologic, in vivo process (Alvarez-Dolado et al. 2003; Willenbring et al. 2004). In this case, the plasticity of gene expression is induced not by microenvironmental effects, but by cytoplasmic and/or nuclear factors. This is directly analogous to the findings in experimental heterokaryons studied by Blau and colleagues two decades ago (Blau et al. 1983).

As Blau and investigators ultimately concluded "differentiation is an actively maintained state" (Blau et al. 1985). Examining all these pathways in aggregate, one comes to realize that plasticity is simply a comparatively macro-level change in function and phenotype arising from the micro-level alterations in gene expression. Just as the early transplantation experiments showing restriction of developmental potential over time implied molecular restriction of gene expression, these more newly described phenomena imply reversibility of these "irreversible" gene restrictions. In the earlier instance, decades had to pass before the mechanistic, molecular underpinnings could be confirmed. However, in these more recent and controversial demonstrations of plasticity, the implied reversibility of gene restrictions was already being studied, in parallel, by other investigators.

3
Gene Restrictions: Irreversible Versus Reversible

In the standard model of cell differentiation, the cell makes a series of simple (usually binary) fate decisions that are irreversible and thus restrict the cells to a particular lineage. Implicit in this model is the concept of commitment; if cell fate decisions are irreversible, once a cell has made a particular fate decision, it is committed to that lineage and cannot alter its fate. In this model of differentiation, cell fate is determined by two separate components: the external microenvironment—the extracellular signals that a cell is exposed to—and an internal cellular memory, that is, to which lineage it has already been restricted.

Classic experiments by Nicole Le Douarin and colleagues showed that during neural crest migration and differentiation cells become both committed and restricted to their lineage. Neural crest cells that are transplanted to more rostral or caudal regions of the neural tube retain their fate programming and thus must be committed to their lineage before any obvious morphological or migratory changes occur (Le Douarin and Dupin 1993).

Outside of development, the most widely studied model of differentiation is the hematopoietic system. Under the hierarchical paradigm, a hematopoietic stem cell (HSC), which is already committed to a hematopoietic fate, further differentiates into a common lymphoid progenitor (CLP) or common myeloid progenitor (CMP). These cells are committed to the lymphoid or myeloid lineages, respectively, but can differentiate into any of the cells of that lineage. These then make further cell fate decisions, which eventually result in their terminal differentiation into T cells or B cells or neutrophils or macrophages and so on. Recent experiments have actually identified cells that appear to fit all the requirements of committed CMPs and CLPs (Akashi et al. 2000; Kondo et al. 1997). When used in bone marrow transplant experiments, the putative CLPs differentiated into mature B-cells, T cells, and natural killer cells but were restricted solely to these lineages: no donor-derived myeloid cells could be found. In vitro experiments using cytokine cocktails that promote myeloid differentiation of HSCs resulted in apoptosis rather than myeloid or even lymphoid differentiation. Likewise, the putative CMP was restricted solely to the myeloid lineage and showed differentiation into all cell types in the myelo-erythroid lineage.

While lineage commitment initially restricts a cell to a particular subset of cell fate decisions, those decisions themselves—such as the decision of the HSC to differentiate into the CMP or CLP—are likely to be mostly affected by the microenvironment. Unlike lineage restriction, microenvironmental effects on cell fate are probably stochastic in nature. While extracellular signals may push a cell toward one particular fate decision or another, some cells in a population will follow the alternate path. Lineage commitment, in this traditional model, however, is theoretically complete.

3.1
Mechanisms of Lineage Restriction

The limiting of a cell to a subset of possible fates has two putative molecular mechanisms. The first, which may be thought of as passive lineage restriction, depends on the subset of proteins actually expressed in the cell. A cell cannot differentiate down a pathway if it does not contain the proteins that can respond to the intracellular and extracellular signals that are required by that pathway.

The second mechanism, which may be thought of as active lineage restriction, depends on the continued silencing of genes that are master regulators of alternate lineages (Jaenisch and Bird 2003). In this model the cell retains a working memory of its ancestry, in the form of epigenetic (i.e., non-DNA-encoded) modifications to the genome that render particular gene sets available or less accessible (restricted) for transcription. According to this epigenetic view of differentiation, the cell makes a series of choices (some of which may have no obvious phenotypic expression and are spoken of as determination events) that lead to the eventual differentiated state. Thus, selective gene repression or derepression at an early stage in differentiation will have a wide-ranging consequence in restricting the possible fate of the cell. As usual, there is evidence that both of these mechanisms are important.

The absence of particular signaling receptors or effectors can prevent the differentiation of a cell down a particular lineage. In the hematopoietic system, the HSC makes a fate decision to differentiate into either the CMP or the CLP. IL-2 promotes differentiation down the myeloid lineage. After commitment to the myeloid lineage, the IL-2β receptor is upregulated in the CMP, whereas after lymphoid commitment, no IL-2βR protein can be detected in the CLP. Lineage restriction at early time points after commitment to the CMP or CLP is due to the absence of the IL-2β receptor. If CLPs are isolated from mice that express the human IL-2β receptor they can be induced to differentiate down the myeloid lineage by treatment with human IL-2 (Kondo et al. 2000).

This conversion of lymphoid committed progenitors to the myeloid fate comes at the expense of the lymphoid lineage and is indicative that CLPs have latent GM lineage differentiation potential that can be initiated through IL-2 signaling. It is important to note, however, that this IL-2-induced myeloid differentiation is somewhat transient, and cultured CLPs "irreversibly" commit to the lymphoid lineage after 2 days. It is likely, therefore, that this mechanism of lineage commitment is important only in the early stages of differentiation of a cell type; after this, more permanent silencing of alternate lineages occurs. Many important transcription factors and signaling molecules have different effects in different cell types—an obvious statement but one which is obviously important when talking about this type of lineage restriction. IL-2 becomes important in the end stages of T cell development. There must therefore be a mechanism to limit the transcriptional response of a cell to a particular signal.

3.2
Lineage Restriction by Chromatin Silencing

Differentiation involves the selective activation and silencing of particular gene expression programs. One potential mechanism to restrict cells to a particular lineage is to irreversibly silence the cell-type-specific genes of the alternate lineages. The classic paper by Weintraub and Groudine in 1976, showing that active genes have a different chromatin structure than silenced genes, was the first evidence that DNA accessibility was important in transcriptional regulation (Weintraub and Groudine 1976).

In mammals, there are two major mechanisms of epigenetic control; methylation of DNA at cytosine and modifications of the histone proteins (Jaenisch and Bird 2003). DNA methylation is associated with gene silencing, especially in imprinting and X-inactivation. After DNA synthesis, the daughter strand is methylated by reference to the parental strand, thus maintaining methylation patterns through mitosis. There are no known DNA demethylases and it is thought to be an extremely stable modification. Experiments using transgenes have shown that DNA methylation is stable over more than 50 divisions.

There is increasing evidence that DNA methylation can also be the cause of gene restriction during differentiation, rather than just an associated effect. Some of the first experiments used 5-aza-2'-deoxycytidine (5-Aza-dC), a nucleotide analog that inhibits DNA methyltransferases, and therefore results in hypomethylation of daughter cells, after division. For example, when fibroblasts were treated with 5-aza-dC they acquired the ability to spontaneously differentiate into a range of different mesenchymal lineages, including chondrocytes, adipocytes, and multinucleated myotubes (Taylor and Jones 1979). Such experiments show that reversal of epigenetic modifications associated with gene silencing also reverse the lineage restriction of a cell, allowing it to differentiate down several unexpected pathways.

More recently, this sort of epigenetic reprogramming has been used to increase the number of viable blastocysts in nuclear transfer experiments (Enright et al. 2003). Treatment of nuclei with combinations of Aza-dC and TSA significantly increase the number of viable blastocysts, potentially implying that removing the chromatin-linked lineage restriction of mature cells is necessary for the formation of the totipotent zygote.

3.3
Post-Translation Modification of Histones

At least 100 different post-translational modifications of the various histone proteins are now known. The types of modifications known include acetylation, methylation, phosphorylation, and ubiquitinization. All of these modifications seem to correlate with the transcriptional state of the chromatin in question: active, silenced or potentiated (Jaenisch and Bird 2003). The best-known histone modification is the acetylation of histone H4. Increased acetylation of H4 correlates with active transcription and the major repressor complexes such as the N-CoR and SMRT complexes contain a variety of histone deacetylases.

An implication of an irreversible chromatin silencing mechanism for gene restriction is that more pluripotent cells will have a chromatin structure in which the genes expressed in all future mature lineages will be in a potentiated state rather than a totally silenced state. Following on from Weintraub and Groudine's experiments, it was shown that in FDCP mix cells, an early myeloerythroid cell line, the β-globin locus is susceptible to DNAse degradation well before significant β-globin transcription occurs, indicating some sort of gene potentiation (Jimenez et al. 1992).

In order for certain genes to be permanently epigenetically repressed, active marks such as acetylation of histone H4 must be removed. Recent experiments have shown that histone deacetylases seem to be important in cell fate and lineage restriction. Hematopoietic stem cells that are grown in the presence of the histone deacetylase inhibitor Trichostatin A (TSA) remain pluripotent and do not differentiate, even if grown in the presence of cytokines that promoted differentiation (Milhem et al. 2004). Additionally, it has been shown that histone deacetylase activity is required for differentiation in ES cells (Lee et al. 2004).

Somatic cell nuclear transfer experiments have shown that the more differentiated a cell is, the less likely it is to form a developing blastocyst. Subsequent reprogramming experiments have shown that nuclei with a more generally open chromatin structure, as evidenced by H4 acetylation and H3 Lys 4 methylation, are more likely to result in successful nuclear transfer (Santos et al. 2003).

3.4
Reversibility of Gene Restrictions

If nonlineage-restricted differentiation events truly occur in nature, then the molecular modifications leading to epigenetic gene restriction must be reversible. There is plenty of experimental evidence that all of the epigenetic means of lineage restriction we have mentioned, such as DNA methylation and histone modifications can be reversed by artificial manipulation. In addition, overexpression of single transcription factors can result in a complete change of fate. For example, overexpression of the transcription factor MyoD in fibroblasts also converts them into multinucleated myotubes (Davis et al. 1987), just as treatment with Aza-dC does. Likewise, overexpression of C/EBPα in mature B cells will directly convert them to mature macrophages, with a clear macrophage phenotype including phagocytosis (Xie et al. 2004).

Other experiments looking at reprogramming of nuclei show that epigenetic modifications are far from irreversible. ES cell cytoplasm will effectively reprogram nuclei, increasing histone acetylation and H3 Lys 4 methylation. Cloning by nuclear transfer is obviously an extreme version of such a process. Collas et al. have provided abundant evidence that nuclear and cytoplasmic extracts can reprogram nuclei, for example from a fibroblast to a T lymphocyte, demonstrating the existence of factors that can reverse epigenetic modifications, if not yet identifying them (Collas 1998, 2003).

There is also some indirect evidence that reversal of epigenetic silencing occurs during normal development. During activation of T cells, the promoter of the IL-2 genes is actively demethylated within 7 h, yet 15 h after activation only 13% of cells have entered S-phase (Bruniquel and Schwartz 2003). In this case, DNA demethylation occurs in a gene-specific, tissue-specific manner, so obviously there is nothing fundamentally irreversible about this epigenetic modification.

Recently, two mechanisms for the demethylation of histones have been discovered. In the first, the human peptidylarginine deiminase 4 (PAD4) converts methyl-arginine residues to citrulline (Cuthbert et al. 2004; Wang et al. 2004). It specifically converts histone H3 methyl-Arg 3 and methyl-Arg 17 to citrulline. Secondly, LSD1, a nuclear homolog of amine oxidases, functions as a histone demethylase and specifically demethylates histone H3 lysine (Shi et al. 2004). Although these modifications are associated with active transcription and not gene silencing, the discovery of mechanisms for active demethylation of histones is an important step.

What does this mean for plasticity? The hierarchical, unidirectional view of differentiation is overwhelmingly true during most of development. As such, these dominant pathways were the first and easiest to elucidate (Theise 2004). Less frequent pathways, however, were often obscured by relative insensitivity of experimental techniques. New approaches, revealing the unexpected plasticity phenomena reported in recent years, as well as nuclear transfer experiments (including the heterokaryon experiments of Blau and the now-documented fusion events for repair of visceral epithelia), demonstrate that other pathways exist. These are now gradually being unveiled by epigenetic researchers.

4
Stochasticity Versus Determinism in Cell Behavior

A long-standing debate has been whether cell behavior is determined or is stochastic, i.e., best described as a statistical process incorporating some degree of random behavior. The two possibilities can be distinguished experimentally, in a reductionist approach, looking at the behavior of individual cells, or with a systems approach, looking at behavior of cells in aggregate. The latter is most often done using computational techniques to generate computer models that, with more or less fidelity, give rise to virtual biologically relevant behaviors.

The balance of the debate has been manifested in studies of the hematopoietic system. The experimental ability to isolate single hematopoietic stem cells and grow them in colony-forming units has allowed for comparison of behaviors between individual cells. While some experiments of this type have indicated a deterministic behavior, the bulk of the data suggests variability of cell differentiation upon initiation of colony formation (Ogawa 1999). For example, diverse combinations of more differentiated cells are identified in individual colonies derived from single cells (Leary et al. 1984). Analysis of colonies derived from paired progenitors also reveals variability in modes of differentiation (Leary et al. 1984; Marley et al. 2003). This work is contrasted with other efforts indicating that inductive factors in the microenvironment (e.g., cytokines, cell-matrix adhesion) lead to constraint of differentiative capacity (Metcalf 1998).

The key word in the paragraph above is "constraint." Does constraint imply determinism? Or is it possible to have intermediate degrees of constraint, yielding behaviors that lie intermediate between complete randomness and those that are rigidly determined? This is where the mathematical modelers have been making a large contribution. Models that incorporate some degree of constrained stochasticity faithfully reflect biological behaviors and generate testable hypotheses (Agur et al. 2002; Deenick et al. 2003; Furusawa and Kaneko 2001; Loeffler and Roeder 2002, 2004; O'Neill and Schaffer 2004; Roeder and Loeffler 2002; Roeder et al. 2003). Indeed, as is so often the case in scientific debates, with data mounting on either side of the question, we find ourselves, with time, coming to an acceptable middle ground. In this particular debate, constraint of stochasticity provides the middle ground between the seemingly opposed ideas of stochasticity and determinism. We will return to this concept of constrained randomness in Sect. 5 of this chapter dealing with Complexity Theory and the implications of a systems analysis for cell behavior, below.

Meanwhile, what are possible sources for stochastic behavior in differentiation of cells? Of course, for blood, the movement of cells through the vascular tree, subject to highly stochastic influences of fluid dynamics, brings them into different microenvironments and therefore exposes them to different inductive influences. Most tissues, however, are not fluid in this manner; the cellular microenvironment in intact. Noninjured adult tissues appears rather stable, at least at the supracellular level. But if we look into the biomolecular dynamics on the scale of the cell and its compartments, we find possible sources for stochasticity.

Work from Peter Quesenberry's laboratory demonstrates that a cell's differentiation capacity is tied to its temporal position in the cell cycle (Colvin et al. 2004). With ex vivo synchronization of cell cycle, isolated hematopoietic stem cells, transplanted at different points in their transit through the first cell cycle, display different reconstituting behaviors. This work details "differentiation hotspots" in the cell cycle at which one either finds long-term reconstitution, short-term reconstitution, or lineage restricted reconstitution (e.g., erythropoiesis, leukopoiesis, lymphopoiesis). It is hypothesized that chromatin remodeling as the cycle proceeds underlies changes in gene expression, reflected for example in changes in expression of adhesion molecules and cytokine receptors. The stochasticity of entry into cell cycle is therefore tied to stochasticity of gene expression and differentiation.

Detailed studies of dynamic changes of chromosomal structure indicate entry points for randomness into gene expression and control (Carmo-Fonseca 2002; Carmo-Fonseca et al. 2002). One example: fluorescent labeling of euchromatin in the interphase nucleus reveals movement that is best modeled as a "random walk" diffusion process (Vazquez et al. 2001). This implies that interactions of genes with the important regulatory proteins in the spatially organized nucleosome, while tightly regulated in so many ways, also have an irreducible stochastic element. Thus, stochastic sequestration of genes within sites within the three-dimensional conformational structure of the interphase chromatin results in stochastic variation of gene expression (Vermaak and Wolffe 1998).

David Hume also locates stochasticity at the level of transcription initiation, redefining transcription as a digital rather than an analog process (Hume 2000). Each one of the multiple DNA templates for many genes is either "on" or "off," depending on whether the preinitiation complex of molecules is in place to lead to transcription. But the assembly of these complexes is experimentally demonstrated to be probabilistic. Hume generalizes to the concept that mRNA production is produced in "pulses," the mean frequency of which is determined by the probability of formation of the preinitiation complex. On this basis, he argues that "it is more meaningful to talk about the probability and frequency of transcription rather than the rate" and describes a "quantal" understanding of production of mRNA and, therefore, of gene expression.

5
Complexity Theory and Emergence of Cellular Phenomena

"Complexity theory" is not actually so complex. It describes the phenomena of interacting individuals which, when they fulfill certain criteria, self-organize into emergent structures. When such emergence arises, the system is found to be adaptive, i.e., it can react and change its organization or behavior, despite alterations in the environment, thus surviving as an entity (Theise 2004).

The most commonly used example is that of the ant colony. Ants have a limited number of ways in which they interact with each other: recognition and response to nine different pheromones and to direct contact. Out of those limited interactions, with no central planning, the highly detailed organizational social structure of the ant colony emerges. If one computer models the interactions of ants on the micro scale, similarly complex virtual ant colonies arise on the macro scale without the programmers having written computer code to directly create such structure. This is what is meant by "self organization."

Any system of interacting individuals, actual or virtual, that fulfills certain criteria gives rise to complex adaptive systems. These are:

1. Large numbers of individuals (though determining how many are necessary is not yet well understood).

2. Means of recognizing effects of other individuals within the system.

3. Homeostatic, negative feedback signaling between interacting individuals.

4. Low level stochasticity (too little and the system is rigid and nonadaptive, too much and the system devolves into figurative or literal chaos). This last criterion is referred to as "quenched disorder."

We have previously described cells and cell lineages as examples of complex adaptive systems and showed how they fulfill all the criteria (Hussain and Theise 2004; Theise 2004; Theise and d'Inverno 2004). In particular, the constrained stochasticity discussed above supports this analysis. Thus, one can expect cells to give rise to emergent self-organization and, of course, they do: from the unfolding of the embryo and fetus, with formation of all tissues and organs necessary for development, and then the adaptive stability displayed throughout postnatal life (Furusawa and Kaneko 2000, 2002). Investigators have moreover begun computer modeling cell–cell interactions and find that they can demonstrate the emergence that is seen in life, gaining insight into physiological processes governing, for example, growth and maintenance of small intestinal crypt/villous lining cells and the fluctuations of clones in leukemias (Paulus et al. 1992; Potten and Loeffler 1990; Roeder et al. 2005). Significant discussion already surrounds conceptualization of immune system diversity and response as adaptive self-organization (Brusic and Petrovsky 2003). The current leading hypothesis regarding consciousness is that it is an emergent phenomenon on the macro scale arising from interactions of neuronal networks on the micro scale (Gell-Mann 2001).

This latter concept hints at an aspect of complex systems that we will now discuss in more detail. We have already stated, on the one hand, that cell–cell interactions give rise emergently to tissues and organs. This is, of course, true for the neuronal networks of the brain and the brain as a whole. Yet, for consciousness investigators, the neuronal networks are not considered the macro-level emergence, but rather, the micro-level interacting individuals. Thus, complex systems can exist as hierarchies. The aggregate self-organization of one system can play the role of an interacting agent in a higher level system, giving rise to higher level emergence. Thus, cells give rise to the emergent phenomena of living, moving people. But people, in turn, interact and give rise emergently to the organization of social structures, such as cities, cultures, and civilizations.

Thus, having turned our attention "upwards" from cells, we may also consider turning our attention in the other direction: cells might be emergent self-organization arising from interacting individuals on a smaller, "lower" scale. What would those interacting individuals be? Biomolecules, of course. And it is clear that biomolecules certainly fulfill most of the criteria for a complex system: they occur in enormous numbers, they interact with each other following defined molecular/chemical rules, and these interactions form homeostatic feedback loops. Do they display quenched disorder?

Recent investigations of individual biomolecular "machines" indicate, surprisingly, that the answer is "yes" (Yanagida and Ishii 2003). One example, of many, comes from the work of Toshio Yanagida, of Osaka University (Kitamura and Yanagida 2003). Observing the interactions of single actin and myosin strands, fluorescently labeled and held in place for observation with "laser tweezers," he has demonstrated that the ATP does not supply the energy for bending of the myosin elbow, resulting in movement, but, instead, the movement is random and constant, in response to Brownian motion of the surrounding fluid. The energy from the release of phosphate from ATP provides the energy to constrain this random movement in a directional, physiological fashion. Similar experiments are showing the same phenomena in other interacting elements of molecular motors such as EGF and EGF-receptor binding (Ichinose et al. 2004), kinesin movement along microtubules (Nishiyama et al. 2002), MMP-1 along collagen (Saffarian et al. 2004), and appears, increasingly, to be a generalizable phenomenon (Ait-Haddou and Herzog 2003).

Thus, there is quenched disorder in the way biomolecules interact and so they, too, fulfill all the criteria of a complex system. The emergent phenomenon is the cell. Our concrete understanding of the nature of the cell and how we explore its behavior is altered by this formulation (Kurakin 2005). On the one hand, cells are indeed "things", i.e., building block-like entities that are the fundamental, indivisible subunit of the body. But, also, on the other hand, they are not things, but ephemeral, ever-changing and adapting molecular organization in space and time. Much in the way that one may consider ant colonies, bee hives, or human cities to be things with their own character and structure, but also, alternatively, as organizations of smaller things. It all depends on the scale of observation and investigation.

This formulation keeps clear several features of cells that are often forgotten when investigators are locked into particular frames of reference and of scale. These features will be the subject of the next two sections of this chapter, as we see how genomic plasticity and the complex nature of cells has implications for the debates about stochasticity vs determinism in cell behavior, as well as the impact of observation on the nature of cells.

6
Cellular Uncertainty: Analogy or Metaphor?

We have previously described cell behavior and differentiation as displaying uncertainty (Theise 2002; Theise and Krause 2001, 2002), echoing earlier statements by Potten and Loeffler (Potten and Loeffler 1990), analogous to that of Werner Heisenberg's famous description of quantum physical processes. We initially based this idea on the truism that, as Richard Lewontin has written: "the inside and the outside codetermine the cell." Paying careful attention to this concept, one may infer that to observe or otherwise interact with a cell necessarily changes the microenvironment and therefore necessarily changes the differentiation state or capacity of that cell. From simple venopuncture to more extreme acts of tissue disaggregation and culture, no scientific experiment leaves a cell unchanged.

This includes some of the most fundamental, basic approaches to cell characterization employed by contemporary cell biologists. These include antibody binding to cell surface molecules, which we often refer to as markers, as though they were merely name tags worn by the cell for our purposes. The activities of some markers, such as CD5 and CD45, have been extensively studied (Lozano et al. 2000; Sasaki et al. 2001). It is clear that while some binding of ligand to these receptors can activate some cell processes, other forms of binding will produce alternate effects. So, before isolation with an anti-marker antibody can be assumed to be merely an isolation process, lacking influence on subsequent differentiation events, the relative inertness of the antibody binding needs to be established. If it has not been established, then the interpretation of such data must take into consideration that possibility. However, most markers are not so well characterized and most do not have such a wide array of specific antibodies available for detection. A prime example of this is CD34: it still remains unclear what this molecule actually does (Krause et al. 1996); thus we have no way to determine what the sequelae of the use of detecting antibodies might actually be.

However, whether our use of Heisenbergian uncertainty is simply a useful metaphor or is a precise analogy remains largely unconsidered. The difference lies in whether the ability to truly determine with certainty what a cell is and will do is an artifact of our current technological limitations or whether it is a fundamental aspect of the cell. As with Heisenberg's initial pronouncement, the question becomes: is it possible to create a perfect machine which would eliminate uncertainty? In the case of physics, the answer was no, uncertainty was not artifact, but a fundamental aspect of the nature of the universe. But could we perhaps develop a perfect MRI machine, for example, by which a cell could be completely characterized, in situ, and yet remain unchanged?

A potential answer to this lies in our analysis of cells as emergent phenomena arising from complex interactions of biomolecules. That analysis mandates the dual consideration, depending on the level of scale of observation, that cells exist both as defined entities (the cell and tissue level perspective) or not as defined entities (from the biomolecular perspective). Thus, as stated above, there is no "thing-ness" to a seeming object that is the emergent self-organization from lower-scale elements. They have no independent, stable existence and thus cannot be pinned down with certainty in all of their particulars at any given moment. There can be no perfect machine to accomplish the task. Thus, Cellular Uncertainty is not mere artifact of technological limitations, but is a fundamental aspect of cell nature. On some level, the cell and, therefore, the body itself, are incompletely knowable and must remain so.

7
Postmodern Biology

The implications of these ideas for those interested in biology from a theoretical or from a pragmatic, biomedical point of view, are profound. From hypothesis formation to design of cell biologic experiments to interpretation of data, little remains unchanged. That any isolated cell population can ever be described as truly homogeneous vs heterogeneous falls by the wayside. Variations within an isolated population are often dismissed or criticized as contamination, but while contaminants need to be guarded against, there will always be a degree of inhomogeneity reflective of uncertainty and stochasticity. The rigid use of experimental data, obtained from reductionist approaches, to describe what is happening within the body is a false approach. There is no cell in the body that acts in isolation from the system; thus, cell behavior deduced from analysis of the cell in isolation is only partially informative. Biological processes arise from simultaneous interactions of all elements of the system rather than in the linear mode inherent in most twentieth century experimental design.

Practically speaking, for those interested in biomedical applications, these perhaps discouraging limitations actually open up a broad range of new possibilities. That cells with the entire genome intact can experimentally become any other cell type opens up an astonishing array of possibilities for cell-based therapies (Theise 2003). Whether cells are embryonic, fetal, or postnatal does not matter as much as how clever we are in figuring out how to manipulate them for desired ends. Also, getting at those other parentheses in our title, the issue is not really about adult stem cells except in so far as these concepts are applicable to all cells, not just those in postnatal life and not only those that display stem cell functioning.

The engineering approach to tissue engineering appears flawed. In treating tissues as an engineering problem about the arrangement of cellular building blocks (literally), it misses the possible opportunities for cells to self-organize into useful tissues, ex vivo (Hussain and Thiese 2004). Putting them where we want them, on carefully constructed scaffolds, may not be as interesting as aggregating them in different conditions, quantities, etc., and seeing what they create on their own.

Finally, recognition that cells are merely emergent phenomena breaks the lock of traditional cell doctrine on ways to analyze and describe the body. Testable and reproducible bodily effects that have no anatomical correlate cannot be explained simply on the basis of cells, per se, and require alternate models for explanation. An example of this is the use of acupuncture to influence physiologic processes (Ma 2004). The organ-related meridians shown to be of testable import for placement of needles and success of therapy do not correspond to any structure identifiably made of cells. In the absence of such a correlate, limiting ourselves to cell doctrine limits us in our ability to understand acupuncture and more thoroughly investigate it. Again, depending on the scale of observation, the nature of the body changes. From the molecular point of view, with interacting biomolecular agents in fluid states, the body might just as readily be conceived as a fluid syncytium, cell walls simply representing semi-permeable partitioning of the fluid compartment. A complexity approach reveals that alternate models may be as valid as standard ones.

Truly, plasticity, stochasticity, uncertainty, and complexity bring biology (at last?) into the postmodern age, appropriate for a new millennium. How quickly we can manifest the unlocked potential of our bodies will depend on how quickly we can unlock the fetters of dogma. We can be assured, however, that as with everything in the postmodern era, change occurs with increasing speed. We will not have to wait as long as we waited from the shift from Newtonian mechanics to relativity (centuries), or even from relativity to string theory (decades). The shifts are happening. We must simply let our minds keep pace with them.

References

Agur Z, Daniel Y, Ginosar Y (2002) The universal properties of stem cells as pinpointed by a simple discrete model. J Math Biol 44:79–86

Ait-Haddou R, Herzog W (2003) Brownian ratchet models of molecular motors. Cell Biochem Biophys 38:191–214

Akashi K, Traver D, Miyamoto T, Weissman IL (2000) A clonogenic common myeloid progenitor that gives rise to all myeloid lineages. Nature 404:193–197

Alvarez-Dolado M, Pardal R, Garcia-Verdugo JM, Fike JR, Lee HO, Pfeffer K, Lois C, Morrison SJ, Alvarez-Buylla A (2003) Fusion of bone-marrow-derived cells with Purkinje neurons, cardiomyocytes and hepatocytes. Nature 425:968–973

Bjornson CR, Rietze RL, Reynolds BA, Magli MC, Vescovi AL (1999) Turning brain into blood: a hematopoietic fate adopted by adult neural stem cells in vivo. Science 283:534–537

Blau HM, Brazelton TR, Weimann JM (2001) The evolving concept of a stem cell: entity or function? Cell 105:829–841

Blau HM, Chiu CP, Webster C (1983) Cytoplasmic activation of human nuclear genes in stable heterocaryons. Cell 32:1171–1180

Blau HM, Pavlath GK, Hardeman EC, Chiu CP, Silberstein L, Webster SG, Miller SC, Webster C (1985) Plasticity of the differentiated state. Science 230:758–766

Bruniquel D, Schwartz RH (2003) Selective, stable demethylation of the interleukin-2 gene enhances transcription by an active process. Nat Immunol 4:235–240

Brusic V, Petrovsky N (2003) Immunoinformatics—the new kid in town. Novartis Found Symp 254:3–13; discussion 13–22, 98–101, 250–252

Carmo-Fonseca M (2002) The contribution of nuclear compartmentalization to gene regulation. Cell 108:513–521

Carmo-Fonseca M, Platani M, Swedlow JR (2002) Macromolecular mobility inside the cell nucleus. Trends Cell Biol 12:491–495

Collas P (1998) Cytoplasmic control of nuclear assembly. Reprod Fertil Dev 10:581–592

Collas P (2003) Nuclear reprogramming in cell-free extracts. Philos Trans R Soc Lond B Biol Sci 358:1389–1395

Colvin GA, Lambert JF, Abedi M, Dooner MS, Demers D, Moore BE, Greer D, Aliotta JM, Pimentel J, Cerny J, Lum LG, Quesenberry PJ (2004) Differentiation hotspots: the deterioration of hierarchy and stochasm. Blood Cells Mol Dis 32:34–41

Cuthbert GL, Daujat S, Snowden AW, Erdjument-Bromage H, Hagiwara T, Yamada M, Schneider R, Gregory PD, Tempst P, Bannister AJ, Kouzarides T (2004) Histone deimination antagonizes arginine methylation. Cell 118:545–553

Davis RL, Weintraub H, Lassar AB (1987) Expression of a single transfected cDNA converts fibroblasts to myoblasts. Cell 51:987–1000

Deenick EK, Gett AV, Hodgkin PD (2003) Stochastic model of T cell proliferation: a calculus revealing IL-2 regulation of precursor frequencies, cell cycle time, and survival. J Immunol 170:4963–4972

Endo T, Bryant SV, Gardiner DM (2004) A stepwise model system for limb regeneration. Dev Biol 270:135–145

Enright BP, Kubota C, Yang X, Tian XC (2003) Epigenetic characteristics and development of embryos cloned from donor cells treated by trichostatin A or 5-aza-2'-deoxycytidine. Biol Reprod 69:896–901

Ferrari G, Cusella-De Angelis G, Coletta M, Paolucci E, Stornaiuolo A, Cossu G, Mavilio F (1998) Muscle regeneration by bone marrow-derived myogenic progenitors. Science 279:1528–1530

Furusawa C, Kaneko K (2000) Complex organization in multicellularity as a necessity in evolution. Artif Life 6:265–281

Furusawa C, Kaneko K (2001) Theory of robustness of irreversible differentiation in a stem cell system: chaos hypothesis. J Theor Biol 209:395–416

Furusawa C, Kaneko K (2002) Origin of multicellular organisms as an inevitable consequence of dynamical systems. Anat Rec 268:327–342

Gell-Mann M (2001) Consciousness, reduction, and emergence. Some remarks. Ann N Y Acad Sci 929:41–49

Harris RG, Herzog EL, Bruscia EM, Grove JE, Van Arnam JS, Krause DS (2004) Lack of a fusion requirement for development of bone marrow-derived epithelia. Science 305:90–93

Hume DA (2000) Probability in transcriptional regulation and its implications for leukocyte differentiation and inducible gene expression. Blood 96:2323–2328

Hussain MA, Theise ND (2004) Post-natal stem cells as participants in complex systems and the emergence of tissue integrity and function. Pediatr Diabetes 5 [Suppl 2]:75–78

Ianus A, Holz GG, Theise ND, Hussain MA (2003) In vivo derivation of glucose-competent pancreatic endocrine cells from bone marrow without evidence of cell fusion. J Clin Invest 111:843–850

Ichinose J, Murata M, Yanagida T, Sako Y (2004) EGF signalling amplification induced by dynamic clustering of EGFR. Biochem Biophys Res Commun 324:1143–1149

Ishikawa F, Drake CJ, Yang S, Fleming P, Minamiguchi H, Visconti RP, Crosby CV, Argraves WS, Harada M, Key LL Jr, Livingston AG, Wingard JR, Ogawa M (2003) Transplanted human cord blood cells give rise to hepatocytes in engrafted mice. Ann N Y Acad Sci 996:174–185

Jaenisch R, Bird A (2003) Epigenetic regulation of gene expression: how the genome integrates intrinsic and environmental signals. Nat Genet 33 Suppl:245–254

Jang YY, Collector MI, Baylin SB, Diehl AM, Sharkis SJ (2004) Hematopoietic stem cells convert into liver cells within days without fusion. Nat Cell Biol 6:532–539

Jimenez G, Griffiths SD, Ford AM, Greaves MF, Enver T (1992) Activation of the beta-globin locus control region precedes commitment to the erythroid lineage. Proc Natl Acad Sci U S A 89:10618–10622

Kitamura K, Yanagida T (2003) Stochastic properties of actomyosin motor. Biosystems 71:101–110

Kondo M, Scherer DC, Miyamoto T, King AG, Akashi K, Sugamura K, Weissman IL (2000) Cell-fate conversion of lymphoid-committed progenitors by instructive actions of cytokines. Nature 407:383–386

Kondo M, Weissman IL, Akashi K (1997) Identification of clonogenic common lymphoid progenitors in mouse bone marrow. Cell 91:661–672

Krause DS, Fackler MJ, Civin CI, May WS (1996) CD34: structure, biology, and clinical utility. Blood 87:1–13

Krause DS, Theise ND, Collector MI, Henegariu O, Hwang S, Gardner R, Neutzel S, Sharkis SJ (2001) Multi-organ, multi-lineage engraftment by a single bone marrow-derived stem cell. Cell 105:369–377

Kurakin A (2005) Self-organization vs Watchmaker: stochastic gene expression and cell differentiation. Dev Genes Evol 215:46–52

Le Douarin NM, Dupin E (1993) Cell lineage analysis in neural crest ontogeny. J Neurobiol 24:146–161

Leary AG, Ogawa M, Strauss LC, Civin CI (1984) Single cell origin of multilineage colonies in culture. Evidence that differentiation of multipotent progenitors and restriction of proliferative potential of monopotent progenitors are stochastic processes. J Clin Invest 74:2193–2197

Lee JH, Hart SR, Skalnik DG (2004) Histone deacetylase activity is required for embryonic stem cell differentiation. Genesis 38:32–38

Loeffler M, Roeder I (2002) Tissue stem cells: definition, plasticity, heterogeneity, self-organization and models—a conceptual approach. Cells Tissues Organs 171:8–26

Loeffler M, Roeder I (2004) Conceptual models to understand tissue stem cell organization. Curr Opin Hematol 11:81–87

Lozano F, Simarro M, Calvo J, Vila JM, Padilla O, Bowen MA, Campbell KS (2000) CD5 signal transduction: positive or negative modulation of antigen receptor signaling. Crit Rev Immunol 20:347–358

Ma SX (2004) Neurobiology of acupuncture: toward CAM. Evid Based Complement Alternat Med 1:41–47

Marley SB, Lewis JL, Gordon MY (2003) Progenitor cells divide symmetrically to generate new colony-forming cells and clonal heterogeneity. Br J Haematol 121:643–648

Metcalf D (1998) Lineage commitment and maturation in hematopoietic cells: the case for extrinsic regulation. Blood 92:345–347; discussion 352

Milhem M, Mahmud N, Lavelle D, Araki H, DeSimone J, Saunthararajah Y, Hoffman R (2004) Modification of hematopoietic stem cell fate by 5aza 2'deoxycytidine and trichostatin A. Blood 103:4102–4110

Newsome PN, Johannessen I, Boyle S, Dalakas E, McAulay KA, Samuel K, Rae F, Forrester L, Turner ML, Hayes PC, Harrison DJ, Bickmore WA, Plevris JN (2003) Human cord blood-derived cells can differentiate into hepatocytes in the mouse liver with no evidence of cellular fusion. Gastroenterology 124:1891–1900

Nishiyama M, Higuchi H, Yanagida T (2002) Chemomechanical coupling of the forward and backward steps of single kinesin molecules. Nat Cell Biol 4:790–797

Ogawa M (1999) Stochastic model revisited. Int J Hematol 69:2–5

O'Neill A, Schaffer DV (2004) The biology and engineering of stem cell control. Biotechnol Appl Biochem 40:5–16

Paulus U, Potten CS, Loeffler M (1992) A model of the control of cellular regeneration in the intestinal crypt after perturbation based solely on local stem cell regulation. Cell Prolif 25:559–578

Petersen BE, Bowen WC, Patrene KD, Mars WM, Sullivan AK, Murase N, Boggs SS, Greenberger JS, Goff JP (1999) Bone marrow as a potential source of hepatic oval cells. Science 284:1168–1170

Potten CS, Loeffler M (1990) Stem cells: attributes, cycles, spirals, pitfalls and uncertainties. Lessons for and from the crypt. Development 110:1001–1020

Roeder I, Kamminga LM, Braesel K, Dontje B, de Haan G, Loeffler M (2005) Competitive clonal hematopoiesis in mouse chimeras explained by a stochastic model of stem cell organization. Blood 105:609–616

Roeder I, Loeffler M (2002) A novel dynamic model of hematopoietic stem cell organization based on the concept of within-tissue plasticity. Exp Hematol 30:853–861

Roeder I, Loeffler M, Quesenberry PJ, Colvin GA, Lambert JF (2003) Quantitative tissue stem cell modeling. Blood 102:1143–1144; author reply 1144–1145

Saffarian S, Collier IE, Marmer BL, Elson EL, Goldberg G (2004) Interstitial collagenase is a Brownian ratchet driven by proteolysis of collagen. Science 306:108–111

Santos F, Zakhartchenko V, Stojkovic M, Peters A, Jenuwein T, Wolf E, Reik W, Dean W (2003) Epigenetic marking correlates with developmental potential in cloned bovine preimplantation embryos. Curr Biol 13:1116–1121

Sasaki T, Sasaki-Irie J, Penninger JM (2001) New insights into the transmembrane protein tyrosine phosphatase CD45. Int J Biochem Cell Biol 33:1041–1046

Shi Y, Lan F, Matson C, Mulligan P, Whetstine JR, Cole PA, Casero RA (2004) Histone demethylation mediated by the nuclear amine oxidase homolog LSD1. Cell 119:941–953

Taylor SM, Jones PA (1979) Multiple new phenotypes induced in 10T1/2 and 3T3 cells treated with 5-azacytidine. Cell 17:771–779

Theise ND (2002) New principles of cell plasticity. C R Biol 325:1039–1043

Theise ND (2003) Liver stem cells: prospects for treatment of inherited and acquired liver diseases. Expert Opin Biol Ther 3:403–408

Theise ND (2004) Perspective: stem cells react! Cell lineages as complex adaptive systems. Exp Hematol 32:25–27

Theise ND, d'Inverno M (2004) Understanding cell lineages as complex adaptive systems. Blood Cells Mol Dis 32:17–20

Theise ND, Krause DS (2001) Suggestions for a new paradigm of cell differentiative potential. Blood Cells Mol Dis 27:625–631

Theise ND, Krause DS (2002) Toward a new paradigm of cell plasticity. Leukemia 16:542–548

Theise ND, Wilmut I (2003) Cell plasticity: flexible arrangement. Nature 425:21

Vazquez J, Belmont AS, Sedat JW (2001) Multiple regimes of constrained chromosome motion are regulated in the interphase Drosophila nucleus. Curr Biol 11:1227–1239

Vermaak D, Wolffe AP (1998) Chromatin and chromosomal controls in development. Dev Genet 22:1–6

Wang Y, Wysocka J, Sayegh J, Lee YH, Perlin JR, Leonelli L, Sonbuchner LS, McDonald CH, Cook RG, Dou Y, Roeder RG, Clarke S, Stallcup MR, Allis CD, Coonrod SA (2004) Human PAD4 regulates histone arginine methylation levels via demethylimination. Science 306:279–283

Weintraub H, Groudine M (1976) Chromosomal subunits in active genes have an altered conformation. Science 193:848–856

Willenbring H, Bailey AS, Foster M, Akkari Y, Dorrell C, Olson S, Finegold M, Fleming WH, Grompe M (2004) Myelomonocytic cells are sufficient for therapeutic cell fusion in liver. Nat Med 10:744–748

Willenbring H, Grompe M (2003) Embryonic versus adult stem cell pluripotency: in liver only fusion matters. J Assist Reprod Genet 20:393–394

Xie H, Ye M, Feng R, Graf T (2004) Stepwise reprogramming of B cells into macrophages. Cell 117:663–676

Yanagida T, Ishii Y (2003) Stochastic processes in nano-biomachines revealed by single molecule detection. Biosystems 71:233–244

Subject Index